AF566936

Atlas of Cerebrovascular Disease

Edited by
PHILIP B. GORELICK, MD, MPH

Director, Section of Cerebrovascular Disease
Rush-Presbyterian-St. Luke's Medical Center
Professor, Rush Medical College
Chicago, Illinois, USA

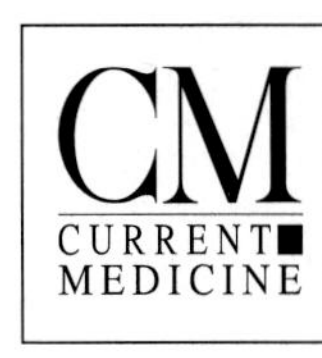

Philadelphia

Current Medicine

DEVELOPMENTAL EDITOR: .... ELIZABETH HOWARD

ASSISTANT EDITOR: .... CHARLENE FRENCH

MANAGING EDITOR: .... LORI BAINBRIDGE

ART DIRECTOR: .... PAUL FENNESSY

DESIGNERS: .... ROBERT LEBRUN AND JERILYN BOCKORICK

ILLUSTRATION DIRECTOR: .... ANN SAYDLOWSKI

ILLUSTRATORS: ...... WIESIA LANGENFELD, ANN SAYDLOWSKI, LARRY WARD, LISA WEISCHEDEL, AND GARY WELCH

PRODUCTION: .... DAVID MYERS AND WENDY FEINSTEIN

TYPESETTING DIRECTOR: .... COLLEEN WARD

Atlas of Cerebrovascular Disease/Edited by Philip B. Gorelick.
p. cm.
Includes bibliographical references and index.
ISBN 1-878132-16-4 (hb:alk.paper)
1. Cerebrovascular disease--Atlases. I. Gorelick, Philip B.
[DNLM: 1. Cerebrovascular Disorders--atlases. WL 17 A8813 1996]
RC388.5.A85 1996
616.8 1--dc20
DNLM/DLC 95-4881
for Library of Congress CIP

PRINTED IN SINGAPORE BY IMAGO PRODUCTIONS (FE) LTD.
2 4 5 3 1

ISBN:1-878132-16-4

To my parents, Ruth and Harold, in recognition for their love and support.

Contributors

HAROLD P. ADAMS, JR, MD
Division of Cerebrovascular Diseases
Department of Neurology
University of Iowa College of Medicine
Iowa City, Iowa, USA

JOSÉ BILLER, MD
Professor and Chairman
Department of Neurology
Indiana University School of Medicine
Indianapolis, Indiana, USA

ROGER A. BILLHARDT, MD
Assistant Professor of Medicine
Rush-Presbyterian-St. Luke's Medical Center
Chicago, Illinois, USA

JULIEN BOGOUSSLAVSKY, MD
Department of Neurology
University of Lausanne
Lausanne, Switzerland

JOHN V. BOWLER, MB, MD
Clinical Neurological Sciences
University of Western Ontario
London, Ontario, Canada

FERNANDO BOZZOLA, MD
Department of Neurology
University of Buenos Aires Medical Center
DF Santojanni Hospital
Buenos Aires, Argentina

MAURA BRAGONI, MD
Department of Neuroscience
University of Rome
Rome, Italy

DALE CHARLETTA, MD
Department of Radiology
Baylor College of Medicine
Houston, Texas, USA

ROBERT M. CROWELL, MD
Neurosurgeon
The Berkshire Medical Center
Pittsfield, Massachusetts
Clinical Professor of Neurosurgery
University of Massachusetts Medical School
Worcester, Massachusetts, USA

JEFFREY C. CURTIN, DO
Assistant Professor of Neurology
Section of Cerebrovascular Disease
Director, Hyperacute Stroke Service
Rush-Presbyterian-St. Luke's Medical Center
Chicago, Illinois, USA

PATRICIA H. DAVIS, MD
Assistant Professor
Department of Neurology
The University of Iowa College of Medicine
Iowa City, Iowa, USA

EDWARD FELDMANN, MD
Associate Professor
Department of Clinical Neurosciences
Brown University School of Medicine
Providence, Rhode Island, USA

GLEN GEREMIA, MD
Associate Professor of Radiology
Rush-Presbyterian-St. Luke's Medical Center
Chicago, Illinois, USA

LARRY B. GOLDSTEIN, MD
Assistant Professor of Medicine (Neurology)
Assistant Research Professor (Center for Health Policy Research and Education)
Duke University
Durham Department of Veterans Affairs Medical Center
Durham, North Carolina, USA

DAVID C. GOOD, MD
Associate Professor of Neurology
Director of Rehabilitation
The Bowman Gray School of Medicine
Wake Forest University
Winston-Salem, North Carolina, USA

PHILIP B. GORELICK, MD, MPH
Director, Section of Cerebrovascular Disease
Rush-Presbyterian-St. Luke's Medical Center
Professor, Rush Medical College
Chicago, Illinois, USA

WILLIAM M. GREENLEE, MD
Assistant Professor of Radiology
Rush-Presbyterian-St. Luke's Medical Center
Chicago, Illinois, USA

VLADIMIR HACHINSKI, MD
Richard and Beryl Ivey Professor and Chairman
Clinical Neurological Sciences
University of Western Ontario
London, Ontario, Canada

L. ANNE HAYMAN, MD
Department of Radiology
Baylor College of Medicine
Houston, Texas, USA

CATHY M. HELGASON, MD
Professor of Neurology
University of Illinois College of Medicine
Chicago, Illinois, USA

ROBERT C. JANZER, MD
Division of Neuropathology
University of Lausanne
Lausanne, Switzerland

L. JAAP KAPPELLE, MD
University Department of Neurology
University Hospital Utrecht
Utrecht, The Netherlands

MICHAEL A. KELLY, MD
Associate Professor of Neurological Sciences
Rush Medical College
Chairman, Division of Neurology
Cook County Hospital
Chicago, Illinois, USA

PHILIP R. LIEBSON, MD
Professor of Medicine
Echocardiography Laboratory
Consultant, Preventive Cardiology
Senior Attending Physician
Rush-Presbyterian-St. Luke's Medical Center
Chicago, Illinois, USA

CARLOS MANGONE, MD
Director, Alzheimer's Center
University of Buenos Aires Medical Center
DF Santojanni Hospital
Buenos Aires, Argentina

JOSEPH C. MASDEU, MD
Professor and Chairman of Neurology
New York Medical College
Adjunct Professor of Neurology
New York University School of Medicine
New York, New York, USA

VINCENT T. MILLER, MD
Department of Neurosciences
Marshfield Clinic
Chippewa Falls, Wisconsin, USA

PANAYIOTIS MITSIAS, MD
Staff Neurologist
Department of Neurology
Henry Ford Hospital
Detroit, Michigan, USA

ALEXANDER L. NEUMANN, BS
Associate Professor of Medicine
Technical Director, Echocardiography Laboratory
Rush-Presbyterian-St. Luke's Medical Center
Chicago, Illinois, USA

CHRISTOPHER S. OGILVY, MD
Assistant Professor of Surgery
Harvard Medical School
Assistant Visiting Neurosurgeon
Director, Cerebrovascular Surgery
Co-Director, Brain Aneurysm/AVM Center
Massachusetts General Hospital
Boston, Massachusetts, USA

THOMAS C. ORIGITANO, MD, PHD
Assistant Professor of Neurological Surgery and Physiology
Loyola University Medical Center
Maywood, Illinois, USA

JAMES T. PATRICK, MD, PHD
Attending Neurologist and Neuroimager
Dent Neurologic Institute
Lucy Dent Imaging Center
Buffalo, New York, USA

NABIH M. RAMADAN, MD
Staff Neurologist
Director, Noninvasive Cerebrovascular Laboratory
Department of Neurology
Henry Ford Hospital
Detroit, Michigan, USA

ANNE MARIE RITTER, MD
Department of Neurosurgery
Medical College of Virginia
Richmond, Virginia, USA

STUART W. ROSENBUSH, MD
Assistant Professor of Medicine
Rush-Presbyterian-St. Luke's Medical Center
Chicago, Illinois, USA

ELLIOT J. ROTH, MD
Medical Director
Rehabilitation Institute of Chicago
Professor and Chairman
Department of Physical Medicine and Rehabilitation
Northwestern University Medical School
Chicago, Illinois, USA

JEFFREY S. SOBLE, MD
Assistant Professor of Medicine
Associate Director, Medical Intensive Care Unit
Rush-Presbyterian-St. Luke's Medical Center
Chicago, Illinois, USA

JAMES C. TORNER, PHD
Professor, Department of Preventive Medicine and Environmental Health
The University of Iowa College of Medicine
Iowa City, Iowa, USA

JANET L. WILTERDINK, MD
Assistant Professor
Department of Clinical Neurosciences
Brown University School of Medicine
Providence, Rhode Island, USA

Preface

Stroke is the premier neurologic disease. It is the third leading cause of death and a major cause of adult disability. It is estimated that there are 500,000 strokes, 150,000 stroke deaths, and 3 million stroke survivors each year in the United States. About 31% of stroke survivors are dependent in their activities of daily living. Furthermore, billions of dollars are spent on stroke worldwide, and the total cost of stroke in the United States is estimated at $30 billion.

Our knowledge of stroke risk factors, diagnosis, and treatment has grown substantially during the past 30 years. This explosion of information surpasses that of any other neurologic disease and has resulted in the identification of treatable stroke risk factors and effective prevention strategies that have stemmed from clinical trials. Thus, stroke remains the most common and preventable neurologic disease.

The *Atlas of Cerebrovascular Disease* addresses all of the facets and complexities of stroke risk factors, diagnosis, and treatment in the 1990s in an easily digestible format that emphasizes illustrative displays with brief, understandable textual commentary. There is information on the latest advances in stroke diagnosis and treatment, as well as discussions of a diverse spectrum of topics including atherosclerotic and nonatherosclerotic stroke mechanisms. The emphasis is on the practical application of information for diagnosis and treatment. Such information will assist internists, general and family practitioners, neurologists, psychiatrists, residents, and medical students in the management of stroke patients. This up-to-date atlas will prove useful to all who diagnose and treat stroke patients.

Philip B. Gorelick
Rush-Presbyterian-St. Luke's Medical Center
Chicago, Illinois

Contents

CHAPTER 6
Neuropathology and Pathophysiology of Intraparenchymal Hemorrhage
Janet L. Wilterdink and Edward Feldmann

CHAPTER 7
Nonatherosclerotic Stroke
Nabih M. Ramadan and Panayiotis Mitsias

CHAPTER 8
Cranial Computed Tomography and Magnetic Resonance Imaging of Cerebrovascular Disorders
Glen Geremia and William M. Greenlee

CHAPTER 9
Diagnosing Cerebrovascular Disease Using Magnetic Resonance Angiography and Conventional Cerebral Angiography
Anne Marie Ritter, L. Anne Hayman, and Dale Charletta

CHAPTER 10
Imaging of Stroke with Single Photon Emission Computed Tomography
Joseph C. Masdeu

CHAPTER 11
Echocardiography in the Assessment of Cerebrovascular Events
Philip R. Liebson, Jeffrey S. Soble, and Alexander L. Neumann

CHAPTER 12
Cardiac Diagnostics in Embolic Stroke and Preoperative Evaluation for Carotid Surgery
Roger A. Billhardt and Stuart W. Rosenbush

CHAPTER 13
Hematologic Evaluation of the Stroke Patient
Maura Bragoni and Edward Feldmann

CHAPTER 14
Management of Medical Complications in Cerebrovascular Disease
James T. Patrick and José Biller

CHAPTER 15
The Use of Antiplatelet Drugs to Prevent Stroke
L. Jaap Kappelle and Harold P. Adams, Jr

CHAPTER 16
Anticoagulation in Cerebrovascular Disease
Vincent T. Miller

CHAPTER 17
Novel Therapeutic Approaches to the Treatment of Ischemic Stroke and Transient Ischemic Attack
Cathy M. Helgason

CHAPTER 18
Carotid Endarterectomy and Novel Surgical Therapies for Cerebral Ischemia
Robert M. Crowell and Christopher S. Ogilvy

CHAPTER 19
Treatment of Aneurysmal Subarachnoid Hemorrhage
Thomas C. Origitano

CHAPTER 20
Management of Intracerebral Hemorrhage
Michael A. Kelly

CHAPTER 21
Basic Principles and Strategies of Rehabilitation in Cerebrovascular Disease
David C. Good

CHAPTER 22
Natural History of Recovery and Influence of Comorbid Conditions on Stroke Outcome
Elliot J. Roth

CHAPTER 23
Commonly Prescribed Medications and Novel Pharmacologic Approaches in Stroke Rehabilitation
Larry B. Goldstein

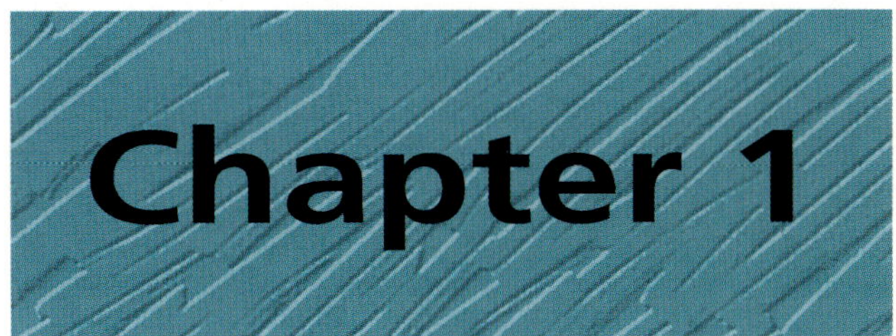

Epidemiology of Cerebral Infarction

JOHN V. BOWLER
VLADIMIR HACHINSKI

Stroke is the third leading cause of death [1] after heart disease and cancer. Stroke mortality in the United States was 150,300 in 1988 while the annual incidence is 500,000, 75% being new cases. Cerebral infarction accounts for about 80% of strokes [2]. There has been a reduction in the incidence of cerebral infarction, due largely to the management of hypertension. As the population ages, the crude incidence is likely to increase because cerebral infarction is primarily a disease of old age (the incidence doubling or tripling with every decade after the fifth) [3].

Table 1.1. Mortality of cerebral infarction taken from selected studies

Study	Location	Years studied	Age range	Year, mortality per 100,000		
Yates [169]	England and Wales	1932–1961	All	1932, 54; 1961, 195		
Stern and Gaskill [173]	Texas	1970–1976	All	Mortality stable at 60 to 110 between 1970 and 1976		
Modan and Wagener [10], Cooper and coworkers [66]	United States	1960–1988	All		White	Black
				1960,	149	280.3
				1986,	58.2	106.5
Ahmed and coworkers [29]	Pennsylvania	1971–1980	All	1971, 61; 1980, 38		
Wylie [7]	England and Wales	1949–1967	All	1950, 69; 1967, 92		
Wender and coworkers [174]	Poland	1977–1985	Over 20 y	1977, 193; 1985, 154		

Table 1.2. Age-standardized stroke mortality rates per 100,000 population in 27 countries by sex, 1985*

Country	Men		Women	
	Rank	Rate	Rank	Rate
Bulgaria	1	249.2	1	155.8
Hungary	2	229.4	2	130.4
Czechoslovakia	3	176.6	4	102.6
Romania†	4	171.5	3	129.2
Yugoslavia†	5	145.1	5	101.2
Singapore	6	136.0	6	92.0
Japan	7	106.9	11	60.4
Scotland	8	99.3	7	77.0
Finland	9	98.1	13	57.3
Poland	10	95.8	10	62.5
Hong Kong	11	94.4	9	63.5
Austria	12	89.9	16	48.5
Northern Ireland	13	84.4	8	66.8
Ireland	14	72.2	12	58.6
England and Wales	15	70.6	14	54.2
Germany	16	68.2	19	38.8
Belgium†	17	64.1	18	41.3
New Zealand	18	62.0	15	49.9
France	19	60.4	26	28.1
Australia	20	60.3	17	44.7
Denmark	21	55.3	20	37.8
Norway	22	54.8	22	34.6
Sweden	23	48.1	24	30.5
Netherlands	24	47.0	23	31.3
United States	25	45.4	21	35.1
Canada	26	39.1	25	28.3
Switzerland	27	37.8	27	20.6

**From* Bonita and coworkers [15]; with permission.
†1984 rates.

Table 1.3. Percentage change per annum in stroke mortality in 27 countries by sex, 1970 to 1985

Country	Men		Women	
	Rank	Change	Rank	Change
Hungary	1	3.9	1	2.1
Poland	2	2.9	2	1.7
Bulgaria	3	2.2	5	-0.5
Yugoslavia	4	0.7	3	-0.3
Romania	5	0.6	4	-0.4
Czechoslovakia	6	0.1	7	-0.8
Denmark	7	-1.2	8	-2.4
Hong Kong	8	-2.3	6	-0.5
Austria	9	-2.3	11	-3.3
Sweden	10	-2.7	16	-4.0
Singapore	11	-2.8	9	-2.6
Netherlands	12	-3.1	15	-4.0
Scotland	13	-3.1	12	-3.4
England and Wales	14	-3.3	10	-3.3
Germany	15	-3.3	14	-3.9
Norway	16	-3.5	17	-4.4
Finland	17	-3.6	22	-5.0
Ireland	18	-3.7	19	-4.7
Northern Ireland	19	-3.8	13	-3.6
New Zealand	20	-3.8	20	-4.7
Switzerland	21	-4.1	23	-5.1
Belgium	22	-4.4	18	-4.5
France	23	-4.5	25	-5.4
Canada	24	-4.6	21	-4.8
Australia	25	-5.4	26	-6.5
United States	26	-5.7	24	-5.2
Japan	27	-7.1	27	-7.0

**From* Bonita and coworkers [15]; with permission.

MORTALITY OF CEREBRAL INFARCTION

Mortality statistics usually present data for all stroke types combined as the distinction between stroke types is notoriously unreliable in mortality data [4]. For all stroke types combined, the mortality worldwide varies 12-fold between 20 and 250 per 100,000 population per annum (Tables 1.1, 1.2, and 1.3).

LIMITATIONS OF MORTALITY DATA

Mortality data, though readily obtainable in many countries, have several flaws that limit their usefulness. Firstly, mortality data can only reflect incidence if the relationship between mortality and incidence remains constant [5]. However, the mortality of cerebral infarction may have decreased, though this may be an artifact of the increasing detection of less severe cases. Medical fashion may influence diagnosis [6,7]. This resulted in many sudden deaths being ascribed to stroke, particularly cerebral hemorrhage, in the early part of this century, especially before the recognition of myocardial infarction, overstating both the total stroke mortality and the proportion of parenchymal hemorrhages [8]. Accurate distinction between cerebral infarction and hemorrhage remains a particular problem in mortality statistics [9]. Changes in the coding of death certificates have caused little change in the apparent mortality [10] (Figure 1.1) in recent times but may explain the whole of the apparent fall in US stroke mortality up to 1925 [11]. Coding of stroke as "ill-defined" has increased and constitutes up to 60% of strokes [10]. Most of these are infarcts and their exclusion from the categories specific for infarction will bias mortality statistics. Changes in the population may pose problems; the slow fall in age-adjusted death rates seen before the introduction of effective antihypertensive medication may be an artifact of age adjustment, diagnostic accuracy, and the northward migration of southern blacks [12]. The accuracy of certification is poor. There is a consistent 40% shortfall in the identification of stroke on death certificates when compared with other data from the same community [8,13], and a 13% to 22% false-positive rate [13,14], mostly due to agonal changes in consciousness [13]. The omission of the diagnosis of stroke on death certificates increases with the time from stroke to death, *ie*, from 30% omission at 1 year, to complete omission at 20 years [13] (Figure 1.2).

INCIDENCE OF CEREBRAL INFARCTION

Much of the international variability in mortality data may be artifactual. While the age-standardized mortality rates vary 10-fold between countries [1,15], population study data vary by a factor of less than four [16]. This falls further with standardization to the same population [17] (Figure 1.3). However, like mortality data, the rise in incidence remains exponential with age (Figure 1.4).

Incidence data are not without problems. By avoiding the use of death certification it becomes theoretically possible to detect all strokes, but the degree to which this occurs depends on the nature of the study. The most thorough and most costly is a door-to-door survey. There is evidence that these surveys produce the highest incidence figures [17]. The quickest and cheapest rely on hospital discharge data with the obvious disadvantage that cases not attending the hospital cannot be detected. Such studies may fail to identify 40% of strokes compared with more exhaustive studies involving family physicians [18]. Studies vary regarding the inclusion of both recurrent and initial stroke. This variation is important as the inclusion of recurrent stroke increases the apparent incidence by about 30% [17]. Changing degrees of diagnostic enthusiasm, often with the patient's age, affect the classification of stroke type. In one study, the declining use of diagnostic investigations with increasing age altered the ratio of cerebral infarcts to unspecified stroke from 3:1 in those aged 55 to 74 years to 1:3 in those aged over 84 years [19]. Changing diagnostic tools are poten-

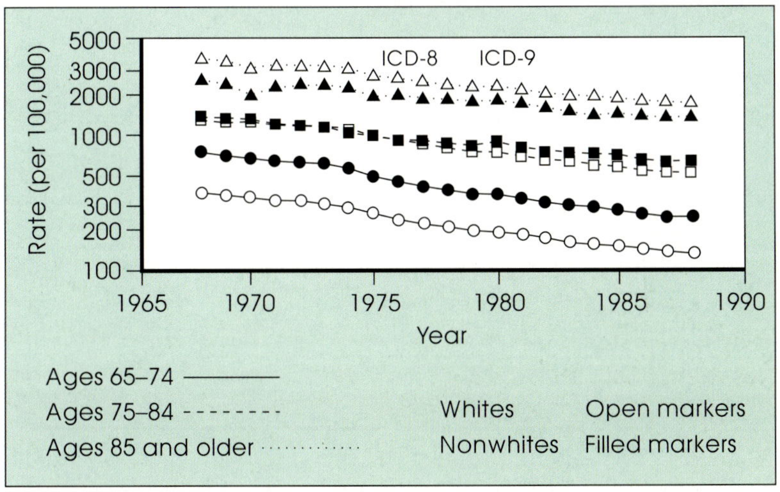

FIGURE 1.1

Graph showing age-specific death rates in the United States from all cerebrovascular accidents for selected years between 1968 and 1988 for those aged 65 years or older (International Classification of Diseases [ICD]-8 430-438, ICD-9 430-438), age adjusted to 1980 US population. (*From* Modan and Wagener [10]; with permission.)

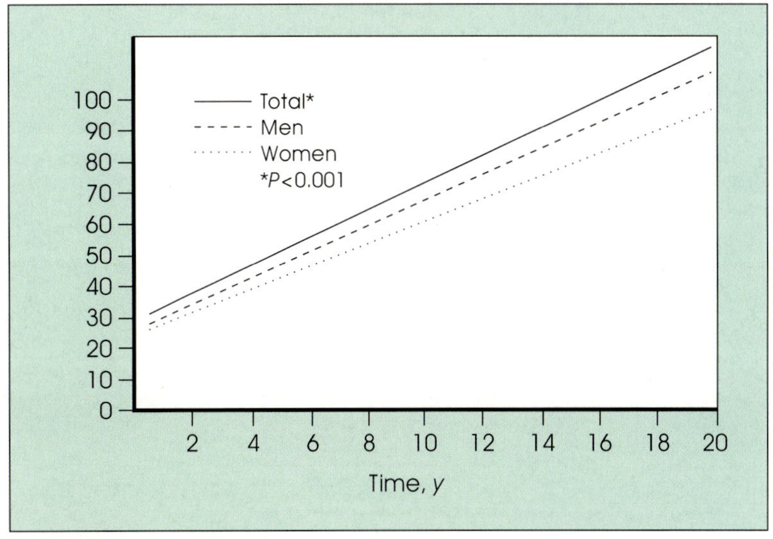

FIGURE 1.2

Death certificate false-negative rate as a function of interval from cerebral infarction to death. (*From* Corwin and coworkers [13]; with permission.)

tially a major confounder in assessing the recent changes in the incidence of stroke, as computed tomography (CT) and magnetic resonance (MR) imaging greatly enhance diagnostic sensitivity and specificity for acute neurologic events. One technique attempting to overcome this is the retrospective rediagnosis of cases from hospital records, excluding the CT data, to make diagnostic methods between current and older data more comparable. This may fail, however, since the physicians at the time would have been influenced in their diagnoses and, quite probably, detection of physical signs by the CT scans [20]. Even a prosaic matter such as record keeping may influence the apparent incidence of stroke and its classification into subtypes when based on doctors' records if the quality of the data recorded varies over time [20].

Regional Variation

Population surveys have produced similar incidence figures in different countries, findings that contrast with mortality data [21,22] (Table 1.4). At most a three- to fourfold variation is seen. Such variations are also seen within countries; there is a threefold north-south difference in the incidence of cerebral infarction in China [23], and variations of similar magnitude in Taiwan [24]. Stroke mortality is greater in the southeastern United States and there is weak evidence of a negative association between longitude in men and women, and between latitude in men, and stroke mortality [25].

CHANGES IN THE MORTALITY OF STROKE

In a comprehensive survey of mortality data for stroke of all types, sufficient data were found from 27 countries to conclude that a decrease in mortality of between 3% and 5% per annum had occurred in most western countries over the period from 1970 to 1985. Japan experienced a greater, and eastern Europe a lesser decline, or an increase in some cases [15]; other data have generally shown a decline in stroke mortality (Table 1.3).

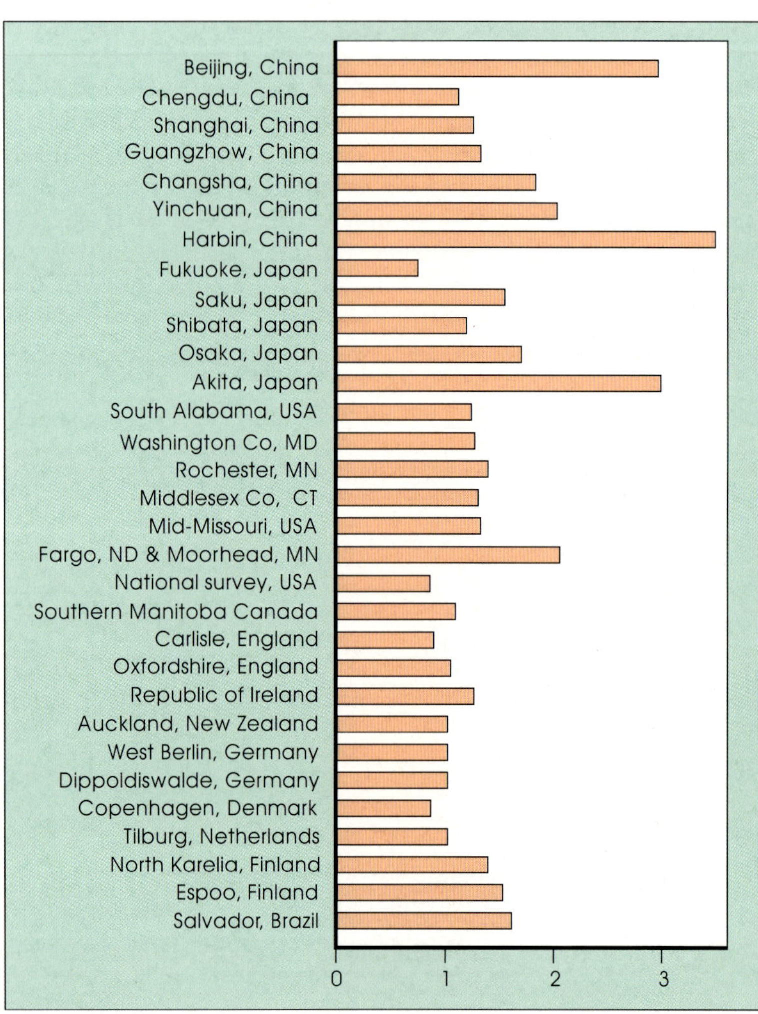

FIGURE 1.3

Incidence ratios, standardized for age for initial stroke in selected communities illustrating the relatively limited variation. (*From* Alter and coworkers [17]; with permission.)

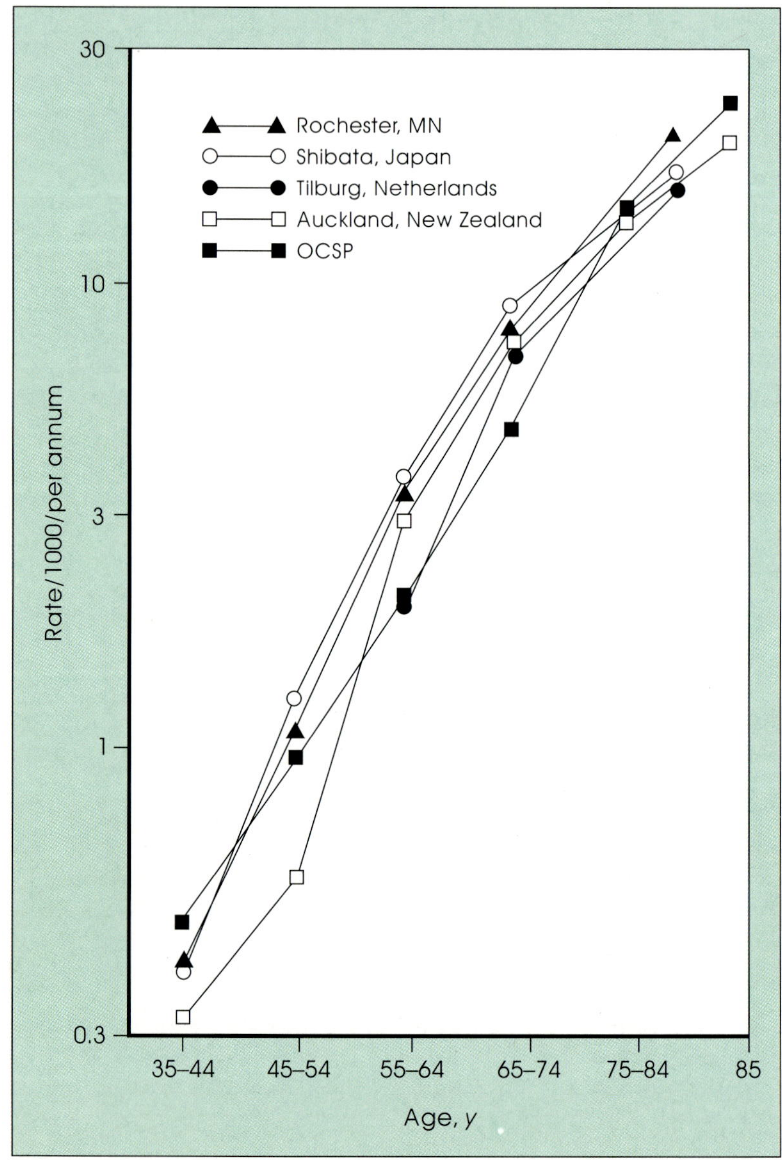

FIGURE 1.4

Data from five studies showing the logarithmic increase in incidence rates with age. OCSP—Oxfordshire Community Stroke Project. (*From* Bamford and coworkers [170]; with permission.)

The decline in men is typically slightly less than the decline in women (Figure 1.5) [15]. Figures vary for the period before this. From 1914 to 1960 mortality in the United States decreased by 44% in white men, 51% in white women, 27% in nonwhite women, and 12% in nonwhite men. Between 1960 and 1975 mortality in these groups fell by 28%, 31%, 33%, and 41%, respectively. The absolute changes were -34, -34, -58, and -71/100,000/per annum, respectively [26] or about 2% per annum between 1950 and 1972 [27,28]. Percentage changes are typically lower in the elderly, and older blacks show the smallest change [27].

Changes in Apparent Stroke Severity and Its Effect on Mortality

While mortality has consistently declined, the changes may not reflect incidence as the case fatality ratio may have fallen. Two explanations, which are not mutually exclusive, are proposed for the fall in the case fatality ratio. The first is that the severity of stroke has truly decreased; the second is that less severe strokes are being diagnosed more often because of increased public and medical awareness and improved diagnostic technology, notably CT and MR scanning. Two studies suggest that an alteration in the nature of the disease has changed the case-fatality ratio [10,29], but neither excludes the increased detection of less severe cases. Other studies have found that changes in case fatality are not a sufficient explanation for the changes in mortality and support a true decrease in incidence [30].

CHANGES IN THE INCIDENCE OF CEREBRAL INFARCTION

Population studies, particularly those that have used standard criteria over a prolonged period, provide a more accurate method of solving this problem. In Rochester, data beginning from the middle of the century has shown an accelerating decline in the incidence of cerebral infarction, the decline between each quinquennium from 1945 to 1949 being 4%, 7%, 12%, 14%, and 22%. The total incidence has declined from 159 per 100,000 between 1945 and 1949 to 83 per 100,000 between 1970 and 1974. CT scanning was too late to affect this data [31], and the decline was not due to increased survival after stroke [31,32]. More recent data from this study [31] and others based in Finland [33] and Japan [34,35] have shown about a 20% decline during the 1980s. CT use increased notably during this time [36].

Table 1.4. Incidence of cerebral infarction from several population surveys and related studies

Study	Location	Years studied	Study type	Age range	Incidence per 100,000
Terent [175]	Soderhamn, Sweden	1975–1978 1983–1986	Prospective community with data from all hospitals, nursing homes, and general practitioners	All	Men, 154; women, 160 Men, 127; women, 199
Sarti and coworkers [14]	Finland	1983–1986	Prospective, detailed case finding	25–74	Men, 34–51; women, 22–30
Bamford and coworkers [170]	Oxfordshire, England	1981–1986	Prospective community with data from all hospitals, nursing homes and general practitioners	All	Men, 150; women, 171; total, 160
Ueda and coworkers [176]	Japan	1961–1981	Prospective community, averaged over 20 years in an aging cohort	Over 40	Men, 305; women, 265; total, 570
Shimamoto and coworkers [34]	Japan	1964–1968 1979–1983	Prospective community but only small numbers	Over 40	**Sex and age / 1961–1968 / 1979–1983** Men 40–69: 520 / 203 Men ≥70: 1220 / 1440 Women 40–69: 240 / 137 Women ≥70: 600 / 740
Kojima and coworkers [44]	Akita, Japan	1975–1981	Akita, Japan, from 1975 to 1981, 109 patients who suffered their first stroke were registered and were monitored for 5 years	All	Men, 213; women, 152

While these studies support a true decline in incidence, at least until recent years, others do not. The Framingham study found no significant change in the incidence of cerebral infarction between 1953 and 1973, though stroke severity on admission decreased [37], suggesting that less severe strokes were detected more often. A study from Göteborg, Sweden, reports similar findings [38]. Data from Denmark have either shown an increase in strokes between the mid 1970s and late 1980s [39] or no change [40].

Despite some inconsistencies, this data can be explained by a decrease in both the incidence and mortality of cerebral infarction, partially offset by an increased awareness of stroke and improved diagnostic techniques. Consequently, less severe infarcts are being detected more often. In some populations this has resulted in apparent stability, or even an increase, in the incidence of cerebral infarction. As the case mix of cerebral infarction has shifted in favor of less severe lesions, the apparent mortality has declined.

Basis of the Decline

The treatment of hypertension is likely to be the major factor in the decline in incidence of cerebral infarction [26,31,33,35,41,42]. However, it may not be a complete explanation [27,36]. In one study [36], the decrease in women preceded the development of effective antihypertensive therapy. The role of competition by other conditions for mortality also needs to be considered [43].

Prevalence of Cerebral Infarction

Prevalence data can only be obtained by means of detailed population surveys, and data regarding this are scant. Details from some studies are given in Table 1.5.

CASE FATALITY RATIO OF CEREBRAL INFARCTION

Typical case fatality rates are 12% at 7 days [31], 7% to 20% at 1 month [2,19,31,44–46], 17% at 6 months [19], and 22% at 1 year [44]. Current figures represent a 50% decrease in in-hospital case fatality [20], though this may be due to the admission of less serious cases. Mortality at 5 years is 44% in men and 36% in women after nonembolic infarcts [45]. After stroke sufficient to produce hemiplegia, mortality is 50% to 70% [47,48]. Additional data are given in Table 1.6.

Time Course

Two peaks of mortality occur after cerebral infarction. The first, between the second and sixth day, is largely due to transtentorial herniation; the second is more diffuse, maximal in the second week, and primarily due to the complications of immobility [2,49], particularly bronchopneumonia, aspiration pneumonia, deep venous thrombosis, and pulmonary embolism. Stroke-associated mortality extends beyond the acute event for at least 2 years [31], and possibly many years, after the original event [50], mainly due to further stroke and other cardiovascular disease.

Factors Affecting Mortality

Stroke severity, best indicated by the presence of impaired consciousness, is the most powerful factor affecting mortality [20,29,51]. Increasing age is another major factor [2,3,14, 45–48,52]. The Oxfordshire Community Stroke Project [2] identified a 30-day case fatality of 7% in those aged under 65 years, increasing to 19% in those over 85 years, though other studies have reported higher

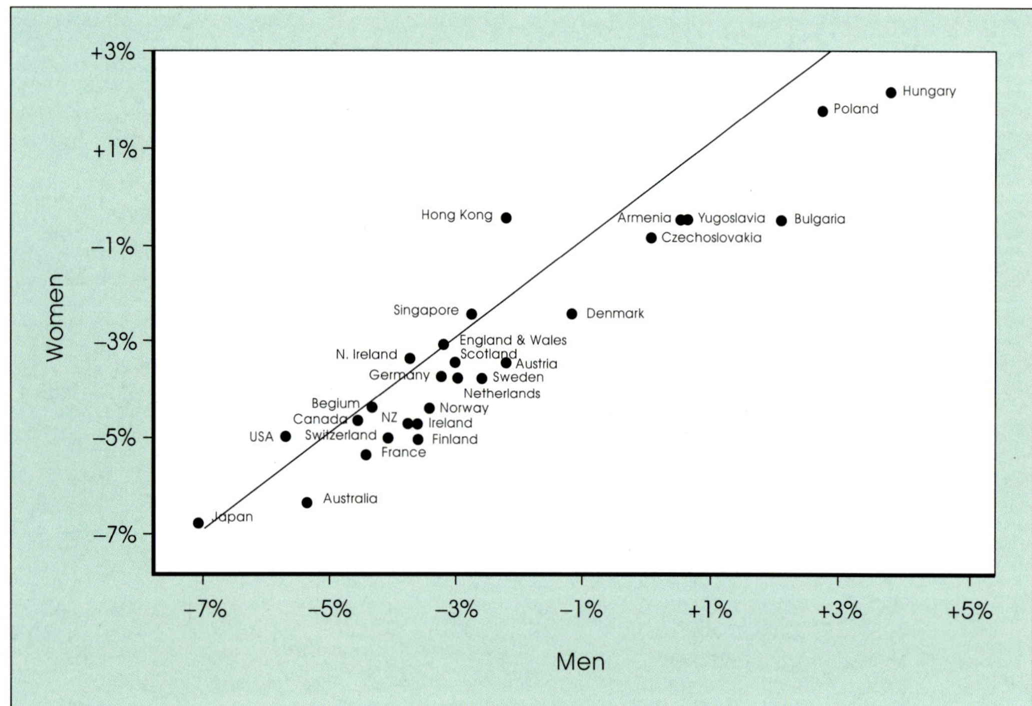

FIGURE 1.5

Scatterplot of the percentage changes in annual standardized stroke mortality rates in men and women from 1970 through 1985 for 27 countries. *Line* indicates equal percentage changes for men and women. NZ—New Zealand. (*From* Bonita and coworkers [15]; with permission.)

Table 1.5. Prevalence data for cerebral infarction from several selected studies

Study	Country	Years studied	Study type and comments	Age range	Prevalence per 100,000
Hu and coworkers [178]	Taiwan	1986	Door-to-door screening and clinical examination for cases screened positive; crude figures, all stroke, 67% thought to be infarcts	Over 35 y	Age range, y: 36–44, 45–54, 55–64, 65–74, 75–84, 85+, Mean Men: 2.6, 4.0, 32.1, 33.5, 49.4, 45.5, 20.6 Women: 0.0, 3.6, 17.3, 33.9, 35.1, 27.8, 11.9 Total: 1.1, 3.8, 26.1, 33.7, 42.5, 37.5, 16.4
Wolf and coworkers [84]	United States	1976	Review article	All	Total, 794 Age < 45, 66 Age >65, 5063
Li and coworkers [82]	China	1983	Population survey based in six cities in China	All	Crude, 459; age-adjusted, 532
Paschalis and coworkers [86]	Greece	1985	Door-to-door survey	Over 20 y	Age range, y — Men — Women 50–59: 775, 826 60–69: 9523, 1010 70+: 3225, 9722 Total: 1627, 1221 Total for both sexes: 1417

Table 1.6. Morbidity and mortality of cerebral infarction taken from several studies

Study	Location	Years	Morbidity, %	Mortality, %	Comments
Howard and coworkers [53]	United States	1969–1973	Not stated	67 after 5 years	Mortality due to: Index stroke, 31% Subsequent stroke, 25% Cardiac disease, 16% Other causes, 29%
Ueda and coworkers [176]	Japan	1961–1981	36.8 severely disabled	Not available	Hypertension, diabetes, and obesity increased the risk of severe disability after age correction
Dalsgaard-Nielson [179]	Denmark	1940–1953	36.5 heavily disabled or worse 19 moderately disabled or better	44.3 during admission	Retrospective review of case records; no definitions of terminology used for disability
Gillum and coworkers [30]	Minnesota, USA	1970–1980	Not available	Sex and Age — 1970 — 1980 Men 30–64, 23, 15 Men 65–74, 17, 20 Women 30–74, 14, 16	Data limited to hospital mortality (without time limit)
Sarti and coworkers [14]	Finland	1983–1986	Not available	Men: 18 thrombotic, 21 embolic, 46 unspecified Women: 18 thrombotic, 31 embolic, 55 unspecified	Population survey; not all cases had computed tomography scans or postmortem examinations; highest figures from the regions of Finland are given

(continued)

figures in the elderly [18,45,46]. Preexisting handicap increases mortality from 8% to 15% in those with no prior handicap and mortality is increased from 22% to 63% in those with a severe prior handicap [2,3]. Cardiac disease is also a major factor affecting mortality [53]. An abnormal electrocardiogram is sufficient to affect the prognosis [54,55], and hypertension and cardiac disease continue to affect mortality for 10 years [45]. An embolic etiology increases the case-fatality ratio from 30% to 42% [14,46,54]. Race may not be a risk factor. Analysis showed that racial variation in stroke risk factors and initial stroke type explained the differences in outcome [55,56]. Early recurrence of cerebral infarction increases the 30-day case fatality rate from 7.4% to 20% [57]. Weaker factors that may increase mortality include smoking and increased cholesterol [58]. Sex as a factor is disputed [46, 52,53].

MORBIDITY OF CEREBRAL INFARCTION

Data regarding functional outcome after cerebral infarction are given in Table 1.6. The elderly do particularly poorly after cerebral infarction [31]. In one large population-based study, 30% of the elderly were moderately or severely handicapped at 6 months after stroke, this figure falling to 16% in younger patients [3]. At 3 to 5 years, between 20% and 40% of survivors of infarction are functionally dependent in activities of daily living while between 22% and 37% are dependent to a lesser degree [44,59]. Psychiatric morbidity is considerable. At 3 years, 25% of survivors have a major depressive illness compared with 6% of the age-matched population, while anxiety is twice as common in stroke patients [59].

Table 1.6. Morbidity and mortality of cerebral infarction taken from several studies (*continued*)

Study	Location	Years	Morbidity, %	Mortality, %	Comments
Sacco and coworkers [55]	New York, USA	1983–1986	Not available	Whites: 25 Blacks: 21 Hispanics: 14	Hospital admissions only, limited to cerebral infarction; data for mortality at 12 months
McGovern and coworkers [20]	Minneapolis, USA	1970–1985	Not available	1970 / 1980 / 1985 Men: 28.8 / 21.0 / 14.2 Women: 26.3 / 22.8 / 12.1	Hospital admission only; cerebral infarcts and primary intracerebral hemorrhage
Kojima and coworkers [44]	Akita, Japan	1975–1981	Functional independence after cerebral infarction at 5 years: fully independent, 60 partially dependent, 7 totally dependent, 30	3-Week mortality, 7, and first year mortality, 22	None
Epstein and coworkers [177]	Israel	1984	Not available	Men, 20 Women, 38	Case fatality ratios at 3 months
Bonita and coworkers [18]	Auckland, New Zealand	1981	Not available	Time / Age, y / Men / Women 1 month / <65 / 25.3 / 30.1 1 month / 85+ / 36.4 / 70.8 1 year / <65 / 30.2 / 31.5 1 year / 85+ / 63.6 / 75.4	None
Malmgren and coworkers [13]	Oxfordshire, England	1983	Handicap (6 months) Age, y / Moderate / Severe <45 / 11.1 / 5.6 45–54 / 23.5 / 5.9 55–64 / 8.9 / 8.9 65–74 / 8.0 / 13.3 75–84 / 11.6 / 8.5 ≥85 / 17.9 / 9.0	Age, y / Mortality at 6 months <45 / 11.1 45–54 / 11.8 55–64 / 22.2 65–74 / 21.3 75–84 / 29.5 ≥85 / 56.7	Community-based study

RISK FACTORS FOR CEREBRAL INFARCTION

Unmodifiable Risk Factors

Age

Age is the single most powerful risk factor for cerebral infarction (Table 1.7), since the increase with age is exponential, doubling or tripling with every decade after the fifth [34,60–64] (Figure 1.4). The decreasing incidence of cerebral infarction is greatest in the elderly [31,36].

Sex

While early data from the Rochester study suggested no difference between the sexes [8], many other studies have identified a higher incidence in men. Mortality rates for men are 23% to 115% higher than for women in all countries [15]. No study has identified a higher incidence in women. One study found a higher incidence in very elderly women, the incidence in men being higher than the incidence in women in younger age groups [65]. Another found that sex differences declined with increasing age [63]. This may reflect the competitive effect of vascular disease in younger men in that those prone to vascular disease of any kind may have died before the eighth decade.

The decline in stroke has selectively benefitted women. Between 1945 and 1949 and 1970 and 1974 the fall in men was from 181 to 105, but in women the fall was from 138 to 69 [31]. The fall may also have begun earlier in women than in men [36], though larger falls in men have been reported [34].

Race

There is a higher incidence of all strokes types and cerebral infarction in blacks [56,62]. The mortality for all strokes in the United States between 1960 and 1986 in blacks was just under twice that of the white population [66]. Maoris have an incidence of stroke 44% higher than the remainder of the New Zealand population [18]. In blacks, the burden falls disproportionately on younger individuals. In the early 1980s, black men aged 35 to 44 years had a stroke mortality rate five times that of whites, while for young black women the rate was 3.57 times that of whites [67]. Conversely, rates for Hispanics and whites in the United States are comparable [56]. Despite this evidence that racial factors are important, a study investigating the incidence of stroke in several countries found no difference in the incidence of cerebral infarction [22]. Risk factors are more common in North American blacks than in whites, and the increased incidence of diabetes and hypertension alone may account for 50% of the extra incidence [68]. Racial effects are also apparent in the change in the incidence of stroke. Between 1960 and 1988 the fall in nonwhites was greater than that in whites [10,26,66].

Family History

There is little information on family history and stroke. A few studies support a role for family history [69–74], but part of the effect of family history is clearly mediated through other hereditary factors such as blood pressure, diabetes, and cholesterol levels [70,73]. Many studies supporting a role for family history did not consider these factors.

Previous Stroke

The recurrence rate for cerebral infarction lies between 10% and 30% [55,75–77] (Figure 1.6). The first 6 months is the period of highest risk [55,77] with an 8.6% recurrence rate [77], while the 1-month recurrence rate is 3.3% [57]. Hypertension, diabetes [57,75], and smoking [77] increase the risk, while an infarct of undetermined cause is associated with a diminished risk. Etiology affects the recurrence rate (Figure 1.7) and curiously atherothrombotic and not cardioembolic events may have the highest recurrence rates [57,75]. Age, race, sex, myocardial

Table 1.7. Risk factors for cerebral infarction

Unmodifiable risk factors	Questionable, rare, or weak modifiable risk factors	Risk factors predominant in the young
Age	AIDS	Mitral valve leaflet prolapse
Sex	Alcohol	Sickle cell disease and other hemoglobinopathies
Race	Fibrinogen and platelets	Migraine
Family history	Lipids	Cocaine abuse
Previous stroke	Exercise	Obstructive sleep apnea
Major modifiable risk factors	Obesity	Intercurrent infection
Atrial fibrillation	Hematocrit	Patent foramen ovale
Hypertension	Water supply	Atrial septal aneurysm
Isolated systolic hypertension	Anticardiolipin antibodies	Systemic lupus erythematosus
Myocardial infarction	Oral contraceptives	
Other heart disease	Pregnancy	
Diabetes mellitus	Homocystinuria	
Transient ischemic attacks	Diet	
Smoking	Socioeconomic status	
	Season	
	Claudication	

infarction, atrial fibrillation, and valvular heart disease do not significantly affect the risk [75,77,78]. Patients with the lowest combination of risk factors have a 2-year risk of 9.5% while the risk in the highest group is 24.5% [75].

Fibrinogen

Increasing fibrinogen levels correlate with an increasing risk of stroke [79,80], but the association may be weaker in women [79]. Fibrinogen levels covary with smoking but even so retain significance after multivariate analysis [80]. β-Thromboglobulin may be a risk factor in younger patients [81].

Modifiable risk factors

Atrial Fibrillation

Atrial fibrillation causes 20% of all infarcts [82] and is associated with a relative risk of death from stroke of 12.25 [83], while the relative risk of stroke varies from 4.1 to 10 [83–86]. The risk of

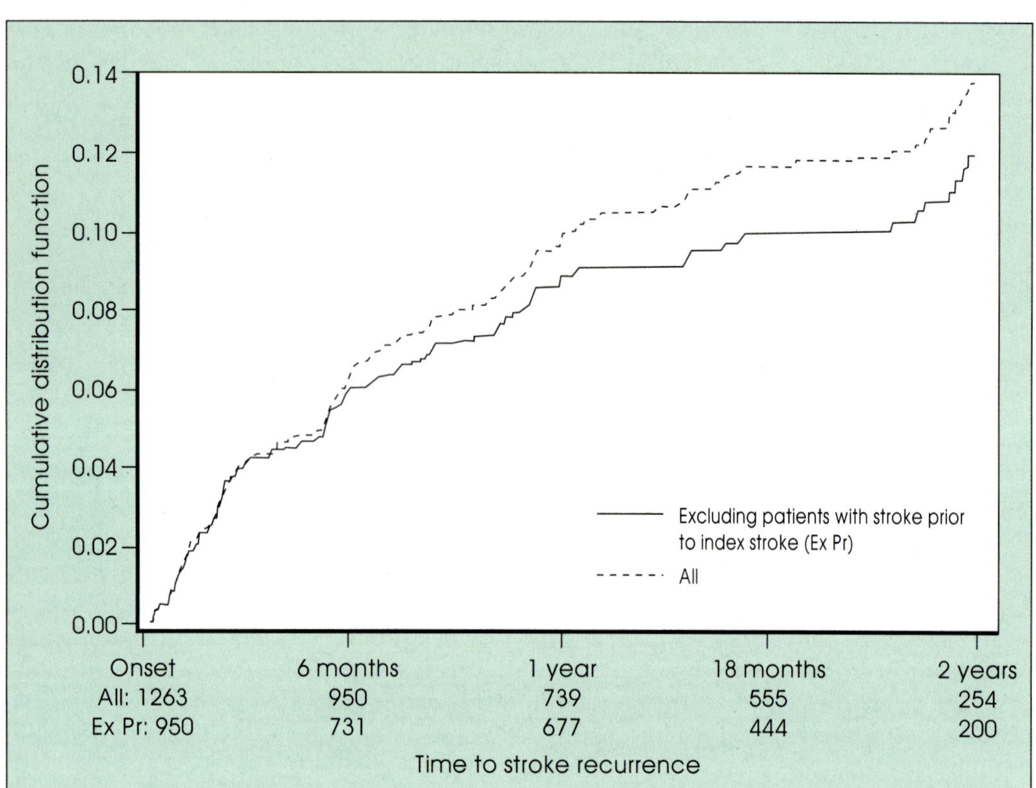

FIGURE 1.6

Stroke recurrence within 2 years by prior stroke status. Numbers below horizontal axis are patients remaining in risk group at end of each interval. (*From* Hier and coworkers [75]; with permission.)

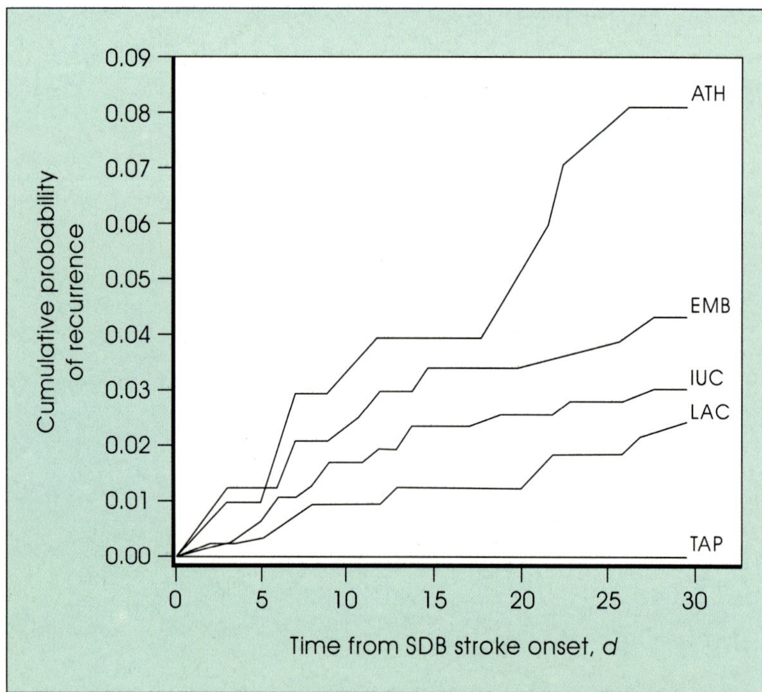

FIGURE 1.7

Kaplan-Meier estimates of probability of early recurrent stroke by index stroke subtype. ATH—atherosclerosis; EMB—cardioembolism; IUC—infarction of undetermined cause; LAC—lacunae; SDB—Stroke Data Bank; TAP—tandem arterial pathology. (*From* Sacco and coworkers [57]; with permission.)

stroke from atrial fibrillation is greatest in the first month when 25% occur, while 41% occur in the first year [87]. The annual rate is 2.7% for the next 5 years and 1% thereafter. Cases with rheumatic heart disease are at an increased risk with a relative risk of 17.9 [87,88]. With increasing age, atrial fibrillation, alone among hypertension and cardiac diseases, retains its potency as a risk factor [85]. As the prevalence of atrial fibrillation rises from 0.5% at age 50 to 8.8% at age 89, the attributable risk of stroke for atrial fibrillation increases from 1.5% to 23.5%. By comparison, the attributable risk of stroke for hypertension decreases from 48.8% to 33.4% [89]. Silent infarcts are found in 20% more of the population with atrial fibrillation than without [90–92], and this is exacerbated by increasing age and left atrial diameter [90]. Atrial fibrillation due to thyrotoxicosis in elderly patients may not be a risk factor as age, and not the presence of atrial fibrillation, determines the risk of stroke in such patients [93].

Hypertension

After age, hypertension is the most powerful risk factor for cerebral infarction. Table 1.8 illustrates aspects of the association. The relationships between both systolic and diastolic blood pressures and the relative risk of stroke are approximately log linear [94] (Figures 1.8 and 1.9). Both the systolic and diastolic pressures are important [58,62,95,96]. The relationship between hypertension and risk is continuous and there may be no practical lower limit [97]. Repeated measurements of systolic blood pressure provide a better guide to stroke risk than single measurements [98]. In those patients with a labile systolic pressure, the highest pressure recorded retains a substantial correlation with the risk of cerebral infarction [99], suggesting that the tendency to use the lowest measured pressure as the true pressure may be incorrect. The effect of hypertension decreases in the elderly. The relative risk for cerebral infarction falls from 3.5 in those aged 50 to 59 years to 1.7 (not significant) in those aged over 80 years, while attributable risk falls from 48.8% to 33.4% over the same age range [89]. In the elderly, diastolic blood pressure becomes less important than systolic [100]. Sex differences are not prominent in analyses of the effects of hypertension on stroke risk [97,101]. Prolonged treatment of diastolic blood pressure to produce a fall of 6 mm Hg decreases the stroke risk by 40% and the benefits accrue within 3 years [94].

Table 1.8. Data supporting hypertension as a powerful risk factor for cerebral infarction

Type of study, comments, and source	Details of risk factor	Effect
Meta-analysis; Oliver [180]	Diastolic pressure	Log-linear relationship to relative risk for stroke over the range <80 to >109 mm Hg; nine times increase in relative risk over this range
Sixteen-year follow-up in longshoremen; blood pressure divided into high and low according to the mean at entry into the study; Paffenbarger and coworkers [153]	Systolic pressure	Relative risk of death from stroke of 3.31 in those with systolic blood pressure above the population mean at entry
Population study in men aged 40–49 at entry followed for 12 years; small numbers of events because of the young age group of the patients; no information about antihypertensive treatment, the relatively weak association between blood pressure at entry and subsequent risk could be due to subsequent treatment; Håheim and coworkers [58]	Systolic pressure Diastolic pressure	Relative risk of stroke 1.37 Relative risk of stroke 1.60
Population survey in those aged 65 and older in northern England; no relationship between blood pressure and stroke incidence in women at all, and only between measured pressure and stroke incidence in men if groups added together; method of analysis could have led to false-negative conclusions; Evans [181]	History of raised pressure in men Systolic blood pressure in men	Standardized incidence ratio of 2.47 Relative risk 1.9; standardized incidence ratio 95% CI 115 to 412
Population study of 5209 individuals followed for 24 years aged 30–62 at entry; Kannel and coworkers [103]	Isolated systolic hypertension (diastolic <95 mm Hg)	Systolic <140, age-adjusted incidence in men 5.3/1000; systolic 7160, incidence in men 21.0/1000; systolic<140, age-adjusted incidence in women 3.8/1000; systolic 7160, incidence in women 9.6/1000
Population study of 1572 Italian men followed up for 25 years; all stroke types included; Menorti and coworkers [61]	Systolic pressure in men	Hazard ratio of 1.02 per mm Hg
Framingham study; data show that diastolic and systolic pressures are of similar importance, that men and women are approximately equally susceptible, and that there is no lower limit to the pressures at which increasing pressure is associated with increased risk; Kannel and coworkers [97]	Systolic and diastolic pressure	Ratio of observed/expected for atherothrombotic brain infarction of 1.69 for hypertensives after exclusion of gout, obesity, and diabetes

(continued)

Table 1.8. Data supporting hypertension as a powerful risk factor for cerebral infarction (*continued*)

Type of study, comments, and source	Details of risk factor	Effect	
		Relative risk	
	Systolic pressure	**Mean**	**Range**
Case control study using computed tomography–proven cerebral infarction; Ellekjaer and coworkers [95]	140–160 mm Hg	2.28	(1.40–3.70)
	160–180 mm Hg	2.65	(1.56–4.51)
	> 180 mm Hg	3.14	(1.74–5.65)
	Diastolic pressure		
	80–90 mm Hg	1.37	(0.86–2.19)
	90–95 mm Hg	1.37	(0.70–2.68)
	> 95 mm Hg	1.79	(1.10–2.92)
		Hazard ratios (risk per additional mm Hg)	
Hypertensive subjects (10,186) followed for a mean of 9 years; probably unrepresentative of hypertension in general as many cases were from hospital clinics and the patients were young with a mean age of 50 years; figures are for all stroke types determined as any mention of stroke on death certificate; Palmer and coworkers [182]	**Untreated systolic pressure**		
	Men	1.014	
	Women	1.009	
	Men	1.026	
	Women	1.010	
	Treated systolic pressure		
	Men	1.018	
	Women	1.021	
	Men	1.035	
	Women	1.028	

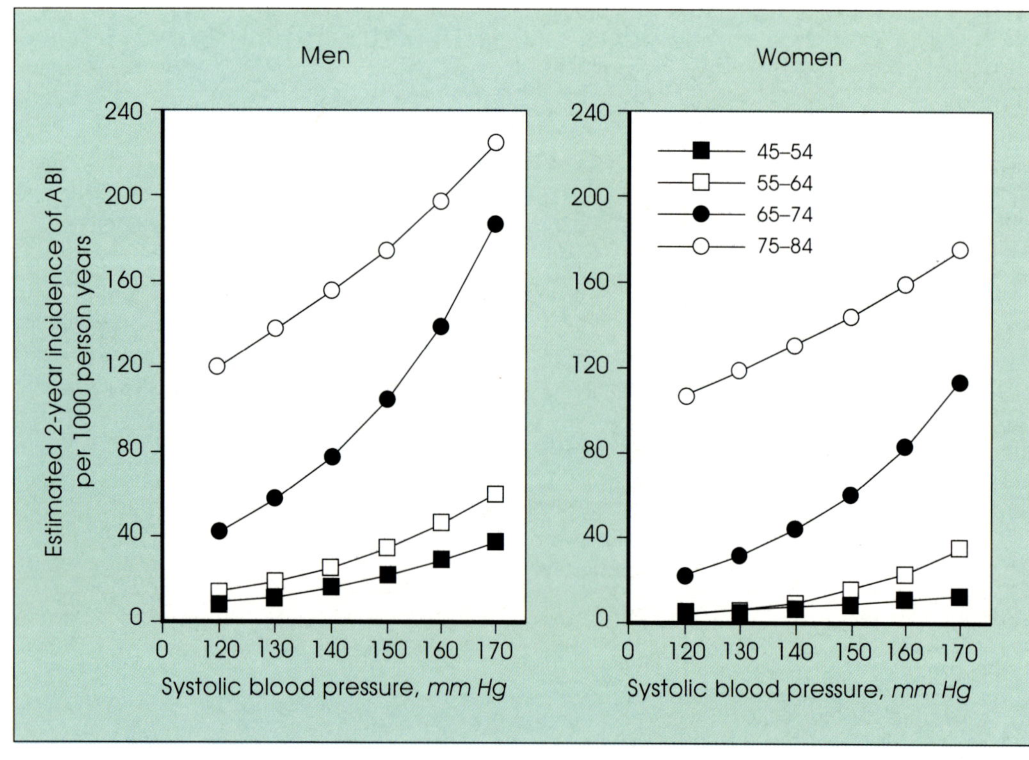

FIGURE 1.8

Incidence of brain infarction according to systolic blood pressure in men and women, ages 45 to 84, whose diastolic pressure is below 95 mm Hg. ABI—atherothrombotic brain infarction. (*From* Wolf and coworkers [171]; with permission.)

Isolated Systolic Hypertension

Isolated systolic hypertension is present in approximately 12% of 65-year-old men and 17% of 65-year-old women, increases with age [102], and has a slightly greater effect in men [100,103]. Treatment of isolated systolic hypertension is effective. A mean reduction in systolic pressure from 155 mm Hg to 143 mm Hg over 5 years produced a 36% fall in incidence [42].

Myocardial Infarction

Cerebral infarction occurs in between 1% and 1.25% of cases within 1 year of myocardial infarction [104,105], though a 5% occurrence has been reported [106]. Nearly all of this occurs in the first month [104–106]. The expected incidence over the same time is 0.1%. Transmural infarcts pose a greater risk than subendocardial infarcts [105]. The presence of other risk factors increases the risk of stroke from 0.29% in the first year with no other factors to 6.76% with four factors. Cerebral infarction after myocardial infarction increases mortality from myocardial infarction from 9% to 31% at 1 year [104]. A history of myocardial infarction is also a risk factor for cerebral infarction, but is of marginal significance when other factors are taken into account [95].

Other Heart Disease

Cardiac disease in general doubles the risk of stroke [84], while left ventricular hypertrophy quadruples it, independent of hypertension, in all subjects except (aged 35–64) men [60, 84,100]. Coronary heart disease increases the relative risk for stroke by 2.9 in those aged 50 to 59 years, this effect decreasing with increasing age. Cardiac failure is associated with a relative risk of 3.9 in those aged 50 to 59, falling dramatically in those over 80 years of age [89]. Illustrative risk ratios for various cardiac conditions are shown in Figure 1.10. Angina in men aged 47 to 55 is associated with a relative risk for cerebral infarction of 2.1 [86]. At least one cardiac source of embolism may be found in 26% of infarcts but the rate of stroke recurrence is low, being 2% in the groups with and without a cardiac source of embolism over the first 30 days [107]. Anticoagulation does not alter the recurrence rate in this group [107].

Diabetes Mellitus

Though variable, the evidence now supports diabetes as a risk factor for stroke. Much of the risk is associated with hypertension [108,109], but diabetes may be second only to systolic blood pressure as a risk factor, even after multivariate analysis [95]. Relative risks from diabetes for cerebral infarction lie in the region of 1.7 to 5.5 [61,84,95,96,101,109,110]. Impaired glucose tolerance may be a risk factor [111,112] and an elevated glycosylated hemoglobin may be found in up to 42% patients with cerebral infarcts not previously known to have diabetes [112].

Transient Ischemic Attacks

In one study based on 184 transient ischemic attacks (TIAs) with a mean follow-up of 3.7 years, 45 patients had a first-ever stroke and 15 more died from stroke. The incidence of stroke was 4.4% in the first month, 8.8% in the first 6 months, and 11.6% in the first year. Over 5 years, the risk was 5.9%/year (Figure 1.11). The relative risk of stroke after TIA is 13.4 in the first 12 months and 7 over the first 7 years [113]. In most studies, the incidence of cardiovascular disease and death at least equals and usually exceeds that due to cerebrovascular disease [114,115].

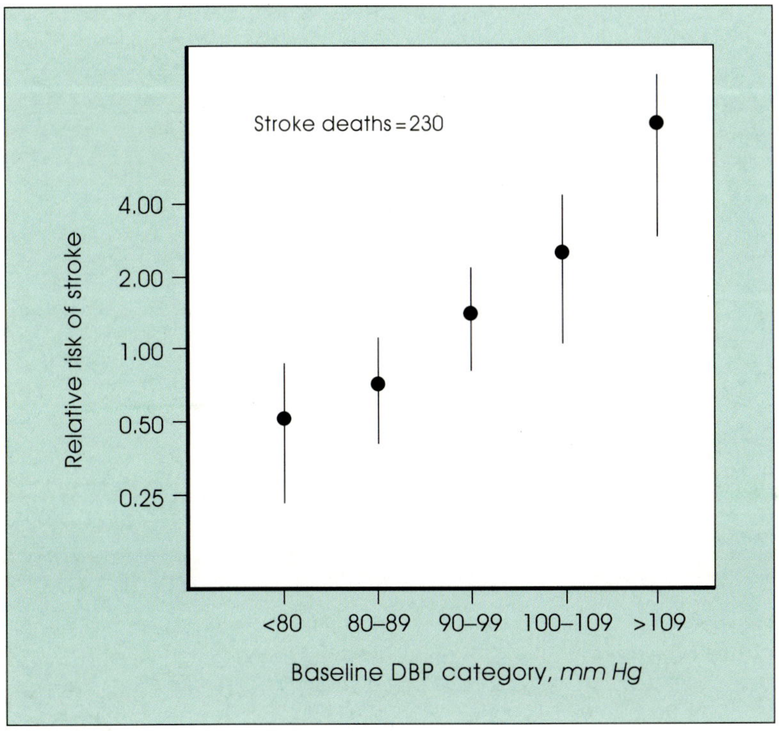

FIGURE 1.9

Relative risks and 95% CIs for death from stroke during 6 years of follow-up by diastolic blood pressure (DBP) at baseline. (*From* MacMahon and coworkers [94]; with permission.)

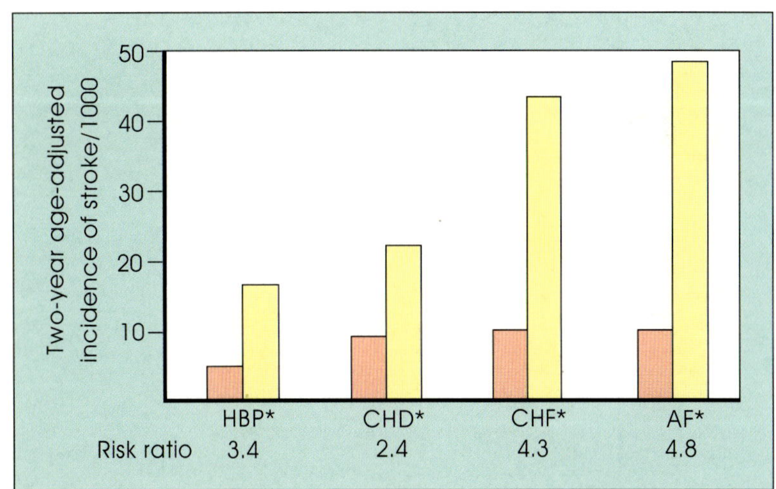

FIGURE 1.10

Bar graph of 2-year age-adjusted incidence of stroke according to presence (*yellow bars*) and absence (*orange bars*) of cardiovascular condition. *Asterisks* indicate *P*<0.001 different from unity. AF—atrial fibrillation; CHD—coronary heart disease; CHF—cardiac failure; HBP—hypertension;. (*From* Wolf and coworkers [89]; with permission.)

Smoking

Despite negative and equivocal studies [60–62,86,95,96,116,117], the evidence now firmly supports smoking as a risk factor [118]. The relative risk for stroke is up to 4.7 [58,101,110]. There is a dose-response relationship, the risk doubling in the heaviest smokers [101,110]. One study has suggested a lesser effect in young women [100], though a large prospective study shows smoking to be a prominent risk factor [119] in this group.

In the Framingham study, cessation of smoking removed the additional risk of stroke within 2 years [101].

Alcohol

The effect of alcohol on cerebral infarction has two aspects, these being sudden heavy (binge) drinking and chronic consumption. There is evidence for an association between sudden heavy drinking and the onset of cerebral infarction in young adults (Figure 1.12) [120–123]. Chronic light alcohol intake is associated with a decreased risk of stroke [110,124,125]. Chronic heavy (180 to over 400 g/wk) consumption is associated with an increased risk (Figure 1.13) [124,126,127]. Lifetime abstinence has been identified with an odds ratio for all stroke (excluding subarachnoid hemorrhage) of 2.36 [126], suggesting a U-shaped association between alcohol intake and stroke risk.

Lipids

Total cholesterol has a weak association with cerebral infarction. In various studies, including two population studies, no additional risk was associated with increased cholesterol levels [58,62,96]. Conversely, data from the Framingham study suggest a weak correlation between cholesterol and triglycerides and the risk of atherothrombotic brain infarction in men under 60 years of age, though triglycerides cease to have a role if cholesterol is included in the statistical model [128]. In one study, hypercholesterolemia was associated with stroke in young women [119]. Triglycerides are not important [58]. Lipoprotein (a) may be an important risk factor [129].

Exercise

Lack of exercise may increase the risk of all stroke in women (relative risk, 1.45) [117], but hypertension and diabetes were not considered in this study. Other work has had negative results [86,95].

Obesity

Most studies that have assessed obesity have found little association between body mass or obesity and the risk of cerebral infarction [58,95,96], though the Framingham study suggested a modest role for relative weight in younger men and older women [100].

Hematocrit

The Framingham study observed a small independent risk for atherothrombotic brain infarction attributable to hematocrit in younger men [100]. Other studies have been negative [60] or have shown a weak correlation abolished by multivariate analysis [130].

Oral Contraceptives

The matter of oral contraceptive use is disputed. The early studies suggesting an association between oral contraceptive use and cerebral infarction were all retrospective case control studies, methodologically weak [131], dated from the late 1970s and early 1980s [131–133] when the dose of estrogen was higher than is now used, or did not consider other risk factors [132].

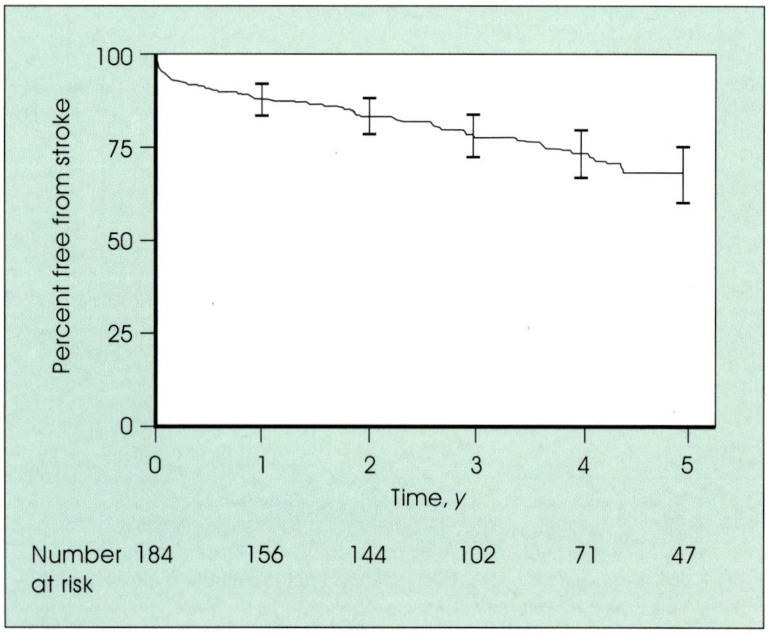

FIGURE 1.11

Kaplan-Meier survival curve showing percentage surviving free from stroke (censoring those dying of other causes) during first 5 years after transient ischemic attack. Error bars indicated 95% CI. (*From* Dennis and coworkers [113]; with permission.)

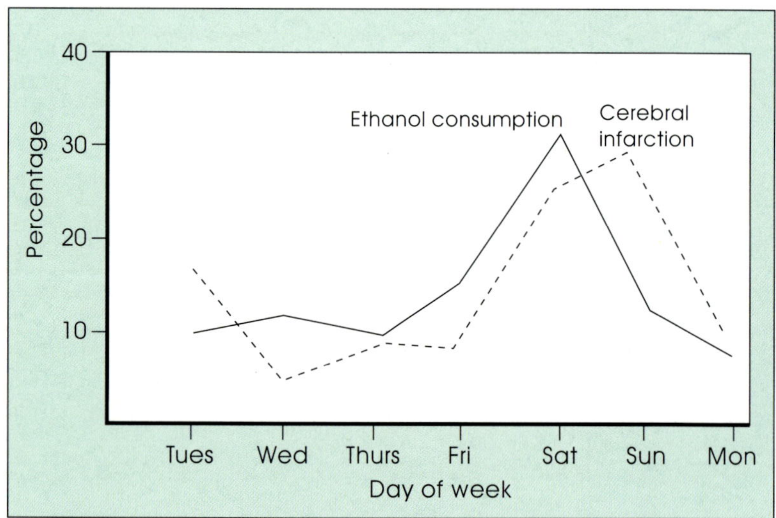

FIGURE 1.12

Distribution of onset of ischemic brain infarction on different weekdays compared with alcohol consumption in the general population. (*From* Hillbom and Kaste [120]; with permission.)

Much of the association may be explained by other risk factors, particularly smoking [119,133], which increased substantially in young women concomitant with increasing use of the oral contraceptive. Stroke in younger women has not increased in a way consistent with an effect of the oral contraceptive [134]. Large prospective studies have not identified an association between oral contraceptive use and cerebral infarction [119,135]. A more recent retrospective case-control study with a full multivariate analysis identified a relative risk of 2.9 with use of oral contraceptive pills containing 50 µg of estrogen. With 30 to 40 µg the relative risk was 1.8, and there was no risk with the progestogen-only preparation [136].

Minor Factors

Soft water has been associated with an increased risk (about 7%) of death from stroke according to death certificates [137], an effect that may be limited to women [138]. Other evidence does not support a role for water hardness in cerebrovascular disease [139], and there is no hypothesis linking the observation to the pathogenesis of stroke. Anticardiolipin antibodies are associated with a relative risk of 2.31 for cerebral infarction [140]. Pregnancy is not associated with a risk of stroke significantly different from nonpregnant women of the same age in western societies [141]. While homozygotes for homocystinuria have long been recognized to be at high risk for stroke, heterozygotes and others with elevated levels of homocysteine are at increased risk for stroke [142,143]. Thirty percent of patients with cerebral ischemic events had homocystine levels above control values (Figure 1.14) [144]. Homocystine is independent of other risk factors [145]. AIDS is a risk factor for cerebral infarction. The precise mechanism is unknown, but an associated central nervous system infection, typically with *Cryptococcus* species, tuberculosis, or varicella zoster, is implicated in half the cases [146]. The age-adjusted mortality of stroke falls with increasing levels of education and income (Figure 1.15) [10]. A decrease in the incidence of cerebral infarction in summer and peak in winter has been reported in several studies and inversely correlated with mean ambient temperature [147,148]. Diurnally, 70% of infarcts occur between midnight and midday (Figure 1.16) [149–151]. An association exists between claudication and cerebral infarction [86]. No evidence supports hyperuricemia as a risk factor. Intercurrent infection may precipitate stroke [152].

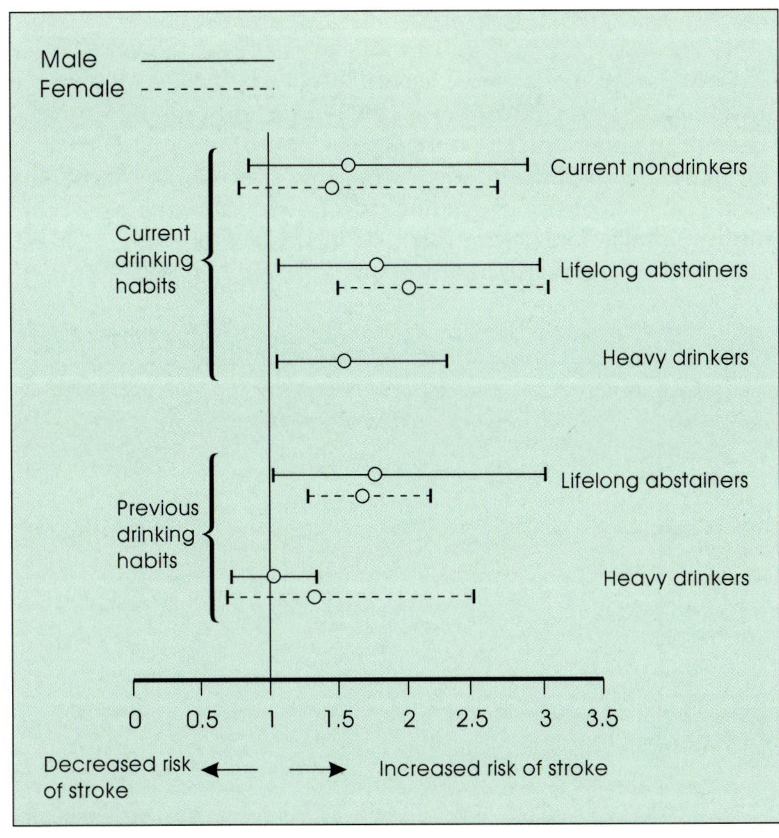

FIGURE 1.13

Graph showing odds ratio of risk of stroke in current and previous drinkers. (*From* Rodgers and coworkers [126]; with permission.)

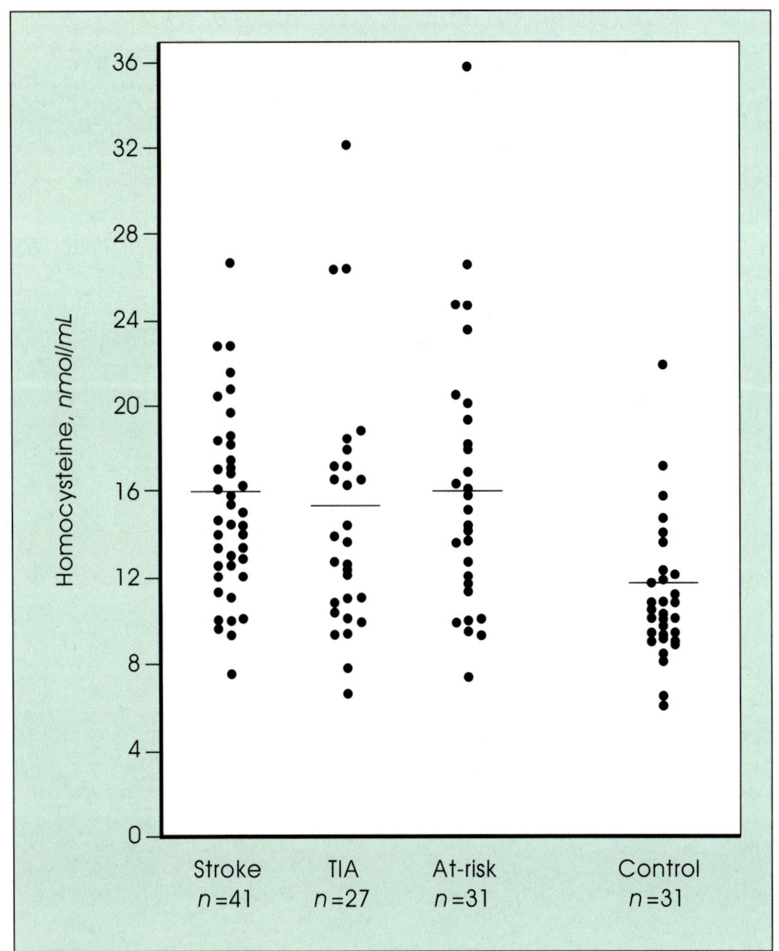

FIGURE 1.14

Scatterplot of plasma homocystine concentration in patients with acute stroke, those with transient ischemic attack (TIA), those at risk for cerebrovascular disease, and controls. (*From* Coull and coworkers [145]; with permission.)

Interactions Between Risk Factors

Risk factors interact multiplicatively rather than by summation, so that the risk of death from stroke increases as the number of risk factors increases, even where these factors are individually of little significance [153,154]. The interaction between blood sugar and blood pressure is shown in Figure 1.17. Risk profiles can be calculated from several readily assessed risk factors (Tables 1.9–1.12) [154].

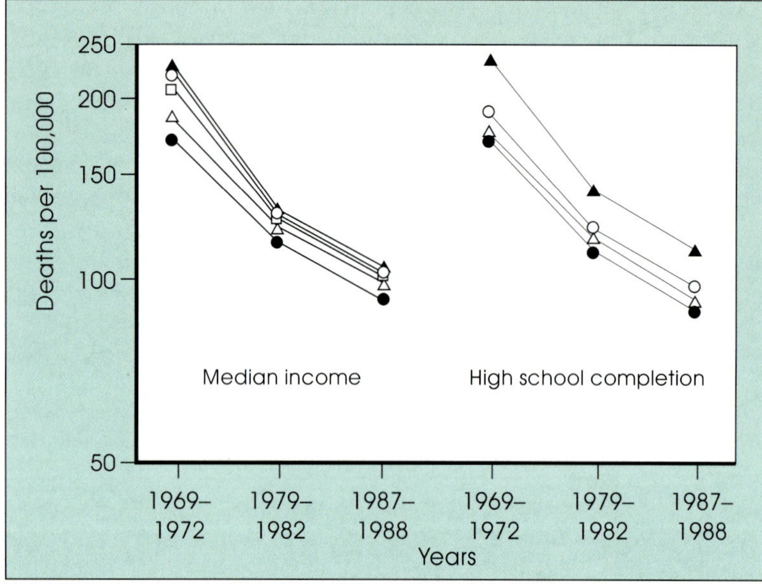

FIGURE 1.15

Graph showing age-adjusted death rates in the United States from stroke, 1968 to 1988, by socioeconomic quintiles. (*From* Modan and Wagener [10]; with permission.)

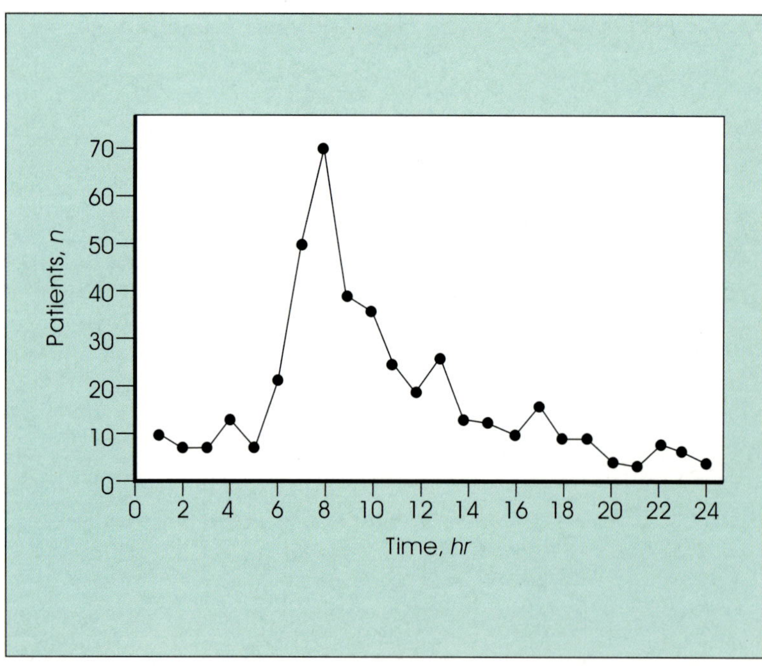

FIGURE 1.16

Graph of circadian variation of observed ischemic stroke onset. Patients with onset of stroke while asleep are omitted. (*From* Argentino and coworkers [151]; with permission.)

Cerebral Infarction in the Young

The etiology of cerebral infarction in the young differs from that in the elderly as atherosclerosis and ischemic heart disease have not usually developed to a sufficient extent in the young to pose a risk of cerebral infarction.

The importance of mitral valve leaflet prolapse (MVLP) as a risk factor for cerebral infarction in the young is disputed [155,156]. It is the sole explanation in 5% to 30% of cases [155,157]. The relative risk may be as high as 9.33, but lower figures have been reported and a problem is posed by the finding of MVLP in 7% of the population, making a diagnosis of stroke due to MVLP one of exclusion. Even making the generous assumption that MVLP explains 30% of cerebral infarcts in the young, the risk of infarction in a patient with MVLP is only one in 6000 per annum [155].

Patent foramen ovale is associated with cerebral infarction [158–160]. In patients aged 15 to 55 with otherwise undiagnosed stroke, the presence of patent foramen ovale, with or without an atrial septal aneurysm, was associated with an odds ratio for stroke of 3.9 (1.5–10). An atrial septal aneurysm alone was associated with an odds ratio of 4.3 (1.3–14.6). Combined, the two produced an odds ratio of 33.3 (4.1–270). The risk attributable to atrial septal aneurysm increased as the excursion of the aneurysm increased [159].

Stroke may be seen in 17% of cases of sickle cell disease [161]. Migraine has a weak association with stroke. Migrainous stroke occurs at a rate of 3.4/100,000 per annum. The prevalence of migraine in the young stroke population is the same as the general population, suggesting that there is no significant long-term risk of nonmigrainous stroke (stroke occurring other than in association with a migraine headache) in these individuals [162]. Drugs, particularly cocaine [163], but also ampheta-

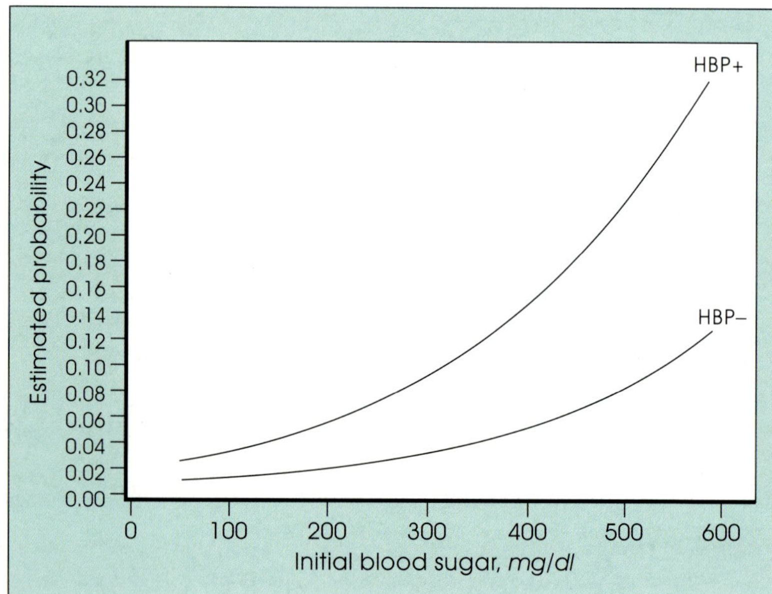

FIGURE 1.17

Relation between initial blood sugar concentration and estimated probability of stroke recurrence by history of hypertension (HBP). (*From* Sacco and coworkers [57]; with permission.)

mine, amphetamine-related drugs, and phencyclidine, are associated with cerebral infarction. Obstructive sleep apnea may give rise to a relative risk for cerebral infarction of 8 (95% CI 1.07–3.56) in those aged 16 to 60 [164]. Stroke may be seen in 15% of patients with systemic lupus erythematosus, usually occurring within the first 5 years after diagnosis [165] and is less commonly seen in association with other vasculitides.

PROTECTIVE FACTORS

Hormone replacement therapy in postmenopausal smokers reduces the risk for all stroke by 28% [117]. Increased leisure exercise may offer some protection from stroke morbidity [58,61] and levels of exercise above sedentary may cut the relative risk of stroke to 0.7 [58], while higher levels of exercise cut the relative risk to 0.5 and less [61,166,167]. There is weak evidence that dietary potassium intake correlates inversely with the risk of stroke-associated death [168]. A decline in the incidence of stroke in Britain during World War II has been attributed to dietary restrictions and suggests that dietary change may decrease risk quickly [169]. Low-fat milk consumption may be beneficial [110], as may be low alcohol intake [110,124,125].

CONCLUSIONS

The mortality from cerebral infarction has decreased mainly as a result of the recognition of the association between hypertension and cerebral infarction and the treatment of hypertension. This represents a major success for epidemiology. The incidence of cerebral infarction has fallen, but the matter remains controversial because of increased awareness of stroke and more sensitive diagnostic tools. Clarification of this point and the identification of other treatable risk factors are matters of major importance in view of the increasing age of the population.

Table 1.9. Variables for the probability of stroke in men aged 55 to 85 years*

Variables	Stroke points										
	0	+1	+2	+3	+4	+5	+6	+7	+8	+9	+10
Age, *y*	54-56	57–59	60–62	63–65	66–68	69–72	73–75	76–78	79–81	82–84	85
Untreated SBP, *mm Hg*	97–105	106–115	116–125	126–135	136–145	146–155	156–165	166–175	176–185	186–195	196–205
Treated SBP, *mm Hg*	97–105	106–112	113–117	118–123	124–129	130–135	136–142	143–150	151–161	162–176	177–205
Diabetes	No		Yes								
Cigarette smoking	No			Yes							
CVD	No				Yes						
AF	No				Yes						
LVH	No					Yes					

**Adapted from* D'Agostino and coworkers [172]; with permission.
AF—atrial fibrillation; CVD—cardiovascular disease; LVH—left ventricular hypertrophy; SBP—systolic blood pressure.

Table 1.10. Ten-year probability of stroke measured by total stroke points in men*

Total points	Probability, %	Total points	Probability, %
1	3	16	22
2	3	17	26
3	4	18	29
4	4	19	33
5	5	20	37
6	5	21	42
7	6	22	47
8	7	23	52
9	8	24	57
10	10	25	63
11	11	26	68
12	13	27	74
13	15	28	79
14	17	29	84
15	20	30	88

**Adapted from* D'Agostino and coworkers [172]; with permission.

Table 1.11. Variables for the probability of stroke in women aged 55 to 84 years*

Variables	Stroke points										
	0	+1	+2	+3	+4	+5	+6	+7	+8	+9	+10
Age, *y*	54–56	57–59	60–62	63–64	65–67	68–70	71–73	74–76	77–78	79–81	82–84
Untreated SBP, *mm Hg*		95–106	107–118	119–130	131–143	144–155	156–167	168–180	181–192	193–204	205–216
Treated SBP, *mm Hg*		95–106	107–113	114–119	120–125	126–131	132–139	140–148	149–160	161–204	205–216
Diabetes	No			Yes							
Cigarette smoking	No			Yes							
CVD	No		Yes								
AF	No						Yes				
LVH	No				Yes						

**Adapted from* D'Agostino and coworkers [172]; with permission.
AF—atrial fibrillation; CVD—cardiovascular disease; LVH—left ventricular hypertrophy; SBP—systolic blood pressure.

Table 1.12. Ten-year probability of stroke measured by total stroke points in women*

Total points	Probability, %	Total points	Probability, %
1	1	15	16
2	1	16	19
3	2	17	23
4	2	18	27
5	2	19	32
6	3	20	37
7	4	21	43
8	4	22	50
9	5	23	57
10	6	24	64
11	8	25	71
12	9	26	78
13	11	27	84
14	13		

**Adapted from* D'Agostino and coworkers [172]; with permission.

REFERENCES

1. Bonita R: Epidemiology of stroke. *Lancet* 1992, 339:342–344.
2. Bamford J, Dennis M, Sandercock P, *et al.*: The frequency, causes, and timing of death within 30 days of a first stroke: the Oxfordshire Community Stroke Project. *J Neurol Neurosurg Psych* 1990, 53:824–829.
3. Malmgren R, Bamford J, Warlow C, *et al.*: Projecting the number of patients with first-ever strokes and patients newly handicapped by stroke in England and Wales. *BMJ* 1989, 298:656–660.
4. Kramer S, Diamond EL, Lilienfeld AM: Patterns of incidence and trends in diagnostic classification of cerebrovascular disease in Washington County, Maryland, 1969–1971 to 1974–1976. *Am J Epidemiol* 1982, 115:398–411.
5. Schoenberg BS: Epidemiology of cerebrovascular disease. *South Med J* 1979, 72:331–336.
6. Netsky MG, Miyaji T: Prevalence of cerebral hemorrhage and thrombosis in Japan: study of the major causes of death. *J Chron Dis* 1976, 29:711–721.
7. Wylie CM: Death statistics for cerebrovascular disease: a review of recent findings. *Stroke* 1970, 1:184–193.
8. Whisnant JP, Fitzgibbons JP, Kurland LT, Sayre GP: Natural history of stroke in Rochester, Minnesota, 1945 through 1954. *Stroke* 1971, 2:11–22.
9. Acheson RM, Fairbairn AS: Record linkage in studies of cerebrovascular disease in Oxford, England. *Stroke* 1971, 2:48–57.
10. Modan B, Wagener DK: Some epidemiological aspects of stroke: mortality/morbidity trends, age, sex, race, socioeconomic status. *Stroke* 1992, 23:1230–1236.
11. Lanska DJ, Mi X: Decline in US stroke mortality in the era before antihypertensive therapy. *Stroke* 1993, 24:1382–1388.
12. Ostfeld A: A review of stroke epidemiology. *Epidemiol Rev* 1980, 2:136–152.
13. Corwin LI, Wolf PA, Kannel WB, McNamara PM: Accuracy of death certification in stroke: the Framingham study. *Stroke* 1982, 13:818–821.
14. Sarti C, Tuomilehto J, Sivenius J, *et al.*: Stroke mortality and case–fatality rates in three geographic areas of Finland from 1983 to 1986. *Stroke* 1993, 24:1140–1147.
15. Bonita R, Stewart AW, Beaglehote R: International trends in stroke mortality. *Stroke* 1990, 32:989–992.
16. Malmgren R, Warlow C, Bamford J, Sandercock P: Geographical and secular trends in stroke incidence. *Lancet* 1987, 2:1196–1200.
17. Alter M, Zhang ZX, Sobel E, *et al.*: Standardized incidence ratios of stroke: a worldwide review. *Neuroepidemiology* 1986, 5:148–158.
18. Bonita R, Beaglehole R, North JD: Event, incidence and case fatality rates of cerebrovascular disease in Auckland, New Zealand. *Am J Epidemiol* 1984, 120:236–243.
19. Jerntrop P, Berglund G: Stroke registry in Malmö, Sweden. *Stroke* 1992, 23:357–361.
20. McGovern PG, Pankow JS, Burke GL, *et al.*: Trends in survival of hospitalized stroke patients between 1970 and 1985: the Minnesota heart survey. *Stroke* 1993, 24:1640–1648.
21. Alter M, Christoferson L, Resch J, *et al.*: Cerebrovascular disease: frequency and population selectivity in an upper midwestern community. *Stroke* 1970, 1:454–465.
22. Aho K, Harmsen P, Hatano S, *et al.*: Cerebrovascular disease in the community: results of a WHO collaborative study. *Bull W H O* 1980, 58:113–130.
23. Perez FI, Gay JR, Taylor RL: WAIS performance of neurologically impaired aged. *Psychol Rep* 1975, 37:1043–1047.
24. Hu HH, Sheng WY, Chu FL, *et al.*: Incidence of stroke in Taiwan. *Stroke* 1992, 23:1237–1241.
25. Fabsitz R, Feinleib M: Geographic patterns in county mortality rates from cardiovascular diseases. *Am J Epidemiol* 1980, 111:315–328.
26. Soltero I, Liu K, Cooper R, *et al.*: Trends in mortality from cerebrovascular diseases in the United States, 1960 to 1975. *Stroke* 1978, 9:549–558.
27. King MJ, Whelton PK, Seidler AJ: Decline in U.S. stroke mortality: Demographic trends and antihypertensive treatment. *Stroke* 1989, 20:14–21.
28. Anderson GL,Whisnant JP: A comparison of trends in mortality from stroke in the United States and Rochester, Minnesota. *Stroke* 1982, 13:804–809.
29. Ahmed OI, Orchard TJ, Sharma R, *et al.*: Declining mortality from stroke in Allegheny county, Pennsylvania: trends in case fatality and severity of disease. *Stroke* 1988, 19:181–184.
30. Gillum RF, Gomez Marin O, Kottke TE, *et al.*: Acute stroke in a metropolitan area, 1970 and 1980. The Minnesota Heart Survey. *J Chron Dis* 1985, 38:891–898.
31. Garraway WM, Whisnant JP, Kurland LT, O'Fallon WM: Changing pattern of cerebral infarction: 1945—1974. *Stroke* 1979, 10:657–663.
32. Garraway WM, Whisnant JP, Drury I: The changing pattern of survival following stroke. *Stroke* 1983, 14:699–703.
33. Tuomilehto J, Bonita R, Stewart A, *et al.*: Hypertension, cigarette smoking, and the decline in stroke incidence in eastern Finland. *Stroke* 1991, 22:7–11.
34. Shimamoto I, Komachi Y, Inada H, *et al.*: Trends for coronary heart disease and stroke and their risk factors in Japan. *Circulation* 1989, 79:503–515.
35. Ueda K, Omae T, Hirota Y, *et al.*: Decreasing trend in incidence and mortality from stroke in Hisayama residents, Japan. *Stroke* 1981, 12:154–160.
36. Broderick JP, Phillips SJ, Shisnant JP, *et al.*: Incidence rates of stroke in the eighties: the end of the decline in stroke? *Stroke* 1989, 20:577–582.
37. Wolf PA, D'Agostino RB, O'Neal MA, *et al.*: Secular trends in stroke incidence and mortality: the Framingham Study. *Stroke* 1992, 23:1551–1555.
38. Harmsen P, Isipogianni A, Wilhelmsen L: Stroke incidence rates were unchanged, while fatality rates declined, during 1971–1987 in Goteborg, Sweden. *Stroke* 1992, 23:1410–1415.
39. Jorgensen HS, Plesner AM, Hubbe P, Larsen K: Marked increase of stroke incidence in men between 1972 and 1990 in Frederiksberg, Denmark. *Stroke* 1992, 23:1701–1704.
40. Lindenstrom E, Boysen G, Nyboe J, Appleyard M: Stroke incidence in Copenhagen, 1976–1988. *Stroke* 1992, 23:28–32.
41. Whisnant JP: The decline of stroke. *Stroke* 1984, 15:160–168.
42. SHEP Cooperative Research Group: Prevention of stroke by antihypertensive drug treatment in older persons with isolated systolic hypertension: final results of the Systolic Hypertension in the Elderly Program (SHEP). *JAMA* 1991, 265:3255–3264.
43. Riggs JE: The decline of mortality due to stroke: A competitive and deterministic perspective. *Neurology* 1991, 41:1335–1338.
44. Kojima S, Omura T, Wakamatsu W, *et al.*: Prognosis and disability of stroke patients after 5 years in Akita, Japan. *Stroke* 1990, 21:72–77.
45. Sacco RL, Wolf PA, Kannel WB, McNamara PM: Survival and recurrence following stroke: the Framingham study. *Stroke* 1982, 13:290–295.
46. Herman B, Leyten AC, van Luijk JH, *et al.*: Epidemiology of stroke in Tilburg, the Netherlands: the population–based stroke incidence register: 2. Incidence, initial clinical picture and medical care, and three–week case fatality. *Stroke* 1982, 13:629–634.
47. Marshall J, Shaw D: The natural history of cerebrovascular disease. *BMJ* 1959, 1:1614–1617.
48. Adams GF, Merrett JD: Prognosis and survival in the aftermath of hemiplegia. *BMJ* 1961, 1:309–314.
49. Silver FL, Norris JW, Lewis AJ, Hachinski VC: Early mortality following stroke: a prospective review. *Stroke* 1984, 15:492–496.
50. Acheson J, Hutchinson EC: The natural history of focal cerebrovascular disease. *Q J Med* 1971, 40:15–23.
51. Kuller L, Anderson H, Peterson D, *et al.*: Nationwide cerebrovascular disease morbidity study. *Stroke* 1970, 1:86–99.

52. Haberman S, Capildeo R, Rose FC: The changing mortality of cerebrovascular disease. *Q J Med* 1978, 47:71–88.

53. Howard G, Evans GW, Murros KE, *et al.*: Cause specific mortality following cerebral infarction. *J Clin Epidemiol* 1989, 42:45–51.

54. Frithz G, Werner I: Studies on cerebrovascular strokes. II. Clinical findings and short–term prognosis in a stroke material. *Acta Med Scand* 1976, 199:133–140.

55. Sacco RL, Hauser WA, Mohr JP: One–year outcome after cerebral infarction in whites, blacks, and Hispanics. *Stroke* 1991, 22:305–311.

56. Sacco RL, Hauser WA, Mohr JP: Hospitalized stroke in blacks and Hispanics in northern Manhattan. *Stroke* 1991, 22:1491–1496.

57. Sacco RL, Foulkes MA, Mohr JP, *et al.*: Determinants of early recurrence of cerebral infarction: the Stroke Data Bank. *Stroke* 1989, 20:983–989.

58. Håheim LL, Holme I, Hjermann I, Leren P: Risk factors of stroke incidence and mortality: a 12–year follow–up of the Oslo study. *Stroke* 1993, 24:1484–1489.

59. Aström M, Asplund K, Aström T: Psychosocial function and life satisfaction after stroke. *Stroke* 1992, 23:527–531.

60. Kagan A, Popper JS, Rhoads GG: Factors related to stroke incidence in Hawaii Japanese men: the Honolulu Heart Study. *Stroke* 1980, 11:14–21.

61. Menotti A, Lanti M, Seccareccia F, *et al.*: Multivariate prediction of the first major cerebrovascular event in an Italian population sample of middle–aged men followed up for 25 years. *Stroke* 1993, 24:42–48.

62. Ostfeld AM, Shekelle RB, Klawans H, Tufo HM: Epidemiology of stroke in an elderly welfare population. *Am J Public Health* 1974, 64:450–458.

63. Lyngborg K, Marquardsen J, Trautner F, *et al.*: Myocardial infarction and cerebral infarction in a Danish suburban community. *Dan Med Bull* 1985, 32:127–131.

64. Chang CC, Chen CJ: Secular trend of mortality from cerebral infarction and cerebral hemorrhage in Taiwan, 1974–1988. *Stroke* 1993, 24:212–218.

65. Alter M, Sobel E, McCoy RC, *et al.*: Stroke in the Lehigh Valley: Incidence based on a community–wide hospital register. *Neuroepidemiology* 1985, 4:1–15.

66. Cooper R, Sempos C, Hsieh S–C, Kovar MG: Slowdown in the decline of stroke mortality in the United States, 1978–1986. *Stroke* 1990, 21:1274–1279.

67. Gillum RF: Stroke in blacks. *Stroke* 1988, 19:1–9.

68. Kittner SJ, White LR, Losonczy KG, Wolf PA: Black–white differences in stroke incidence in a national sample: the contribution of hypertension and diabetes. *JAMA* 1990, 264:1267–1270.

69. Brass LM, Isaacsohn JL, Merikangas KR, Robinette CD: A study of twins and stroke. *Stroke* 1992, 23:221–223.

70. Kiely DK, Wolf PA, Cupples LA, *et al.*: Familial aggregation of stroke: the Framingham study. *Stroke* 1993, 24:1366–1371.

71. Brass LM, Shaker LA: Family history in patients with transient ischemic attacks. *Stroke* 1991, 22:837–841.

72. Khaw K–T, Barrett–Connor EB: Family history of stroke as an independent predictor of ischemic heart disease in men and stroke in women. *Am J Epidemiol* 1986, 123:59–66.

73. Diaz JF, Hachinski VC, Pederson LL, Donald A: Aggregation of multiple risk factors for stroke in siblings of patients with brain infarction and transient ischemic attacks. *Stroke* 1986, 17:1239–1242.

74. Alter M, Kluznik J: Genetics of cerebrovascular accidents. *Stroke* 1972, 3:41–48.

75. Hier DB, Foulkes MA, Swiontoniowski M, *et al.*: Stroke recurrence within 2 years after ischemic infarction. *Stroke* 1991, 22:155–161.

76. Terent A: Survival after stroke and transient ischemic attacks during the 1970s and 1980s. *Stroke* 1989, 20:1320–1326.

77. Burn J, Dennis M, Bamford J, *et al.*: Long–term risk of recurrent stroke after a first–ever stroke: the Oxfordshire community stroke project. *Stroke* 1994, 25:333–337.

78. Shuper A, Mukamel M, Mimouni M, Steinherz R: Noonan's syndrome and neurofibromatosis. *Arch Dis Child* 1987, 62:196–198.

79. Kannel WB, Wolf PA, Castelli WP, D'Agostino RB: Fibrinogen and risk of cardiovascular disease: the Framingham study. *JAMA* 1987, 258:1183–1186.

80. Wilhelmsen L, Svardsudd K, Korsan Bengtsen K, *et al.*: Fibrinogen as a risk factor for stroke and myocardial infarction. *N Engl J Med* 1984, 311:501–505.

81. Scharf RE, Hennerici M, Bluschke V, *et al.*: Cerebral ischemia in young patients: is it associated with mitral valve prolapse and abnormal platelet activity? *Stroke* 1982, 13:454–458.

82. Yamanouchi H, Shimada H, Kuramoto K: Subtypes and proportions of cerebrovascular disease in an autopsy series in a Japanese geriatric hospital. *Klin Wochenschr* 1990, 68:1173–1177.

83. Onundarson PT, Thorgeirsson G, Jonmundsson E, *et al.*: Chronic atrial fibrillation—epidemiologic features and 14 year follow–up: a case control study. *Eur Heart J* 1987, 8:521–527.

84. Wolf PA, Kannel WB, Verter J: Current status of risk factors for stroke. *Neurol Clin* 1983, 1:317–343.

85. Wolf PA, Abbott RD, Kannell WB: Atrial fibrillation: a major contributor to stroke in the elderly: the Framingham Study. *Arch Intern Med* 1987, 147:1561–1564.

86. Harmsen P, Rosengren A, Tsipogianni A, Wilhelmsen L: Risk factors for stroke in middle–aged men in Goteborg, Sweden. *Stroke* 1990, 21:223–229.

87. Petersen P, Godtfredsen J: Risk factors for stroke in chronic atrial fibrillation. *Eur Heart J* 1988, 9:291–294.

88. Brandt J, Welsh KA, Breitner JCS, *et al.*: Hereditary influences on cognitive functioning in older men: a study of 4000 twin pairs. *Arch Neurol* 1993, 50:599–603.

89. Wolf PA, Abbott RD, Kannel WB: Atrial fibrillation as an independent risk factor for stroke: the Framingham Study. *Stroke* 1991, 22:983–988.

90. Feinberg WM, Seeger JF, Carmody RF, *et al.*: Epidemiologic features of asymptomatic cerebral infarction in patients with nonvalvular atrial fibrillation. *Arch Intern Med* 1990, 150:2340–2344.

91. Kempster PA, Gerraty RP, Gates PC: Asymptomatic cerebral infarction in patients with chronic atrial fibrillation. *Stroke* 1988, 19:955–957.

92. Petersen P, Madsen EB, Brun B, *et al.*: Silent cerebral infarction in chronic atrial fibrillation. *Stroke* 1987, 18:1098–1100.

93. Petersen P, Hansen JM: Stroke in thyrotoxicosis with atrial fibrillation. *Stroke* 1988, 19:15–18.

94. MacMahon S, Cutler JA, Stamler J: Antihypertensive drug treatment: potential, expected, and observed effects on stroke and on coronary heart disease. *Hypertension* 1989, 13(suppl):I–45–I–50/

95. Ellekjaer EF, Wyller TB, Sverre JM, Holmen J: Lifestyle factors and risk of cerebral infarction. *Stroke* 1992, 23:829–834.

96. Aronow WS, Starling L, Etienne F, *et al.*: Risk factors for atherothrombotic brain infarction in persons over 62 years of age in a long–term health care facility. *J Am Geriatr Soc* 1987, 35:1–3.

97. Kannel WB, Wolf PA, Verter J, McNamara PM: Epidemiologic assessment of the role of blood pressure in stroke: the Framingham study. *JAMA* 1970, 214:301–310.

98. Keli S, Bloemberg B, Kromhout D: Predictive value of repeated systolic blood pressure measurements for stroke risk: the Zutphen Study. *Stroke* 1992, 23:347–351.

99. Kannel WB, Dawber TR, Sorlie P, Wolf PA: Components of blood pressure and risk of atherothrombotic brain infarction: the Framingham study. *Stroke* 1976, 7:327–331.

100. Wolf PA, Belanger AJ, D'Agostino RB: Management of risk factors. *Neurol Clin* 1992, 10:177–191.

101. Wolf PA, D'Agostino RB, Kannel WB, *et al.*: Cigarette smoking as a risk factor for stroke: the Framingham Study. *JAMA* 1988, 259:1025–1029.

102. Wilking SVB, Belanger A, Kannel WB, *et al.*: Determinants of isolated systolic hypertension. *JAMA* 1988, 260:3451–3455.

103. Kannel WB, Wolf PA, McGee DL, *et al.*: Systolic blood pressure, arterial rigidity, and risk of stroke: the Framingham study. *JAMA* 1981, 245:1225–1229.

104. Tanne D, Goldbourt U, Zion M, *et al.*: Frequency and prognosis of stroke/TIA among 4808 survivors of acute myocardial infarction. *Stroke* 1993, 24:1490–1495.

105. Dexter DD Jr, Whisnant JP, Connolly DC, O'Fallon WM: The association of stroke and coronary heart disease: a population study. *Mayo Clin Proc* 1987, 62:1077–1083.

106. Nakaoka T, Sada T, Kira Y, *et al.*: Risk factors for the complication of cerebral infarction in Japanese patients with acute myocardial infarction. *Jpn Heart J* 1989, 30:635–643.

107. Broderick JP, Phillips SJ, O'Fallon WM, *et al.*: Relationship of cardiac disease to stroke occurrence, recurrence, and mortality. *Stroke* 1992, 23:1250–1256.

108. Roehmholdt ME, Palumbo PJ, Whisnant JP, Elveback LR: Transient ischemic attack and stroke in a community–based diabetic cohort. *Mayo Clin Proc* 1983, 58:56–58.

109. Barrett–Connor E, Khaw K: Diabetes mellitus: an independent risk factor for stroke. *Am J Epidemiol* 1988, 128:116–123.

110: Jamrozik K, Broadhurst RJ, Anderson CS, Stewart–Wynne EG: The role of lifestyle factors in the etiology of stroke: a population–based case–control study in Perth, Western Australia. *Stroke* 1994, 25:51–59.

111. Kase CS, Wolf PA, Chodosh EH, *et al.*: Prevalence of silent stroke in patients presenting with initial stroke: the Framingham Study. *Stroke* 1989, 20:850–852.

112. Riddle MC, Hart J: Hyperglycemia, recognized and unrecognized, as a risk factor for stroke and transient ischemic attacks. *Stroke* 1982, 13:356–359.

113. Dennis M, Bamford J, Sandercock P, Warlow C: Prognosis of transient ischemic attacks in the Oxfordshire Community Stroke Project. *Stroke* 1990, 21:848–853.

114. Rhoads GG, Popper JS, Kagan A, Yano K: Incidence of transient cerebral ischemic attack in Hawaii Japanese men: the Honolulu Heart Study. *Stroke* 1980, 11:21–26.

115. Muuronen A, Kaste M: Outcome of 314 patients with transient ischemic attacks. *Stroke* 1982, 13:24–31.

116. Nomura A, Comstock GW, Kuller L, Tonascia JA: Cigarette smoking and strokes. *Stroke* 1974, 5:483–486.

117. Lindenstrom E, Boysen G, Nyboe J: Lifestyle factors and risk of cerebrovascular disease in women: the Copenhagen city heart study. *Stroke* 1993, 24:1468–1472.

118. Shinton R, Beevers G: Meta–analysis of relation between cigarette smoking and stroke. *BMJ* 1989, 298:789–794.

119. Petitti DB, Wingerd J, Pellegrin F, Ramcharan S: Risk of vascular disease in women: smoking, oral contraceptives, noncontraceptive estrogens and other factors. *JAMA* 1979, 242:1150–1154.

120. Hillbom M, Kaste M: Ethanol intoxication: a risk factor for ischemic brain infarction in adolescents and young adults. *Stroke* 1981, 12:422–425.

121. Hillbom M, Kaste M: Alcohol abuse and brain infarction. *Ann Med* 1990, 22:347–352.

122. Lee K: Alcoholism and cerebrovascular thrombosis in the young. *Acta Neurol Scand* 1979, 59:270–274.

123. Taylor JR, Combs–Orme T: Alcohol and strokes in young adults. *Am J Psych* 1985, 142:116–118.

124. Palomaki H, Kaste M: Regular light–to–moderate intake of alcohol and the risk of ischaemic stroke: is there a beneficial effect? *Stroke* 1993, 24:1828–1832.

125. Klatsky AL, Armstrong MA, Friedman GD: Alcohol use and subsequent cerebrovascular disease hospitalizations. *Stroke* 1989, 20:741–746.

126. Rodgers H, Aitken PD, French JM, *et al.*: Alcohol and stroke. A case–control study of drinking habits past and present. *Stroke* 1993, 24:1473–1477.

127. Gill JS, Shipley MJ, Tsementzis SA, *et al.*: Alcohol consumption—a risk factor for hemorrhagic and non–hemorrhagic stroke. *Am J Med* 1991, 90:489–497.

128. Kannel WB, Gordon T, Dawber TR: Role of lipids in the development of brain infarction: the Framingham study. *Stroke* 1974, 5:679–685.

129. Shintani S, Kikuchi S, Hamaguchi H, Shilgai T: High serum lipoprotein (a) levels are an independent risk factor for cerebral infarction. *Stroke* 1993, 24:965–969.

130. Kannel WB, Gordon T, Wolf PA, McNamara P: Hemoglobin and the risk of cerebral infarction: the Framingham Study. *Stroke* 1972, 3:409–420.

131. Fogelholm R, Aho K: Ischemic cerebrovascular disease in young adults. I. Smoking habits, use of oral contraceptives, relative weight, blood pressure, and electrocardiographic findings. *Acta Neurol Scand* 1973, 49:415–427.

132. Lidegaard O: Cerebrovascular deaths before and after the appearance of oral contraceptives. *Acta Neurol Scand* 1987, 75:427–433.

133. Layde PM, Ory HW, Beral V, Kay CR: Incidence of arterial disease among oral contraceptive users. *J R Coll Gen Pract* 1983, 33:75–82.

134. Handin RI: Thromboembolic complications of pregnancy and oral contraceptives. *Prog Cardiovasc Dis* 1974, 16:395–405.

135. Stampfer MJ, Willett WC, Colditz GA, *et al.*: A prospective study of past use of oral contraceptive agents and risk of cardiovascular diseases. *N Engl J Med* 1988, 319:1313–1317.

136. Lidegaard O: Oral contraception and risk of cerebral thromboembolic attack results of a case–control study. *BMJ* 1993, 306:956–963.

137. Pocock SJ, Shaper AG, Cook DG, *et al.*: British regional heart study: geographic variations in cardiovascular mortality and the role of water quality. *BMJ* 1980, 2:1243–1249.

138. Biorck G, Bostrom H, Widstrom A: On the relationship between water hardness and death rates in cardiovascular disease. *Acta Med Scand* 1965, 178:239–252.

139. Comstock GW, Cauthen GM, Helsing KJ, Goldberg EL: Stroke–associated deaths in Washington County, Maryland, with special reference to water hardness. *Stroke* 1979, 10:199–205.

140. The antiphospholipid antibodies in stroke study (APASS) group: Anticardiolipin antibodies are an independent risk factor for first ischemic stroke. *Neurology* 1993, 43:2069–2073.

141. Wiebers DO, Whisnant JP: The incidence of stroke among pregnant women in Rochester, Minn, 1955 through 1979. *JAMA* 1985, 254:3055–3057.

142. Boers GHJ, Smals AGH, Trijbels FJM, *et al.*: Heterozygosity for homocystinuria in premature peripheral and cerebral occlusive vascular disease. *N Engl J Med* 1985, 313:709–715.

143. Brattstrom LE, Hardebo JE, Hultberg BL: Moderate homocysteinemia—a possible risk factor for arteriosclerotic cerebrovascular disease. *Stroke* 1984, 15:1012–1016.

144. Kelly PA, Faulkner AJ, Burrow AP: The effects of the GABA agonist muscimol upon blood flow in different vascular territories of the rat cortex. *J Cereb Blood Flow Metab* 1989, 9:754–758.

145. Coull BM, Matinow MR, Beamer N, *et al.*: Elevated plasma homocyst(e)ine concentration as a possible independent risk factor for stroke. *Stroke* 1990, 21:572–576.

146. Engstrom JW, Lowenstein DH, Bredesen DE: Cerebral infarctions and transient neurologic deficits associated with acquired immunodeficiency syndrome. *Am J Med* 1989, 86:528–532.

147. Shinkawa A, Ueda K, Hasuo Y, *et al.*: Seasonal variation in stroke incidence in Hisayama, Japan. *Stroke* 1990, 21:1262–1267.

148. Christie D: Stroke in Melbourne, Australia: an epidemiological study. *Stroke* 1981, 12:467–469.

149. Marler JR, Price TR, Clark GL, *et al.*: Morning increase in onset of ischemic stroke. *Stroke* 1989, 20:473–476.

150. Marshall J: Diurnal variation in occurrence of strokes. *Stroke* 1977, 8:230–231.

151. Argentino C, Toni D, Rasura M, *et al.*: Circadian variation in the frequency of ischemic stroke. *Stroke* 1990, 21:387–389.
152. Ameriso SF, Wong VL, Quismorio FP Jr, Fisher M: Immunohematologic characteristics of infection–associated cerebral infarction. *Stroke* 1991, 22:1004–1009.
153. Paffenbarger RS, Laughlin ME, Gima AS, Black RA: Work activity of longshoremen as related to death from coronary heart disease and stroke. *N Engl J Med* 1970, 282:1109–1115.
154. Wolf PA, D'Agostino RB, Belanger AJ, Kannel WB: Probability of stroke: A risk profile from the Framingham study. *Stroke* 1991, 22:312–318.
155. Hart RG, Easton JD: Mitral valve prolapse and cerebral infarction. *Stroke* 1982, 13:429–430.
156. Wolf PA, Sila CA: Cerebral ischemia with mitral valve prolapse. *Am Heart J* 1987, 113:1308–1315.
157. Jones HR Jr, Naggar CZ, Seljan MP, Downing LL: Mitral valve prolapse and cerebral ischemic events. A comparison between a neurology population with stroke and a cardiology population with mitral valve prolapse observed for five years. *Stroke* 1982, 13:451–453.
158. Jeanrenaud X, Kappenberger L: Patent foramen ovale and stroke of unknown origin. *Cerebrovasc Dis* 1991, 1:184–192.
159. Cabanes L, Mas JL, Cohen A, *et al.*: Atrial septal aneurysm and patent foramen ovale as risk factors for cryptogenic stroke in patients less than 55 years of age: a study using transesophageal echocardiography. *Stroke* 1993, 24:1865–1873.
160. Ranoux D, Cohen A, Cabanes L, *et al.*: Patent foramen ovale: is stroke due to paradoxical embolism? *Stroke* 1993, 24:31–34.
161. Portnoy BA, Herion JC: Neurological manifestations in sickle–cell disease with a review of the literature and emphasis on the prevalence of hemiplegia. *Ann Intern Med* 1972, 76:643–652.
162. Henrich JB: The association between migraine and cerebral vascular events: an analytical review. *J Chronic Dis* 1987, 40:329–335.
163. Daras M, Tuchman AJ, Marks S: Central nervous system infarction related to cocaine abuse. *Stroke* 1991, 22:1320–1325.
164. Palomaki H: Snoring and the risk of ischemic brain infarction. *Stroke* 1991, 22:1021–1025.
165. Futrell N, Millikan C: Frequency, etiology, and prevention of stroke in patients with systemic lupus erythematosus. *Stroke* 1989, 20:583–591.
166. Wannamethee G, Shaper AG: Physical activity and stroke in British middle aged men. *BMJ* 1992, 304:597–601.
167. Shinton R, Sagar G: Lifelong exercise and stroke *BMJ* 1993, 307:231–234.
168. Khaw K–T, Barrett–Conner E: Dietary potassium and stroke—associated mortality. *N Engl J Med* 1987, 316:235–240.
169. Yates PA: A change in the pattern of cerebrovascular disease. *Lancet* 1964, 1:65–69.
170. Bamford J, Sandercock P, Dennis M, *et al.*: A prospective study of acute cerebrovascular disease in the community: the Oxfordshire Community Stroke project. 1. Methodology, demography and incident cases of first–ever stroke. *J Neurol Neurosurg Psych* 1988, 51:1373–1380.
171. Wolf PA, Cobb JL, D'Agostino RB: Epidemiology of stroke. In *Stroke: Pathophysiology, Diagnosis and Management, 2nd ed.* Edited by Barnett HJM, Mohr JP, Stein BM, Yatsu FM. New York: Churchill Livingstone; 1992:3–27.
172. D'Agostgino RB, Wolf PA, Belanger AJ, Kannel WB: Stroke risk profile: Adjustment for antihypertensive medication: the Framingham study. *Stroke* 1994, 25:40–43.
173. Stern MP, Gaskill SP: Secular trends in ischemic heart disease and stroke mortality from 1970 to 1976 in Spanish–surnamed and other white individuals in Bexar County, Texas. *Circulation* 1978, 58:537–543.
174. Wender M, Lenart Jankowska D, Pruchnik D, Kowal P: Epidemiology of stroke in the Poznan district of Poland. *Stroke* 1990, 21:390–393.
175. Terent A: Increasing incidence of stroke among Swedish women. *Stroke* 1988, 19:598–603.
176. Ueda K, Fujii I, Kawano H, *et al.*: Severe disability related to cerebral stroke: incidence and risk factors observed in a Japanese community, Hisayama. *J Am Geriatric Soc* 1987, 35:616–622.
177. Epstein L, Rishpon S, Bental E, *et al.*: Incidence, mortality, and case–fatality rate of stroke in northern Israel. *Stroke* 1989, 20:725–729.
178. Hu HH,Chu FL, Chiang BN, *et al.*: Prevalence of stroke in Taiwan. *Stroke* 1989, 20:858–863.
179. Dalsgaard–Nielsen T: Survey of 1000 cases of apoplexia cerebri. *Acta Psych Neurol Scand* 1955, 169–185.
180. Oliver MF: Might treatment of hypercholesterolaemia increase non–cardiac mortality? *Lancet* 1991, 1:1529–1531.
181. Evans JG: Blood pressure and stroke in an elderly English population. *J Epidemiol Community Health* 1987, 41:275–282.
182. Palmer AJ, Bulpitt CJ, Fletcher AE, *et al.*: Relation between blood pressure and stroke mortality. *Hypertension* 1992, 20:601–605.

Chapter 2

Epidemiology of Aneurysmal Subarachnoid Hemorrhage and Intraparenchymal Hemorrhage

PATRICIA H. DAVIS
JAMES C. TORNER

While hemorrhagic stroke accounts for only 10% to 15% of total stroke, the mortality and morbidity rates are higher than for ischemic stroke so that the public health impact from this subtype of stroke is significant. Incidence rates for intraparenchymal hemorrhage (ICH) and subarachnoid hemorrhage (SAH) remained unchanged during the 1980s (Figure 2.1) so that identification of risk factors and development of strategies for prevention are badly needed. Because these subtypes of stroke are less common, epidemiologic studies have been more difficult to perform than for ischemic stroke. There are clearly differences in the epidemiologic features between these two subtypes, *eg*, a younger age of onset and female preponderance for SAH as compared with ICH in most studies [1]. In addition, risk factors are not the same for the two subtypes of hemorrhagic stroke. With the widespread use of neuroimaging procedures, accuracy of diagnosis has improved, and recently, more studies have considered SAH and ICH separately. In this chapter, we will consider the diagnostic criteria and accuracy of diagnosis, etiologic categories, risk factors, prognostic factors, and strategies for prevention for both ICH and SAH. The epidemiology of ICH [2] and SAH [1,3] has been previously reviewed.

DIAGNOSTIC CRITERIA

The diagnostic criteria for ICH and SAH used in the Monitoring Trends and Determinants of Cardiovascular Disease (MONICA) project are listed in Table 2.1 [4]. Use of computed tomography (CT) scanning has greatly improved the accuracy of diagnosis of ICH, and Drury and coworkers [5] estimated that 25% of patients with ICH were incorrectly diagnosed as having cerebral infarcts in the pre–CT scan era. Use of the radiologic and laboratory criteria may be associated with potential misdiagnoses according to the timing of the test. Use of CT scan in ICH may incorrectly classify cases of early spontaneous intrainfarct hemorrhage as ICH [6], and if done after 2 weeks when the hematoma may be hypodense or isodense, can incorrectly classify an ICH as a cerebral infarct [7]. Figures 2.2 and 2.3 delineate the features of hemorrhagic infarction that differentiate it from ICH (Figures 2.4 and 2.5). The CT scan is more sensitive than the magnetic resonance (MR) image for early detection of blood [8], but MR imaging may be more sensitive for older hemorrhages (Figure 2.4). Because of expense or lack of availability of CT scanning for epidemiologic studies, a clinical score, the Guy's Hospital Score, has been devised to differentiate ICH from cerebral infarct. Depending on the population studied, it has a sensitivity of from 81% to 92% and a specificity of 78% to 82% [9].

For diagnosis of SAH, the timing of the tests is also important. For CT scanning, the sensitivity is 95% for the same day, 90% the second day, and drops to 50% at 1 week [10]. A lumbar puncture done earlier than 12 hours after the ictus may be too soon to detect xanthochromia. While Vermeulen and Van Gijn

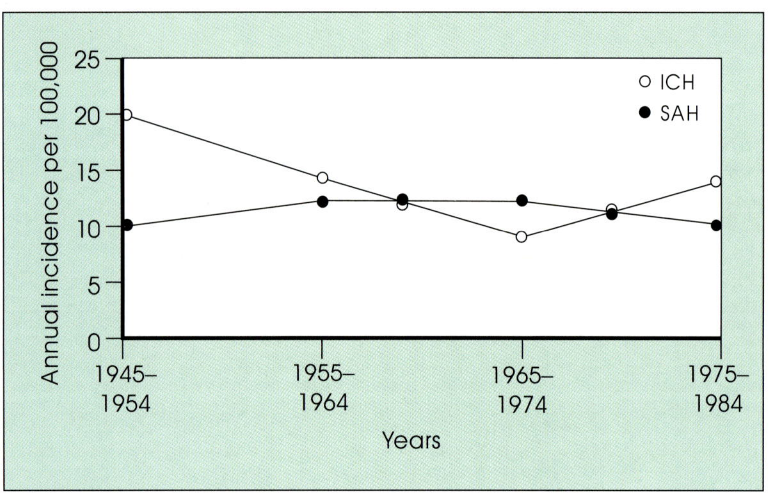

FIGURE 2.1

Incidence rates for intraparenchymal (ICH) and subarachnoid hemorrhage (SAH) have not declined over time in Rochester, MN. (*Data from* Broderick and coworkers [30].)

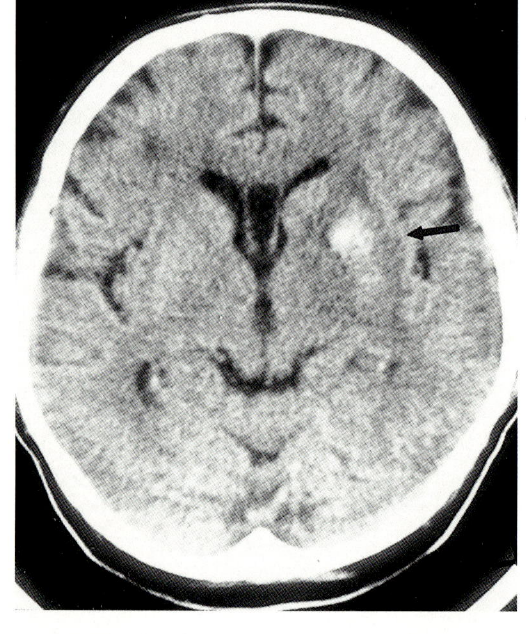

FIGURE 2.2

Computed tomographic scan showing typical patchy appearance of hemorrhagic infarction in the left basal ganglia (*arrow*).

Table 2.1. Diagnostic criteria for intraparenchymal hemorrhage and subarachnoid hemorrhage (MONICA study)*

Intraparenchymal hemorrhage	Subarachnoid hemorrhage
Usually sudden onset during activities	Abrupt onset of severe headache or unconsciousness or both
Often rapidly developing coma, but small hemorrhage presents no disturbance of consciousness	Signs of meningeal irritation (stiff neck, Kernig's and Brudzinski's signs)
CSF often but not always bloody or xanthrochromic	Focal neurologic deficits usually not present
Often severe hypertension present	At least one of the following must be present in addition to the typical symptoms:
Hemorrhage must be confirmed by necropsy or CT scan	Necropsy reveals recent subarachnoid hemorrhage and an aneurysm or AVM
	CT scan with blood in the Sylvian fissure, between the frontal lobes, or in the basal cisterns or cerebral ventricles
	CSF bloody (> 2000 red blood cells and an aneurysm or AVM found on angiography)
	CSF bloody and xanthochromic and the possibility of an intracerebral hemorrhage excluded by necropsy or CT scan

**Data from* Asplund and coworkers [4]. AVM—arteriovenous malformation; CSF—cerebrospinal fluid; CT—computed tomography; MONICA—Monitoring Trends and Determinants of Cardiovascular Disease.

[10] would advocate delaying the lumbar puncture until 12 hours after the ictus, other clinicians would advocate an immediate lumbar puncture for early diagnosis. Between 12 hours and 2 weeks, if spectrophotometry is used, xanthochromia is present in all patients; this figure declines to 70% at 3 weeks and 40% at 4 weeks [10]. Several recent studies have documented a delay in diagnosis because both patients and their physicians fail to recognize symptoms [11–14].

While mortality data are less accurate than morbidity data, death certificate diagnosis of SAH is the most reliable of all stroke subtypes [1]. Comparison of death certificate diagnosis with hospital diagnosis in Baltimore showed an agreement of 66% for ICH and 72% for SAH [15]. Using data from the Minnesota Heart Study, Iso and coworkers [16] noted that the positive predictive value of a diagnosis of ICH improved from 59% in 1970 to 82% in 1980 when death certificate and physician diagnosis were compared. They attributed this improvement to use of CT scanning and concluded that ICH could be accurately separated from cerebral infarction using death certificate data.

ETIOLOGY

The etiologic causes of ICH are outlined in Table 2.2. The contribution of hypertension to ICH appears to be declining over time [17], and more recent studies show that 50% to 60% of ICHs are hypertension related [18,19]. The etiology may be affected by age according to a study of 100 consecutive cases of ICH [20]. For those aged < 40 years, the location was lobar and etiology was arteriovenous malformation (AVM); for those aged 40 to 69 years, the location was deep and the etiology was hypertension; and for those aged ≥ 70 years, the location was lobar and the etiology was hypertension and, possibly, amyloid angiopathy. However, Broderick and coworkers [2] found that hypertension was nearly as common in lobar as in deep, cerebellar, or pontine hemorrhages, and that the association of hypertension with lobar hemorrhages did not decrease with age. MR imaging is more sensitive than CT scanning in determining the underlying etiology (Figure 2.6).

Aneurysmal subarachnoid hemorrhage may be associated with other disorders as shown in Table 2.3 and must be differ-

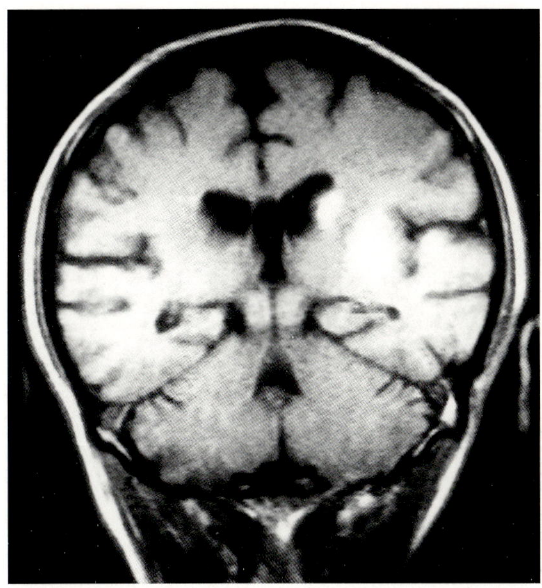

FIGURE 2.3

T1-weighted magnetic resonance image of the same patient as in Figure 2.2 showing more widespread areas of hemorrhage within the infarction than seen on the computed tomography scan.

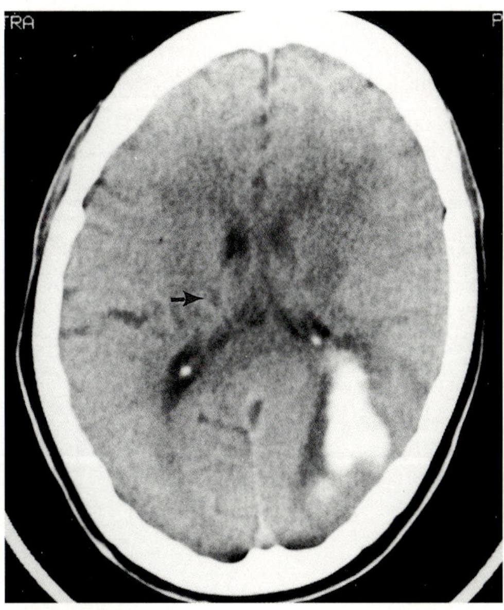

FIGURE 2.4

Computed tomographic scan of an intraparenchymal hemorrhage with a homogenous area of increased density surrounded by edema in the left occipital lobe. A small area of low density (*arrow*) is seen in the right thalamus. This scan was done several weeks after the acute event.

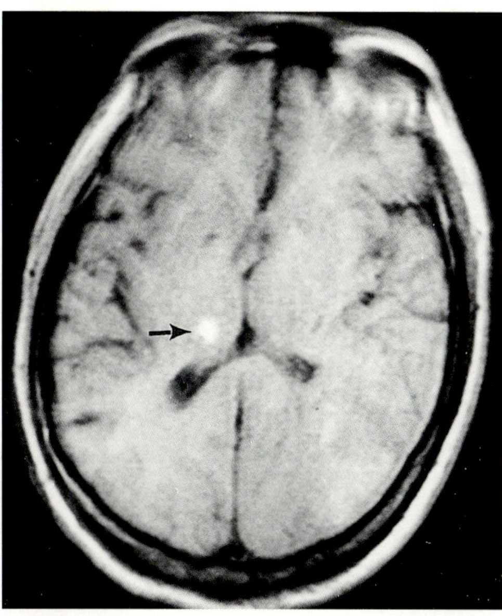

FIGURE 2.5

T1-weighted magnetic resonance image of the same patient as in Figure 2.4 showing that the lesion in the right thalamus *(arrow)* is also a hemorrhage that is not demonstrated on the computed tomography scan.

Table 2.2. Etiology of intracerebral hemorrhage

Hypertension (50%–60%)	Cerebral amyloid angiopathy (includes familial syndromes, Icelandic and Dutch types)	Myeloproliferative disorders (multiple myeloma, acute and chronic myelogenous leukemia, essential thrombocythemia)
Arteriovenous malformation, aneurysm	Coagulopathy (deficiency of factors VII, VIII, IX, XIII, von Willebrand's factor, afibrinogenemia, idiopathic thrombocytopenic purpura, thrombotic thrombocytopenic purpura, disseminated intravascular coagulation, uremia)	Eclampsia
Bleeding into a tumor		Moyamoya syndrome
Anticoagulant use		Acute elevation of blood pressure or reperfusion of ischemic area (prolonged migraine, exposure to cold, dental pain, postendarterectomy)
Fibrinolytic agents		
Sympathomimetic drugs		
Vasculitis		

entiated from nonaneurysmal causes. An initial normal angiogram should be repeated in 7 to 10 days if an aneurysm is suspected. If the hemorrhage is confined to the perimesencephalic area, the risk of an aneurysm or rebleeding is low and a second angiogram is not necessary [22].

DESCRIPTIVE STUDIES

According to the National Hospital Discharge Survey of 1990, 25,000 patients were discharged from short-term, nonfederal hospitals in the United States with SAH, 71,000 with ICH, and 23,000 with other or unspecified intracranial hemorrhage [23]. Population-based incidence rates for SAH are six to 16 per 100,000 and for ICH are 13 to 23 per 100,000 (Figure 2.7) [24]. As a percent of stroke, hemorrhagic stroke accounts for 10% to 15% (Figure 2.8) [25]. The highest reported rates of hemorrhagic stroke are in Finland and Japan [25–27]. ICH is nearly equally distributed in men and women [23]. The incidence of SAH in the United States is higher in women (Figure 2.9). This sex ratio is not consistently observed in other populations [26]. While SAH increases linearly with age, ICH increases exponentially (Figure 2.10). Recent studies also indicate that blacks have a higher risk of ICH and SAH than whites [28].

The mortality rate from stroke has declined progressively since the 1950s (Figure 2.11). Similarly, there has been a decline in mortality associated with cerebral hemorrhage and SAH [23,29]. The case-fatality rate appears to have declined since 1970. The rate of cerebral hemorrhage mortality was 20.2 per 100,000 (International Classification of Disease [ICD] 8:431) in 1970, 12.6 in 1975, and 8.8 in 1981 (ICD 9:431–432). There is reason to believe the rate of decline has slowed. In 1990, the mortality rate was 8.4 per 100,000. Similar trends have been noted elsewhere. The declining mortality may be due to changes in classification of stroke, diagnostic methods for stroke, recurrence rates, case-fatality rates, and incidence rates. Changes in incidence rates may be related to treatment of hypertension, a decrease in coronary heart disease, or decline of other risk factors. However, the incidence of intracerebral hemorrhage does not appear to be declining. In population-based data from Rochester, MN, there is stabilization of rates of ICH and SAH that has not changed since data collection began in 1945 [5,30]. Similar data can be observed in the number of discharge diagnoses with ICH or SAH from the National Hospital Discharge Survey (Figure 2.12) [23]. The failure of rates to decline may be due to changes in diagnosis and classification. The use of CT has changed the detection of intracerebral blood

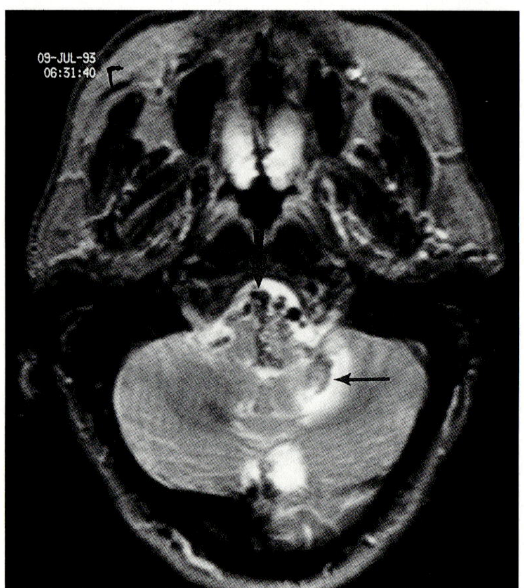

FIGURE 2.6

T2-weighted magnetic resonance image of a patient with a left cerebellar hemorrhage (*small arrow*). The multiple flow voids demonstrate that the etiology is a large arteriovenous malformation (*large arrow*).

Table 2.3. Etiology of subarachnoid hemorrhage

Aneurysmal	Nonaneurysmal
Polycystic kidney disease	Trauma
Ehlers-Danlos syndrome	Perimesencephalic hemorrhage
Coarctation of the aorta	Spinal or cerebral arteriovenous malformation
Moyamoya syndrome	Bleeding diathesis
Tuberous sclerosis	Infectious (meningitis, cortical thrombophlebitis)
Kleinfelter syndrome	
Fibromuscular dysplasia	

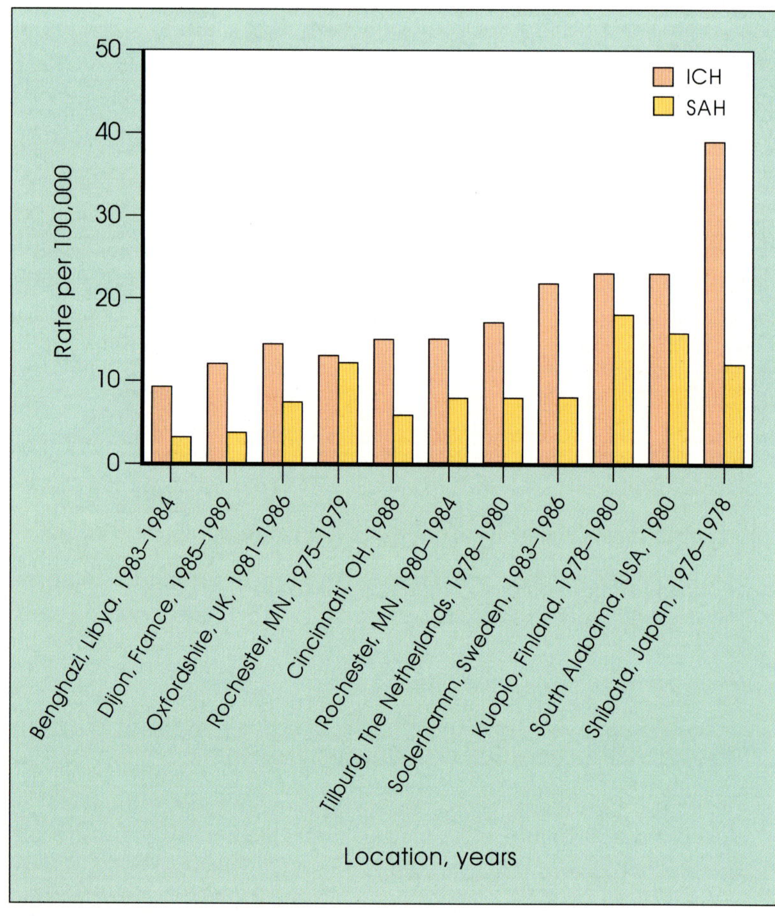

FIGURE 2.7

Incidence rates for intraparenchymal (ICH) and subarachnoid (SAH) hemorrhage from various worldwide locations. (*Data from* Broderick and coworkers [24].)

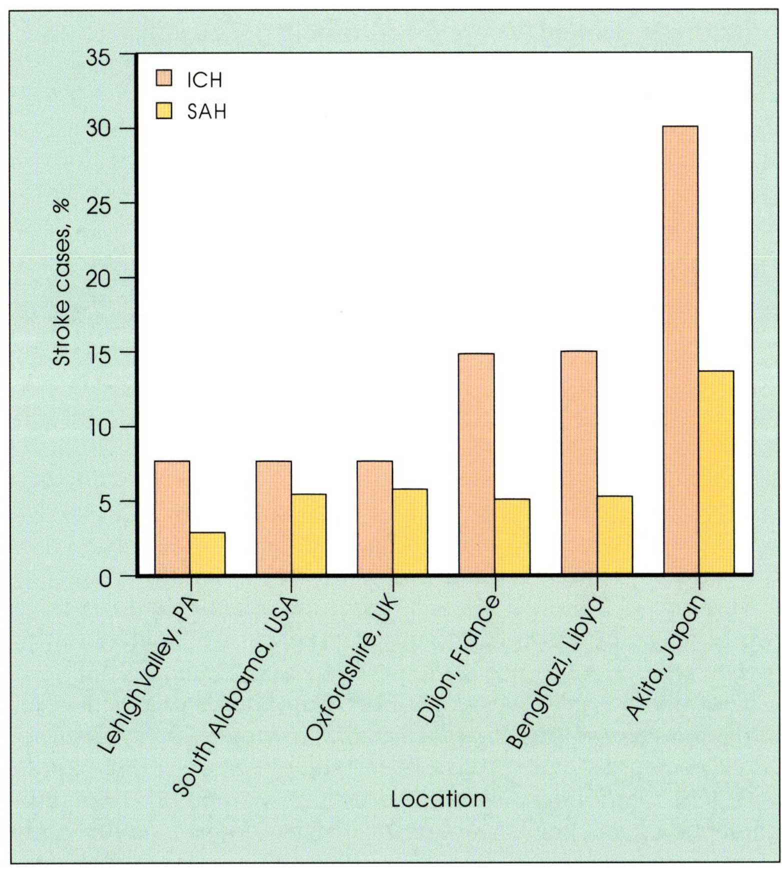

FIGURE 2.8

This figure demonstrates the percentage of total stroke made up by intraparenchymal (ICH) and subarachnoid (SAH) hemorrhage in different geographic locations. (*Data from* Davis and Hachinski [25].)

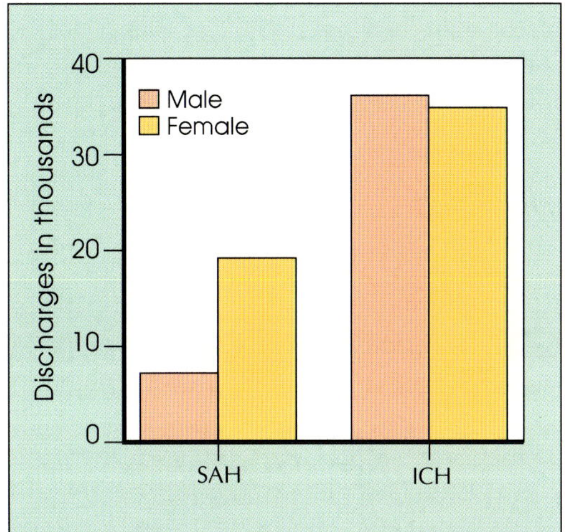

FIGURE 2.9

Data from the National Hospital Discharge Survey that shows an equal sex distribution for intraparenchymal hemorrhage (ICH) and a female preponderance for subarachnoid hemorrhage (SAH).

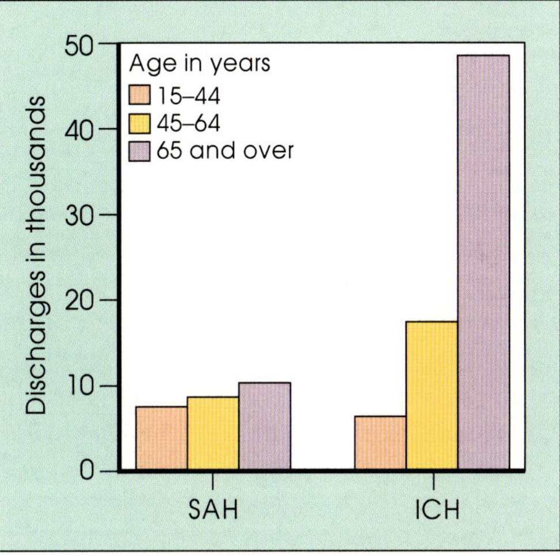

FIGURE 2.10

There is a linear increase with age for subarachnoid hemorrhage (SAH) and an exponential increase for intraparenchymal hemorrhage (ICH). (*Data from* National Hospital Discharge Survey [23].)

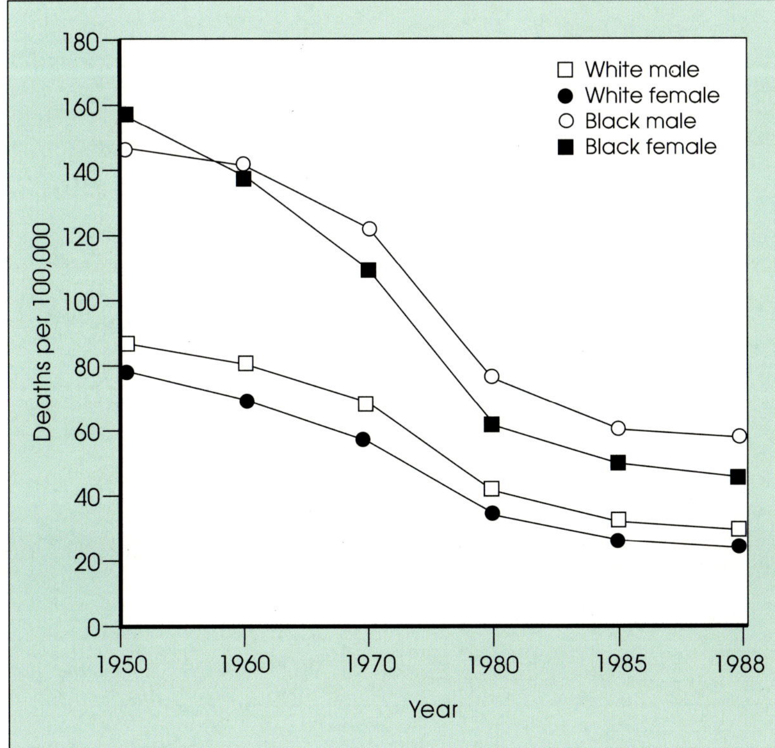

FIGURE 2.11

Trends in cerebrovascular disease age-adjusted death rates showing that mortality rates for cerebrovascular disease have declined since 1950. (*Data from* Monthly Vital Statistics Report [29].)

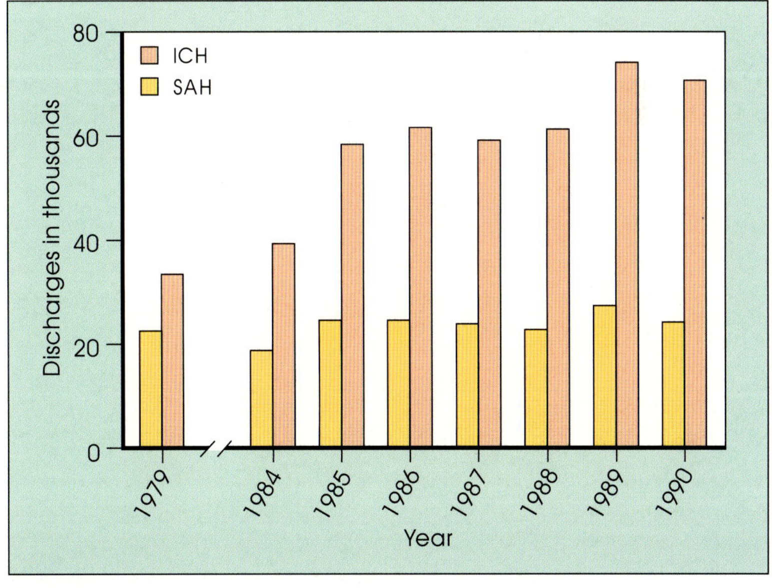

FIGURE 2.12

Data from the National Hospital Discharge Survey showing that discharge diagnoses for intraparenchymal (ICH) and subarachnoid (SAH) hemorrhage have not changed over time.

and may account for increases in incidence [5]. The age distribution and etiology of ICH may also have changed. Investigators have also questioned the further effectiveness of antihypertensives in reducing the occurrence of hemorrhagic stroke [30–32]. There also may be an associated change in risk factors such as anticoagulant and thrombolytic therapy.

RISK FACTORS

Determination of risk factors for ICH and SAH has been difficult because these subtypes of stroke occur less frequently than ischemic stroke. Prospective studies suffer from very small numbers of cases and retrospective studies are hampered by the higher 30-day mortality in these subtypes so that surrogates are often required to provide information. Longstreth and coworkers [33] have demonstrated that agreement between SAH cases and their surrogates is high.

Intraparenchymal Hemorrhage

Risk factors for intraparenchymal hemorrhage are outlined in Table 2.4 [18,34–44]. Few studies have been done since the advent of widespread CT scanning [18,34]. The best established risk factors are age, hypertension, use of anticoagulants, low serum cholesterol, and heavy alcohol intake. Four case-control studies have found hypertension to be a significant risk factor with a relative risk from 3.4 to 4.8 [18,34–36]. Inzitari and coworkers found that the association of leukoaraiosis with ICH could be explained by the associated hypertension [35]. Data from Rochester, MN, showed an increase in the incidence rate of ICH from 1960 through 1964 that could be accounted for by increased use of anticoagulants with a 45% higher incidence rate in patients receiving anticoagulation therapy [5]. A study from Holland demonstrated that the relative risk of ICH was 7.6 in those patients over age 50 years receiving anticoagulants but was unrelated to the degree of anticoagulation [45]. There are two prospective studies reporting an inverse association of serum cholesterol and ICH in men. In the Honolulu Heart Study, the relative risk of the lowest quintile of cholesterol was 2.55 and there was no interaction with blood pressure [43], while in the Multiple Risk Factor Intervention Trial, the relative risk was 3.0 but the increased risk was confined to men with diastolic blood pressures of at least 90 mm Hg [44]. Four recent case-control studies have found heavy alcohol intake to be a risk factor for intracerebral hemorrhage [34,36–38] which, in two of the studies, remained significant even after adjustment for concurrent hypertension [36,38]. Two prospective studies have found an association of alcohol intake with ICH after multivariate adjustment in populations of Japanese origin [39,40].

Less definite risk factors include drug abuse, previous cerebral infarct, previous lacunar infarct, coronary artery disease, and diabetes [18]. There have been multiple case series reported with ICH temporally related to drug use, particularly sympathomimetic agents, including cocaine (alkaloid and hydrochloride form), amphetamines, phenylpropanolamine, ephedrine, and pseudephedrine [46–48]. In one study, drug use occurred in 7%

Table 2.4. Risk factors for intraparenchymal hemorrhage

Factor	Type of study	Cases, *n*	RR	CI or *P* value	CT	Study
Hypertension	Case-control	154	3.9	2.7–5.7	Yes	Brott and coworkers [18]
	Case-control	73	4.8	$P < 0.001$	Yes	Calandre and coworkers [34]
	Case-control	116	4.2	$P < 0.001$	Yes	Inzitari and coworkers [35]
	Case-control	24	3.4	1.0–11.6	Yes	Monforte and coworkers [36]
Ethanol use						
> 100 g/d	Case-control	24	13.3	1.5–11.9	Yes	Monforte and coworkers [36]
≥ 3 drinks/d	Case-control	28	6.8	1.5–31.4	NS	Klatsky and coworkers [37]
> 80 g/d	Case-control	73	7.2	$P < 0.001$	Yes	Calandre and coworkers [34]
> 400 g/wk	Case-control	91	2.5	1.0–6.1	82%	Gill and coworkers [38]
≥ 1.9 drinks/d	Cohort	30	3.0	$P < 0.05$	No	Tanaka and coworkers [39]
> 40 oz/mo	Cohort	—	2.4	0.9–6.2	NS	Donahue and coworkers [40]
Smoking	Cohort	53	1.5	0.8–2.8	NS	Kawachi and coworkers [41]
	Case-control	104	Men 1.8	0.9–3.7	82%	Gill and coworkers [42]
			Women 1.3	0.5–3.4		
Low cholesterol						
< 189 mg/dL	Cohort	77	2.6	1.6–4.1	NS	Yano and coworkers [43]
< 160 mg/dL	Cohort	79	3.0	$P=0.05$	NS	Iso and coworkers [44]

CT—computed tomography; NS—not stated.

of ICH cases [48] but no case-control studies have been published. Mechanisms include acute hypertension, vasculitis, and infectious aneurysms with intravenous use. Brott and coworkers [18] found a relative risk of 22 for a previous cerebral infarction, 8.2 for coronary artery disease, and 2.9 for diabetes, but no multivariate analysis was performed and the control group was drawn from a different population. Inzitari and coworkers [35] found lacunar infarct on CT scan still a significant risk factor even after multivariate adjustment.

With only limited data available, smoking does not appear to be a risk factor for ICH. In one case-control study, the relative risk was increased but did not reach significance [42]. Two prospective studies have examined smoking as a risk factor but one grouped all hemorrhagic strokes together [49], and one showed a nonsignificant increase in risk [41]. Shinton and Beevers [50] concluded that smoking had no clear association with ICH after a meta-analysis of four studies that contrasted with the findings for the other subtypes of stroke. Further studies of smoking as a risk factor are needed.

Recent use of thrombolytic therapy in the setting of acute myocardial infarction has also been associated with increased risk of ICH while the overall risk of stroke is not increased [51]. In a community-based study, the relative risk after multivariate adjustment for hemorrhagic stroke was 3.6 (1.7–8.0 CI) while it was 0.4 for ischemic stroke (0.2–0.9 CI) [52]. Table 2.5 outlines those factors associated with increased risk of intracerebral bleeding in the setting of thrombolytic therapy [53-60]. While ICH is an uncommon complication of thrombolytic therapy, it is frequently lethal with mortality rates of 40% to 50% [52].

Subarachnoid Hemorrhage

In looking at risk factors for subarachnoid hemorrhage, two components have to be considered: factors that promote aneurysm formation and factors that lead to the rupture of aneurysms. At present, with no good screening test for unruptured aneurysms, it is difficult to separate these two. As with ICH, there was limited information in the past about risk factors, with prospective studies suffering from small numbers of cases, and case-control studies were not population-based and did not include those patients who died prior to hospitalization, thereby causing considerable bias. Age and the female gender are well-established risk factors for SAH in most populations [3]. Several recent case-control studies [33,61–63] have confirmed smoking and alcohol use as risk factors. Smoking appears to be the most important factor, having the highest relative risk and a dose-response relationship as delineated in Table 2.6 [33,41,42, 61–66]. Smoking could exert its effect by promoting atherosclerosis that increases the stress in the Circle of Willis, release of proteolytic enzymes by the macrophages in the lungs, and transient elevation of blood pressure. The finding by Longstreth and coworkers [33] that the risk was greatest in the 3 hours after smoking a cigarette would support the last mechanism. As shown in Table 2.7, alcohol use was a less important risk factor [33,38,40,41,62] with some studies supporting chronic use and others acute use. Alcohol use or withdrawal elevates blood pressure, increases cerebral blood flow, and affects coagulation. Two prospective studies support hypertension as a risk factor for SAH [64,66], but case-control studies have found conflicting results [33,61,62]. Since the acute event elevates blood pressure, this risk factor may be difficult to study if using case-control methodology. While two cohort studies completed in the 1960s found an increased risk of SAH with former or current use of oral contraceptives [3], recent case-control studies have not supported either former [33,61,67] or current use [67] as a risk factor for SAH, and this may in part be due to lower doses of estrogen. Drug abuse has also been linked to SAH although this is less frequent than ICH [45,46]. A recent review of 53 cases of cocaine-induced SAH found underlying aneurysms in 85% and postulated that induced acute hypertension was the mechanism of rupture [68]. Longstreth and coworkers [33] also found that the recent use of stimulant drugs was a significant risk factor. Knekt and coworkers [64] found an inverse relationship with body mass index. Diabetes does not appear to be a significant risk factor for SAH [64,69].

PROGNOSIS AND NATURAL HISTORY

While it was initially believed that active bleeding due to ICH usually lasted less than an hour after onset, a recent study with early CT scanning has shown that the volume of the hematoma over the first 12 hours increased by a mean of 107% and this was associated with clinical worsening [70].

Data from Rochester, MN [5] has shown improvement in 30-day mortality rates due to ICH in part because of improved detection by CT scanning of small hemorrhages associated with a

Table 2.5. Factors associated with increased risk of intraparenchymal hemorrhage with thrombolytic therapy

Factor	Study
Age	De Jaegere and coworkers [53], Anderson and coworkers [54]
Hypertension	Anderson and coworkers [54]
Amyloid angiopathy	Kase and coworkers [55], Leblanc and coworkers [56], Wijdicks and Jack [57]
Subcutaneous heparin	Risk increased in ISIS-3 not GISSI-2, Ridker and coworkers [58]
Previous stroke or transient ischemic attack	Gore and coworkers [59]
t-PA > streptokinase	ISIS-3, Ridker and coworkers [58]
Dose of t-PA	Gore and coworkers [59]
Previous oral anticoagulant	De Jaegere and coworkers [53]
Body weight < 70 kg	De Jaegere and coworkers [53]
Female sex	GISSI-2, Maggioni and coworkers [60]

GISSI—Gruppo Italiano per lo Studio della Sopravvivenza nell'Infarto Miocardico-2; ISIS-3—International Study of Infarct Survival-3.

Table 2.6. Smoking as a risk factor for aneurysmal subarachanoid hemorrhage

Cases, *n*	RR		CI		Population-based	Study
149	Heavy 11.1		5–25		Yes	Longstreth and coworkers [33]
	Light 4.1		2.3–7.3			
	Former 1.8		1.0–3.2			
115	Heavy 5.4		3.0–9.7		Yes	Bonita [61]
	Light 3.3		2.0–5.3			
	Former 1.0		—			
278	**Men**	**Women**	**Men**	**Women**	No	Juvela and coworkers [62]
	Light 1.1	Light 1.2	0.3–3.3	0.5–2.7		
	Moderate 2.2	Moderate 3.6	0.8–5.5	1.2–9.6		
	Heavy 9.6	Heavy 2.0	5.1–18.2	0.95–4.1		
217	Men 2.2		1.3–3.5		No	Morris and coworkers [63]
	Women 1.9		1.4–2.6			
187	Men 2.4		1.6–3.7		Yes	Knekt and coworkers [64]
	Women 2.5		1.5–4.1			
114	Men 2.7		1.3–5.7		Yes	Fogelholm and Murros [65]
	Women 3.0		0.9–11.5			
108	Former 2.3		1.1–3.6		Cohort (women)	Kawachi and coworkers [41]
	Current 4.9		2.9–8.1			
104	Men 4.5		2.4–8.4		No	Gill and coworkers [42]
	Women 2.5		1.4–4.5			
36	1.7		*P*=0.03		Cohort	Sacco and coworkers [66]

Table 2.7. Alcohol intake as a risk factor for aneurysmal subarachanoid hemorrhage

Chronic

Amount	Cases, *n*	RR	CI	Population-based	Study
5–14 g/d	28	3.7	1.0–13.8	Cohort (women)	Kawachi and coworkers [41]
> 2 drinks/d	149	2.2	0.9–5.1	Case-control	Longstreth and coworkers [33]
1–14 oz/mo	NS	2.8	0.9–8.6	Cohort (Men)	Donahue and coworkers [40]
15–39 oz/mo	NS	3.5	1.1–12.0		
≥ 40 oz/mo	NS	3.8	1.1–13.3		
10–90 g/wk	193	0.67	0.4–1.1	Case-control	Gill and coworkers [38]
100–390 g/wk		0.47	0.3–0.8		
≥ 390 g/wk		1.31	0.6–2.9		

Acute (within 24 hours of the event)

Amount	Cases, *n*	RR		CI		Population-based	Study
		Men	**Women**	**Men**	**Women**		
1–40 g	278	0.3	0.4	0.1–0.8	0.2–0.8	Case-control	Juvela and coworkers [62]
41–120 g		2.5	6.4	1.1–5.5	2.3–17.9		
> 120 g		4.5		1.5–12.9			

NS—not stated.

good prognosis (Figure 2.13). Table 2.8 outlines the results from more recent studies [19,29,71–77]. Several authors [71,73,78] have developed multivariate models to determine the important predictors of 30-day mortality due to ICH. Broderick and coworkers [72] found that the volume of the hemorrhage (0–29 cc, 30–60 cc, 61 or more cc), determined by an easily clinically applied method, and the Glasgow Coma Scale (GCS) (≥9, ≤8) predicted mortality with a sensitivity of 96% and a specificity of 98% in 188 cases in greater Cincinnati, OH, although they have not validated this on other data sets. Tuhrim and coworkers [73], using 94 cases from the Stroke Data Bank (SDB) found that GCS scores (≥9, ≤8), pulse pressure (≤ 40, 41–65, >65), hemorrhage size (<27 cc, 27–72 cc, >72 cc), and presence of intraventricular hemorrhage (IVH) were significant prognostic factors. When they applied this model to the main phase of the SDB, survival was accurately predicted in 94% at 30 days [73]. These findings of GCS, hemorrhage size, and presence of IVH as prognostic factors were confirmed in other studies [78–80]. Conflicting results have been obtained concerning the effect of the location of hemorrhage on mortality. Schutz and coworkers [20] found the highest mortality in putaminal hemorrhages, followed by thalamic and then lobar hemorrhages. Other researchers found that the mortality rate at 1 year was the same for lobar hemorrhages as it was for basal ganglia hemorrhages [71]. Using the 237 patients with ICH enrolled in the SDB, Massaro and coworkers [81] concluded that there was no difference in 30-day mortality between lobar and deep hemorrhages. Working with the same data set, others found the highest mortality rate in caudate hemorrhages and the lowest in cerebellar hemorrhages [19]. Two studies have confirmed that the use of anticoagulants is associated with a worse outcome following ICH [20,80].

Several studies have examined functional outcomes following ICH. At 1 year, functional independence has varied from 27% [44] to 55% [71]. Complications following ICH include pneumonia (15.5%), urinary tract infection (15%), arrhythmia (8.4%), and seizures (8.0%) [19]. Risk of recurrence is low (four of 120 cases at 1 year) [71], particularly for hypertensive hemorrhage, but is higher for hemorrhage due to amyloid angiopathy [82].

While 70% of patients are in good neurologic condition following a subarachnoid hemorrhage (SAH) from a ruptured cerebral aneurysm, less than 60% have a good recovery and only one third have an uneventful clinical course [83]. Secondary events play a major role in determining outcome. The major causes of death and disability from SAH are direct consequences of the initial hemorrhage, recurrent hemorrhage, cerebral ischemia, and medical complications [83,84]. Death

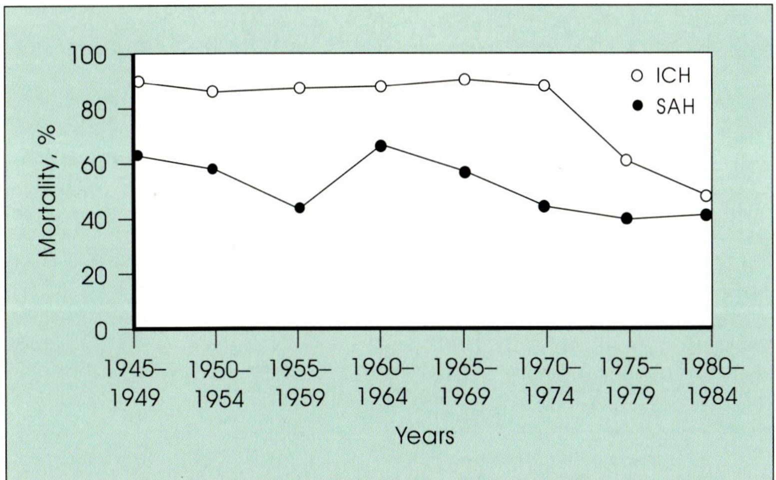

FIGURE 2.13

There has been a decline in the case-fatality rate for intraparenchymal (ICH) but not subarachnoid (SAH) hemorrhage over time in Rochester, MN. (*Data from* Broderick and coworkers [30].)

Table 2.8. Thirty-day mortality due to intraparenchymal hemorrhage

Location	Study years	Cases, *n*	30-day mortality, %	Study
Rochester, MN	1980–1984	< 80	42	Broderick and coworkers [30]
Holland	1986–1989	157	43	Franke and coworkers [71]
Cincinnati, OH	1988	188	44	Broderick and coworkers [72]
Stroke Data Bank	1983–1986	225	29	Tuhrim and coworkers [73]
Bordeaux, France	late 1980s	166	31	Daverat and coworkers [74]
Umbria, Italy	1986–1989	37	38	Ricci and coworkers [75]
Oxfordshire, UK	1981–1984	66	52	Bamford and coworkers [76]
Quebec, Canada	1981–1988	1195	49	Mayo and coworkers [77]

following subarachnoid hemorrhage occurs in phases by cause. The predominating causes are the initial hemorrhage and associated progressive decline from the initial effects, recurrent hemorrhage, focal ischemic deficits primarily from vasospasm, hydrocephalus, and medical complications such as pulmonary embolus, bronchopneumonia, sepsis, and renal complications [83,84]. The phases of mortality have been described by Weir and coworkers [85]. The initial hemorrhage is responsible for the early deaths. As much as 20% of SAH cases die before getting medical attention [86]. Of patients admitted in coma, 70% will die [83].

Several prognostic factors have been demonstrated in large prospective studies. Neurologic status is the major determinant of outcome. Tables 2.9 and 2.10 list predictors in order of importance [83,87–89]. Advanced age is also a prognostic indicator for mortality, hydrocephalus, and cerebral ischemia. A normal CT scan or one that reveals a thin SAH layer is a favorable factor for prognosis. Aneurysm location also predicts outcome. Intraventricular hemorrhage is associated with hydrocephalus and is not a risk factor for cerebral ischemia. Posterior circulation aneurysms have a poor prognosis; middle cerebral

Table 2.9. Prognostic factors in subarachnoid hemorrhage: International Study on Timing of Aneurysm Surgery*

Mortality	Clinical hydrocephalus	Focal ischemic deficit
Consciousness level (+)	CT–hydrocephalus (+)	CT–SAH–thick layer (+)
Age (+)	CT–intraventricular hemorrhage (+)	CT–Normal (-)
CT–SAH–thin layer (-)	CT–SAH (+)	Age (+)
Admission systolic blood pressure (+)	Consciousness level (+)	Admission systolic blood pressure (+)
Number of medical conditions (+)	Pre-SAH hypertension (+)	Consciousness level (+)
CT–intracerebral hemorrhage (+)	Age (+)	CT–intraventricular hemorrhage (-)
Site: middle cerebral	Site: posterior circulation (+)	CT–SAH–diffuse layer (+)
CT–SAH–diffuse layer (+)	Postoperative hypertension (+)	Time of CT scan (+)
Site: basilar (+)		Motor response (+)
		Site: vertebral (-)
		CT–decreased density (+)

**Data from* Kassel and coworkers [83] and Graff-Rodford and coworkers [87].
CT—computed tomography; SAH—subarachnoid hemorrhage.
+,increases risk; -,decreases risk.

Table 2.10. Prognostic factors in subarachnoid hemorrhage for recurrent hemorrhage*

Acute (conservative)	Chronic	Antifibrinolytic therapy (acute)
Admission systolic blood pressure	Aneurysm size	Interval to angiography
Interval to treatment	Site: anterior cerebral–anterior communicating artery	Site: middle cerebral
Neurologic grade	Admission systolic blood pressure	Sex
Prior medical conditions		Site: Internal carotid–posterior communicating artery
Age		Admission systolic blood pressure
		Gastrointestinal hemorrhage
		Neurologic grade

**Data from* Torner and coworkers [88, 89].

aneurysms have a more favorable outcome. As for rebleeding, the time of treatment, the blood pressure, and the neurologic status have an effect on acute events. Chronic rebleeding appears to be related to the aneurysm's location and size and to blood pressure. These factors must be considered in relation to other factors that are more specific to the pathophysiologic response to SAH.

PREVENTION OF HEMORRHAGIC STROKE

Blood Pressure Control

Hypertension is a common risk factor for hemorrhagic stroke. Clinical trials demonstrated in the 1960s that stroke was prevented by control of severe hypertension [90]. Further trials investigated whether lower levels of blood pressure could also be controlled to prevent stroke and coronary heart disease. In a review by Collins and coworkers [91] the aggregate effect by the antihypertensive trials was a 42% reduction in stroke incidence with an average reduction in diastolic blood pressure of 6 mm Hg. (Figure 2.14). Most of the trials achieved a reduction between 5 and 10 mm Hg of diastolic blood pressure with a reduction of stroke incidence of 25% or more in all but two studies. In 1991, the trial of Systolic Hypertension in the Elderly Program demonstrated a reduction in stroke of 37% in men and women 60 years of age or over [92]. However, there is little information on stroke subtype in the studies. Since 80% of strokes are ischemic in origin, the effect on hemorrhagic stroke is only presumed. The sample size of ICH and SAH events that have been reported are small. The evidence that antihypertensive medications have had an effect on ICH and SAH incidence has been ecological. Even though a higher percentage of hypertension is controlled, there has been little change in the incidence of ICH and SAH in the past decade [30,32,93–95]. Changes in diagnosis by CT and patterns of ICH may also contribute to the lack of change in incidence [5]. The control of hypertension may have an effect on stroke mortality, which has been declining. Although blood pressure control cannot be conclusively associated with ICH and SAH incidence, it has the largest impact on stroke prevention.

Smoking Cessation

The evidence that smoking cessation reduces risk for SAH is indirect. In the case-control study done by Longstreth and coworkers [33], former smokers had a lower relative risk compared with light or moderate smokers. In addition, the time since the last cigarette demonstrated an inverse relationship of risk for SAH. In a large prospective study of 117,006 women, it was observed that former smokers also had a lower relative risk than current smokers and that the duration since quitting was associated with a decreased risk of SAH [41].

Unruptured Aneurysms

The prevalence of unruptured aneurysms is probably between 0.5% to 1.0% [96,97]. Twenty percent of patients with ruptured intracranial aneurysms have multiple aneurysms. The annual risk of rupture is between 1% and 2% per year [96,98]. Size of the aneurysm appears to be a risk factor for future rupture. Aneurysms of less than 3 mm are unlikely to cause hemorrhage [99,100]. Wiebers and coworkers [101] found that aneurysms above 10 mm were at risk, with the risk increasing by size. (Figure 2.15) The critical size, mostly in series of ruptured aneurysms examined retrospectively, was between 5 and 7 mm [102–105]. In most series, the reason for angiography was neurologic symptoms (*eg*, referent to the aneurysm, cerebral ischemia, or intracranial tumors). Patients who are symptomatic may be at higher risk than those discovered incidentally [106]. The natural history of these conditions also needs to be considered.

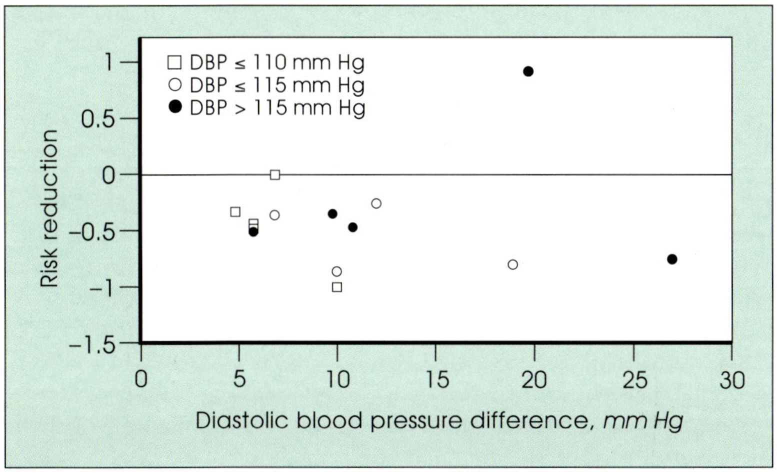

FIGURE 2.14

Risk reduction for stroke according to the initial diastolic blood pressure (DBP) and the average reduction in DBP. (*Data from* Collins and coworkers [91].)

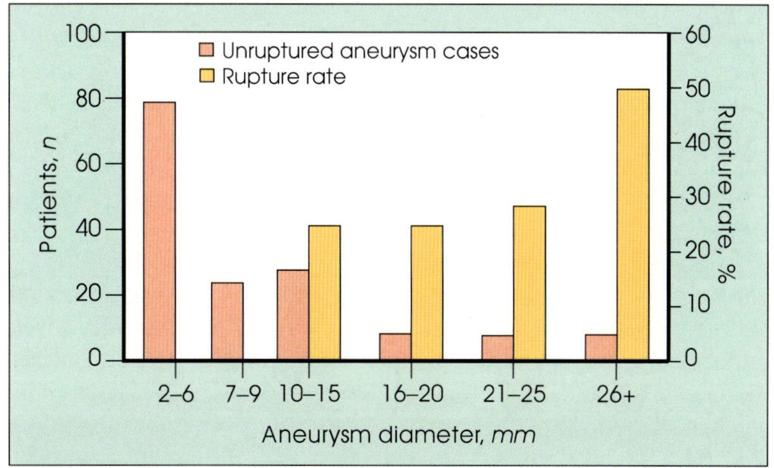

FIGURE 2.15

Risk of rupture increases for unruptured aneurysms over 10 mm in size. (*Data from* Wiebers and coworkers [101].)

Screening of High-Risk Populations

Possible high-risk groups would be those with familial cases and heritable disorders. The risk of angiographic complications has resulted in the recommendation that screening not be done [107]. ter Berg and coworkers [108] in a review of familial intracranial aneurysms, suggest that screening might be done in families of two or more affected members whose age is between 35 and 65 years. It is recommended that digital subtraction angiography be performed. The benefit of screening with MR angiography still needs to be determined [109].

Surgery

Several clinical series of surgical treatment for unruptured aneurysms have been reported [110–116]. There are no reports of postoperative hemorrhage in these series. Mortality rate has ranged from 0% to 7% and morbidity from 0% to 15%. In the series of Wirth and coworkers [116] there was a relationship of operative morbidity to aneurysm size and accessibility. There was no relationship of age to morbidity. There is little consensus as to the minimal size or other criteria for surgery.

Few studies have been conducted to determine the natural history of aneurysms that are incompletely clipped. Feuerberg and coworkers [117] examined 715 patients operated on between 1970 and 1980. Twenty-seven patients (3.8%) showed incomplete obliteration on follow-up angiography. One patient rebled during 266 person-years of follow-up. However, in another case series reported by Lin and coworkers [118], 19 patients (approximately 1% of cases before 1982) were readmitted for regrowth of aneurysms; 17 had a recurrent hemorrhage.

Coils

In the past 5 years, aneurysm occlusion has been attempted by using platinum coils to achieve thrombosis of the aneurysm. Several clinical series [119–121] of various sample sizes have reported occlusion and complication rates associated with the procedure. In a series of 71 patients, Casasco and coworkers [120] reported a total occlusion rate of 85% with a mean follow-up of 13 months. Size of the aneurysm was related to occlusion rate. Two patients had SAH during the procedure due to perforation of the aneurysmal sac. Two patients with posttreatment enlargements bled after treatment.

A larger multicenter study of 120 patients was conducted using the Guglielmi detachable coil [121]. Candidates included patients who were poor surgical candidates or surgical failures. Fifty-seven percent presented with intracranial hemorrhage. Complete occlusion occurred in 81% of small-necked aneurysms and 19% of wide-necked aneurysms. One patient had rupture during the procedure and one patient died at 18 months of SAH from a giant aneurysm (partially occluded). These preliminary reports suggest that coils can promote thrombosis and occlusion in a majority of cases.

Balloons

Balloon embolization was described by Serbinenko [122] in 1974. Several clinical series (Level V) have been reported with selection criteria of different patients [123,124]. In a series of 84 patients, Higashida and coworkers [125] reported an occlusion rate of 77% with multiple embolizations required in 12%. Treatment failures included subarachnoid hemorrhage (12%), stroke (11%), balloon rupture (1%), valve leakage (1%), myocardial infarction (1%), and pulmonary embolus (1%).

Polymer Embolization

Researchers in 1992 [126] reported a case series of six patients who were not surgical candidates and had direct infusion of a cellulose acetate polymer. The polymer has the advantage of conforming to the shape of the aneurysm and hardens within 5 minutes of application. Three of eight aneurysms were 100% occluded. One patient bled from a residual neck of the aneurysm 3 months after initial infusion.

CONCLUSIONS

With the more widespread use of neuroimaging, diagnostic accuracy for ICH and SAH has improved. This has made temporal trends difficult to assess because of the detection of smaller hemorrhages. The etiology of ICH is diverse, and the role of hypertension as a causative factor may be declining over time. With the aging of the population, amyloid angiopathy may become of greater importance. In younger age groups the increasing use of illicit drugs, in particular cocaine, may cause increasing numbers of hemorrhagic stroke. While the outcome has improved, incidence rates for SAH and ICH have not changed during the 1980s. Several recent case-control studies of SAH have demonstrated that smoking is the major risk factor, with alcohol use of lesser importance. This is unlike ICH in which smoking does not appear to be a significant risk factor, although hypertension, alcohol use, anticoagulant use, and low serum cholesterol are consistent risk factors, despite limited data.

The major prognostic factors for ICH include GCS, hemorrhage size, and the presence of intraventricular blood; for SAH, neurologic status, age, aneursym location, and thickness of SAH on CT scan are important factors. Strategies for prevention of hemorrhagic stroke include blood pressure control and screening for unruptured aneurysms, but these are of unproven value. The role of surgery for unruptured aneurysms is not well-defined because no clinical trials have been performed. For SAH, smoking cessation appears to be associated with a decreased risk. Further studies to better elucidate the risk factors for hemorrhagic stroke and to determine if modification of these factors will reduce the risk are needed.

REFERENCES

1. Torner JC: Epidemiology of subarachnoid hemorrhage. *Sem Neurol* 1984, 4:354–369.
2. Frankowski RF: Epidemiology of stroke and intracerebral hemorrhage. In *Intracerebral Hematomas*. Edited by Kaufman HH. New York: Raven Press; 1992:1–11.
3. Longstreth WT, Koepsell TD, Yerby MS, *et al.*: Risk factors for subarachnoid hemorrhage. *Stroke* 1985, 16:377–385.
4. Asplund K, Tuomilehto J, Stegmar B, *et al.*: Diagnostic criteria and quality control of the registration of stroke events in the MONICA project. *Acta Med Scand* 1988, 728(suppl):26–39.
5. Drury I, Whisnant JP, Garraway WM: Primary intracerebral hemorrhage: impact of CT on incidence. *Neurology* 1984, 653–657.
6. Bogousslavsky J, Regli F, Uske A, *et al.*: Early spontaneous hematoma in cerebral infarct: is primary cerebral hemorrhage overdiagnosed? *Neurology* 1991, 41:837–840.
7. Dennis MS, Bamford JM, Molyneux AJ, *et al.*: Rapid resolution of signs of primary intracerebral hemorrhage in computed tomograms of the brain. *BMJ* 1987, 295:379–381.
8. Feldmann E: Intracerebral hemorrhage. *Stroke* 1991, 22:684–691.
9. Sandercock PAG, Allen CMC, Corston RN, *et al.*: Clinical diagnosis of intracranial hemorrhage using Guy's Hospital score. *BMJ* 1985, 291:1675–1677.
10. Vermeulen M, van Gijn J: The diagnosis of subarachnoid hemorrhage. *J Neurol Neurosurg Psychiatry* 1990, 53:365–372.
11. Bassi P, Bandera R, Loiero M, *et al.*: Warning signs in subarachnoid hemorrhage. *Acta Neurol Scand* 1991, 84:277–281.
12. Edner G, Ronne-Engstrom E: Can early admission reduce aneurysmal rebleeds? A prospective study on aneurysmal incidence, aneurysmal rebleeds, admission and treatment delays in a defined region. *Br J Neurosurg* 1991, 5:601–608.
13. Hauerberg J, Anderson BB, Eskesen V, *et al.*: Importance of the recognition of a warning leak as a sign of a ruptured intracranial aneurysm. *Acta Neurol Scand* 1991, 83:61–64.
14. Ferro JM, Lopes J, Melo TP, *et al.*: Investigation into the causes of delayed diagnosis of subarachnoid hemorrhage. *Cerebrovasc Dis* 1991, 1:160–164.
15. Garland FC, Lilienfeld AM, Garland CF: Declining trends in mortality from cerebrovascular disease at ages 10-65 years: a test of validity. *Neuroepidemiology* 1989, 8:1–23.
16. Iso H, Jacobs DR, Goldman L: Accuracy of death certificate diagnosis of intracranial hemorrhage and nonhemorrhagic stroke: the Minnesota Heart Survey. *Am J Epidemiol* 1990, 132:993–998.
17. Furlan AJ, Whisnant JP, Elveback LR: The decreasing incidence of primary intracerebral hemorrhage: a population-based study. *Ann Neurol* 1979, 5:367–373.
18. Brott T, Thalinger K, Hertzberg V: Hypertension as a risk factor for spontaneous intracerebral hemorrhage. *Stroke* 1986, 17:1078–1083.
19. Hier DB, Babcock DJ, Foulkes MA, *et al.*: Influence of site on course of intracerebral hemorrhage. *J Stroke Cerebrovasc Dis* 1993, 3:65–74.
20. Schutz H, Bodeker R, Damian M, *et al.*: Age-related spontaneous intracerebral hematoma in a German community. *Stroke* 1990, 21:1412–1418.
21. Broderick J, Brott T, Tomsick T, *et al.*: Lobar hemorrhage in the elderly: the undiminishing importance of hypertension. *Stroke* 1993, 24:49–51.
22. Rinkel GJE, Wijdicks EFM, Vermuelen M, *et al.*: The clinical course of perimesenencephalic nonaneurysmal subarachnoid hemorrhage. *Ann Neurol* 1991, 29:463–468.
23. Vital and Health Statistics: *Detailed Diagnosis and Procedures, National Hospital Discharge Survey,* 1990, Series 13: data from the National Health Survey No. 113. DHHS Publication No. (PHS):92-1774.
24. Broderick JP, Brott T, Tomsick T, *et al.*: Intracerebral hemorrhage more than twice as common as subarachnoid hemorrhage. *J Neurosurg* 1993, 78:188–191.
25. Davis PH, Hachinski V: Epidemiology of cerebrovascular disease. In *Neuroepidemiology: A Tribute to Bruce Schoenberg.* Edited by DW Anderson. Boca Raton: CRC Press; 1991:27–53.
26. Sarti C, Tuomilehto J, Salomaa V, *et al.*: Epidemiology of subarachnoid hemorrhage in Finland from 1983 to 1985. *Stroke* 1991, 22:848–853.
27. Kiyohara Y, Ueda K, Hasuo Y, *et al.*: Incidence and prognosis of subarachnoid hemorrhage in a Japanese rural community. *Stroke* 1989, 20:1150–1155.
28. Broderick JP, Brott T, Tomsick T, *et al.*: The risk of subarachnoid and intracerebral hemorrhages in blacks as compared with whites. *N Engl J Med* 1992, 326:733–736.
29. Monthly Vital Statistics Report. National Center for Health Statistics. 1983–1990, vols. 31–38.
30. Broderick JP, Phillips SJ, Whisnant JP, *et al.*: Incidence rates of stroke in the eighties: the end of the decline in stroke? *Stroke* 1989, 20:577–582.
31. Ingall TJ, Whisnant JP, Wiebers DO, *et al.*: Has there been a decline in subarachnoid hemorrhage mortality? *Stroke* 1989, 20:718–724.
32. Harmsen P, Tsipogianni A, Wilhelmsen L: Stroke incidence rates were unchanged while fatality rates declined during 1971-1987 in Goteborg, Sweden. *Stroke* 1992, 23:1410–1415.
33. Longstreth WT, Nelson LM, Koepsell TD, *et al.*: Cigarette smoking, alcohol use, and subarachnoid hemorrhage. *Stroke* 1992 23:1242–1249.
34. Calandre L, Arnal C, Ortega JF, *et al.*: Risk factors for spontaneous cerebral hematomas: case-control study.*Stroke* 1986, 17:1126–1128.
35. Inzitari D, Giordano GP, Ancona AL, *et al.*: Leukoaraiosis, intracerebral hemorrhage, and arterial hypertension. *Stroke* 1990, 21:1419–1423.
36. Monforte R, Estruch R, Graus F, *et al.*: High ethanol consumption as risk factor for intracerebral hemorrhage in young and middle-aged people. *Stroke* 1990, 21:1529–1532.
37. Klatsky AL, Armstrong MA, Friedman GD: Alcohol use and subsequent cerebrovascular disease hospitalizations. *Stroke* 1989, 20:741–746.
38. Gill JS, Shipley MJ, Tsementzis SA, *et al.*: Alcohol consumption–a risk factor for hemorrhagic and non-hemorrhagic stroke. *Am J Med* 1991, 90:489–497.
39. Tanaka H, Ueda Y, Hayashi M, *et al.*: Risk factors for cerebral hemorrhage and cerebral infarction in a Japanese rural community. *Stroke* 1982, 13:62–73.
40. Donahue RP, Abbott RD, Reed DW, *et al.*: Alcohol and hemorrhagic stroke: the Honolulu Heart Program. *JAMA* 1986, 255:2311–2314.
41. Kawachi I, Colditz GA, Stampfer MJ, *et al.*: Smoking cessation and decreased risk of stroke in women. *JAMA* 1993, 269:232–236.
42. Gill JS, Shipley MJ, Tsementzis SA, *et al.*: Cigarette smoking: a risk factor for hemorrhagic and nonhemorrhagic stroke. *Arch Intern Med* 1989, 149:2053–2057.
43. Yano K, Reed DM, MacLean CJ: Serum cholesterol and hemorrhagic stroke in the Honolulu Heart Program. *Stroke* 1989, 20:1460–1465.
44. Iso H, Jacobs DR, Wentworth D, *et al.*: Serum cholesterol levels and six-year mortality from stroke in 350,977 men screened for the Multiple Risk Factor Intervention Trial. *N Engl J Med* 1989, 320:904–910.
45. Franke CL, de Jonge J, van Swieten JC, *et al.*: Intracerebral hematomas during anticoagulant treatment. *Stroke* 1990, 21:726–730.
46. Levine SR, Brust JCM, Futrell N, *et al.*: A comparative study of the cerebrovascular complications of cocaine: alkaloidal versus hydrochloride—a review. *Neurology* 1991, 41:1173–1177.
47. Kaku DA, Lowenstein DH: Emergence of recreational drug abuse as a major risk factor for stroke in young adults. *Ann Intern Med* 1990, 113:821–827.
48. Sloan MA, Kittner SJ, Rigamonti D, *et al.*: Occurrence of stroke associated with use or abuse of drugs. *Neurology* 1991, 41:1358–1364.
49. Abbott RD, Yin Yin MA, Reed DW, *et al.*: Risk of stroke in male cigarette smokers. *N Engl J Med* 315:717–720.

50. Shinton R, Beevers G: Meta-analysis of relation between cigarette smoking and stroke. *BMJ* 1989, 298:789–794.
51. Vaitkus PT, Berlin JA, Schwartz JS, *et al.*: Stroke complicating acute myocardial infarction: a meta-analysis of risk modification by anti-coagulation and thrombolytic therapy. *Arch Intern Med* 1992, 152:2020–2024.
52. Longstreth WT, Litwin PE, Weaver WD, *et al.*: Myocardial infarction, thrombolytic therapy, and stroke: a community-based study. *Stroke* 1993, 24:587–590.
53. De Jaegere PP, Arnold AA, Balk AH, *et al.*: Intracranial hemorrhage in association with thrombolytic therapy: incidence and clinical predictive factors. *J Am Coll Cardiol* 1992, 19:289–294.
54. Anderson JL, Karagounis L, Allen A, *et al.*: Older age and elevated blood pressure are risk factors for intracerebral hemorrhage after thrombolysis. *Am J Cardiol* 1991, 68:166–170.
55. Kase CS, O'Neal AM, Fischer M, *et al.*: Intracranial hemorrhage after use of tissue plasminogen activator for coronary thrombolysis. *Ann Intern Med* 1990, 112:17–21.
56. Leblanc R, Haddad G, Robitaille Y: Cerebral hemorrhage from amyloid angiopathy and coronary thrombolysis. *Neurosurgery* 1992, 31:586–590.
57. Wijdicks EFM, Jack CR Jr: Intracerebral hemorrhage after fibrinolytic therapy for acute myocardial infarction. *Stroke* 1993, 24:554–557.
58. Ridker PM, Hebert PR, Fuster V, *et al.*: Are both aspirin and heparin justified as adjuncts to thrombolytic therapy for acute myocardial infarction? *Lancet* 1993, 341:1574–1577.
59. Gore JM, Sloan M, Price TR, *et al.*: Intracerebral hemorrhage, cerebral infarction, and subdural hematoma after acute myocardial infarction and thrombolytic therapy in the thrombolysis in myocardial infarction study. *Circulation* 1991, 83:448–459.
60. Maggioni AP, Franzosi MG, Santoro E, *et al.*: The risk of stroke with acute myocardial infarction after thrombolytic and antithrombotic therapy. *N Engl J Med* 1992, 327:1–6.
61. Bonita R: Cigarette smoking, hypertension and the risk of subarachnoid hemorrhage: a population-based case-control study. *Stroke* 1986, 17:831–835.
62. Juvela S, Hillbom M, Numminen H, *et al.*: Cigarette smoking and alcohol consumption as risk factors for aneurysmal subarachnoid hemorrhage. *Stroke* 1993, 24:639–646.
63. Morris KM, Shaw DM, Foy PM: Smoking and subarachnoid hemorrhage: a case-control study. *Br J Neurosurg* 1992, 6:429–432.
64. Knekt P, Reunanen A, Aho K, *et al.*: Risk factors for subarachnoid hemorrhage in a longitudinal population study. *J Clin Epidemiol* 1991, 44:933–939.
65. Fogelholm R, Murros K: Cigarette smoking and subarachnoid hemorrhage: a population-based case-control study. *J Neurol Neurosurg Psych* 1987, 50:78–80.
66. Sacco RL, Wolf PA, Bharucha NE, *et al.*: Subarachnoid and intracerebral hemorrhage: natural history, prognosis, and precursive factors in the Framingham Study. *Neurology* 1984, 34:847–854.
67. Thorogood M, Mann J, Murphy M, *et al.*: Fatal stroke and use of oral contraceptives: findings from a case-control study. *Am J Epidemiol* 1992, 136:35–45.
68. Oyesiku NM, Colohan ART, Barrow DL, *et al.*: Cocaine-induced aneurysmal rupture: an emergent negative factor in the natural history of intracranial aneurysms? *Neurosurgery* 1993, 32:518–526.
69. Adams HPA Jr, Putnam SF, Kassell NF, *et al.*: Prevalence of diabetes mellitus among patients with subarachnoid hemorrhage. *Arch Neurol* 1984, 41:1033–1035.
70. Broderick JP, Brott TR, Tomsick T, *et al.*: Ultra-early evaluation of intracerebral hemorrhage. *J Neurosurg* 1990, 72:195–199.
71. Franke CL, van Swieten JC, Algra A, *et al.*: Prognostic factors in patients with intracerebral haematoma. *J Neurol Neurosurg Psych* 1992, 55:653–657.
72. Broderick JP, Brott TG, Duldner JE, *et al.*: Volume of intracerebral hemorrhage: a powerful and easy-to-use predictor of 30-day mortality. *Stroke* 1993, 24:987–993.
73. Tuhrim S, Dambrosia JM, Price TR, *et al.*: Intracerebral hemorrhage: external validation and extension of a model for prediction of 30-day survival. *Ann Neurol* 1991, 29:658–663.
74. Daverat P, Castel JP, Dartigues JF, *et al.*: Death and functional outcome after spontaneous intracerebral hemorrhage: a prospective study of 166 cases using multivariate analysis. *Stroke* 1991, 22:1–6.
75. Ricci S, Celani MG, La Rosa F, *et al.*: SEPIVAC: A community-based study of stroke incidence in Umbria, Italy. *J Neurol Neurosurg Psych* 1991, 54:695–698.
76. Bamford J, Dennis M, Sandercock P, *et al.*: The frequency, causes and timing of death within 30 days of a first stroke: the Oxfordshire Community Stroke Project. *J Neurol Neurosurg Psych* 1990, 53:824–829.
77. Mayo NE, Goldberg MS, Levy AR, *et al.*: Changing rates of stroke in the province of Quebec, Canada: 1981-1988. *Stroke* 1991, 22:590–595.
78. Portenoy RK, Lipton RB, Berger AR, *et al.*: Intracerebral hemorrhage: a model for the prediction of outcome. *J Neurol Neurosurg Psych* 1987, 50:976–979.
79. Helweg-Larsen S, Sommer W, Strange P, *et al.*: Prognosis for patients treated conservatively for spontaneous intracerebral hematomas. *Stroke* 1984, 15:1045–1048.
80. Radberg JA, Olsson JE, Radberg CT: Prognostic parameters in spontaneous intracerebral hematomas with special reference to anticoagulant treatment. *Stroke* 1991, 22:571–576.
81. Massaro AR, Sacco RL, Mohr JP, *et al.*: Clinical discriminators of lobar and deep hemorrhages: the Stroke Data Bank. *Neurology* 1991, 41:1881–1885.
82. Kase CS: Diagnosis and management of intracerebral hemorrhage in elderly patients. *Clin Geriatr Med* 1991, 7:549–567.
83. Kassell NF , Torner JC , Haley EC, *et al.*: The International Cooperative Study on the Timing of Aneurysm Surgery, part 1: overall management results. *J Neurosurg* 1990, 73:18–36.
84. Haley EC, Kassell NF, Torner JC, *et al.*: A randomized controlled trial of high-dose intravenous nicardipine in aneurysmal subarachnoid hemorrhage: a report of the Cooperative Aneurysm Study. *J Neurosurg* 1993, 78:537–547.
85. Weir B, Grace M, Hansen J, *et al.*: Time course of vasospasm in man. *J Neurosurg* 1978, 48:173–178.
86. Phillips LH, Whisnant JP, O'Fallon WM, *et al.*: The unchanging pattern of subarachnoid hemorrhage in a community. *Neurology* 1980, 30:1034–1040.
87. Graff-Radford NR, Torner JC, Adams HP, *et al.*: Factors associated with hydrocephalus after subarachnoid hemorrhage: a report of the Cooperative Aneurysm Study. *Arch Neurol* 1989, 46:744–752.
88. Torner JC, Nibbelink DW, Burmeister LF: Statistical comparisons of end results of a randomized treatment study. In *Aneurysmal Subarachnoid Hemorrhage. Report of the Cooperative Study.* Edited by Sahs AL, Nibbelink DW, Torner JC. Baltimore: Urban & Schwarzenberg; 1981:249–276.
89. Torner JC, Kassell NF, Wallace RB, *et al.*: Preoperative prognostic factors for rebleeding and survival in aneurysm patients receiving antifibrinolytic therapy: report of the cooperative aneurysm study. *Neurosurgery* 1981, 9:506–513.
90. Hypertension Detection and Follow-Up Program Cooperative Group: Five-year findings of the hypertension detection and follow-up program, III: reduction in stroke incidence among persons with high blood pressure. *JAMA* 1982, 247:633–638.
91. Collins R, Peto R, MacMahon S, *et al.*: Blood pressure, stroke, and coronary heart disease. Part 2: short-term reductions in blood pressure: overview of randomized drug trials in their epidemiological context. *Lancet* 1990, 335:827–838.

92. SHEP Cooperative Research Group: Prevention of stroke by antihypertensive drug treatment in older persons with isolated systolic hypertension: final results of the Systolic Hypertension in the Elderly Program (SHEP). *JAMA* 1991, 265:3255–3264.
93. Phillips SJ, Whisnant JP, O'Fallon WM, *et al.*: A community blood pressure survey: Rochester, Minnesota, 1986. *Mayo Clin Proc* 1988, 63:691–699.
94. Klag MJ, Whelton PK, Seidler AJ: Decline in US stroke mortality: demographic trends and antihypertensive treatment. *Stroke* 1989, 20:14–21.
95. Cooper R, Sempos C, Hsieh S-C, *et al.*: Slowdown in the decline of stroke mortality in the United States, 1978–1986. *Stroke* 1990, 21:1274–1279.
96. Rosenorn J, Eskesen V, Schmidt K: Unruptured intracranial aneurysms: an assessment of the annual risk of rupture based on epidemiological and clinical data. *Br J Neurosurg* 1988, 2:369–378.
97. Atkinson JLD, Sundt TM, Houser OW, *et al.*: Angiographic frequency of anterior circulation intracranial aneurysms. *J Neurosurg* 1989, 70:551–555.
98. Jane JA, Kassell NF, Torner JC, *et al.*: The natural history of aneurysms and arteriovenous malformations. *J Neurosurg* 1985, 62:321–323.
99. Locksley HB: Natural history of subarachnoid hemorrhage, intracranial aneurysms, and arteriovenous malformations: based on 6,368 cases in the Cooperative Study. In *Intracranial Aneurysms and Subarachnoid Hemorrhage. A Cooperative Study.* Edited by Sahs AL, Perret GE, Locksley HB, *et al.* Philadelphia: JB Lippincott; 1969:37–108.
100. McCormick WF, Acosta-Rua GJ: The size of intracranial saccular aneurysms: an autopsy study. *J Neurosurg* 1970, 33:422–427.
101. Wiebers DO, Whisnant JP, Sundt TM, *et al.*: The significance of unruptured intracranial saccular aneurysms. *J Neurosurg* 1987, 66:23–29.
102. Cromptom MR: Mechanism of growth and rupture in cerebral berry aneurysms. *BMJ* 1966, 1:1138–1142.
103. Ferguson GG: Physical factors in the initiation, growth, and rupture of human intracranial saccular aneurysms. *J Neurosurg* 1972, 37:666–667.
104. Kassell NF, Torner JC: Size of intracranial aneurysms. *Neurosurgery* 1983, 12:291–297.
105. Ojemann RG: Management of the ruptured intracranial aneurysm. *N Engl J Med* 1981, 304:725–726.
106. Wiebers DO, Whisnant JP, O'Fallon WM: The natural history of unruptured intracranial aneurysms. *N Engl J Med* 1981, 304:696–698.
107. Levey AS, Paulker SG, Kassirer JP: Occult intracranial aneurysms in polycystic kidney disease: when is cerebral arteriography indicated? *N Engl J Med* 1983, 308:986– 994.
108. ter Berg HW, Dippel DW, Limburg M, *et al.*: Familial intracranial aneurysms: a review. *Stroke* 1992, 23:1024–1030.
109. Ross JS, Masaryk TJ, Modic MT, *et al.*: Intracranial aneurysms: evaluation by MR angiography. *AJNR* 1990, 11:449–456.
110. Eskeen V, Rosenorn N, Schmidt K, *et al.*: Clinical features and outcome in 48 patients with unruptured intracranial saccular aneurysms: a prospective consecutive study. *Br J Neurosurg* 1987, 1:47–52.
111. Heiskanen O: Risks of surgery for unruptured intracranial aneurysms. *J Neurosurg* 1986, 65:451–453.
112. Jain KK: Surgery of intact intracranial aneurysms. *J Neurosurg* 1974, 40:495–498.
113. Salazar JL: Surgical treatment of asymptomatic and incidental intracranial aneurysms. *J Neurosurg* 1980, 53:20–21.
114. Samson DS, Hodosh RM, Clark WK: Surgical management of unruptured asymptomatic aneurysms. *J Neurosurg* 1977, 46:731–734.
115. Nishimoto A, Ueta K, Onbe H, *et al.*: Nationwide Cooperative Study of intracranial aneurysm surgery in Japan. *Stroke* 1985, 16:48–52.
116. Wirth FP, Laws ER, Piepgras DS: Surgical treatment of incidental intracranial aneurysms. *Neurosurgery* 1983, 12:507–511.
117. Feuerberg I, Lindquist C, Lindquist M, *et al.*: Natural history of postoperative aneurysm rests. *J Neurosurg* 1987, 66:30–34.
118. Lin T, Fox AJ, Drake CG: Regrowth of aneurysm sacs from residual neck following aneurysmal clipping. *J Neurosurg* 1989, 70:556–560.
119. Guglielmi G, Vinuela F, Dion J, *et al.*: Electrothrombosis of saccular aneurysms via endovascular approach. Part 2: preliminary clinical experience. *J Neurosurg* 1991, 75:8–14.
120. Casasco AE, Aymard A, Gobin P, *et al.*: Selective endovascular treatment of 71 intracranial aneurysms with platinum coils. *J Neurosurg* 1993, 79:3–10.
121. Guglielmi G, Vinuela F, Duckwiler G, *et al.*: Endovascular treatment of posterior circulation aneurysms by electrothrombosis using electrically detachable coils. *J Neurosurg* 1992, 77:515–524.
122. Serbinenko FA: Balloon catheterization and occlusion of major cerebral vessels. *J Neurosurg* 1974, 41:125–145.
123. Fox AJ, Vinuela F, Pelz DM, *et al.*: Use of detachable balloon for proximal artery occlusion in the treatment of unclippable cerebral aneurysms. *J Neurosurg* 1987, 66:40–46.
124. Romodanov A, Scheglov VI: Intravascular occlusion of saccular aneurysms of the cerebral arteries by means of a detachable balloon catheter. In *Advances and Technical Standards in Neurosurgery, vol. 9.* Edited by Krayenbuhl H. Zurich: Springer-Verlag; 1982:25–48.
125. Higashida RT, Halbach VV, Barnwell SL *et al.*: Treatment of intracranial aneurysms with preservation of parent vessel: results of percutaneous balloon embolization in 84 patients. *AJNR* 1990, 11:633–640.
126. Kinugasa K, Mandai S, Terai Y, *et al.*: Direct thrombosis of aneurysms with cellulose acetate polymer. Part 2: Preliminary clinical experience. *J Neurosurg* 1992, 77:501–507.

Chapter 3

Epidemiology of Vascular Dementia

PHILIP B. GORELICK
CARLOS MANGONE
FERNANDO BOZZOLA

In the broadest use of the term, *vascular dementias* describe dementias resulting from cerebral blood vessel disease [1,2]. In most cases there is thromboembolic cerebrovascular disease, traditional cardiovascular disease risk factors such as hypertension, and abrupt onset of dementia coinciding with cerebral infarction. As explained by Fisher [3], vascular dementia is "a matter of strokes large and small." There has recently been a resurgence of interest in vascular dementia [4]. Old concepts are being challenged and new hypotheses are being tested [5–7]. Such research initiatives are furthering our knowledge about this important disease entity. In this chapter we review important epidemiologic advances that have enhanced our understanding of vascular dementia and are leading to the early detection and prevention of this devastating disease.

MAGNITUDE OF THE PROBLEM

Dementia is a health problem largely associated with advanced age. The prevalence of dementia is highest in the elderly, which is the most rapidly expanding segment of our population [8]. If current health trends of diminishing age-specific mortality persist, the number of elderly will continue to increase in an unprecedented manner in the coming decades. Figure 3.1 summarizes estimates of the absolute numbers of elderly in the United States and worldwide and those with dementia in the United States in the coming years. By the year 2040 it is estimated that one in 30 Americans will have dementia! Furthermore, it is estimated that the elderly in developing countries will constitute approximately 70% of the world's aged in the 21st century.

AT THE TURN OF THE CENTURY AND NOW

Epidemiologic concepts about dementia have changed since the early part of the 20th century as the proportion of elderly in the population has grown dramatically. In the early part of the 20th century the percentage of elderly in the population was relatively small (Figure 3.2) [8,9], and failure of cerebral function and cognition was commonly attributed to "hardening of the arteries" because it was assumed that arteriosclerosis reduced cerebral blood flow and so impaired cognition [10]. Degenerative dementia as described by Alzheimer was recognized but considered uncommon. Furthermore, Alzheimer, who was considered by many to be one of the pioneers in delineating cerebrovascular disease in the early 1900s and in distinguishing this condition from other diseases, made astute clinical and pathologic observations about arteriosclerotic and other senile processes [11] that were not again underscored until some 50 years later by Fisher [12].

In the 1960s and 1970s clinical and epidemiologic concepts of vascular dementias and Alzheimer's disease were critically reassessed. It was apparent then that Alzheimer's disease was the leading cause of progressive and irreversible dementia and that vascular dementia was the second most common cause. During the 1970s the term *multi-infarct dementia* was coined by Hachinski and coworkers [13] to denote progressive loss of cognitive functions and impairment of social skills when there is a clinical history of a dementia syndrome characterized by abrupt onset, stepwise deterioration, fluctuating course, and focal neurologic signs caused by cerebral infarction. The term *vascular dementia* has recently been popularized since it has a broader denotation and takes into account subtypes of the disease [5,6].

Finally, Binswanger's controversial role in defining vascular dementia in the late 1800s must be acknowledged [14]. Although many consider Binswanger to have been one of the pioneers in delineating cerebrovascular diseases, the neuropathologic evidence that he presented for the vascular dementia syndrome, subcortical arteriosclerotic encephalopathy (Binswanger's disease), was scant, and to this day the clinical, neuroradiologic, neuropathologic, and pathophysiologic features remain controversial.

DIAGNOSTIC CRITERIA

Clinical criteria for vascular dementia have evolved over time and are listed chronologically in Tables 3.1 and 3.2 according to Roth [15], Mayer-Gross and coworkers [16], the *Diagnostic and*

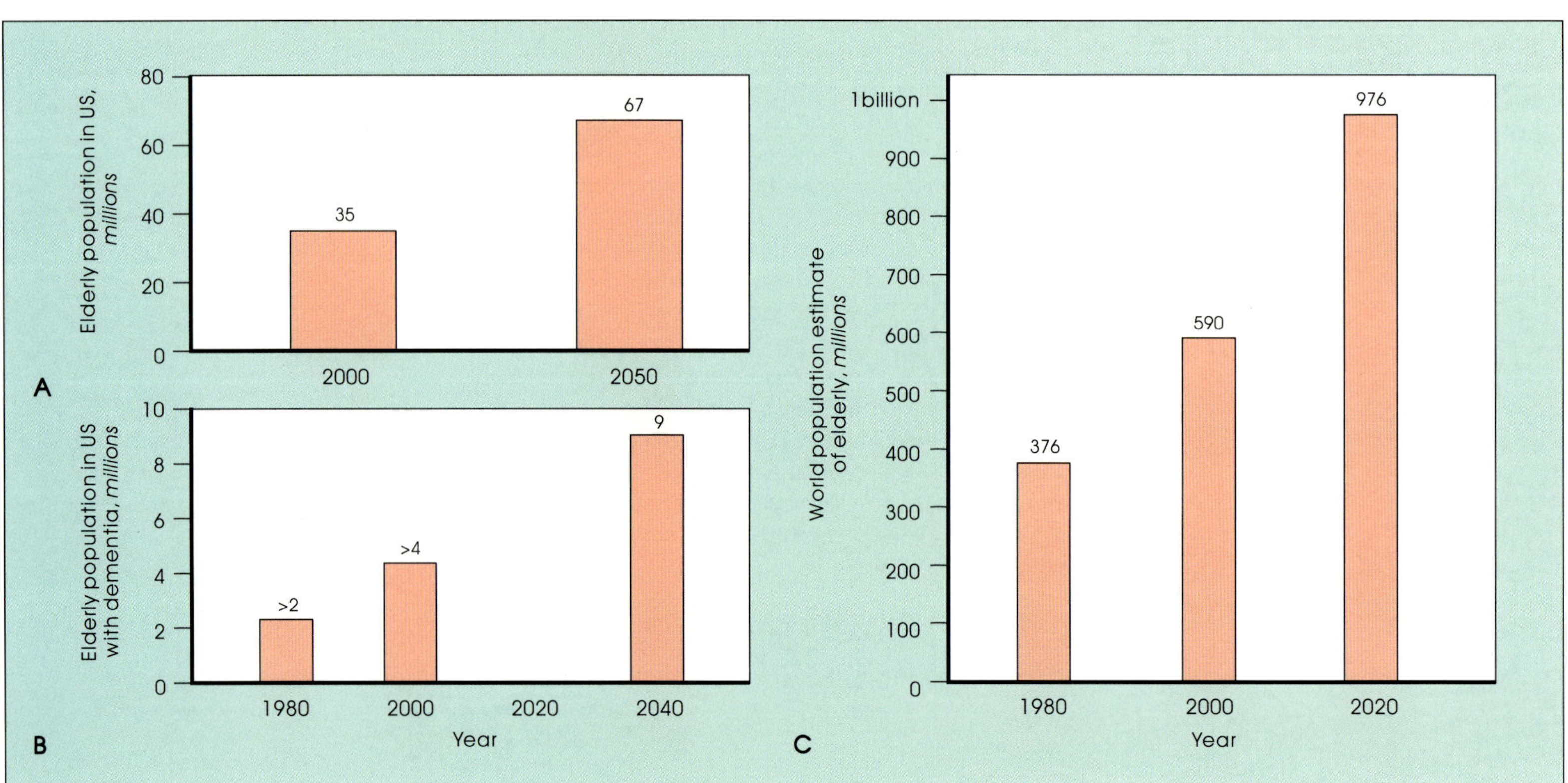

FIGURE 3.1

Demographic estimates for the elderly. **A**, Absolute numbers of elderly (> 65 years) in the United States by year. **B**, Absolute numbers of elderly in the United States with dementia by year. **C**, World population estimate of elderly (≥ 60 years) by year. By 2020, developing countries will represent 70% of the world's elderly.

Statistical Manual of Mental Disorders, 3rd edition revised (DSM-IIIR) [17], the State of California Alzheimer's Disease Diagnostic and Treatment Centers [18], and the NINDS-AIREN Work Shop [19]. Generally, most modern criteria require the following key components to establish a diagnosis of vascular dementia: the presence of dementia, the presence of stroke, and a temporal relationship between dementia and stroke [6]. Furthermore, most modern criteria define dementia by the presence of impairment in several cognitive domains including memory (Table 3.3) [20].

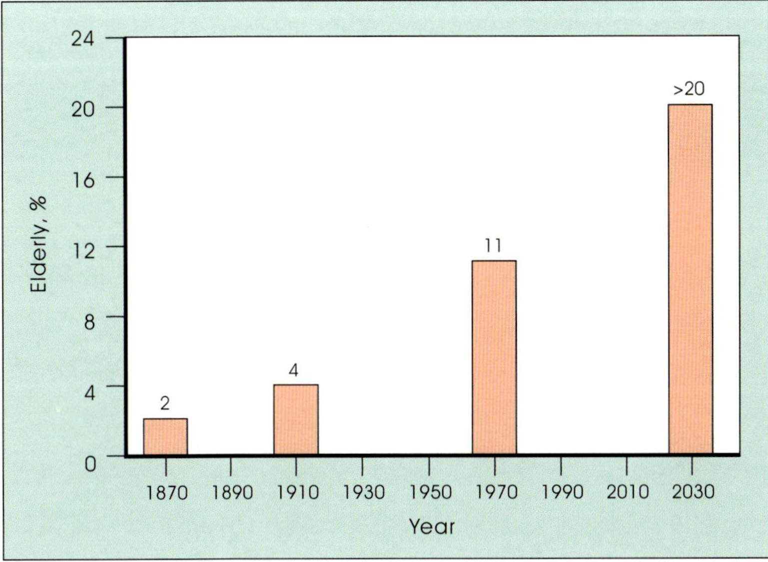

FIGURE 3.2

Demographic estimates of the percentage of elderly from the turn of the century to the future.

Critics have charged that diagnostic criteria such as those of the DSM-IIIR lack sufficient sensitivity and specificity, evidence to validate the criteria, and uniform, operationally defined diagnostic terms [21–23]. More recently, proposed diag-

Table 3.1. Early diagnostic criteria for vascular dementia

Arteriosclerotic psychosis*

- Focal signs and symptoms indicative of cerebrovascular disease
- Fluctuating or remittent course with any one of the following features:
  - Emotional incontinence
  - Preservation of insight
  - Epileptiform seizures

Arteriosclerotic psychosis†

- Symptoms make their appearance following a number of strokes
- Sixty to 70 years of age of onset
- History of hypertension
- Memory disturbance, restlessness, emotionality, and wandering at night
- Somatic complaints
- Maintenance of creative and intellectual powers
- Cooling of emotions and diminishment of drive and initiative
- Preservation of judgment and basic personality until the late stages of the disease
- Emotional incontinence
- Depression
- Epileptiform seizure
- Neurologic lesions and fluctuating course of disease

**Data from* Roth [15].
†*Data from* Mayer-Gross and coworkers [16].

Table 3.2. Modern diagnostic criteria for vascular dementia*

Multi-infarct dementia according to the DSM-IIIR

- Dementia (includes impairment in short- and long-term memory; impairment or disturbance in at least abstract thinking, judgment, higher cortical function, or personality; disturbance that interferes with work or usual social activities; and an organic factor or factors judged to be etiologically related to the disturbance)
- Stepwise deteriorating course with "patchy" distribution of deficits
- Focal neurologic signs and symptoms
- Significant cerebrovascular disease judged to be etiologically related to the disturbance

Probable ischemic vascular dementia according to the ADDTC

- Dementia (deterioration sufficient to interfere with conduct of patient's customary affairs of life)
- Evidence of two or more ischemic strokes by history, neurologic signs, or neuroimaging studies; or occurrence of a single stroke with a clearly documented temporal relationship to the onset of dementia
- Evidence of at least one infarct outside the cerebellum by computed tomography or T_1-weighted magnetic resonance imaging

Definite ischemic vascular dementia according to the ADDTC

- Clinical evidence of dementia
- Pathologic confirmation of multiple infarcts, some outside of the cerebellum

Probable vascular dementia according to the NINDS-AIREN Work Shop

- Dementia (cognitive decline from a previously higher level of functioning manifested by impairment of memory and of two or more cognitive domains, *eg*, orientation, attention, language, visuospatial functions, executive functions, motor control, and praxis)
- Cerebrovascular disease
- Relationship between the above two disorders, manifested or inferred by the presence of one or more of the following:
  - Onset of dementia within 3 months following a recognized stroke
  - Abrupt deterioration in cognitive functions or fluctuating, stepwise progression of cognitive deficits

Definite vascular dementia according to the NINDS-AIREN Work Shop

- Clinical criteria for probable vascular dementia
- Histopathologic evidence of cerebrovascular disease
- Absence of neurofibrillary tangles and neuritic plaques exceeding those expected for age
- Absence of other clinical or pathologic disorder capable of producing dementia

**Data from* the Diagnostic and Statistical Manual of Mental Disorders (DSM-IIIR) [17], Chui and coworkers [18], and Roman and coworkers [19]; with permission.
ADDTC—Alzheimer's Disease Diagnostic and Treatment Centers (California).

nostic criteria [18,19] are undergoing clinical and pathologic validation [6].

The Hachinski Score (Table 3.4) [13] has been used to differentiate vascular from degenerative dementia. Those with scores of 7 or higher are thought to have vascular dementia while those with scores of 4 or lower are considered to have degenerative dementia. The scale is weighted to identify stroke. Thus, low Hachinski Scores generally rule out cerebrovascular disease, but high scores do not exclude coexistent degenerative dementia (*eg*, Alzheimer's disease).

Table 3.3. Cognitive domains*

Attention	Psychomotor retardation
Language and verbal output	Neuropsychiatric features
Memory	Praxis
Visuospatial abilities	Calculation
Executive functions	Orientation

**From* Cummings and Benson [20]; with permission.

Table 3.4. The Hachinski Score for the differentiation of vascular and degenerative dementia*

Feature	Point value
Abrupt onset	2
Stepwise deterioration	1
Fluctuating course	2
Nocturnal confusion	1
Relative preservation of personality	1
Depression	1
Somatic complaints	1
Emotional incontinence	1
History of hypertension	1
History of strokes	2
Evidence of associated atherosclerosis	1
Focal neurologic symptoms	2
Focal neurologic signs	2

**From* Hachinski and coworkers [13]; with permission.

Table 3.5. Classification of vascular dementia

Anatomic	Etiologic*
Deep hemisphere infarcts or hemorrhages	Atherosclerosis
Superficial cortical infarcts or hemorrhages	Fibromuscular dysplasia
Combined deep and superficial infarcts or hemorrhages	Atrial fibrillation
Subarachnoid hemorrhage	Lupus erythematosus
	Aneurysmal subarachnoid hemorrhage

*The reader is referred to Cummings and Benson [20] for a comprehensive listing of the etiologic classification of vascular dementia.

CLASSIFICATION

Vascular dementia may be classified according to the site of cerebral infarction or stroke, or by the cause of the underlying lesion (Table 3.5) [20]. By the anatomic classification, vascular dementias due to cerebral infarcts may be divided into deep infarcts caused by occlusions of small penetrating arteries (lacunae), superficial cortical infarcts caused by occlusion of major intracranial or extracranial arteries or small arterioles, and a combination of deep and superficial infarcts. The etiologic classification includes a comprehensive list of thrombotic (*eg*, atherosclerosis, fibromuscular dysplasia, lupus erythematosus), embolic (*eg*, atrial fibrillation, atrial myxoma), and other causes (*eg*, subarachnoid

Table 3.6. Prevalence of vascular dementia according to EURODEM collaborators*†

	Age, y						
Population	30–59	60-64	65–69	70–74	75–79	80–84	85–89
Finland (entire country)							
Women	0.0%	0.5%		2.9%		6.2%	
Men	0.04%	1.5%		3.2%		3.6%	
Appignano, Italy							
Women	—	0.0%		2.2%		9.2%	
Men	—	0.0%		4.8%		16.3%	
Lund, Sweden							
Women	0.0%	0.0%		2.6%		7.0%	
Men	0.0%	1.6%		4.6%		4.8%	
Cambridge, UK							
Women	—	—	—	—	1.5%	2.8%	
Men	—	—	—	—	1.8%	3.5%	
Cambridgeshire, UK							
Women	—	—	—	2.2%	3.3%	—	—

**From* Rocca and coworkers [26]; with permission.
†In this table mixed dementia was combined with vascular dementia.
EURODEM—European Community Concerted Action Epidemiology and Prevention of Dementia.

Table 3.7. Incidence of vascular dementia according to several international studies*†

Population	Age, y	Incidence
Lund, Sweden	Women ≤80	11.0%
	Men ≤80	13.4%
	Women ≤90	25.1%
	Men ≤90	29.8%
Finland	55–64	3.7/100,000
	65–74	42/100,000
	75–84	205/100,000
	≥85	556/100,000
Rochester, Minnesota	>29	28/100,000

**From* Gorelick and Mangone [2]; with permission.
†In this table mixed dementia was combined with vascular dementia.

hemorrhage) of stroke [20]. Identification of specific vascular mechanisms that contribute to cognitive impairment is important to our understanding of vascular dementia [24]. Overall, cerebral infarcts are the most common cause of vascular dementia.

PREVALENCE AND INCIDENCE

In the United States and Europe vascular dementia is second to Alzheimer's disease as the leading cause of dementia [2]. It is estimated that Alzheimer's disease accounts for 50% to 60% of cases, vascular dementia for about 10% to 20% of cases, and mixed vascular and degenerative dementias for a major proportion of the remaining progressive and irreversible dementias. Overall, the frequency of vascular dementia rises exponentially with age, and men are at greater risk for vascular dementia while women are at greater risk for Alzheimer's disease [6]. Interestingly, vascular dementia appears to be more prevalent in the Orient, a region of the world with high stroke rates [25]. Although this latter trend is not well established in developing countries because there is a paucity of epidemiologic research on dementias of late life, it is anticipated that vascular dementia will be important in those developing countries with high stroke rates. Thus, among populations with high stroke rates there may be a double burden of dementia with a universal rate for Alzheimer's disease and an excess rate for vascular dementia [8].

Prevalence data for vascular dementia from the European Community Concerted Action Epidemiology and Prevention of Dementia (EURODEM) collaborative reanalysis are presented in Table 3.6 [26]. Of 23 surveys of dementia, five met the DSM-III or equivalent inclusion criteria for the reanalysis. Incidence data from several international studies are presented in Table 3.7 [27–30].

SECULAR TRENDS

Time-trend data suggest that vascular dementia may be declining. Age-specific incidence rates in Lundby, Sweden, during the time periods of 1947 to 1956 and 1957 to 1972 and the age-adjusted incidence rates in Rochester, Minnesota, from 1960 to 1974 show declines in dementia due to cerebrovascular disease [27,28,31]. This decline parallels the decline in stroke mortality during the 1960s and 1970s.

SURVIVAL

Patients with progressive dementias appear to have increased mortality when survival rates are corrected for expected survival of age- and sex-matched controls [32–35]. These findings for vascular dementia, Alzheimer's disease, and mixed dementias are reviewed in Figure 3.3. Overall, survival trends show that

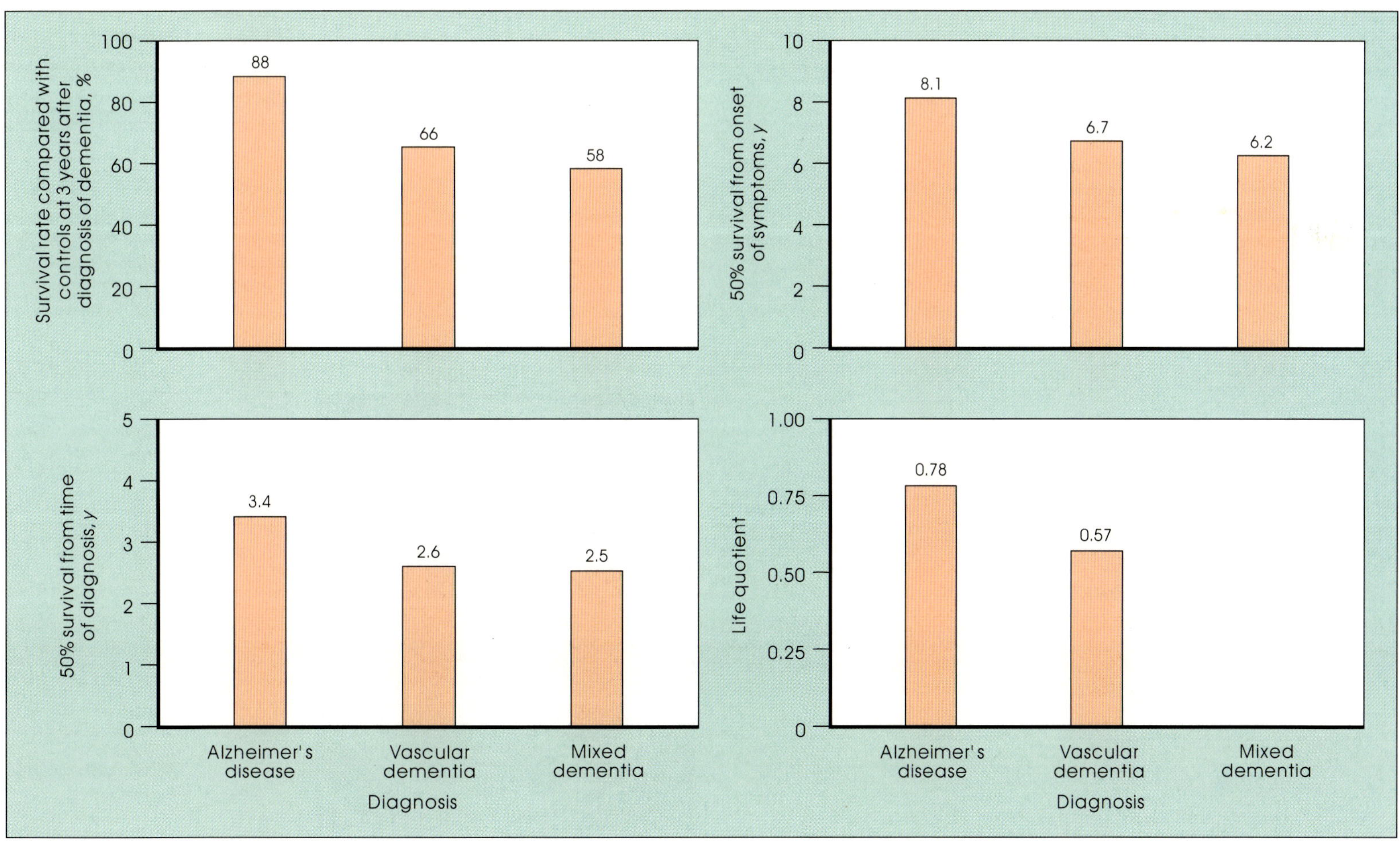

FIGURE 3.3

Survival in patients with Alzheimer's disease, vascular dementia, and mixed dementia. *Life quotient* is the estimated survival divided by the expected survival.

patients with vascular dementia or mixed dementia have shorter survival rates than those with Alzheimer's disease.

RISK FACTORS

Until recently, formal epidemiologic study of risk factors for vascular dementias received little attention because it was assumed that risk factors for dementia associated with stroke would be the same as those for ischemic and other cerebrovascular diseases [36]. The important clinicopathologic correlations of Tomlinson and coworkers [37] included several salient points about dementia associated with stroke: 1) vascular dementia is related to volume of cerebral hemisphere tissue infarcted and possibly to the location of infarction; 2) stroke is common among the aged; and 3) the presence of stroke does not necessarily mean that there is vascular dementia (Table 3.8). More recent studies have suggested that the following factors might be associated with vascular dementia: 1) history of hypertension, neurologic symptoms, and bilateral cerebral infarction [38]; 2) multiple infarcts, cerebral volume loss, and cerebral atrophy [39]; and 3) infarct number, site (*eg*, thalamus or angular gyrus), and the presence of cortical atrophy or hydrocephalus (Table 3.9) [40].

It is well established that stroke patients and patients with vascular dementia have a high prevalence of risk factors for cardiovascular disease such as hypertension, heart disease, diabetes mellitus, and cigarette smoking [41]. However, it remains to be determined which clinical factors distinguish patients with multi-infarcts and dementia from those with multi-infarcts without dementia. We carried out a case-control study to determine which medical, demographic, and neurologic factors were predictors of multi-infarct patients with dementia (cases) and multi-infarct patients without dementia (controls) [42,43]. There were 61 cases and 86 controls. The findings are summarized in Table 3.10. Key demographic and medical factors that predicted case-control status were advanced age, lower educational attainment, history of recent cigarette smoking, myocardial infarction, and systolic blood pressure level [42]. Key computed tomographic (CT) factors were left hemisphere infarction and diffuse enlargement of the left lateral ventricle [43].

Our results are both consistent with prior studies and plausible. Age is a well-established risk factor for dementia [8] and education has also been recognized more recently as a possible risk factor (Orgogozo JM. Paper presented at the NINDS/AIREN International Work Shop on Vascular Dementia; 1991; Bethesda) [44–49]. It is uncertain whether education exerts its effect through direct mechanisms or through more indirect associations with other socioeconomic-related factors (*eg*, occupation). History of myocardial infarction and recent cigarette smoking are strongly associated with stroke and could be related to vascular dementia by any of a number of pathophysiologic mechanisms that are reviewed in detail elsewhere [42,50,51]. Systolic blood pressure level may need to be elevated in chronic hypertensives with multi-infarcts to maintain cerebral perfusion and cognition [42,52]. Left cortical infarction is our key CT

Table 3.8. Possible risk factors for vascular dementia*

Factor	Comment
Volume of cerebral infarction	Dementia noted at 50 mL cerebral volume loss and definitely present by 100 mL cerebral volume loss
Site of cerebral infarction	Damage to eloquent brain loci such as the thalamus or angular gyrus region could lead to dementia

**Data* from Tomlinson and coworkers [37]; with permission.

Table 3.9. Factors associated with vascular dementia

Study	Factors
Ladurner and coworkers [38]	History of hypertension and neurologic symptoms; bilateral cerebral infarcts
Loeb and coworkers [39]	Multiple cerebral infarcts; volume of cerebral tissue loss; cerebral atrophy
Tatemichi and coworkers [40]	Infarct number; infarct site; cortical atrophy

Table 3.10. Putative risk factors for dementia associated with multi-infarcts

Medical and demographic factors*

Advanced age	History of myocardial infarction
Lower educational attainment	Systolic blood pressure level
History of recent cigarette smoking	

Computed tomographic factors

Left hemisphere infarction
Diffuse enlargement of the left lateral ventricle

*All factors were positively associated with case status except systolic blood pressure level, which was negatively associated with case status.

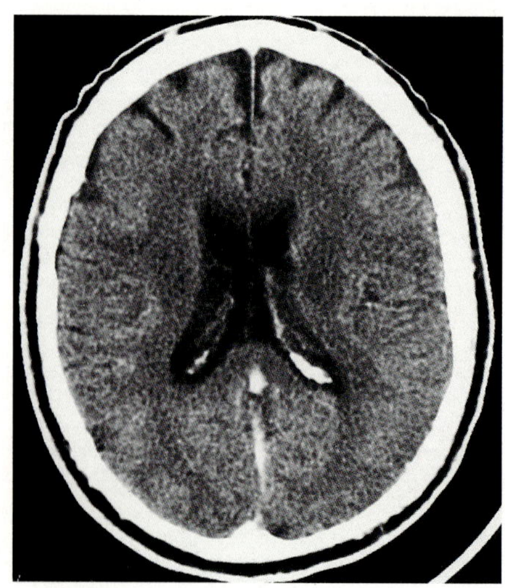

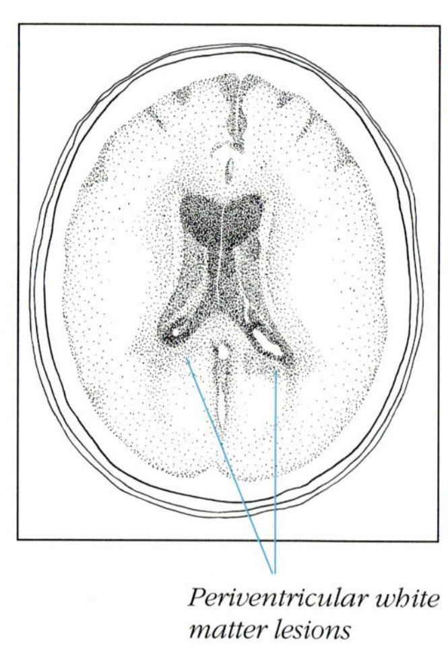

FIGURE 3.4

Computed tomographic scan and accompanying line drawing depict periventricular subcortical white matter lucencies associated with dementia.

predictor of dementia associated with stroke and probably relates to the left hemisphere's important role in language function [53]. Enlargement of the left lateral ventricle can be explained by left cortical or subcortical infarcts, which were prevalent in our study [43].

There is controversy about the role of radiologically diagnosable subcortical white matter changes on CT and magnetic resonance (MR) images in vascular and other dementias [53,54]. On CT the lesions appear as periventricular zones of lucency that have been termed leukoaraiosis: rarefaction or thinning of the white matter (Figure 3.4). Table 3.11 summarizes the appearance of these lesions on T2-weighted MR images (Figure 3.5), and Table 3.12 shows some of the pathologic correlates of the subcortical lesions [53]. Some studies have shown a relation between subcortical white matter changes and dementia while others have shown no correlation [53]. The presence of white matter changes on CT may be a better predictor of dementia than their presence on MR scans [54]. Furthermore, such changes may be observed in Alzheimer's disease [55] and could represent incomplete infarction of the white matter associated with hypotensive episodes in these patients.

PREVENTION OF VASCULAR DEMENTIA

As stroke leads to vascular dementia, the prevention of stroke will lead to a substantial reduction of vascular dementia. Treatable risk factors for stroke (*eg*, hypertension, heart disease, cigarette smoking) and measures aimed at the primary prevention of stroke are well established and are reviewed in the first chapter of this atlas. The use of carotid endarterectomy and antithrombotics should prove to reduce the incidence of vascular dementia as these treatments serve as secondary ischemic stroke preventatives. As we learn more about specific risk factors for vascular dementia, targeted primary and secondary prevention strategies can be bolstered [2,42]. Furthermore, a search for pharmacologic agents that enhance the microcirculation or "ischemic penumbra," or enhance failing memory circuits in established stroke or vascular dementia may prove to be beneficial [56].

Evidence is emerging that vascular dementia may be more common than previously supposed [57]. The possibilities of primary and secondary prevention of stroke suggest that vascular dementia may be more amenable to prevention and treatment than any other form of dementing illness.

Table 3.11. Location and appearance of white matter lesions on T2-weighted magnetic resonance images

Hyperintense thick rims surrounding the lateral ventricles	Unified or multifocal subcortical patches
Caps around the poles of the lateral ventricles	Confluent subcortical patches

**From* Chimowitz and coworkers [53]; with permission.

Table 3.12. Pathologic correlates of subcortical lesions

Necrosis	Arteriolar sclerosis
Diffuse demyelination	Dilation of the ventricular system
Gliosis	Dilated perivascular spaces (ètat criblé)
Small subcortical infarcts	Vascular ectasia

**From* Chimowitz and coworkers [53]; with permission.

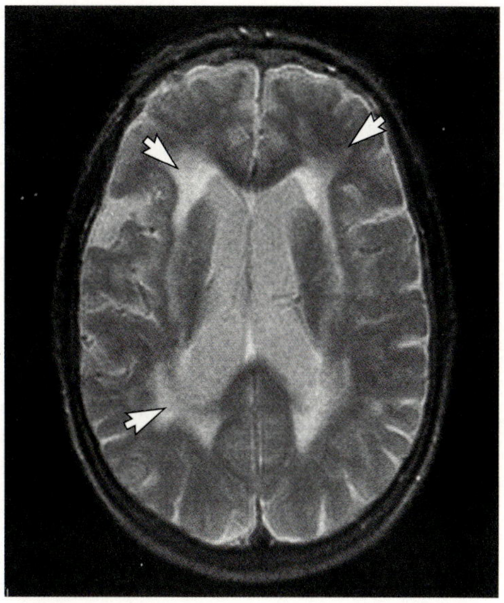

FIGURE 3.5

T2-weighted magnetic resonance image of periventricular white matter lesions (*arrows*) capping the ventricles.

REFERENCES

1. Scheinberg P: Dementia due to vascular disease: a multifactorial disorder. *Stroke* 1988, 19:1291–1299.
2. Gorelick PB, Mangone C: Vascular dementias in the elderly. *Clin Geriatr Med* 1991, 7:599–615.
3. Fisher CM: Dementia in cerebrovascular disease. In *Cerebral Vascular Disease.* Edited by Siekert R, Whisnant J. New York: Grune and Stratton; 1968:232–236.
4. Hachinski VC: The decline and resurgence of vascular dementia. *Can Med Assoc J* 1990, 142:107–111.
5. Gorelick PB, Roman GC: Vascular dementia: in search of answers. *Neuroepidemiology* 1991, 10:225–227.
6. Gorelick PB, Roman GC: Vascular dementia: a time to "seize the moment." *Neuroepidemiology* 1993, 12:139–140.
7. Tatemichi TK: How acute brain failure becomes chronic: a view of the mechanisms of dementia related to stroke. *Neurology* 1990, 40:1652–1659.
8. Brody JA, Cohen DC: Epidemiologic aspects of Alzheimer's disease: facts and fragments. *J Aging Health* 1989, 1:139–149.
9. Mortimer JA: The epidemiology of dementia: international comparisons. In *Epidemiology and Aging: An International Perspective.* Edited by Brody JA, Maddox GL. New York: Springer; 1988:150–164.
10. Marshall J: Vascular and multi-infarct dementia: do they exist? In *Vascular and Multi-Infarct Dementia.* Edited by Meyer JS, Lechner H, Marshall J, *et al.* Mount Kisco, NY: Futura; 1988:1–3.
11. Alzheimer A (translated by Forstl H, Beats B): A contribution concerning the pathologic anatomy of mental disturbance in old age. *Alzheimer Dis Assoc Dis* 1991, 5:69–70.

12. Fisher CM: Senile dementia: a new explanation of its causation. *Can Med Assoc J* 1951, 65:1–7.
13. Hachinski VC, Lassen NA, Marshall J: Multi-infarct dementia: a cause of mental deterioration in the elderly. *Lancet* 1974, 2:207–210.
14. Olszewski J: Subcortical arteriosclerotic encephalopathy: review of the literature on the so-called Binswanger's disease and presentation of two cases. *World Neurol* 1965, 3:359–375.
15. Roth M: The natural history of mental disorder in old age. *J Ment Sc* 1955, 101:281–301.
16. Slater E, Roth M: Mental diseases in the aged. In *Clinical Psychiatry*, 3rd ed. Edited by Mayer-Gross W, Slater E, Roth M. Baltimore: Williams & Wilkins; 1969:593–596.
17. American Psychiatric Association: *Diagnostic and Statistical Manual of Mental Disorders*, 3rd ed. (Revised). Washington, DC: American Psychiatric Association; 1987:100–123.
18. Chui HC, Victoroff JI, Margolin D, *et al.*: Criteria for the diagnosis of ischemic vascular dementia proposed by the State of California Alzheimer's Disease Diagnostic and Treatment Centers. *Neurology* 1992, 42:473–480.
19. Roman GC, Tatemichi TK, Erkinjuntti T, *et al.*: Vascular dementia: diagnostic criteria for research studies: report of the NINDS-AIREN International Work Shop. *Neurology* 1993, 43:250–260.
20. Cummings JL, Benson DF: Mental status examination. In *Dementia: A Clinical Approach*, 2nd ed. Edited by Cummings JL, Benson DF. Boston: Butterworth-Heinemann; 1992:19–44.
21. Liston EH, LaRue A: Clinical differentiation of primary degenerative and multi-infarct dementia: a critical review of the evidence: Part I. Clinical studies. *Biol Psychiatry* 1983, 18:1451–1465.
22. Liston EH, LaRue A: Clinical differentiation of primary degenerative and multi-infarct dementia: a critical review of the evidence: Part II. Pathological studies. *Biol Psychiatry* 1983, 18:1467–1484.
23. Liston EH, LaRue A: DSM-III diagnosis of multi-infarct dementia. *Compr Psychiatry* 1986, 27:54–59.
24. Hachinski VC: Multi-infarct dementia: a reappraisal. *Alzheimer Dis Assoc Dis* 1991, 5:64–68.
25. Udea K, Hasuo Y, Fujishima M: Prevalence and etiology of dementia in a Japanese community. *Stroke* 1992, 23:798–803.
26. Rocca WA, Hofman A, Brayne C, *et al.*: The prevalence of vascular dementia in Europe: facts and fragments from 1980-1990 studies. *Ann Neurol* 1991, 30:817–824.
27. Hagnell O, Lanke J, Rorsman B, *et al.*: Current trends in the incidence of senile and multi-infarct dementia: a prospective study of a total population followed over 25 years: the Lundby Study. *Arch Psychiatr Nervenkcr* 1983, 233:423–438.
28. Rorsman B, Hagnell O, Lanke J: Mortality and age psychosis in the Lundby Study: death risk of senile and multi-infarct dementia: changes over time in a prospective study of a total population followed over 25 or 15 years. *Neuropsychobiology* 1985, 14:13–16.
29. Molsa PK, Martilla RJ, Rinne UK: Epidemiology of dementia in a Finnish population. *Acta Neurol Scand* 1982, 65:541–552.
30. Schoenberg BS, Kokman E, Okazaki H: Alzheimer's disease and other dementing illnesses in a defined United States population: incidence rates and clinical features. *Ann Neurol* 1987, 22:724–729.
31. Kokman E, Chandra VJ, Schoenberg BS: Trends in incidence of dementing illness in Rochester, Minnesota, in three quinquennial periods, 1960-1974. *Neurology* 1988, 38:975–980.
32. Barclay LL, Zemcov A, Blass JP, *et al.*: Survival in Alzheimer's disease and vascular dementia. *Neurology* 1985, 35:834–840.
33. Hier DB, Warach J, Gorelick PB, *et al.*: Predictors of survival in clinically diagnosed Alzheimer's disease and multi-infarct dementia. *Arch Neurol* 1989, 46:1213–1216.
34. Martin DC, Miller JK, Kapoor W, *et al.*: A controlled study of survival with dementia. *Arch Neurol* 1987, 44:1122–1126.
35. Molsa PK, Martilla RJ, Rinne UK: Survival and cause of death in Alzheimer's disease and multi-infarct dementia. *Acta Neurol Scand* 1986, 74:103–107.
36. Evans JG: The epidemiology of the dementias in the elderly. In *Epidemiology and Aging: An International Perspective.* Edited by Brody JA, Maddox GL. New York: Springer; 1988:36–53.
37. Tomlinson BE, Blessed G, Roth M: Observations of the brains of demented old people. *J Neurol Sci* 1970, 11:205–242.
38. Ladurner G, Iliff LD, Lechner H: Clinical factors associated with dementia in ischemic stroke. *J Neurol Neurosurg Psychiatry* 1982, 45:97–101.
39. Loeb C, Gandolfo C, Bino G: Intellectual impairment and cerebral lesions in multiple cerebral infarcts: a clinical-computed tomography study. *Stroke* 1988, 19:560–565.
40. Tatemichi TK, Foulkes MA, Mohr JP, *et al.*: Dementia in stroke survivors in the Stroke Data Bank Cohort: prevalence, incidence, risk factors and computed tomographic findings. *Stroke* 1990, 21:858–866.
41. Meyer JS, McClintic WL, Rogers RL, *et al.*: Aetiologic considerations and risk factors for MID. *J Neurol Neurosurg Psychiatry* 1988, 51:1489–1497.
42. Gorelick PB, Brody JA, Cohen D, *et al.*: Risk factors for dementia associated with multiple cerebral infarcts: a case-control analysis in predominantly African American hospital based patients. *Arch Neurol* 1993, 50:714–720.
43. Gorelick PB, Chatterjee A, Patel D, *et al.*: Cranial computed tomographic observations in multi-infarct dementia: a controlled study. *Stroke* 1992, 23:804–811.
44. Gurland BJ: The borderlands of dementia: the influence of sociocultural characteristics on rates of dementia occurring in the senile. In *Clinical Aspects of Alzheimer's Disease and Senile Dementia.* Edited by Miller NE, Cohen GD. New York: Raven Press; 1981:61–84.
45. Mortimer JA: Do psychosocial risk factors contribute to Alzheimer's disease? In *Etiology of Dementia of Alzheimer's Type.* Edited by Henderson AS, Henderson JH. New York: John Wiley and Sons, Ltd; 1988:39–52.
46. Evans DA, Beckett LA, Albert MS, *et al.*: Level of education and change in cognitive function in a community population of older persons. *Ann Epidemiol* 1993, 3:71–77.
47. Zhang M, Katzman R, Salmon D, *et al.*: The prevalence of dementia and Alzheimer's disease in Shanghai, China: impact of age, gender and education. *Ann Neurol* 1990, 27:428–437.
48. Korczyn AD, Kahana E, Galper Y: Epidemiology of dementia in Ashkelon, Israel. *Neuroepidemiology* 1991, 10:100.
49. Talemichi TK, Desmond DW, Mayeux R, *et al.*: Dementia after stroke: baseline frequency, risks and clinical features in a hospitalized cohort. *Neurology* 1992, 42:1185–1193.
50. Wolf PA: Cigarettes, alcohol and stroke. *N Engl J Med* 1986, 315:1087–1089.
51. Rogers RL, Meyer JS, Judd BW, *et al.*: Abstention from cigarette smoking improves cerebral perfusion among elderly chronic smokers. *JAMA* 1985, 253:2970–2974.
52. Liu CK, Miller BL, Cummings JL, *et al.*: A quantitative MRI study of vascular dementia. *Neurology* 1992, 42:138–143.
53. Chimowitz MI, Awad IA, Furlan AJ: Periventricular lesions on MRI: facts and theories. *Stroke* 1989, 20:963–967.
54. Mirsen TR, Lee DH, Wong CJ, *et al.*: Clinical correlates of white-matter changes on magnetic resonance imaging scans of the brain. *Arch Neurol* 1991, 48:1015–1021.
55. Brun A, Englund E: A white matter disorder in dementia of the Alzheimer type: a pathoanatomical study. *Ann Neurol* 1986, 19:253–262.
56. Cohen MM, de Toledo-Morrell L, Morrell F: Pharmacologic treatment of multi-infarct dementia. Edited by Chopra JS, Jagannathan K, Sawhney IMS, *et al.* New York: Elsevier; 1990:83–90.
57. Skoog I, Nilsson L, Palmertz B, *et al.*: A population-based study of dementia in 85-year-olds. *N Engl J Med* 1993, 328:153–158.

Chapter 4

Pathophysiology and Neuropathology of Ischemic Stroke Subtypes

JULIEN BOGOUSSLAVSKY
ROBERT C. JANZER

Cerebral infarction is not a single disease, and the differentiation of several clinical, pathophysiologic, and etiologic subtypes may be critical for adequate management of patients.

The most common mechanism of ischemic stroke is embolic, either from an atheromatous arterial lesion (artery-to-artery thromboembolism) or from the heart (cardioembolism). Less commonly, in situ occlusion of an extracranial or a cerebral artery may be incriminated in the absence of embolism: first, when the occluded artery is a small perforating branch without collateral supply (*ie*, lacunar infarct) [1]; and second, when large-artery occlusion may produce hemodynamic failure in the corresponding territory because of lack of functioning anastomoses (hemodynamic infarction). Finally, abnormalities of the blood itself may also lead to ischemic stroke (coagulation disorders, hyperviscosity, anemia, leukemias and related disorders). Figure 4.1 shows the relative frequency of ischemic stroke pathophysiologic subtypes from a population-based stroke center [2].

In whites, artery-to-artery embolism (Figure 4.2) is linked mainly to the development of extracranial atherosclerosis, while intracranial atherosclerosis plays a major role in Asians, and to a lesser extent in blacks. However, this distinction is valid mainly for the anterior circulation, while recent studies have shown that intracranial vertebral artery or basilar artery atherosclerosis is also an important cause of posterior circulation infarcts in whites [3]. The main sites of atherosclerosis development are depicted in Figure 4.3.

For practicing physicians, one of the most useful ways to address the various forms of ischemic stroke is through their topographic subtypes because there is a link between topography, etiology, and pathophysiology of cerebral infarcts.

MIDDLE CEREBRAL ARTERY SUPERFICIAL TERRITORY INFARCTS

Superficial branches of the middle cerebral artery (MCA) originate distal to the origin of the lenticulostriate arteries. As they course in the subarachnoid space, they are called *pial* branches. They supply the cortical-subcortical territory of the MCA after the MCA trunk divides into two (upper and lower) or three

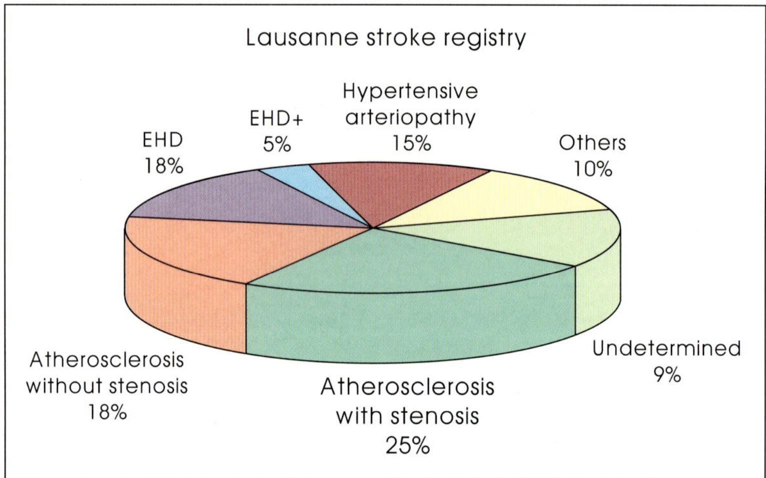

FIGURE 4.1

Frequency of etiology of cerebral infarcts (Lausanne Stroke Registry).

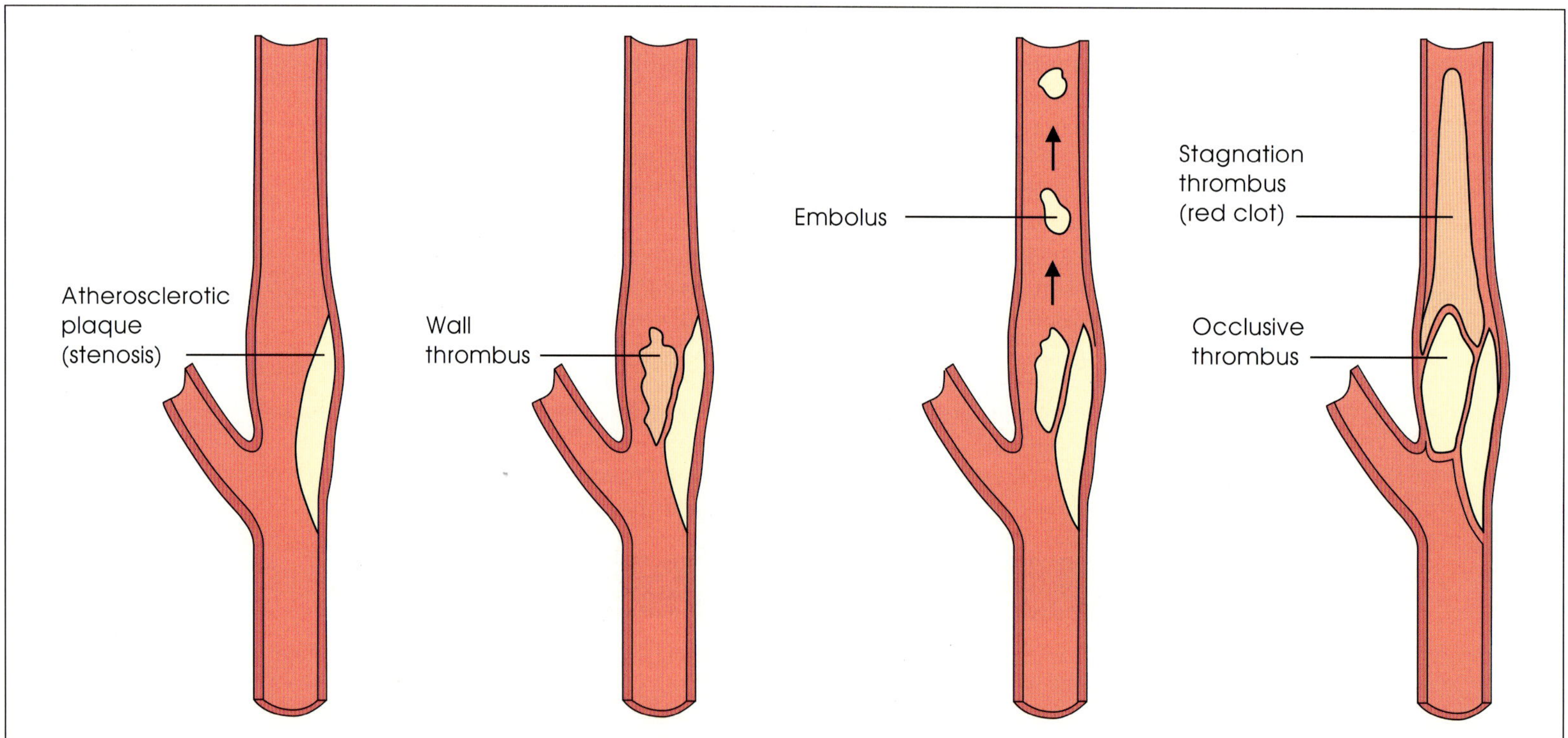

FIGURE 4.2

Mechanism of artery-to-artery thromboembolism.

(upper, middle, and lower) divisions which, in their turn, divide into several branches (Figure 4.4). MCA pial territory infarcts (Figure 4.5) may be partial when only a distal branch is occluded, or they may be rather large when the occlusion is more proximal at the level of the MCA bifurcation or trifurcation and the collateral system is not adequate. Because one characteristic of the pial artery network is to have extensive anastomoses, multiple distal emboli are usually necessary to lead to infarction. Actually, at least half of the patients with MCA pial territory infarct may show angiographic evidence for distal occlusion, suggesting embolism [2], and most of the angiographically normal cases may be due to delayed performance of angiography because these occlusions tend to disappear early. The presumed cause of embolism is large-artery disease (≥ 50% internal carotid artery [ICA] or MCA stenosis or occlusion in one third of the patients and cardiac disease in one quarter of the

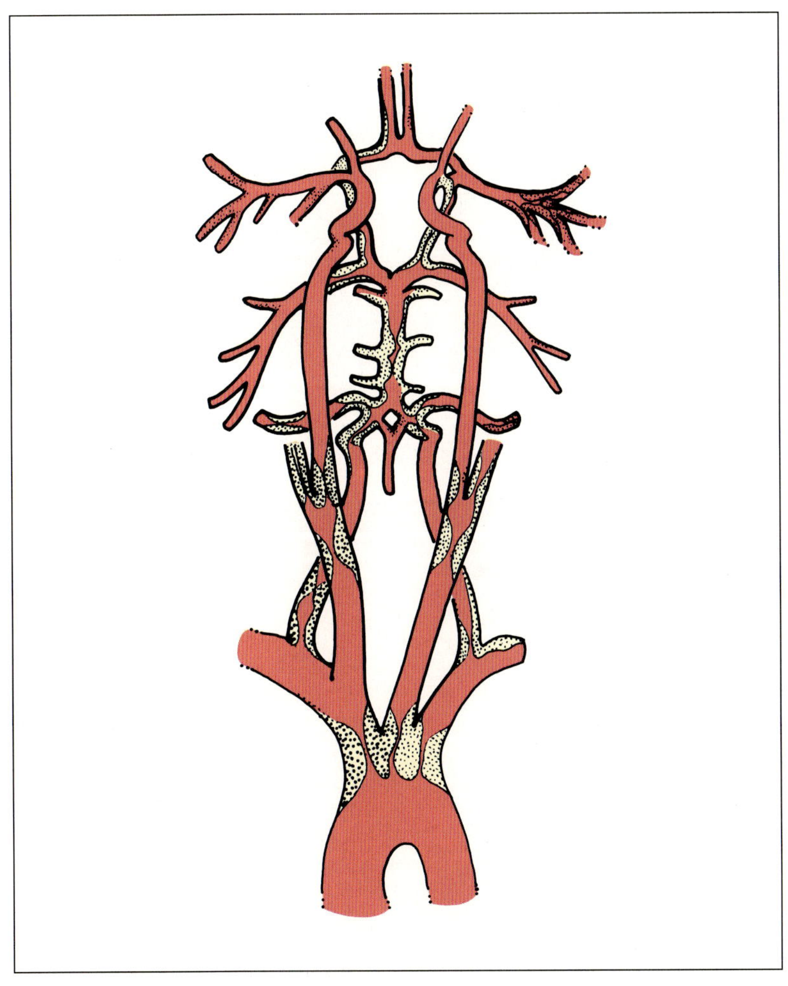

FIGURE 4.3

Sites of developing atheromatosis.

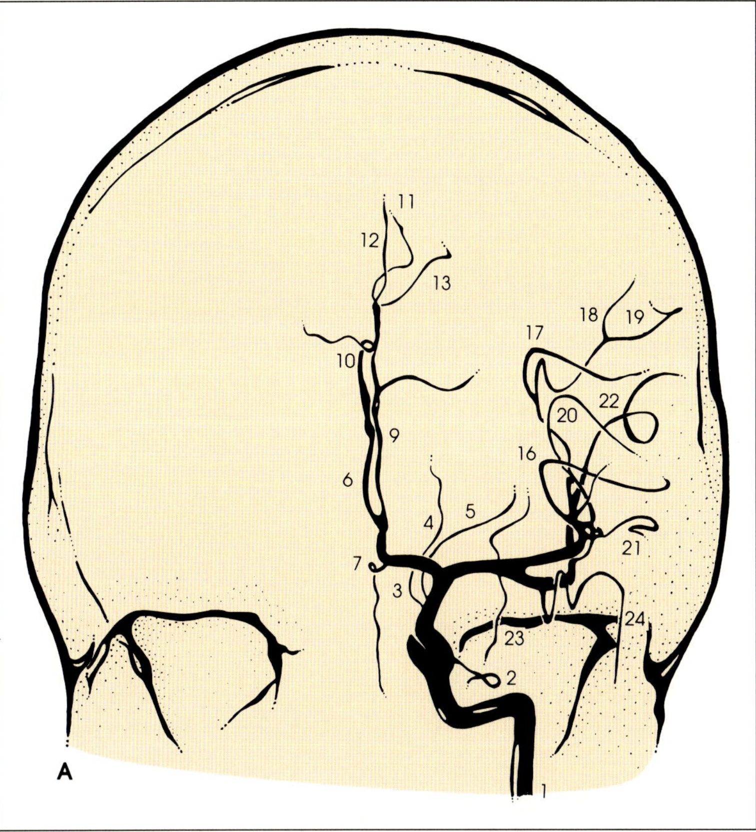

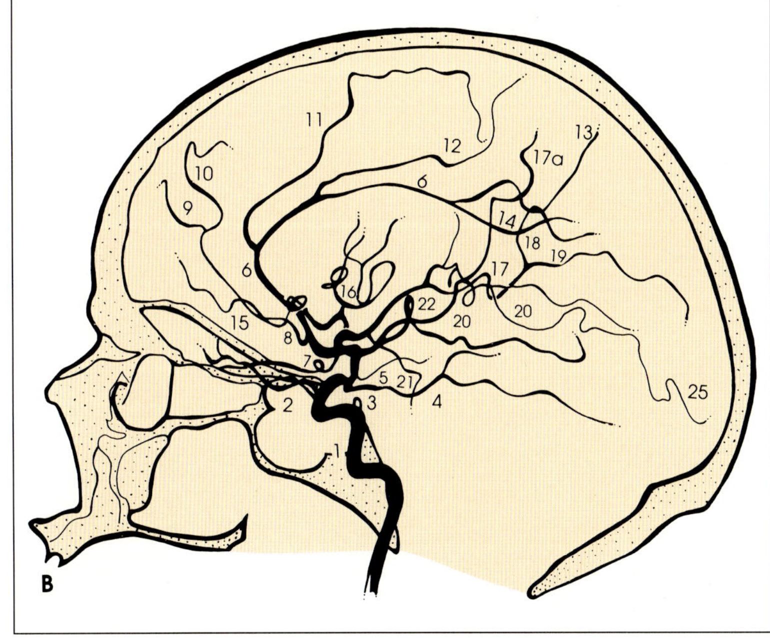

FIGURE 4.4

Cerebral arteries (carotid system): frontal (**A**) and lateral (**B**) views. (*Adapted from* Bogousslavsky and Hommel [35]; with permission.)

patients) [4]. Interestingly, potential cardiac sources of embolism are particularly common with infarcts in the territory of the lower division of the MCA, which are also associated with more disability than infarcts in the territory of the upper division [4].

Because most of the frontal, temporal, and parietal lobes are supplied by the MCA pial branches (Figure 4.5), the neurologic picture may be variable according to the location of the infarct (Figure 4.6) (Tables 4.1, 4.2, and 4.3). It can even be misleading when isolated motor hemiparesis or sensory stroke may wrongly suggest a deeper lesion, or when aphasia is associated with unexpected sparing of speech areas.

INFARCTS IN THE TERRITORY OF THE DEEP PERFORATORS FROM THE CAROTID SYSTEM

In contrast to the pial arterial network, the deep perforators from the distal ICA or the MCA trunk are terminal branches that perforate the basal part of the cerebral hemispheres (Figures 4.4 and 4.7). For that reason, occlusion of one or several perforators is always associated with an infarct—usually small—in the corresponding territory. These small deep infarcts are often called "lacunar," but it should be remembered that lacunes may be caused by nonischemic processes, such as small hemorrhage

FIGURE 4.5

A–**F**, Anatomic structures in the cerebral hemispheres relevant to stroke syndromes and superficial (pial) arterial territories.

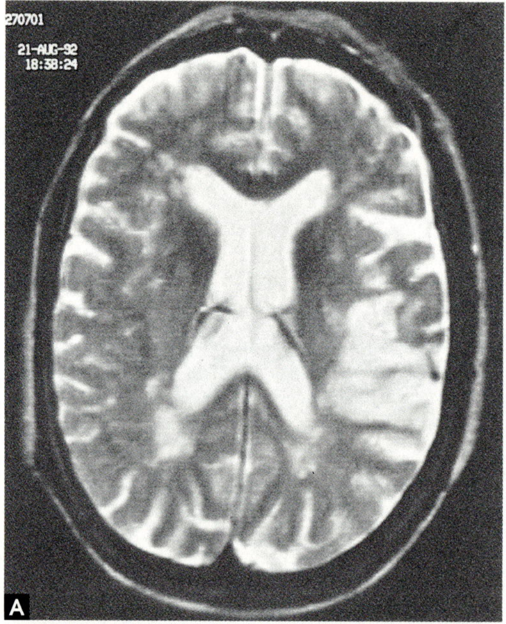

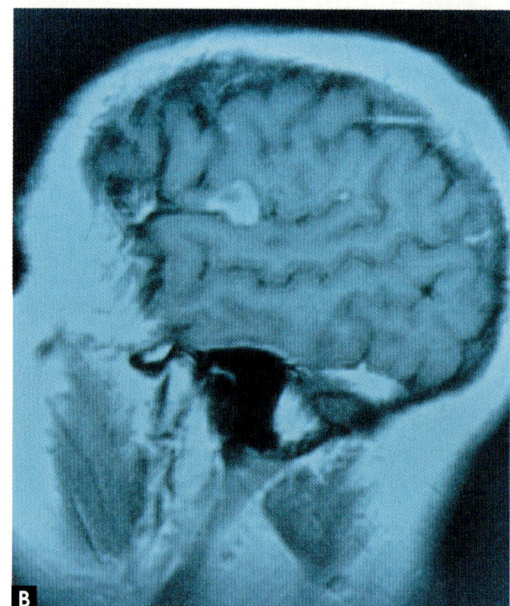

FIGURE 4.6

Types of superficial middle cerebral artery infarcts on magnetic resonance imaging. **A**, Left anterior parietal artery territory infarct with conduction aphasia and right hemisensory loss. **B**, Frontal-opercular infarct with isolated contralateral lower facial palsy (**C**). (*continued*)

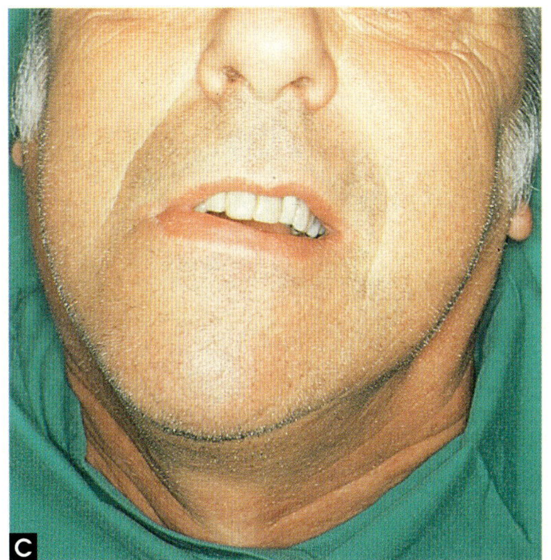

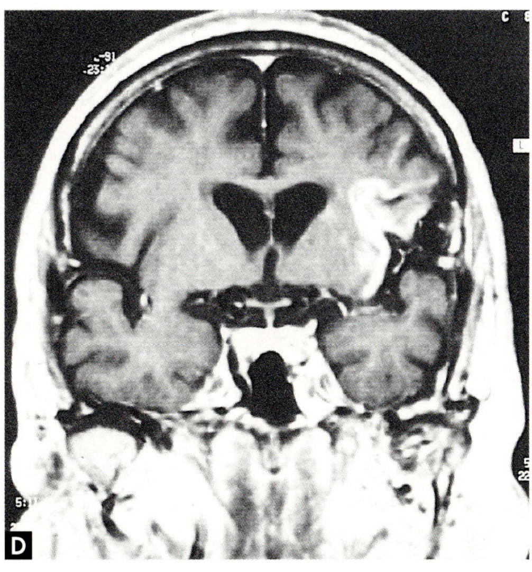

FIGURE 4.6

(*continued*) **D**, Left frontal-insular infarct with Broca's aphasia and slight right hemiparesis.

Table 4.1. Middle cerebral artery pial branches syndromes

Prefrontal artery	Precentral artery	Central sulcus artery	Anterior parietal artery	Upper posterior parietal/ angular gyrus artery	Lower posterior parietal/ temporal arteries
Frontal syndrome	Hemiparesis with proximal predominance (abduction-elevation) Premotor syndrome of Luria	Faciobrachial hemiparesis predominating distally, distal monoparesis of upper limb Cheiro-oral sensory loss	Pseudothalmic hemisensory loss (Foix-Chavany-Lévy syndrome)	Lateral hemianopia or lower-quadrant anopia Cortical sensation dysfunction	Lateral hemianopia or upper-quadrant anopia
Left: transcortical motor aphasia	Left: minor variant of Broca's aphasia, agraphia	Left: cortical dysarthria (phonetic disintegration syndrome of Ombredane et Durand)	Left: conduction aphasia, Ideomotor apraxia, phonologic agraphia/alexia	Left: Wernicke's aphasia variants (*eg,* anomic aphasia, transcortical sensory aphasia), lexical alexia with agraphia, apraxia, Gertsmann's syndrome, auto-topagnosia, (optic ataxia), leftward eye-tracking impairment	Left: Wernicke's aphasia asymbolia for pain
Right: motor hemineglect			Right: postrolandic motor hemineglect	Right: hemineglect and other visuospatial disturbances, asomatognosia, constructive apraxia, unilateral left apraxia, optic ataxia, bilateral eye-tracking impairment	Right: Acute confusional state, spatial hemineglect, spatial delirium
		Bilateral: faciolinguopharyngeo masticatory diplegia (Foix-Chavany-Marie syndrome)		Bilateral: Balint's syndrome (visual disorientation, simultanagnosia, optic ataxia, visual fixation impairment), altitudinal neglect	Bilateral: pure word deafness, cortical deafness, rejection behavior (Denny Brown-Chamber's syndrome)

or nonischemic dilatation of periarteriolar space (Figure 4.8) [5]. It is widely accepted that lacunar infarcts are usually due to in situ occlusion of the corresponding small perforator by a microatheromatous or lipohyalinotic process associated with chronic arterial hypertension. This assumption appears correct for very small lacunar infarcts (< 0.3–0.5 cm) associated with occlusion of *one* single perforator, but these infarcts are usually *asymptomatic* [1]. Although small-artery disease probably remains a leading etiology, in larger (0.5–1.5 cm or larger)—and *symptomatic*—small deep infarcts, other potential causes may also be considered, since more than one third of these patients may have a potential cardiac source of embolism or large-artery

Table 4.2. Critical areas involved in ischemic aphasia

Area	Result
Broca's area (foot of F_3)	Transient decrease of speech output
Supplementary motor area or underlying white matter pathways toward perisylvian speech zones	Transcortical motor aphasia
Lower motor cortex	Cortical dysarthria (phonetic disintegration syndrome of Ombredane and Durand)
Opercular-insular region with subcortical involvement including the medial-subcallosal fasciculus	Classic Broca's aphasia
Posterior part of T_1	Wernicke's aphasia
Supramarginal gyrus and/or underlying white matter	Conduction aphasia, phonological agraphia/alexia
Angular gyrus	Isolated anomia, lexical agraphia/alexia
Parieto-occipital junction (posterior-temporal isthmus region)	Transcortical sensory aphasia
Posterior-parahippocampal gyrus and collateral isthmus	Isolated impaired verbal learning

Table 4.3. Clinical features of infarction in the right hemisphere

Frontal infarction
- Impersistence
- Persistence
- Hemineglect (motor)
- Reduplicate phenomena

Parietal infarction
- Constructive apraxia
- Dressing apraxia
- Unilateral left apraxia
- Hemineglect (spatial)
- Anosognosia
- Visuospatial disturbances
- Topographic disorientation
- Optic ataxia
- Impairment of bilateral horizontal, smooth eye tracking

Temporal infarction
- Nonverbal memory dysfunction
- Amusia without aphasia
- Acute confusional state or agitated delirium and other psychiatric variants

Occipital infarction
- Palinopia
- Prosopagnosia

Large infarction
- Response-to-next-patient stimulation

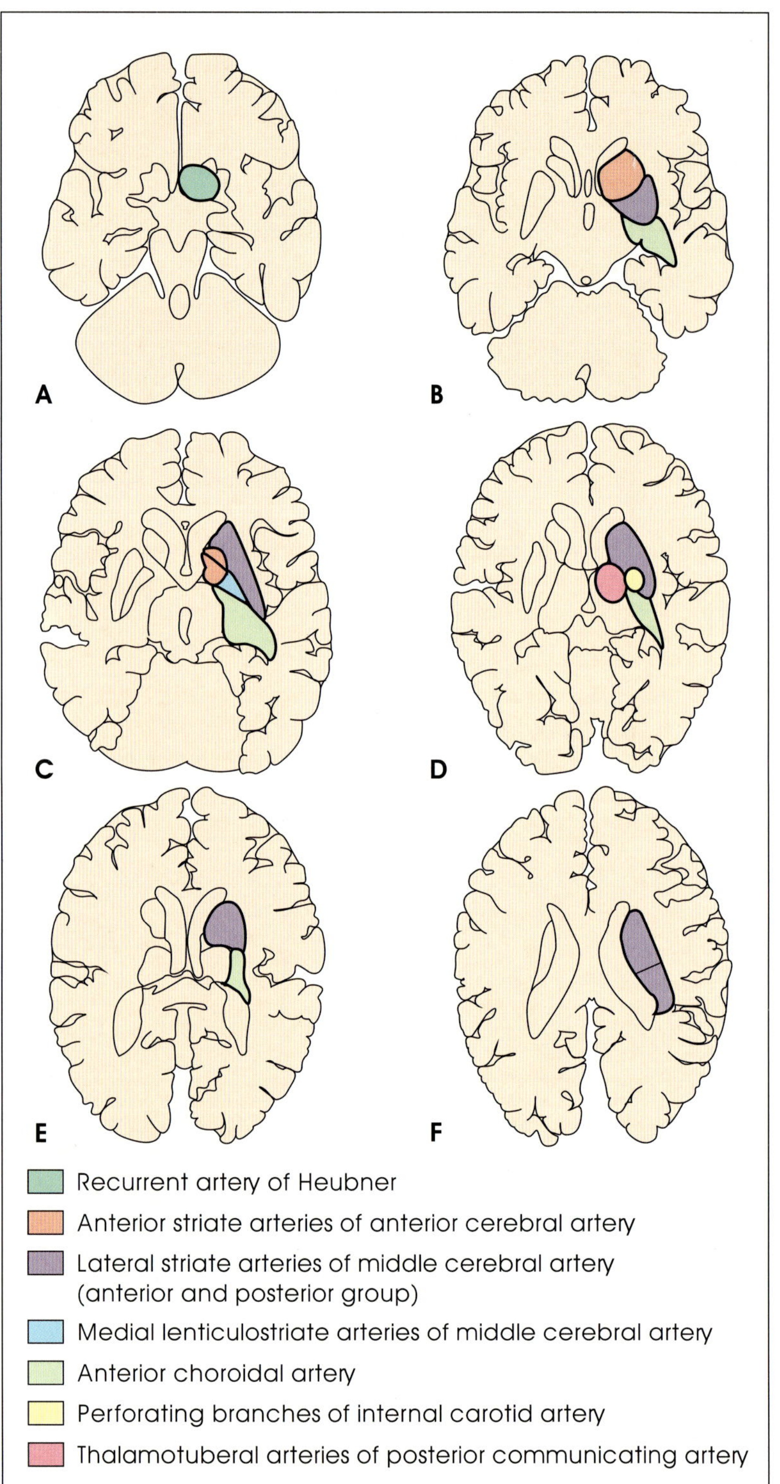

FIGURE 4.7

A–F, Template of the subcortical arterial territories (carotid system). (*Adapted from* Bogousslavsky and Hommel [37]; with permission.)

disease (≥ 50% ICA stenosis or occlusion), often in the absence of concomitant hypertension [5]. Embolism to the MCA trunk is a particularly common cause of complete lenticulostriate territory infarction (known as large striatocapsular infarcts or extended infarcts of the lentiform nucleus), by occluding the lenticulostriate arteries at their origin while collateral circulation explains sparing of the superficial pial territory (Figure 4.9) [6].

While it is unclear if large-artery or cardiac disease is just coincidental in many patients with small deep infarct, it is likely that atherosclerosis of the MCA trunk (or of the basilar artery for small paramedian infarcts in the brain stem), which can occlude the origin of deep perforators, has largely been overlooked as a potential etiology of small deep infarcts [7,8]. Moreover, hypertension does not seem to be the only factor associated with small-artery disease leading to lacunar infarction; diabetes mellitus should also be considered [5].

Clinical manifestations are largely dependent on the size of infarct. The larger infarcts may produce combined motor, sensory, and neuropsychologic dysfunction not markedly different from superficial MCA territory infarcts (Figure 4.10). Smaller infarcts have often been linked to isolated contralateral motor or sensory disturbances ("lacunar syndromes"). However, the four main classic lacunar syndromes (pure motor hemiparesis, pure sensory stroke, ataxic hemiparesis, and sensorimotor stroke) should be considered suggestive of lacunar infarction, which is defined as a small deep infarct from hypertensive small-vessel disease only when face-arm-leg involvement is present [9]. In our opinion, the use of terms such as lacune, lacunar infarct, or lacunar syndrome should always be accompanied with a precise definition of the terms.

The artery of Heubner from the anterior cerebral artery (ACA) and the anterior choroidal artery from the carotid siphon are not only perforators because they also supply cortical territories (Table 4.4) (Figures 4.4, 4.7, 4.11). Thus, their system of supply can be compared with that of the MCA, and their etiologic spectrum of infarction is similar [10,11].

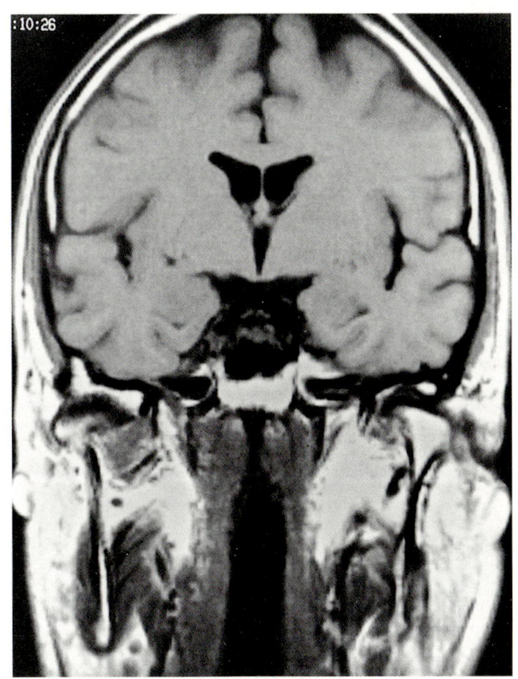

FIGURE 4.8

Cribled state magnetic resonance imaging in an asymptomatic patient.

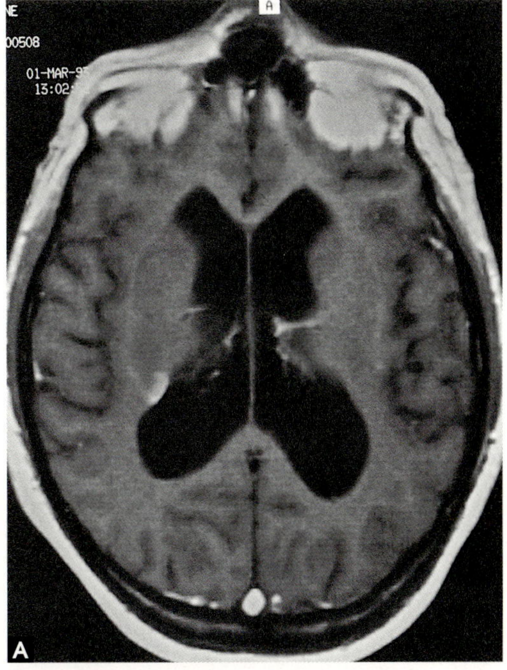

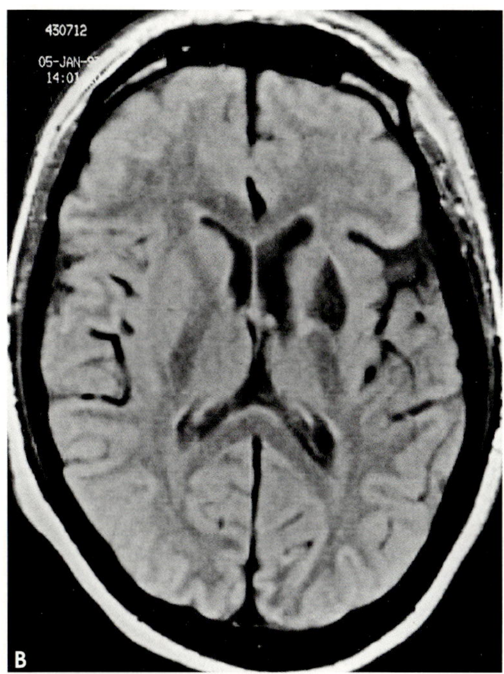

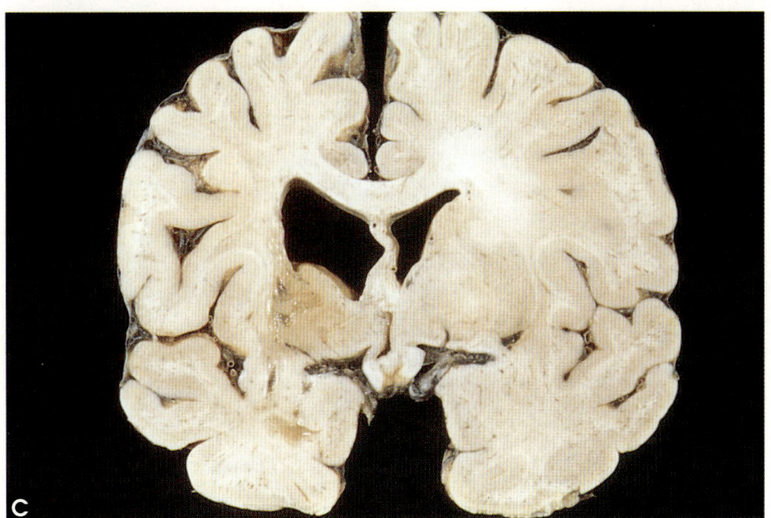

FIGURE 4.9

Lenticulostriate infarcts. **A**, Small lacunar. **B**, Large striatocapsular infarcts. **C**, Lacunar infarcts in striatum (pathology).

ANTERIOR CEREBRAL ARTERY TERRITORY INFARCTS

Although the ACA (Figures 4.4, 4.5) originates from the carotid siphon at the same level as the MCA, ACA territory infarcts are between 20 and 30 times less common than MCA territory infarcts. However, etiologic patterns do not differ between MCA and ACA territory infarcts [11].

Infarcts in the territory of Heubner's artery or in the territory of the anterior striate branches are usually discussed together with lenticulostriate infarcts in general [5]; their neurologic picture is not specific. In ACA pial territory infarcts, the association of crural hemiparesis, mutism at onset, transcortical motor aphasia, frontal tasks impairment, mood disturbance, incontinence, grasp reflex, and unilateral left apraxia may help to localize the infarct before computed tomography (CT) or magnetic resonance (MR) imaging, but proportional (arm-leg-arm) hemiparesis or hemisensory defect, hemineglect, or confusional state may be misleading (Table 4.5). Simultaneous bilateral ACA territory infarction (Figure 4.12) may occur in relation to a common origin of both ACAs. Akinetic mutism with incontinence and bilateral grasp reflex is suggestive of this type of infarct, which is uncommon (< 10%).

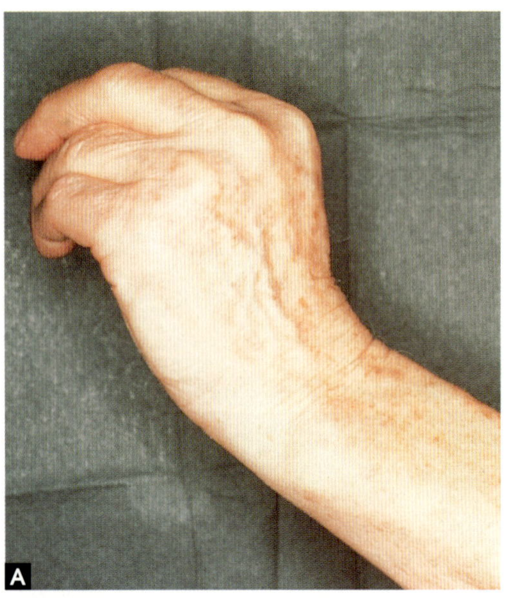

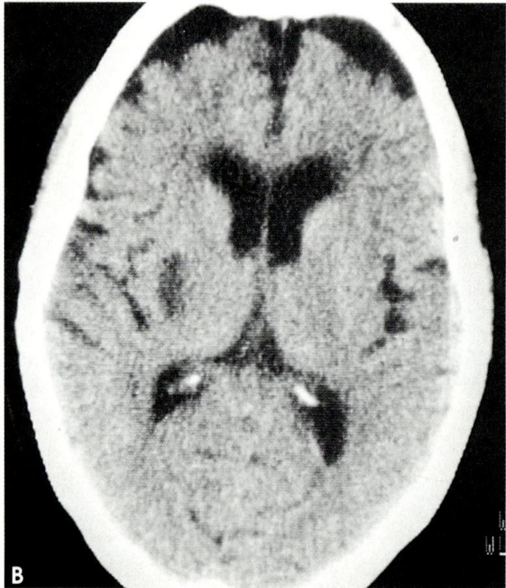

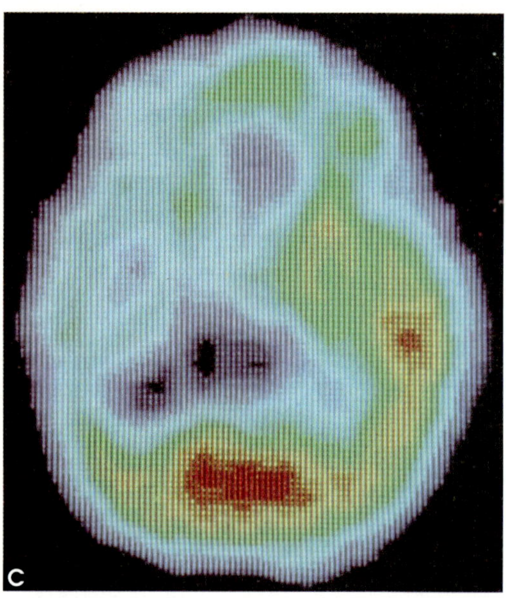

FIGURE 4.10

Examples of subcortical infarct. **A**, Atypical distal upper limb palsy with deep infarct. **B** and **C**, Single photon emission tomography shows extensive subcortical and cortical hypoperfusion in a patient with small left anterior choroidal artery infarct, moderate hemiparesis, and aphasia.

Table 4.4. Neurologic syndromes of anterior choroidal artery territory infarcts

- Hemiplegia, hemianesthesia, hemianopia and variants
- Pure motor hemiparesis
- Pure sensory stroke
- Ataxic hemiparesis
- Hypesthetic ataxic hemiparesis
- Hemiataxia and ipsilateral hemisensory defect
- Quadruple homonymous sectoranopia
- Neuropsychologic disturbances that may be associated:
  - Left: dysphasia, apraxia (constructive), dysmnesia
  - Right: hemineglect
  - Bilateral: acute pseudobulbar mutism

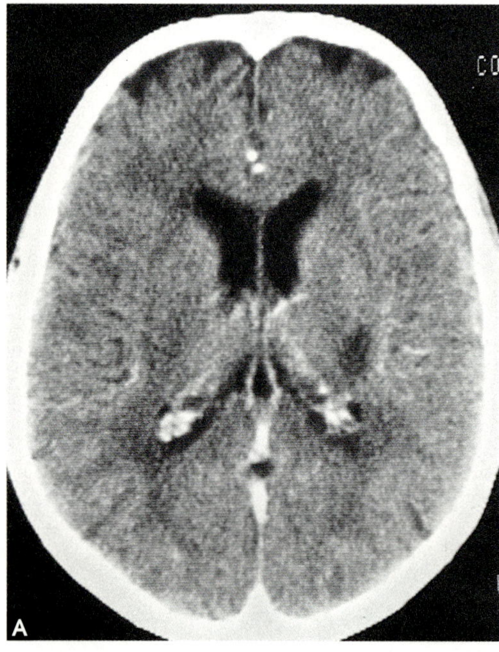

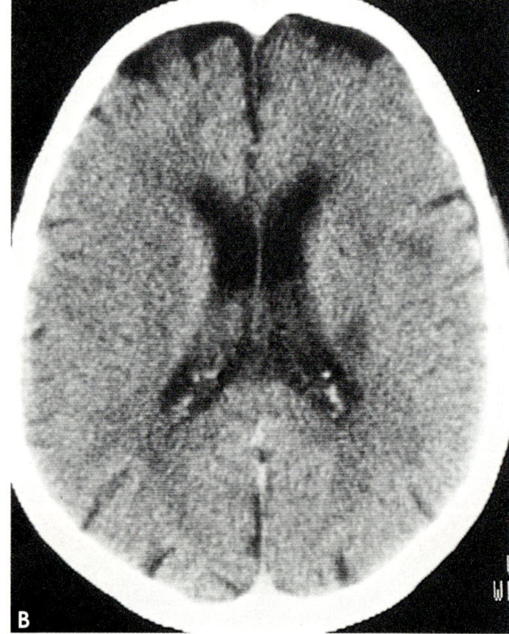

FIGURE 4.11

Anterior choroidal artery territory infarct. **A**, First level. **B**, Second level.

BORDER ZONE CEREBRAL INFARCTS

Infarction may develop at the level of the collateral border zone between two main pial arterial territories. These extraterritorial infarcts are commonly called *watershed* or *distal field* infarcts. They usually occur between the ACA and MCA territories (anterior watershed infarcts), or between the MCA and posterior cerebral artery (PCA) territories (posterior watershed infarcts) (Figure 4.13). In the former, hemiparesis, predominating in the lower limb, with transcortical motor aphasia when lesion is on the left, is the most common neurologic finding when the infarct predominates in the subcortical white matter, mimicking ACA territory infarction [12]. However, when the infarct is limited to the cortex, proximal brachial hemiparesis is present because the

Table 4.5. Neurologic features of anterior cerebral artery territory infarct

Hemiparesis	Right infarct
Crural predominance	Initial mutism
Brachiofacial (with deep extension of infarct)	Left motor/spatial neglect
Hemihypesthesia	Abulia, apathy (euphoria, disinhibition)
Same distribution as hemiparesis	Acute confusional state (frontal syndrome)
Contralateral grasp reflex	Ipsilateral grasp reaction
Urinary (fecal) incontinence	Bilateral infarct
Left infarct	Bilateral hemiparesis including pseudoparaplegia, akinetic mutism, severe mood disturbances, long-lasting incontinence
Initial mutism	
Transcortical motor aphasia or minor variants (right motor neglect)	
Unilateral left apraxia	
Abulia, apathy (euphoria, disinhibition), frontal syndrome (impaired conflictual tasks)	

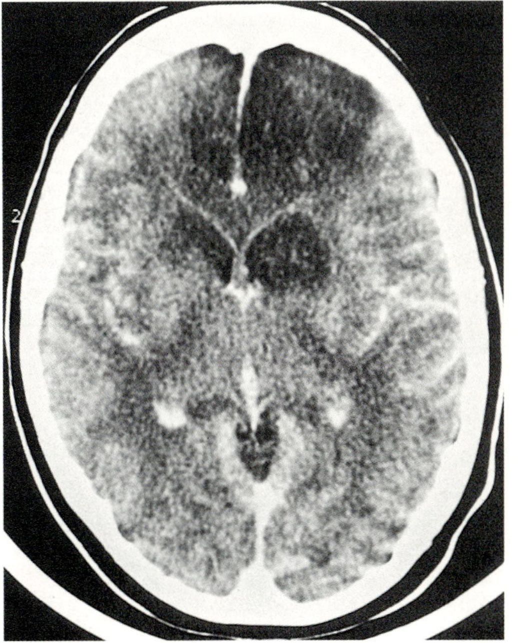

FIGURE 4.12

Computed tomography of bilateral anterior cerebral artery territory infarct.

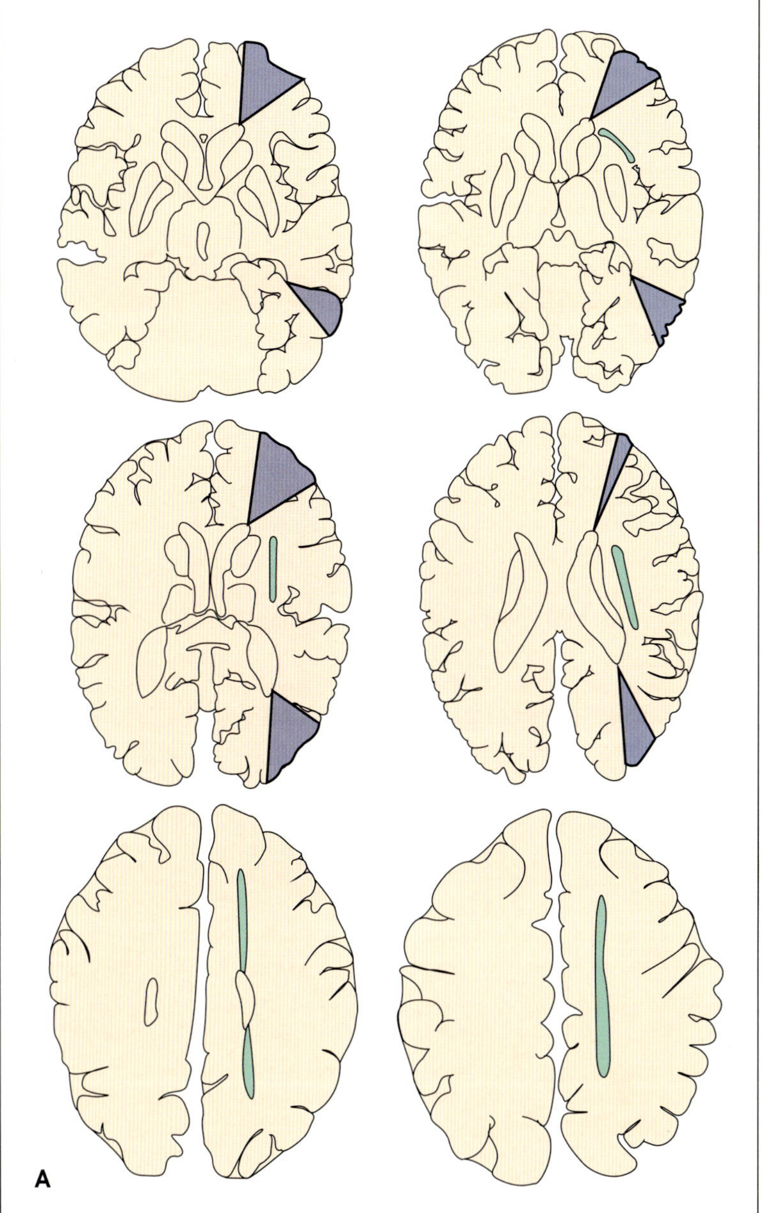

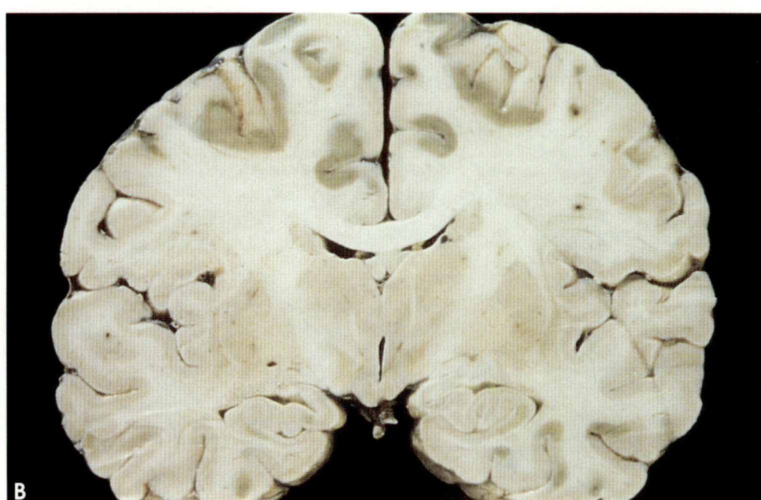

FIGURE 4.13

Border zone ischemia. **A**, Border-zone areas in the cerebral hemispheres. **B**, Combined anterior-posterior watershed infarcts (pathology).

junction of the ACA and MCA territories is at the level of the arm-shoulder representation on the motor strip; thus, in bilateral anterior watershed cortical infarcts, a picture of bibrachial paralysis ("man-in-the-barrel") may occur. Posterior watershed infarcts yield a neurologic picture that is similar to that of posterior MCA pial territory infarcts, except for a more common occurrence of transcortical sensory aphasia (Table 4.6) [12].

Bilateral watershed infarcts often have a symmetrical pattern. They usually develop in relation to episodes of severe hypotension, cardiocirculatory distress, prolonged hypoxemia, or bilateral severe carotid disease [13]. Unilateral watershed infarcts are also associated with some degree of hemodynamic failure (hypotension, bradycardia, high hematocrit level) in patients with ipsilateral carotid occlusion or tight stenosis [11]. They are good examples of hemodynamic infarcts, though microemboli may also account for some border zone infarcts.

An infarction between the deep and superficial (pial) territories of the MCA is uncommon. It is sometimes called a subcortical watershed or internal watershed infarct [14,15]. However, the term watershed may be inappropriate because it implies a border zone between two pial territories at the level of their collateral network. In fact, no such collaterals exist between the deep perforators (which are end arteries) and the pial branches of the MCA system. For this reason, the term *subcortical junctional* or *border zone infarct* seems more appropriate [16]. Hemiparesis with or without hemisensory dysfunction is the most common neurologic disturbance. As for watershed infarcts, hemodynamic failure associated with severe disease of the ipsilateral ICA is the usual etiology.

Table 4.6. Superficial watershed infarcts

Anterior watershed infarcts ACA and MCA
Hemiparesis with crural predominance (when infarct extends subcortically), hemiparesis with proximal brachial predominance (when infarct is mainly cortical, bilateral form of brachial diplegia or man-in-the-barrel syndrome), hemihypesthesia of same distribution
Left: transcortical motor aphasia (often after initial mutism)
Right: Motor hemineglect, apathy, euphoria, (anosognosia)
Posterior watershed infarcts MCA and PCA
Cortical hemihypesthesia with faciobrachial predominance
Lateral hemianopia or upper-quadrant anopia
Left: transcortical sensory aphasia or isolated anomia
Right: spatial hemineglect anosognosia

ACA—anterior cerebral artery; MCA—middle cerebral artery; PCA—posterior cerebral artery.

CENTRUM OVALE INFARCTS

The centrum ovale, which contains the core of the hemispheric white matter, receives its blood supply from the superficial MCA system through perforating medullary branches, which course from the convexity toward the lateral ventricles (Figure 4.14). There are two groups of infarcts: 1) large infarcts, which are associated with severe carotid disease and with neurologic-neuropsychologic dysfunction not different from superficial MCA infarcts; and 2) small infarcts, which are associated with hypertension or diabetes and with partial motor or sensory disturbances (such as monoparesis), usually of progressive onset [17].

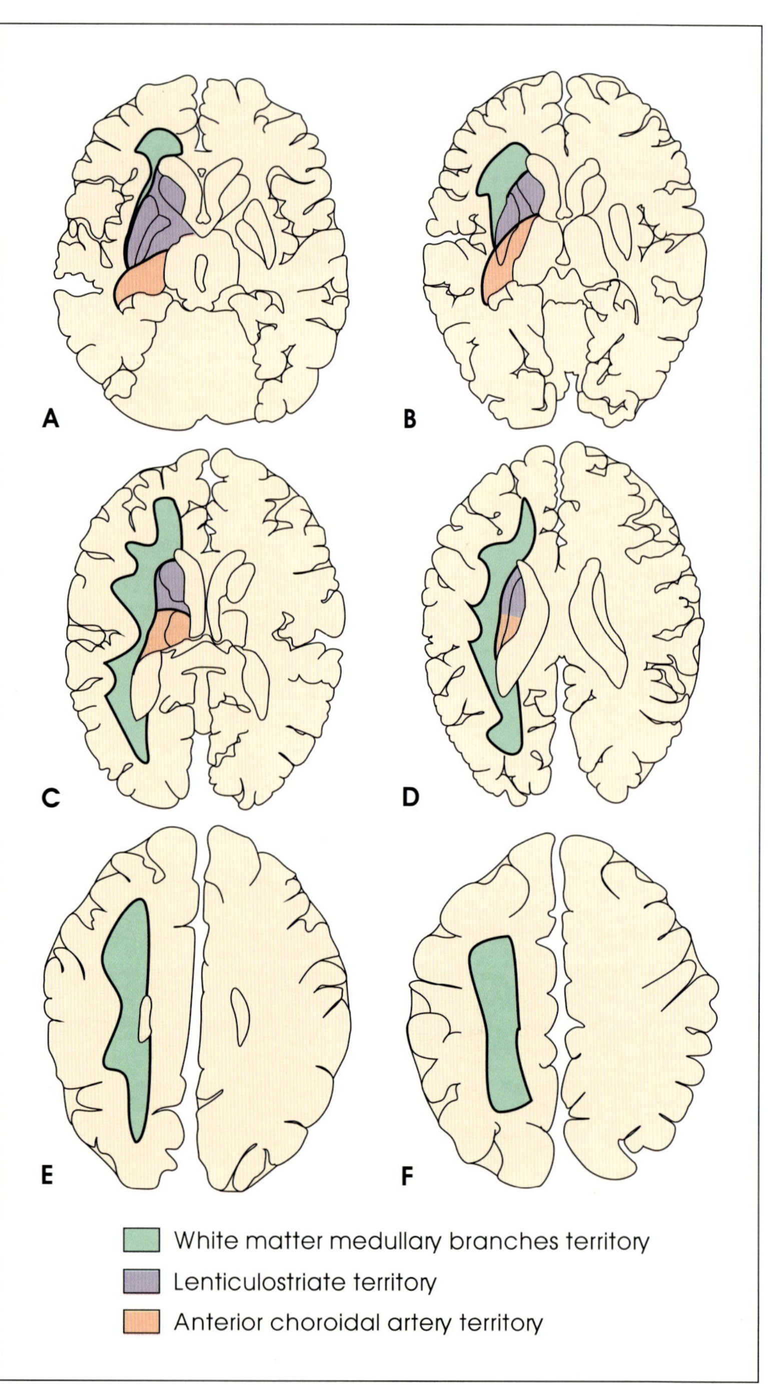

FIGURE 4.14

A–F, White matter medullary branch territory.

These infarcts are usually overlooked in the classifications of subcortical infarcts. Thus, as depicted in Table 4.7, we propose to classify subcortical infarcts in the carotid system into four main territory groups [16,18].

LARGE SUPRATENTORIAL INFARCTS

Entire MCA, and MCA and ACA Territory Infarcts

These often lethal infarcts are commonly associated with acute carotid occlusion and subsequent embolic occlusion of the ACA and MCA trunks at their origin from the carotid siphon (Figure 4.15). This type of acute carotid occlusion may be cardioembolic or due to an intraluminal clot or dissection, while atheromatous stenosis is uncommon. Infarction of the whole hemisphere may develop in patients who have a fetal origin of the PCA from the carotid siphon. It should be remembered that large infarcts—often hemorrhagic—combining involvement of the ACA and MCA territories can be of venous origin (superior sagittal sinus with cortical venous thrombosis).

Large Subcortical Infarction

Subcortical infarcts encompassing the territory of the deep perforators but also the subcortical part of the MCA pial territory are usually associated with ICA occlusion. Sparing of the cortex may be seen on CT scan, probably in relation to a preserved collateral network in the pial arterioles.

POSTERIOR CEREBRAL ARTERY SUPERFICIAL TERRITORY INFARCTS

The superficial (pial) branches of the PCA include the hippocampal, medial temporo-occipital, splenial, internal occipital (or parieto-occipital), and calcarine arteries (Figure 4.16). The posterior choroidal branches have an internal temporal pial network, but they are usually considered with the deep branches to the thalamus. Infarcts limited to the territory of just one branch of the PCA are the most common type of PCA pial territory infarction (uniterritorial), often involving the calcarine artery territory. Isolated mediotemporal involvement is rare. The most common biterritorial infarct combines calcarine and internal occipital arteries territory involvement [19]. Subtotal or total PCA pial territory infarction is not rare with occlusion of the P_2 segment of the PCA trunk just after the origin of the thalamogeniculate and posterior choroidal branches.

The neurologic manifestations are dominated by visual symptoms, which may be simple (hemianopia) or complex (alexia, achromatopsia, agnosia, visual memory impairment) (Table 4.8)

Table 4.7. Four territory groups of subcortical infarcts in the carotid system

Deep perforator territory
From the middle cerebral artery (MCA) trunk
Anterior choroidal artery
Heubner's artery
Posterior communicating artery
Perforating medullary branches territory
From the superficial MCA branches
Border zone
Between the territory of deep perforators and the superficial territory
Combined territories

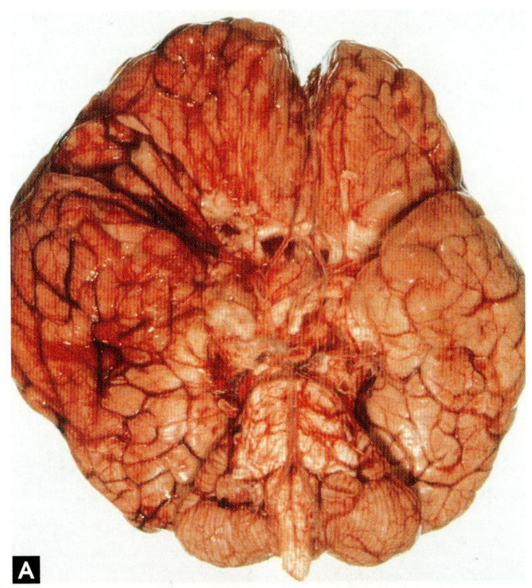

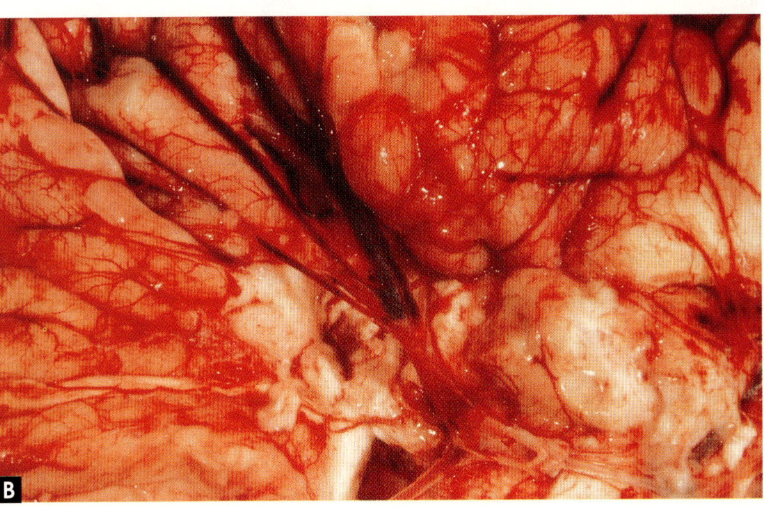

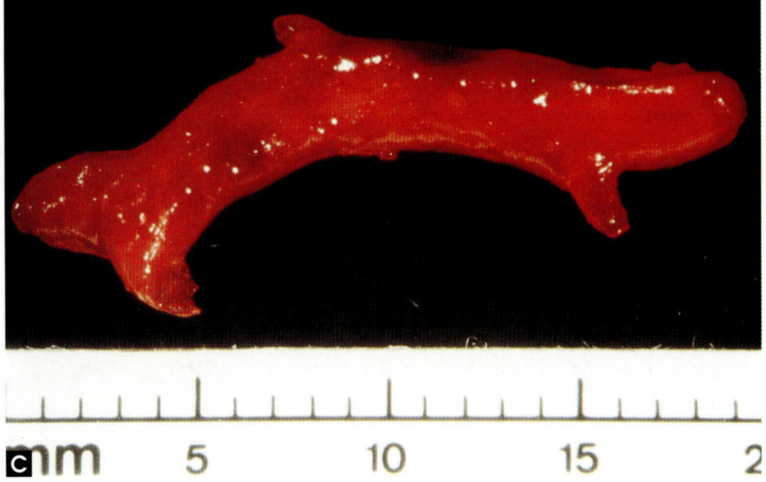

FIGURE 4.15

Embolic occlusion of anterior cerebral artery (ACA) and middle cerebral artery (MCA) trunks (neuropathology). **A**, Acute infarction with swelling and congestion of the entire territory of ACA and MCA. **B**, Detail of *A*. **C**, Embolus of cardiac origin, prepared from specimen shown in *A* and *B*.

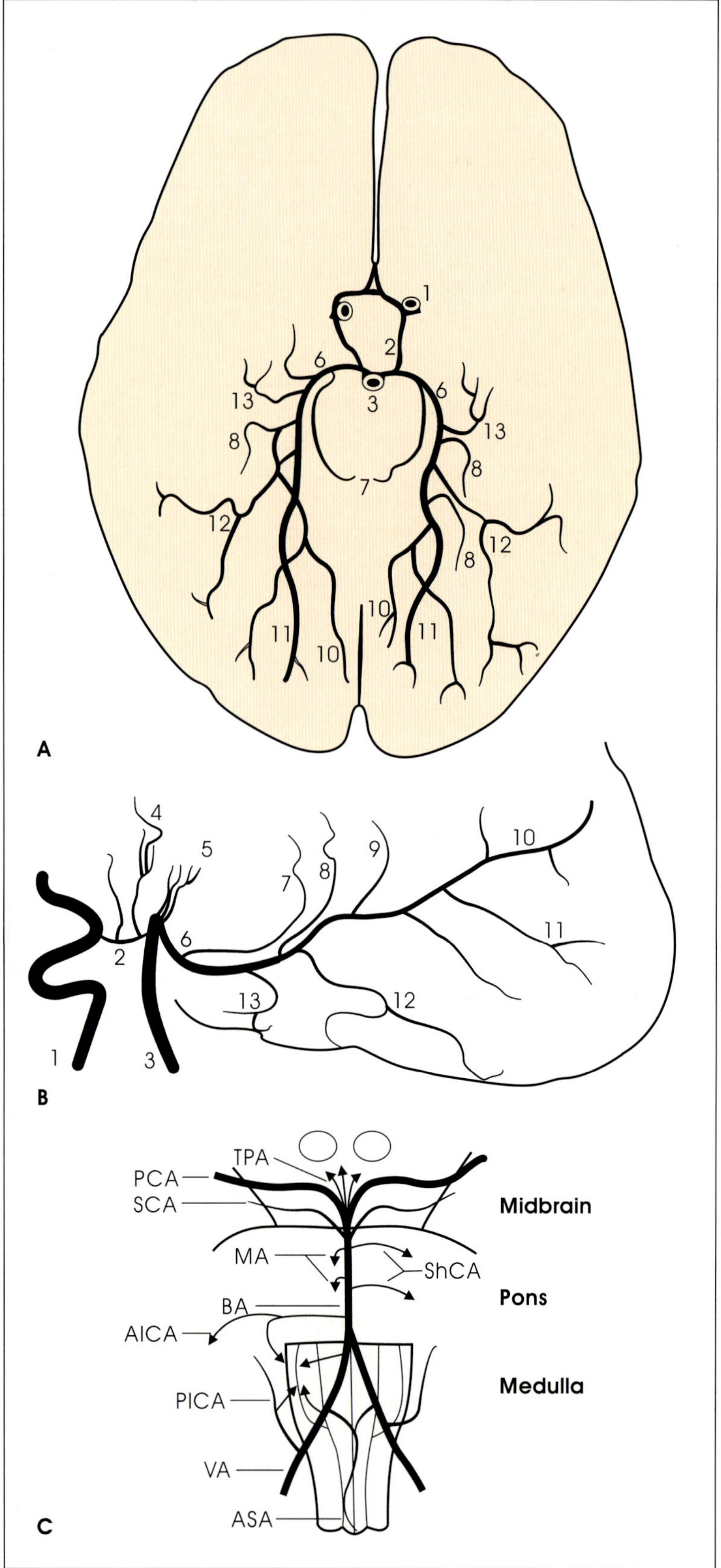

FIGURE 4.16

Cerebral arteries (vertebrobasilar system): lateral (**A**), transverse (**B**) views, and basal arteries (**C**). (*Adapted from* Bogousslavsky and Hommel [35]; with permission.)

Table 4.8. Neurologic features of posterior cerebral artery territory infarct

Structure involved	Neurologic dysfunction
Midbrain (crus cerebri)	Hemiplegia
Thalamus	*See* Table 4-11
Paramedian territory	
Inferolateral territory	
Posterior choroidal territory	
Medial temporal lobe	Memory disturbances
Occipital lobe	Lateral hemianopia or other homonymous lateral visual field cut
	Visual hallucinations, metamorphopsia, monocular diplopia
	Impairment of movement perception, astereopia
	Left tactile: visual anomia, left hand diagnostic apraxia (posterior callosal involvement)
	Left:dysmnesia (for verbal material), transient global amnesia, pure alexia, optic aphasia (visual anomia), transcortical sensory aphasia, hemiachromatopsia, color anomia, visual hemineglect. acute confusional state, acute delirium
	Right: dysmnesia (for nonverbal material), transient global amnesia, visual hemineglect, palinopsia (prosopagnosia?), impaired mental imagery (Charcot-Wilbrandt syndrome)
	Bilateral: bilateral hemianopia, sometimes with tubular vision and/or cortical blindness, Anton's syndrome, altitudinal hemianopia, prosopagnosia, visual-object agnosia, Klüver-Bucy syndrome, amnesia

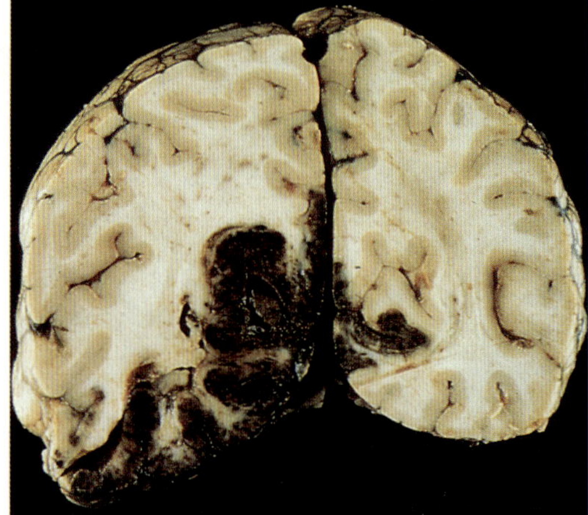

FIGURE 4.17

Bilateral occipital infarcts due to compression of the posterior cerebral artery at the tentorium by diffuse brain edema (pathology).

[19,20]. In pathologic series, PCA infarction is often due to compression by edema during temporal lobe herniation (Figure 4.17). In a clinical setting, the etiology is usually embolic, mainly from the heart vertebrobasilar atherosclerosis [20]. The high prevalence of embolic occlusion of the PCA explains why occipital infarcts may be bilateral in over 5% of the cases, with cortical blindness or double hemianopia often sparing macular vision (the reason for this sparing remains unclear, but may be related to specific anatomic features of the vascular supply to the occipital pole). In these cases, memory disturbances may be related to involvement of the posterior part of the parahippocampal gyrus.

THALAMIC INFARCTS

The arterial supply to the thalamus may be divided into four main groups corresponding to rather characteristic infarcts (Table 4.9) (Figures 4.18, 4.19) [21,36,37]:

1) The paramedian (or thalamoperforate) branches from the P_1 segment of the PCA. They also supply the most rostral paramedian part of the midbrain (vertical gaze dysfunction, disturbed consciousness, amnesia, and other neurobehavioral dysfunction). Because a single pedicle can supply both sides in up to one third of the cases, bilateral paramedian infarction is particularly common.
2) The inferolateral (or thalamogeniculate) branches from the P_2 segment of the PCA, supplying the ventrolateral mass of the thalamus (hemisensory disturbances, hemiataxia-hemisensory dysfunction).
3) The posterior choroidal arteries (one lateral and one medial group) from the P_2 segment of the PCA. These arteries supply the posterior part of the thalamus and also contribute to the supply of the geniculate bodies and medial temporal lobe together with the anterior choroidal artery (mainly visual hemifield disturbances such as horizontal sectoranopia). The most distal branches also supply the extreme rostral part of the thalamus, but clinical-radiologic correlations are lacking in infarct cases.
4) The tuberothalamic (or polar) branches originate from the posterior communicating artery so that they are literally at the interface between the carotid and vertebrobasilar systems. They supply the anterolateral part of the thalamus (neuropsychologic dysfunction such as dysphasia, amnesia, neglect). Not rarely, these branches may be lacking and their territory is taken over by the paramedian branches.

Table 4.9. Thalamic infarcts

Inferolateral territory infarcts	Paramedian territory infarcts
Hemihypesthesia and partial variants (including cheiro-oral syndrome), pain	Decreased consciousness–hallucinosis
Mild hemiparesis or ataxia (sometimes ataxic hemiparesis, painful ataxic hemiparesis, hypesthetic ataxic hemiparesis, or hemiataxia with hemihypesthesia)	Moderate hemiparesis, asterixis, ataxia, astasia, action-induced dystonia
Asterixis	Upgaze limitation, vertical one-and-a-half syndrome
No neuropsychological disturbances	Left: dysphasia, dysmnesia, hemineglect
	Right: hemineglect, dysmnesia for nonverbal material, confusional state
Tuberothalmic territory infarcts	Bilateral: mitral coma, severe amnesia, confusional state, dysphasia, neglect, loss of self-psychic activation, ataxia, upgaze/downgaze/vertical gaze palsy
Left: dysphasia (hemineglect)	
Right: hemineglect, mild hemiparesis or hemihypesthesia	
	Posterior-choroidal territory infarcts
	Visual field cut: horizontal homonymous sectoranopia
	Upper- or lower-quadrant-anopia
	Mild hemiparesis/hemihypesthesia/speech disturbances
	Blepharospasm

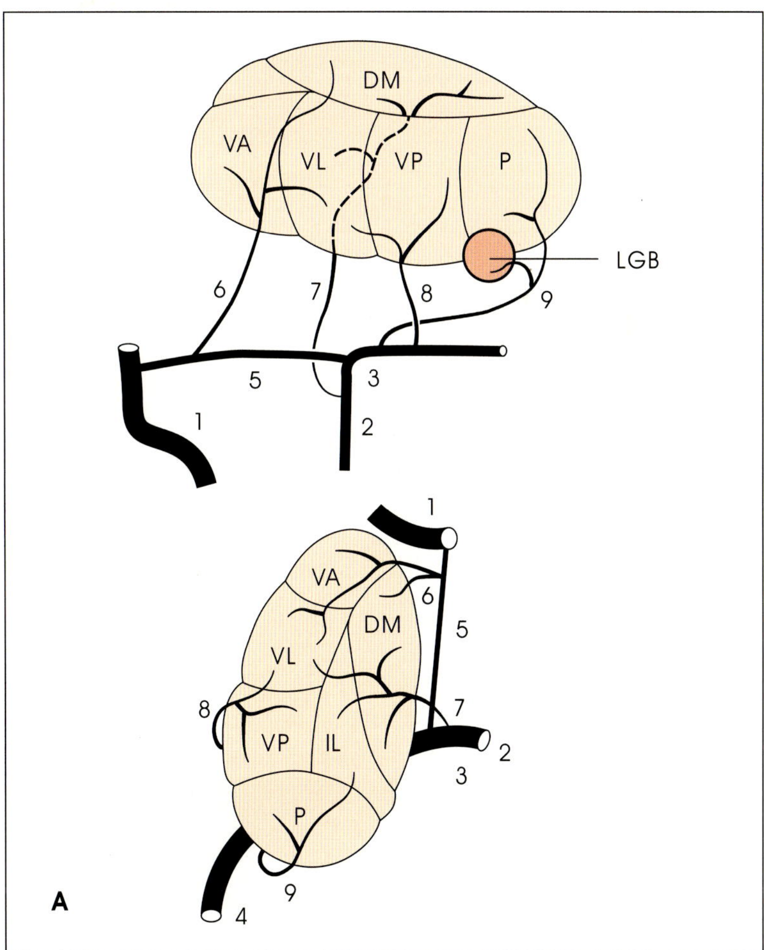

FIGURE 4.18

Thalamic territories. **A**, Arterial branches. (*continued*)

The etiology of thalamic infarcts is varied. Small-vessel disease associated with hypertension or diabetes accounts for not more than one third of the cases, while cardioembolism and artery-to-artery embolism accounts for at least 25% to 30%. Other causes (arteritis, migraine, and so on) may also be responsible, more commonly than in other infarcts.

This etiologic pattern may be related in part to the fact that although thalamic arteries are perforators, they have reciprocal anastomoses, contrary to the lenticulostriate perforators. Thus, simultaneous occlusion of several perforators (from embolism) may be necessary to lead to infarct, while single perforator occlusion due to in situ small-vessel disease may not be synonymous with infarction.

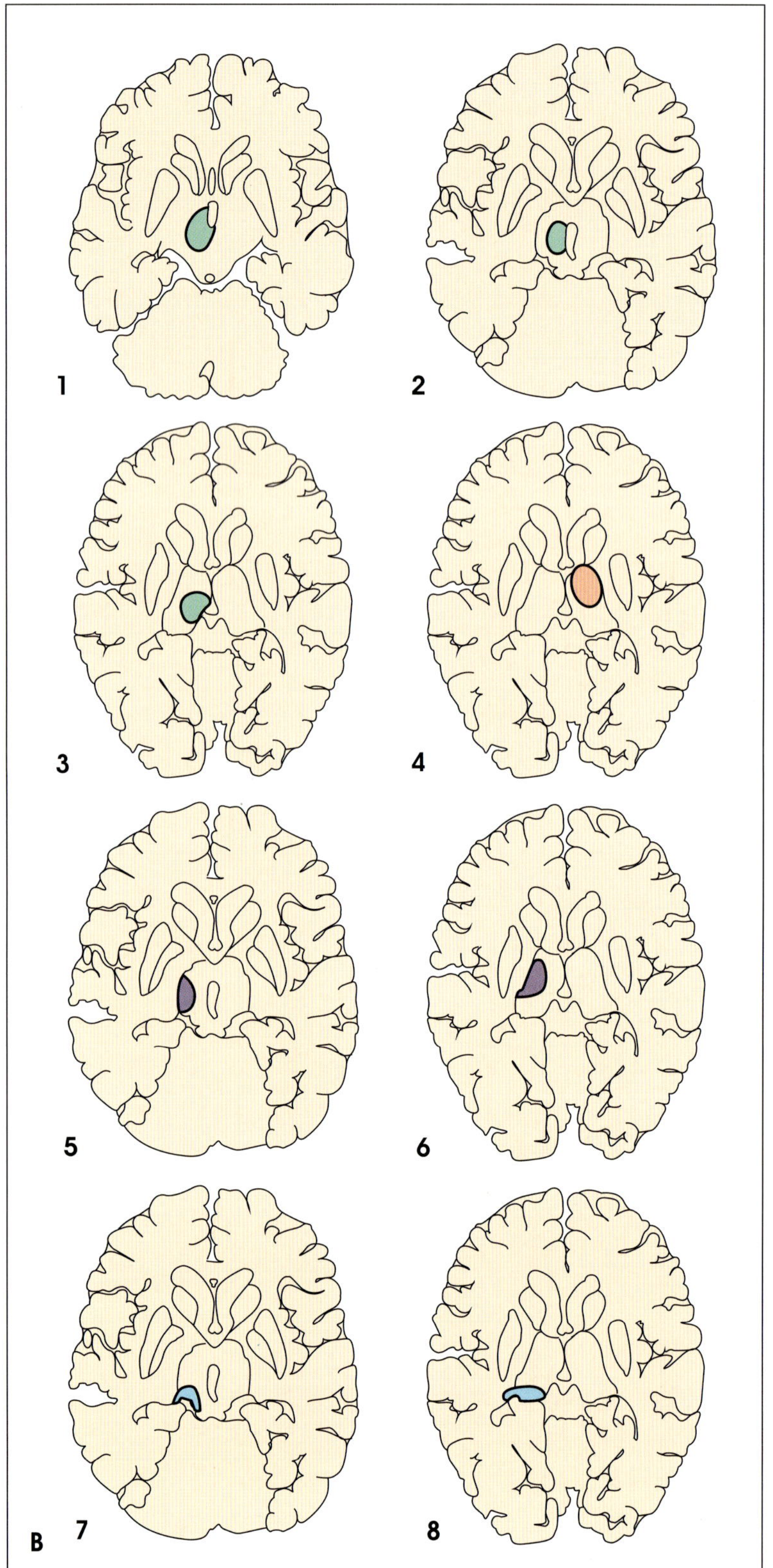

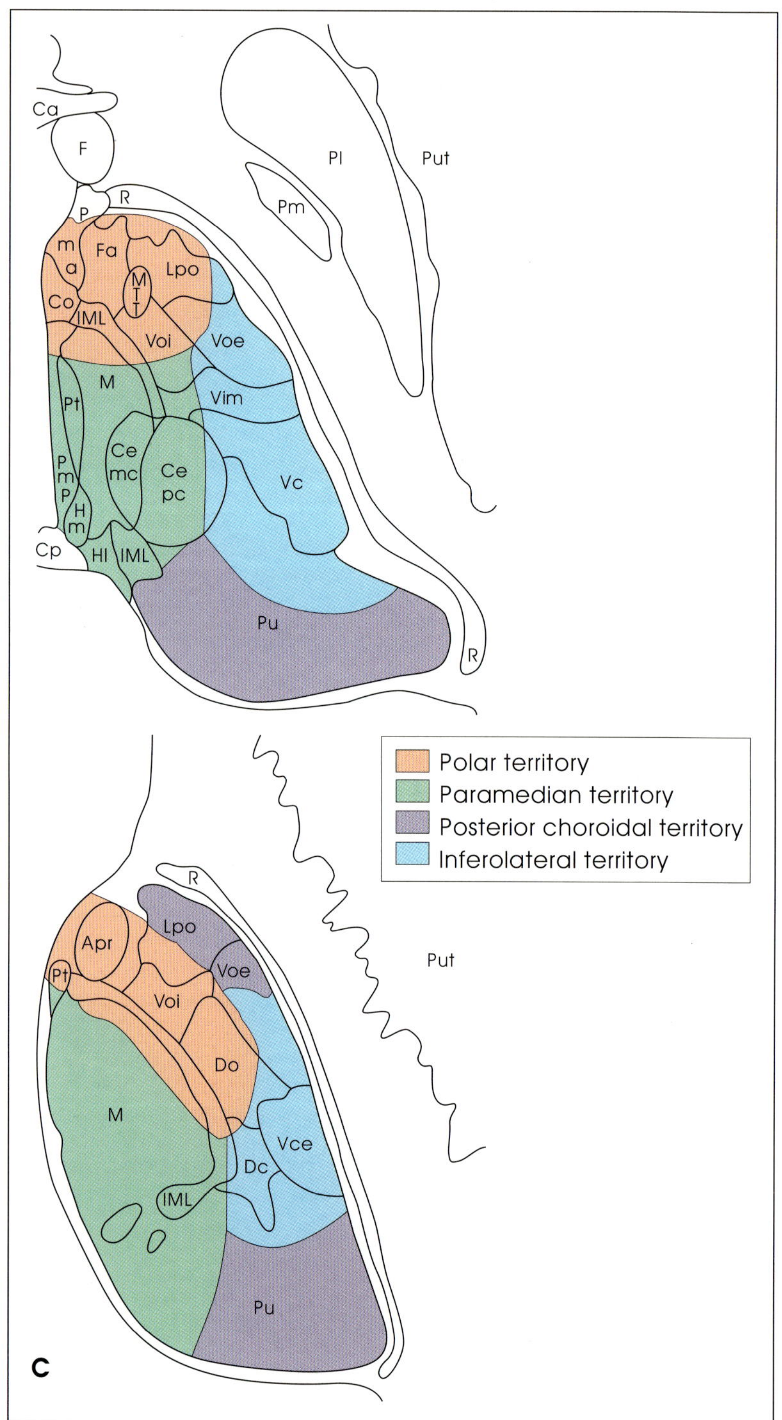

FIGURE 4.18

(*continued*) **B**, Templates of territories shown by computed tomography and magnetic resonance imaging. **1–3**, Paramedian territory. **4**, Polar territory. **5** and **6**, Inferolateral territory. **7** and **8**, Posterior choroidal territory. **C**, Detailed relation between territories and nuclear subgroups. (*Adapted from* Bogousslavsky and Hommel [35]; with permission.)

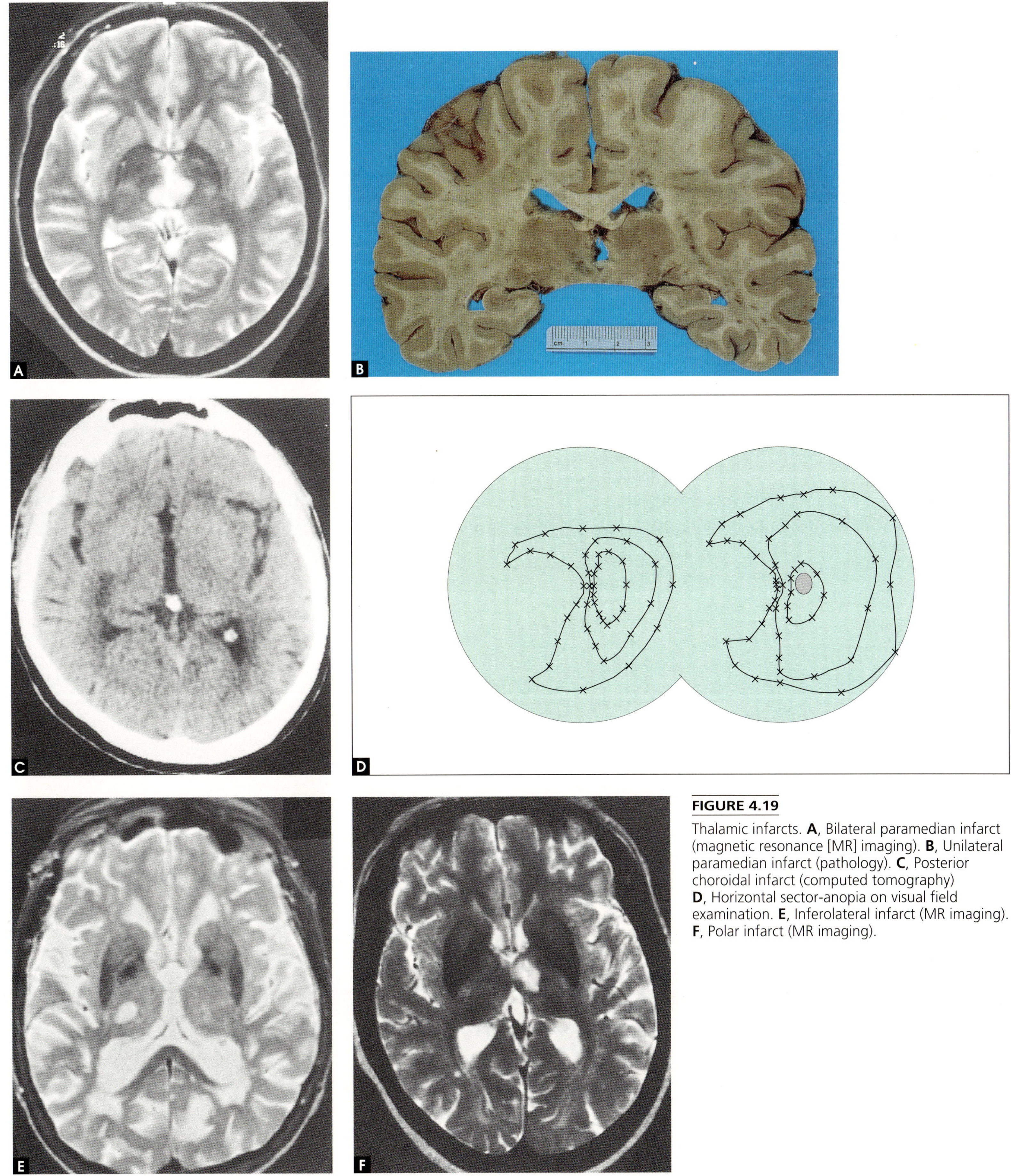

FIGURE 4.19

Thalamic infarcts. **A**, Bilateral paramedian infarct (magnetic resonance [MR] imaging). **B**, Unilateral paramedian infarct (pathology). **C**, Posterior choroidal infarct (computed tomography) **D**, Horizontal sector-anopia on visual field examination. **E**, Inferolateral infarct (MR imaging). **F**, Polar infarct (MR imaging).

TOTAL AND SUBTOTAL POSTERIOR CEREBRAL ARTERY TERRITORY INFARCTS

Superficial and deep PCA territory infarction combines occipital, internal temporal, thalamic and midbrain involvement. The blood supply of the PCA to the midbrain comes from two sources: first, the paramedian branches from the P_1 segment (see thalamic infarcts); and second, the intermediolateral and lateral branches from the P_2 segment, which supply the rostral part of the cerebral peduncles (including corticospinal tract). Thus, two patterns of PCA trunk occlusion may exist [22]: 1) P_1 occlusion: involvement of midbrain, (rostral paramedian and lateral-intermediolateral), thalamic (except tuberothalamic), and pial territories; and 2) P_2 occlusion: same except sparing of the paramedian thalamic–paramedian rostral midbrain territory.

The combination of hemiplegia, hemihypesthesia, and hemianopia may mimic MCA or anterior choroidal artery territory infarction. P_1 and P_2 occlusion is nearly always embolic, either from the heart or from basilar atherosclerosis.

BRAIN STEM INFARCTS

Midbrain, pontine, and medullary infarcts usually develop in characteristic territories, in relation to a stereotyped blood supply system, which includes (from medial to lateral side) paramedian perforating branches and short circumferential arteries directly from the basilar artery, and large circumferential arteries, which are in fact the three cerebellar arteries—the superior cerebellar artery (SCA), the anterior inferior cerebellar artery (AICA), and the

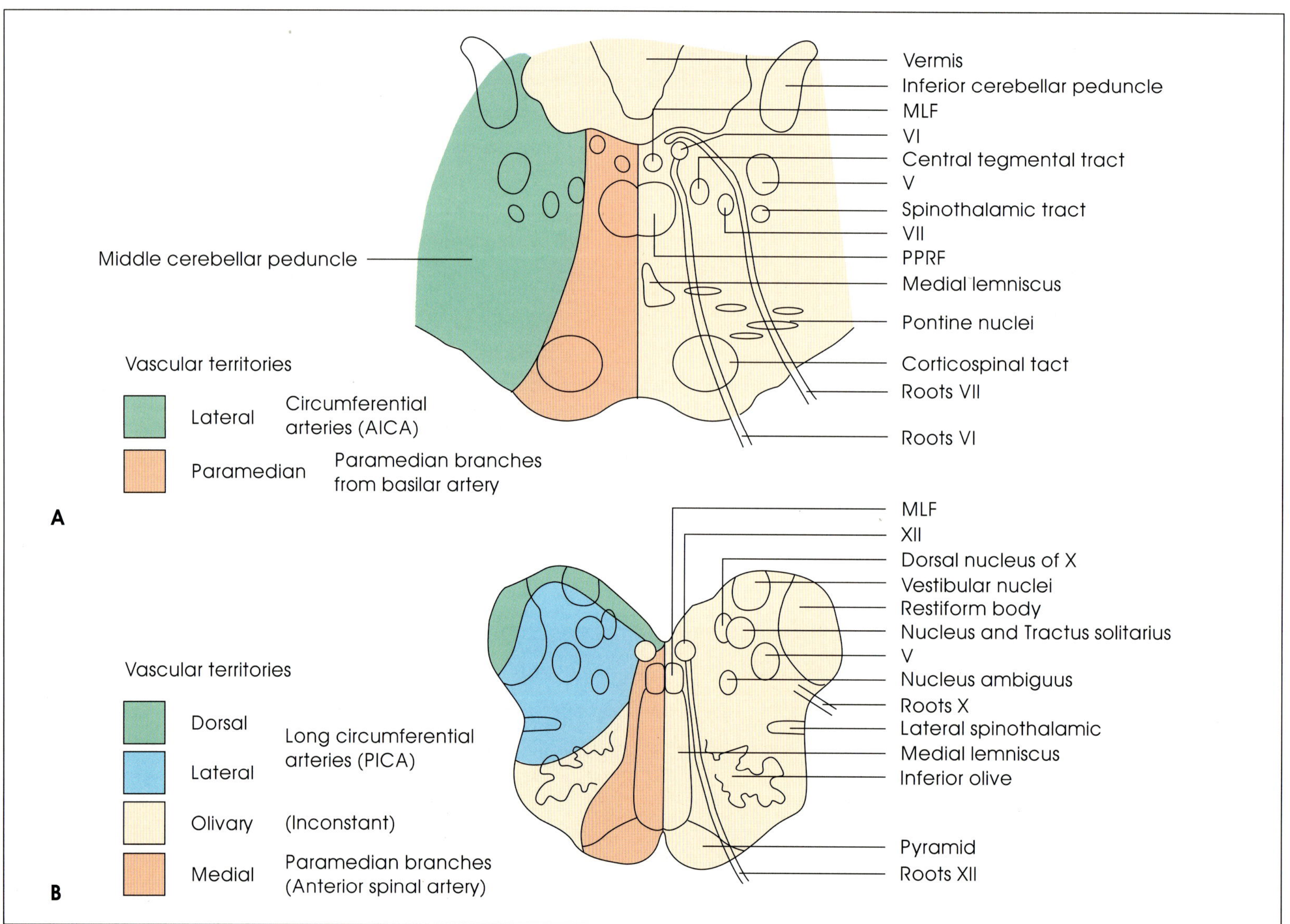

FIGURE 4.20

Brain stem territories. **A**, Pons. **B**, Medullary. *(continued)*

posterior inferior cerebellar artery (PICA), and supply the dorsal brain stem as well as their cerebellar territory (Figure 4.20). Most of the clinically relevant brain stem infarcts involve the paramedian and lateral (short circumferential branches) territories (Figure 4.21). Thus, they may be associated with small-vessel disease (lacunar infarction), but also with basilar artery (for the pons and midbrain) or vertebral artery (for the medulla) disease that obstructs the mouth of these small arteries (branch disease) (Figure 4.22) [3]. Embolism is not a usual cause of isolated brain stem infarction because small emboli tend not to lodge in the proximal and middle parts of the basilar artery but at its tip (where they may occlude the PCAs or their branches and the SCAs). Large emboli, which may stop more proximally in the basilar artery, lead to large infarcts not limited to the brain stem. The neurologic manipulations caused by brain stem infarcts are multiple (Table 4.10) (Figures 4.23, 4.24).

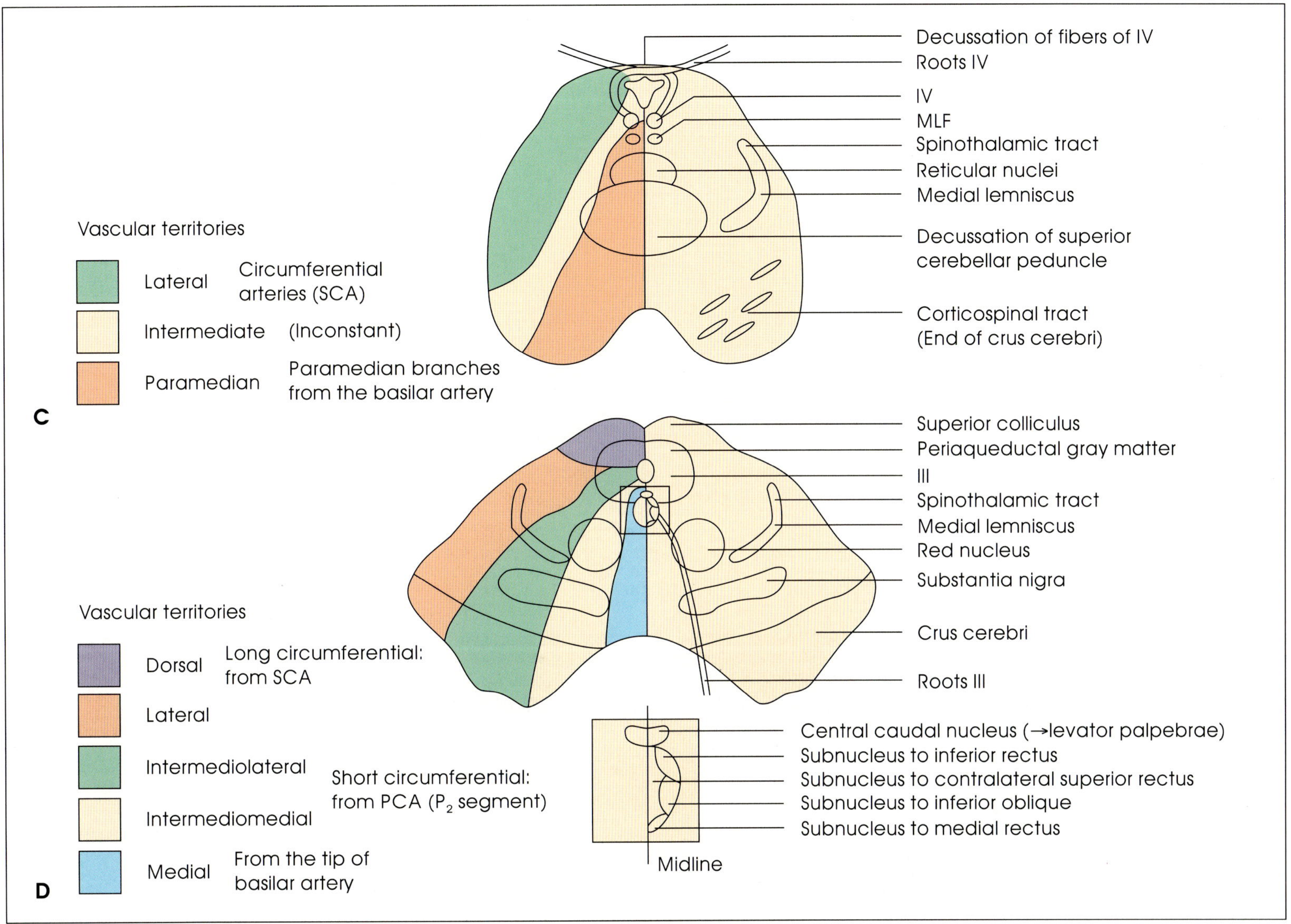

FIGURE 4.20

(continued) **C**, Lower midbrain. **D**, Upper midbrain. *(continued)*

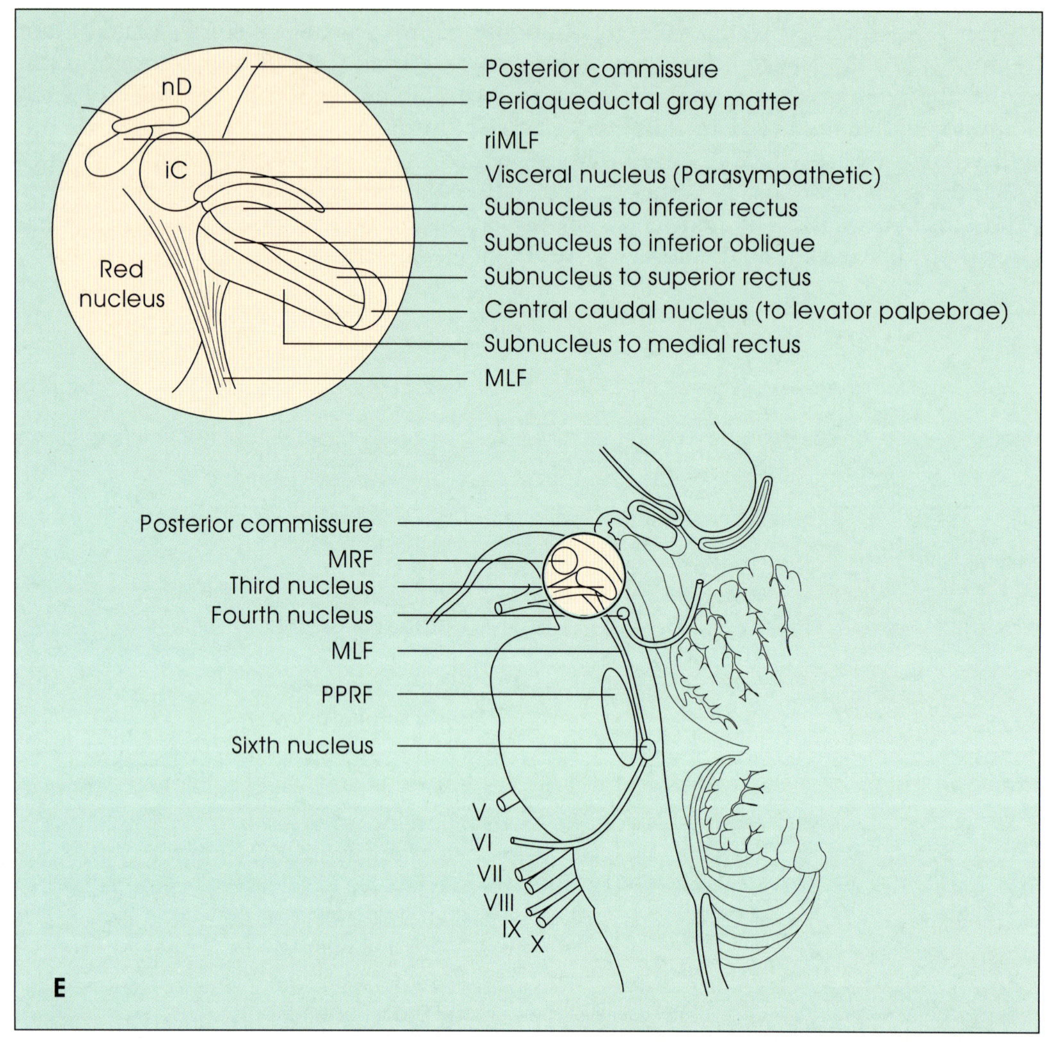

FIGURE 4.20

(*continued*) **E**, Sagittal view. (*Adapted from* Bogousslavsky and Hommel [35]; with permission.)

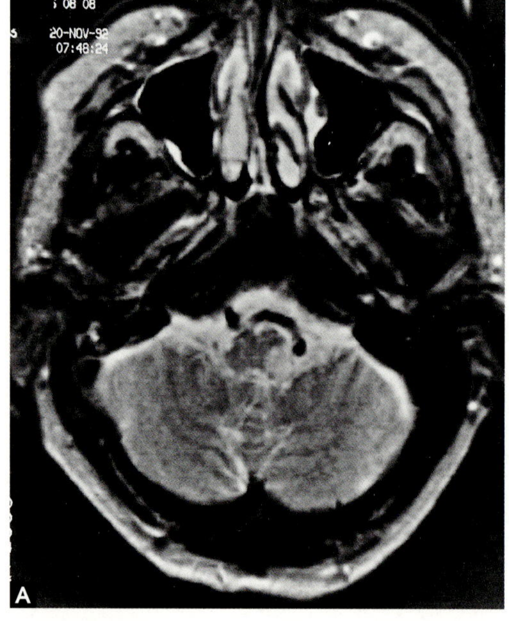

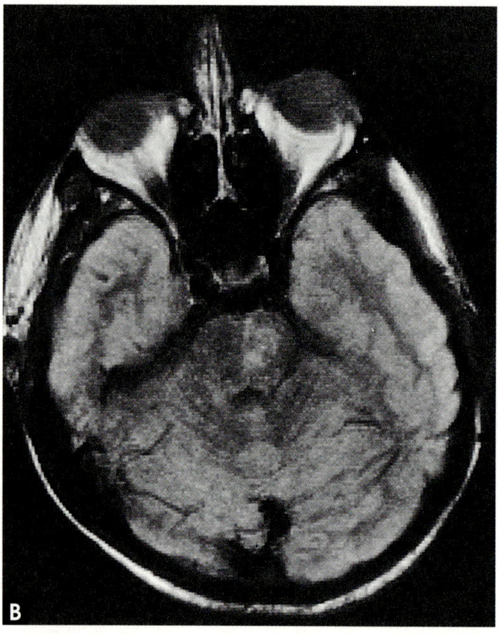

FIGURE 4.21

Brain stem infarcts (magnetic resonance imaging). **A**, Lateral medullary infarct. **B**, Pontine infarct.

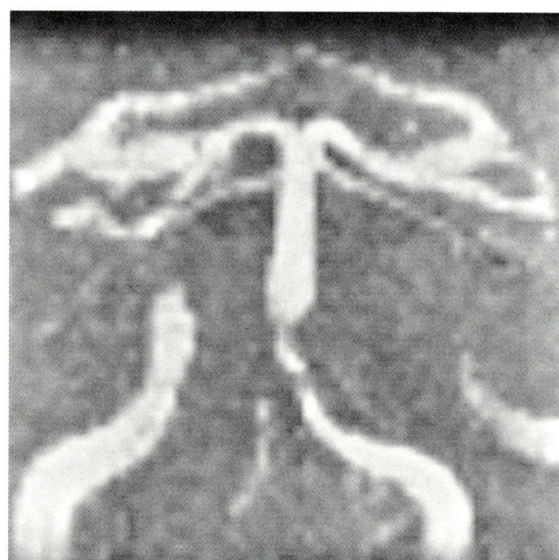

FIGURE 4.22

Magnetic resonance angiography showing basilar artery stenosis.

Table 4.10. Clinical features in medullary infarcts and basilar occlusion

Lateral medullary infarction	Medial medullary infarction (Dejerine's syndrome)	Basilar artery occlusion	Perforating artery occlusion
Blurred vision, difficulties of fixation, oblique diplopia, and sometimes tilting of the visual world with 90° to 180° inversion, vertigo, nausea and vomiting, hiccups, difficulty in swallowing, hoarseness of the voice, dysarthria and altered taste, nystagmus, cardiac sinusal bradycardia, fever, sleep apnea, urine retention Ipsilateral to the lesion Facial pain Facial hypesthesia Facial weakness Facial anhydrosis Gait and limb ataxia Lateropulsion Palatal palsy Horner's syndrome Vocal cord paralysis Hemiplegia or hemiparesis (Opalski's lower medullary syndrome) Contralateral to the lesion Pain and temperature hypesthesia Sometimes Babinski's sign or hypersudation Hemiparesis (Babinski-Nageotte syndrome)	Ipsilateral to the lesion Weakness and wasting of the tongue Contralateral to the lesion Hemiplegia and tactile-proprioceptive sensory loss Combined lateral and medial or medullary or medullary and pontine infarctions Babinski-Nageotte syndrome	"Locked-in" syndrome Sudden onset, often preceeded with TIAs, dizziness, headaches, tetraplegia, decerebrate response, bilateral extensor responses, facial diplegia, trismus, lingual and pharyngeal palsy, dysarthria, hoarseness of the voice, horizontal gaze palsy, ocular bobbing (the patient is fully alert and communication is possible using a code with the eyes opening and vertical gaze) Partial syndromes Internuclear ophthalmoplegia, horizontal one-and-a-half syndrome, conjugate horizontal gaze palsy, six-nerve palsy, ptosis, palatal myoclonus, sensory motor deficits Midbrain and top of the basilar occlusion Sudden onset, coma and abnormalities of alertness, memory impairments, akinetic mutism, third nerve palsy, mydriasis or fixed midpositioned pupils, corectopia, vertical gaze disturbances, hemiplegia or tetraplegia, bilateral extensor responses, peduncular hallucinosis, chorea, or hemiballism	Pure motor stroke, ataxic hemiparesis, pure sensory stroke, dysarthria, and clumsy hand

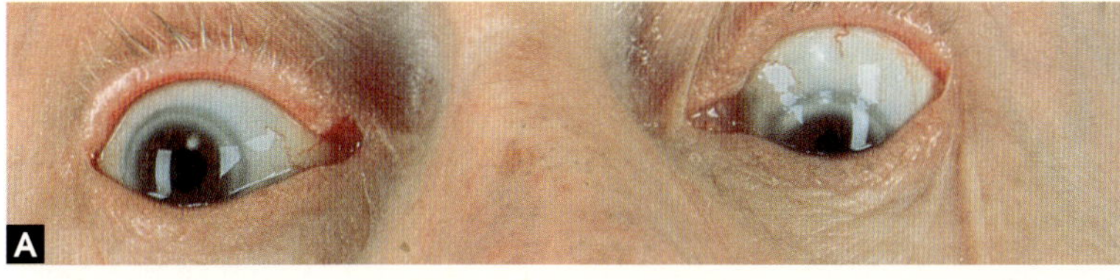

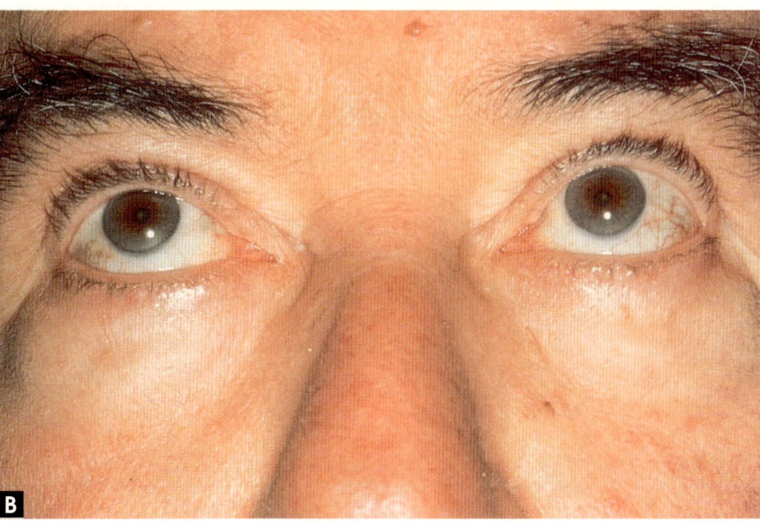

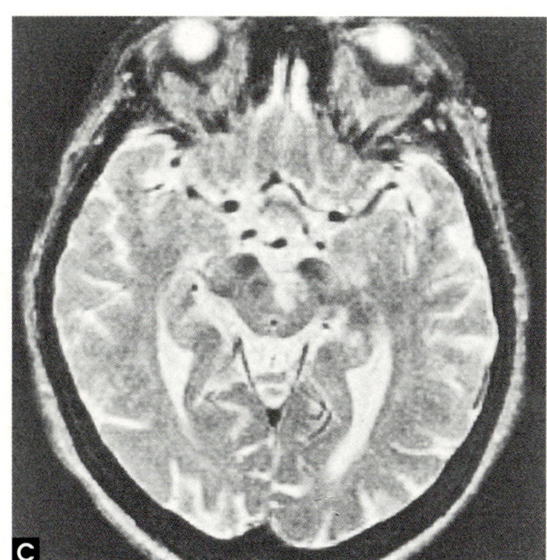

FIGURE 4.23

Eye movement disorders in midbrain infarcts. **A**, Nuclear third-nerve syndrome (ptosis, third-nerve palsy, contralateral upgaze limitation). **B**, Vertical one-and-a-half syndrome (upgaze palsy). **C**, Midbrain infarct (magnetic resonance imaging). (*continued*)

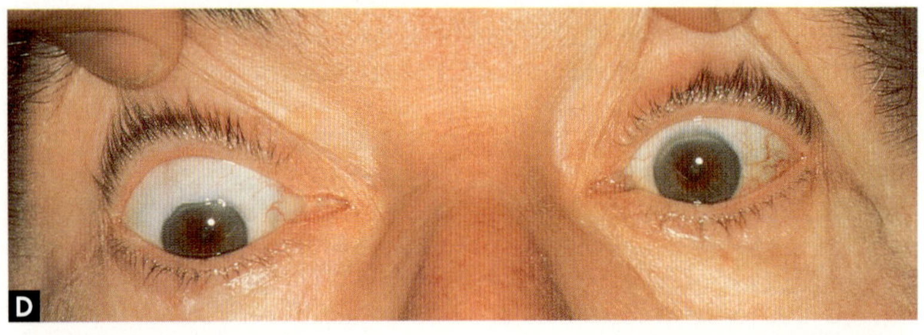

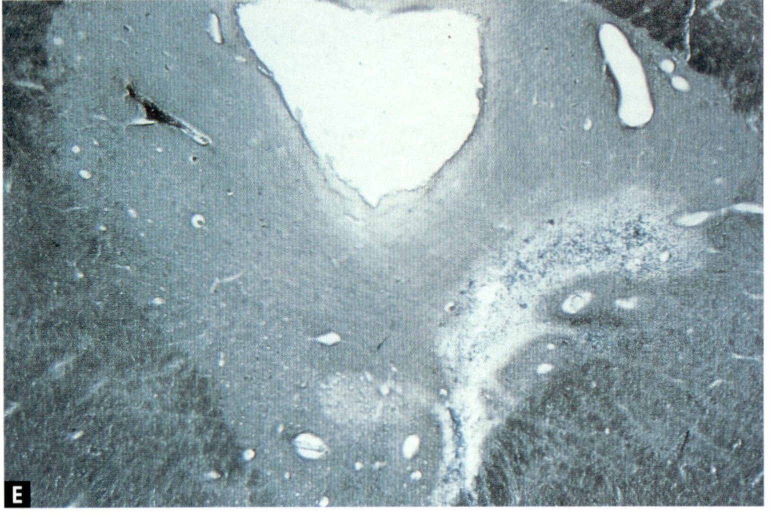

FIGURE 4.23

(*continued*) **D**, Unilateral downgaze palsy in extreme rostral midbrain infarct (**E**).

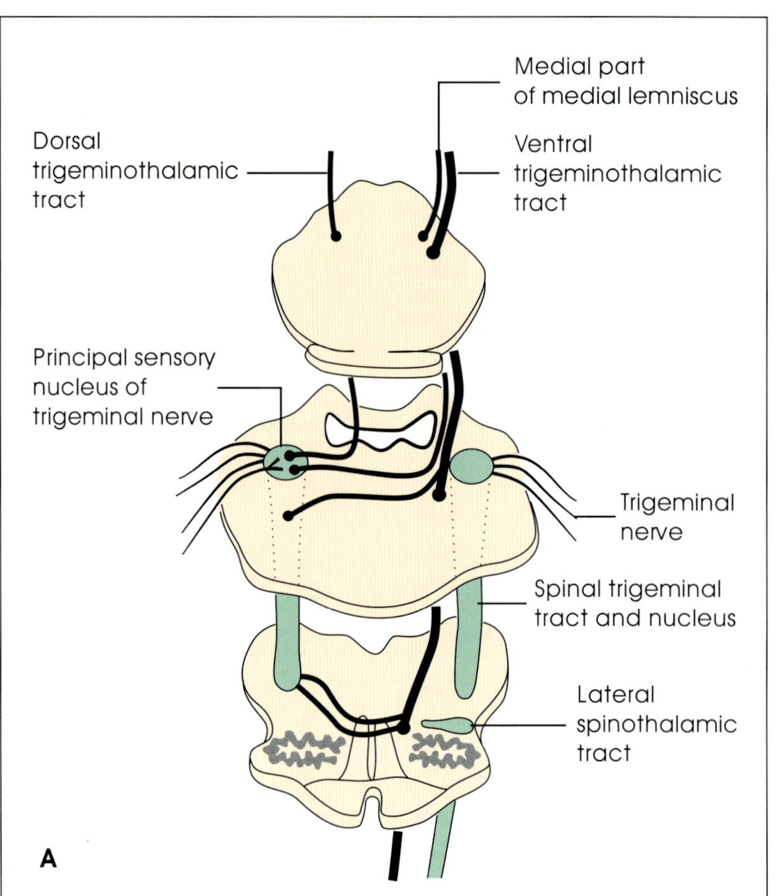

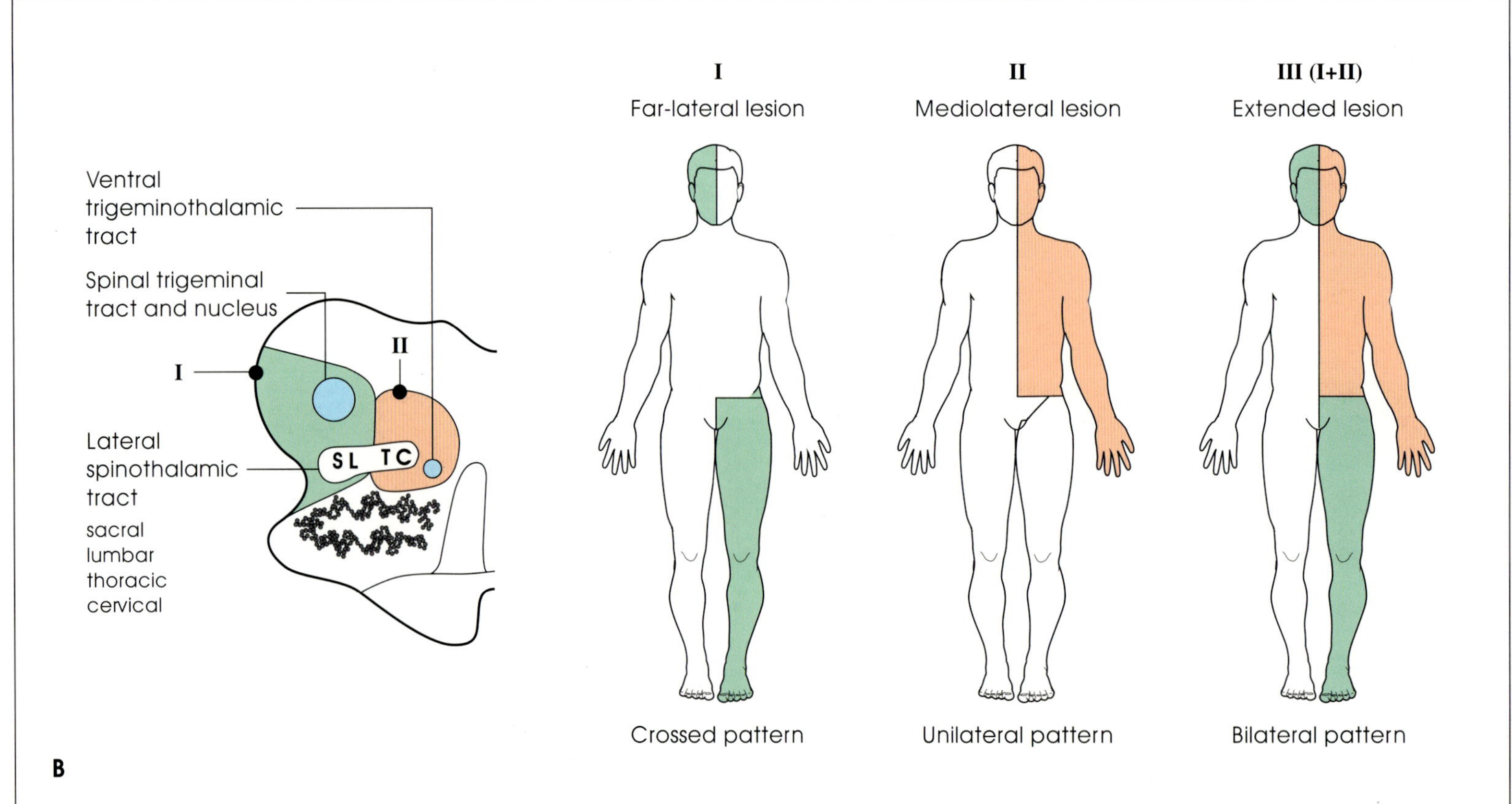

FIGURE 4.24

Sensory tract syndromes in lower brain stem infarcts. **A**, Anatomy. **B**, Syndromes.

CEREBELLAR INFARCTS

PICA Territory Infarcts

PICA territory infarcts are the most common type of symptomatic cerebellar infarcts (over 50% in clinical practice) (Table 4.11) (Figures 4.25, 4.26), [21,22]. Most cases seem related to atheromatous occlusion of the vertebral artery, less commonly the PICA itself [1]. Cardioembolism may account for more than one third of autopsy cases, but its prevalence is not well known in patients.

AICA Territory Infarcts

AICA territory infarcts are the less common type of cerebellar infarcts. Infarction of the lateral part of the lower pons is usual in association with cerebellar involvement [23]. Contrary to PICA and SCA territory infarcts, cardioembolism seems an uncommon cause, and basilar-AICA atherosclerosis may explain most of the cases.

SCA Territory Infarcts

In SCA territory infarcts, clinically relevant brain stem (midbrain) involvement is less common than in AICA territory infarct [22,24]. Cardioembolism is a classic cause, but basilar-SCA atherosclerosis may be at least as common.

Other Cerebellar Infarcts

Large cerebellar infarcts are usually PICA territory infarcts in patients with AICA aplasia. They are typically responsible for a rapid deterioration, tonsillar herniation, and death in the absence of surgical intervention [22,25].

Watershed cerebellar infarcts may occur at the border zone between PICA, SCA, and AICA territories (Figure 4.27). Their clinical diagnosis remains controversial since the overlap of the cerebellar arteries may be particularly variable. An association with hemodynamic failure has been postulated, but definite proof is still lacking.

Small cerebellar infarcts have been reported in presumed cerebellar border zones, but also within the main cerebellar territories. The concept of lacunar infarct in the cerebellum may deserve more detailed study, which is now lacking.

Venous cerebellar infarcts are usually large, with a pseudotumoral course.

Table 4.11. Topographic syndromes and causes of cerebellar infarcts

Territory	Syndrome	Causes
PICA and mPICA	Pseudovestibular syndrome with rotatory vertigo, trunk ataxia, nystagmus and mild dysmetria	Cardioembolism
lPICA	Unsteadiness, limb ataxia, ipsilateral axial lateropulsion, absence of trunk ataxia, and dysarthria	Cardioembolism and vertebral atherosclerosis equally
AICA	Association of cerebellar dysfunction with signs of lateropontine involvement	Atherosclerosis of basilar artery
SCA	Cerebellar dysarthria associated with vertigo or unsteadiness, limb or trunk ataxia, nystagmus	Cardioembolism and vertebral atherosclerosis equally

AICA—anterior inferior cerebellar artery; lPICA—lateral branch of posterior inferior cerebellar artery; mPICA—medial branch posterior inferior cerebellar artery; SCA—superior cerebellar artery.

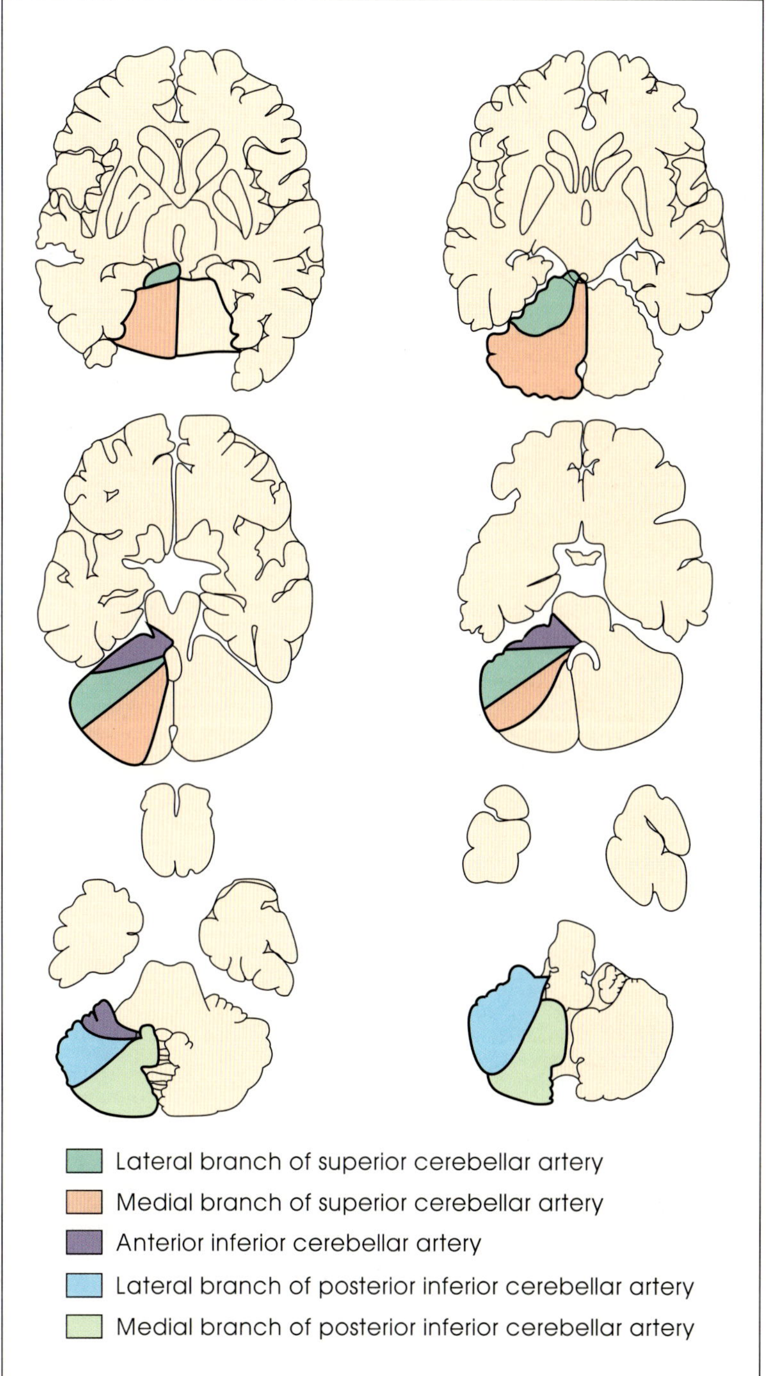

FIGURE 4.25

Arterial territories of the cerebellum.

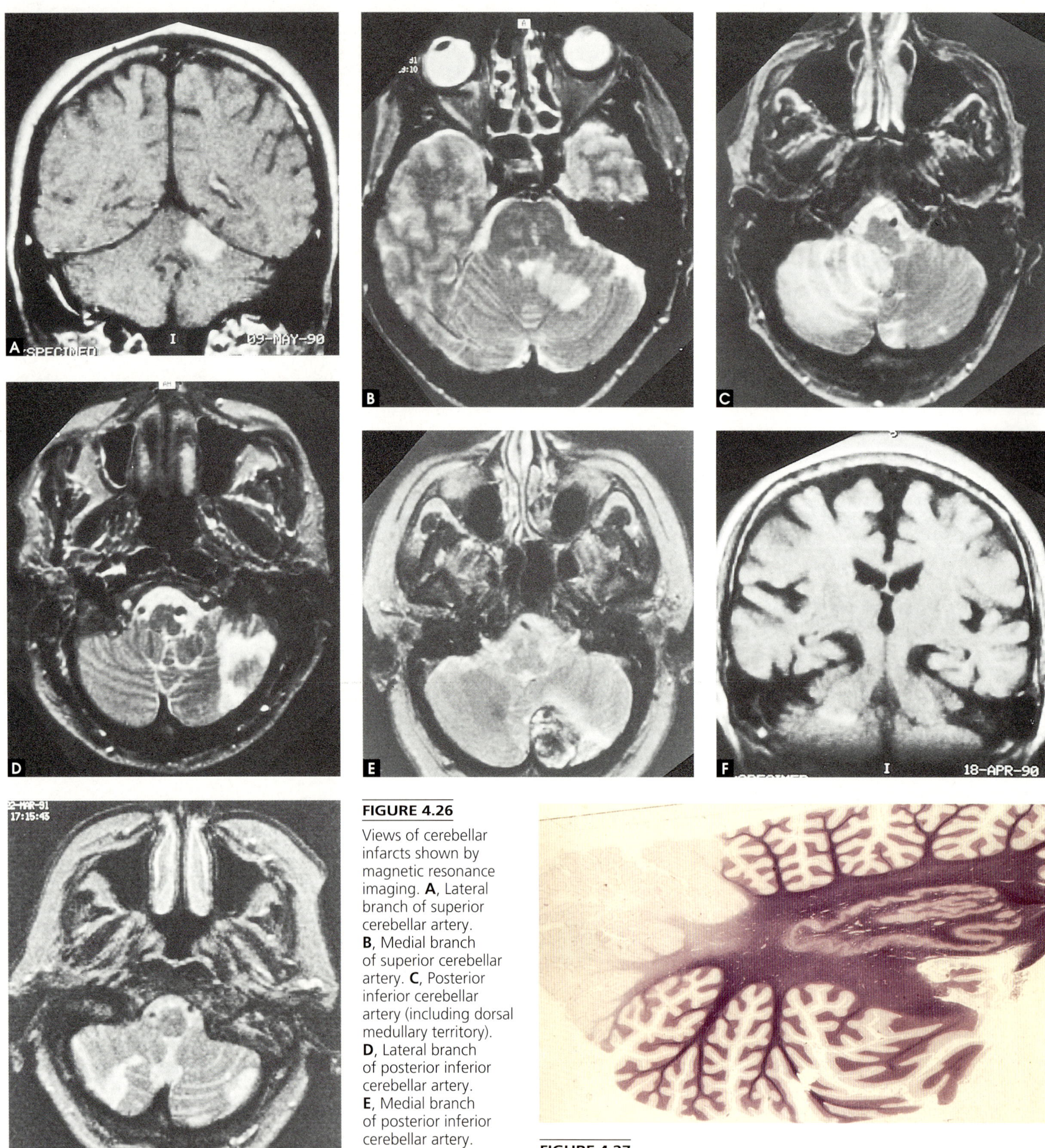

FIGURE 4.26

Views of cerebellar infarcts shown by magnetic resonance imaging. **A**, Lateral branch of superior cerebellar artery. **B**, Medial branch of superior cerebellar artery. **C**, Posterior inferior cerebellar artery (including dorsal medullary territory). **D**, Lateral branch of posterior inferior cerebellar artery. **E**, Medial branch of posterior inferior cerebellar artery. **F**, Anterior inferior cerebellar artery. **G**, Bilateral watershed.

FIGURE 4.27

Watershed cerebellar infarct. Microscopic slide (Luxol-Nissl stain) showing pale area corresponding to neuron and myelin loss.

MULTIPLE INFARCTS

Extended Vertebrobasilar Infarcts

The most common form of extended vertebrobasilar infarcts may be the "top-of-the-basilar syndrome" in which embolism at the basilar artery–PCA junction may produce midbrain, superior cerebellar, thalamic, and distal PCA territory infarction [3,26].

Little attention has been given to other extended or multilevel infarcts in the vertebrobasilar system, with variable combinations of brain stem, cerebellar, thalamic, temporal, and occipital involvement.

Simultaneous Multiple Infarcts

Bilateral supratentorial infarcts, and carotid territory plus vertebrobasilar territory infarcts usually suggest cardioembolism, often associated with septicemia (Figure 4.28), when they occur during the same stroke. Two simultaneous infarcts in one cerebral hemisphere (Figure 4.29) are associated with severe ICA disease (75%) (Table 4.12), while the prevalence of potential cardiac sources of embolism does not differ from that found in ischemic strokes in general [27].

Other Multiple Infarcts

In some patients, recurrence of infarcts after previously asymptomatic or paucisymptomatic infarcts may lead to unusual neurologic dysfunction (Figure 4.30) [5,28]. Repeated lacunar infarcts or cardioembolic infarcts may be the most common types of these repeated strokes. Multifocal arteritic processes may account for a smaller proportion of multiple, mostly hemorrhagic infarcts (Figure 4.28).

NEUROPATHOLOGIC ASPECTS

Tissue necrosis distal to the occlusion involves neurons, nerve fibers, glial cells, and mesenchymal cells of the vessel wall [29]. Cell death usually develops quickly, due to the rapid irreversible consequences of energy failure, but it can also be delayed, depending upon partial reperfusion [30,31].

Morphologically, the hallmarks of a fresh ischemic infarct are coagulation necrosis and associated edema (Figure 4.31). One should distinguish between combined cytotoxic and vasogenic edema within the core of frank infarction and perifocal edema

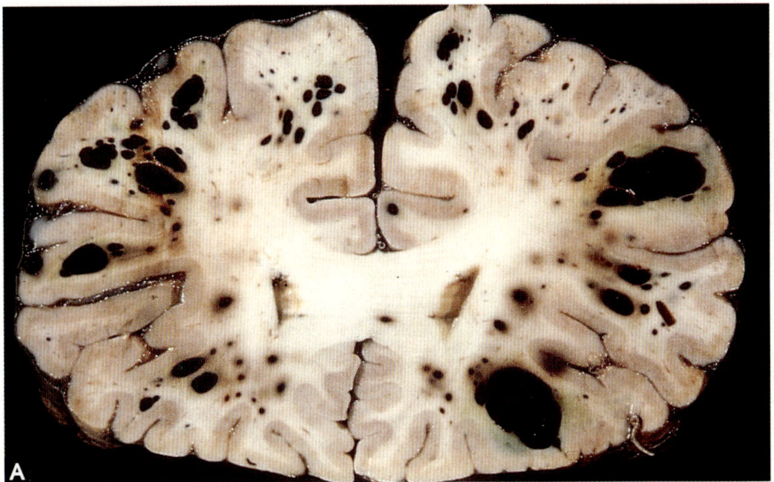

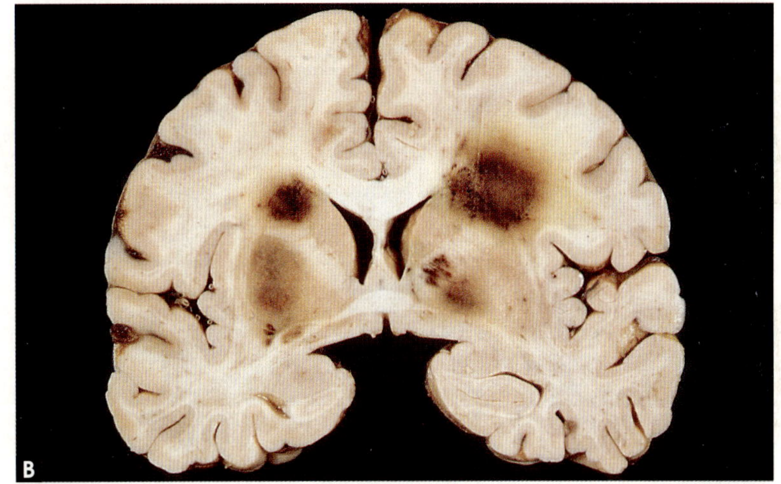

FIGURE 4.28

Multifocal infarcts (pathology). **A**, Multiple small hemorrhagic infarcts due to septic emboli. **B**, Multiple large hemorrhagic infarcts due to aspergillus arteritis.

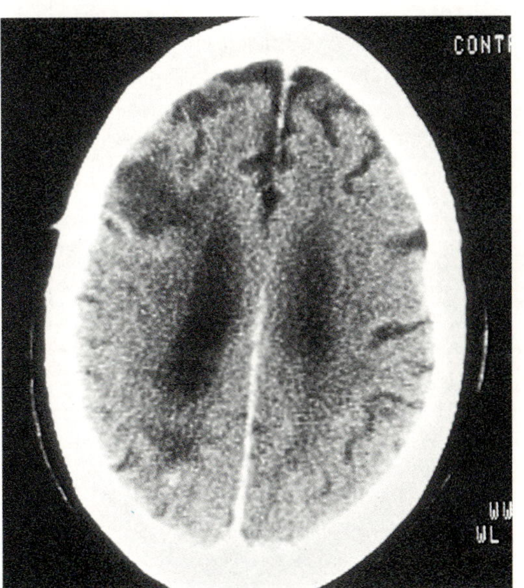

FIGURE 4.29

Double infarct in one cerebral hemisphere shown by computed tomography.

Table 4.12. Clinical syndromes suggesting internal carotid artery occlusion from simultaneous double ipsilateral infarction

Optic nerve and brain
Opticocerebral syndrome
Anterior or deep MCA and posterior MCA
Pure hemiplegia-hemianopia syndrome
Conduction aphasia with hemiparesis
Anterior MCA and posterior watershed
Acute transcortical mixed aphasia isolation-of-speech area

MCA—middle cerebral artery.

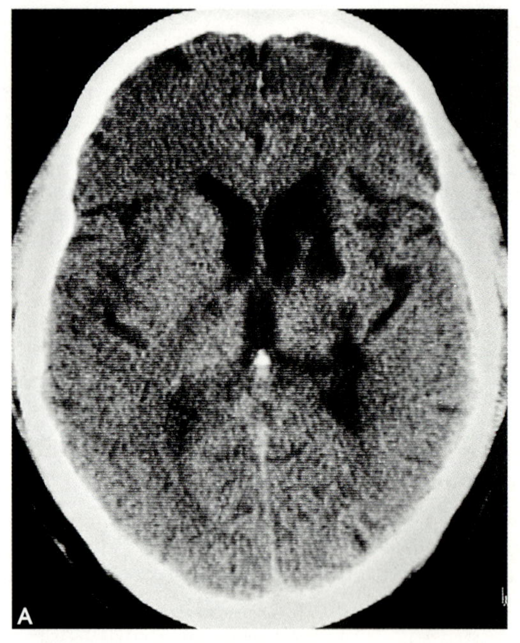

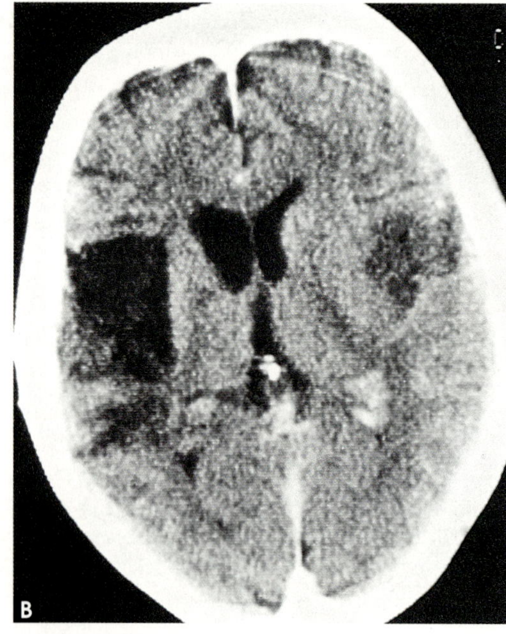

FIGURE 4.30

Examples of multiple cerebral infarcts. **A**, Multiple deep infarcts in a patient with loss of psychic self-activation (aspontaneity, apathy, loss of drive reversible by external stimulation, flattened mood). **B**, Computed tomography scan in acute pseudobulbar syndrome (the patient had an infarct with slight and reversible hemiparesis, but developed a contralateral opercular infarct 6 months later, with bilateral corticonuclear palsy).

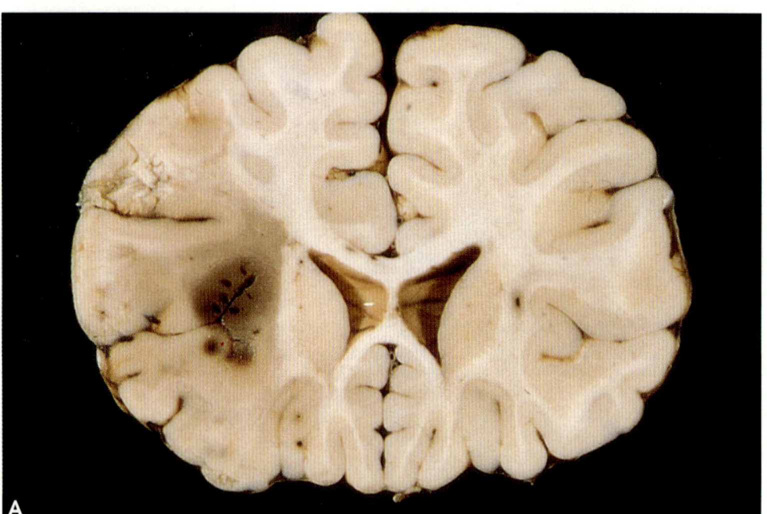

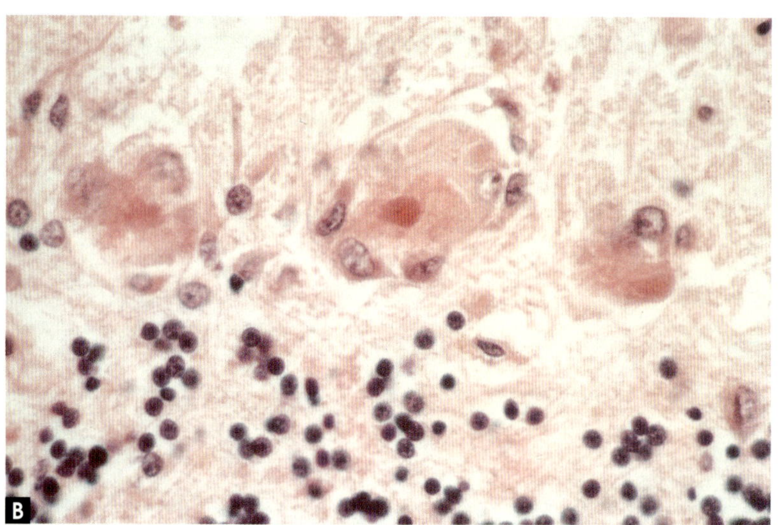

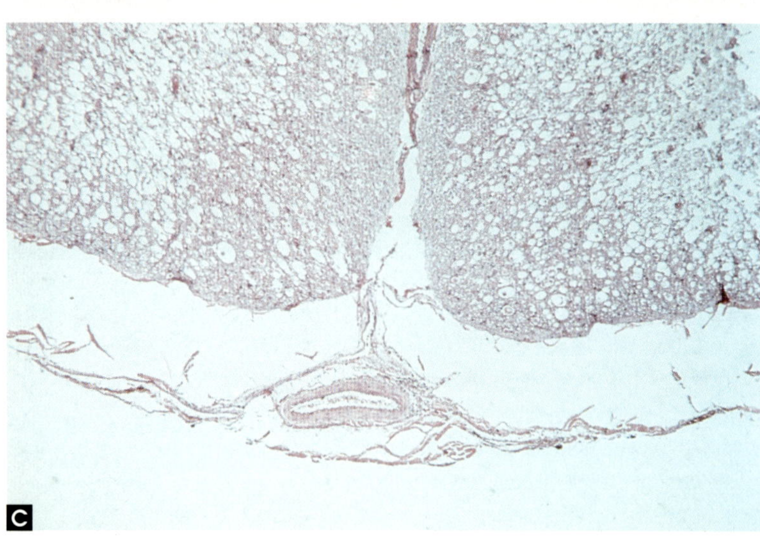

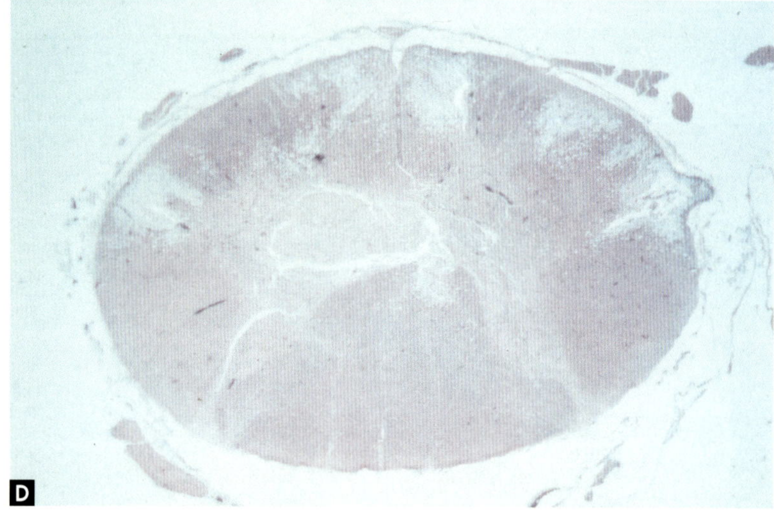

FIGURE 4.31

Neuropathology of fresh ischemic infarct (stage I). **A**, Macroscopic aspect. **B**, Ischemic cell damage (eosinophilic degeneration) of Purkinje's cells (hematoxyline-eosine stain). **C**, Spinal cord infarction with perifocal spongiform–edematous tissue changes (HE-stain). **D**, Detail of *C*.

that corresponds to reversible damage within the neighboring tissue (so-called penumbra). Morphologically, the irreversible ischemic cell change is characterized by eosinophilic homogenization of the cytoplasm and loss of the nucleolus and nuclear membrane (Figure 4.31B). There is actually some controversy about a possible role of a programmed cell death pathway, which might also be activated by ischemia. After 2 to 3 days, the first significant morphologic signs of the infarct's organization become visible. The organization is mainly achieved by activated microglia and blood-derived monocytes transforming themselves into macrophages (Figure 4.32). Capillary endothelial proliferation in the border zones of the infarct and reactive astrogliosis form the other reactive elements in this phase. Generally, neurons rapidly disappear by a process called lique-

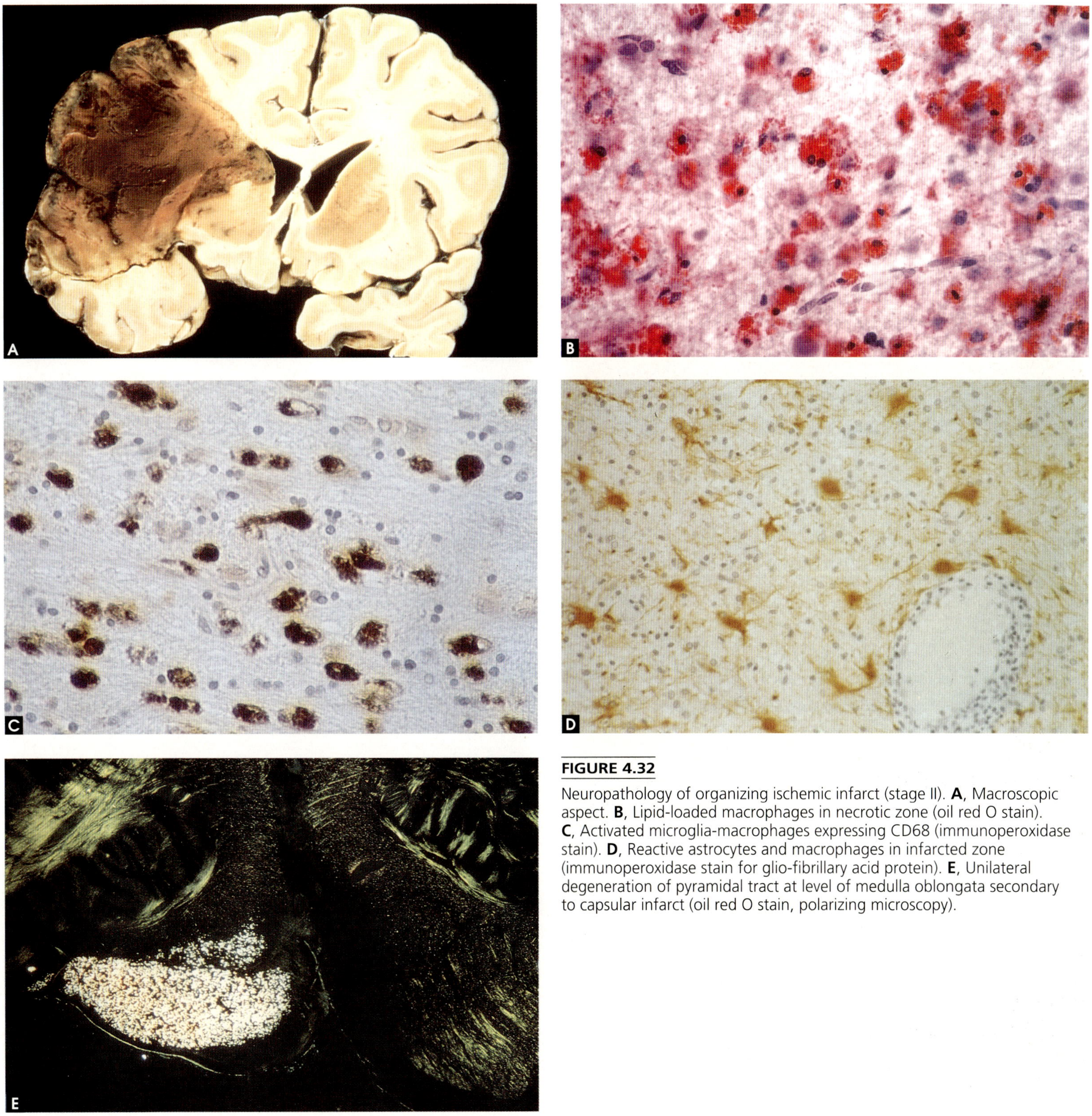

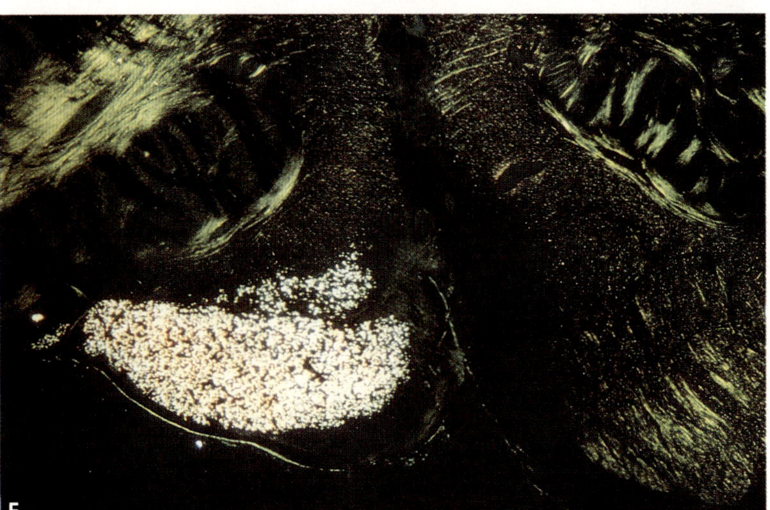

FIGURE 4.32

Neuropathology of organizing ischemic infarct (stage II). **A**, Macroscopic aspect. **B**, Lipid-loaded macrophages in necrotic zone (oil red O stain). **C**, Activated microglia-macrophages expressing CD68 (immunoperoxidase stain). **D**, Reactive astrocytes and macrophages in infarcted zone (immunoperoxidase stain for glio-fibrillary acid protein). **E**, Unilateral degeneration of pyramidal tract at level of medulla oblongata secondary to capsular infarct (oil red O stain, polarizing microscopy).

faction necrosis. Macroscopically, the infarct is well delimited because there is no more edema. It is characterized by a yellowish color due to lipid-loaded macrophages. The signs of organization become prominent about 1 week after a stroke. They persist during several weeks or months and can still be detected years later. The process of anterograde degeneration, corresponding to a partial or subtotal deafferentiation of the regions in which the interrupted connections project, can easily be demonstrated for several months in postmortem investigations (Figure 4.32) [32].

The final organization of an ischemic infarct is characterized by a total reabsorption of the necrotic tissue and accumulation of fluid in the newly formed cystic defect, the end-stage liquefaction necrosis. The cast is usually surrounded by a glial scar.

The morphologic correlation of arterial hypotension or shock in the absence of a major local vessel pathology are border zone infarcts, discussed earlier in this chapter. The infarcts start as multiple microinfarcts, which can become confluent. Prolonged arterial hypotension followed by reperfusion, such as in cardiac arrest with successful resuscitation, can give rise to a typical symmetrical localization of microinfarcts in brain tegmentum, tectal brain stem nuclei, and spinal cord (Figure 4.33) [33]. If prolonged arterial hypotension is complicated by markedly increased intracranial pressure due to diffuse brain edema, the infarcted cortical tissue will display a particular perish pattern, similar to the perinatal lesion known as ulegyria [34]. The parenchymal consequences of global ischemia, oligemia, or generalized brain hypoxia affect the brain, which have led to the concept of selective vulnerability.

Generally, the neurons are the most vulnerable cells, followed by oligodendrocytes, astrocytes, and mesenchymal cells of the vessel wall. But, in different regions of the brain, even the different neuronal populations have different sensitivities. Most neuronal cell types that are selectively vulnerable to an ischemic-hypoxic insult (pyramidal neurons of hippocampal CA1 and subiculum, Purkinje's cells, neurons in neocortical layers three and five, medium-sized neurons of striatum, neurons of lateral reticular nucleus of thalamus, septal neurons, and somatostatin neurons of the dentate hilus) have high amounts of glutamate receptors (kainate, *N*-methyl-D-aspartate, and alpha-amino-3-hydroxy-5-methyl-4-isoxazoleproprionic acid). Although most of the neurochemical data are based on experimental models, there is increasing evidence that these concepts are also valid in human stroke or in diffuse anoxic-ischemic encephalopathy (Figure 4.33), which provides the basis for a rational therapeutic neuroprotective approach in ischemic brain disease.

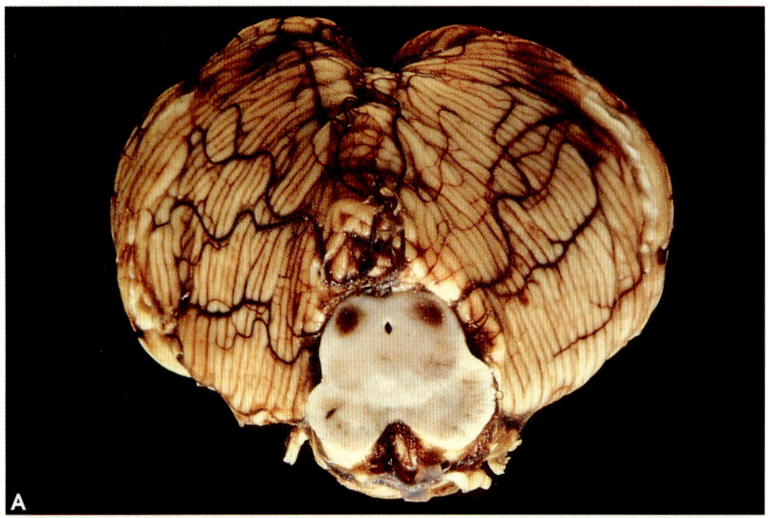

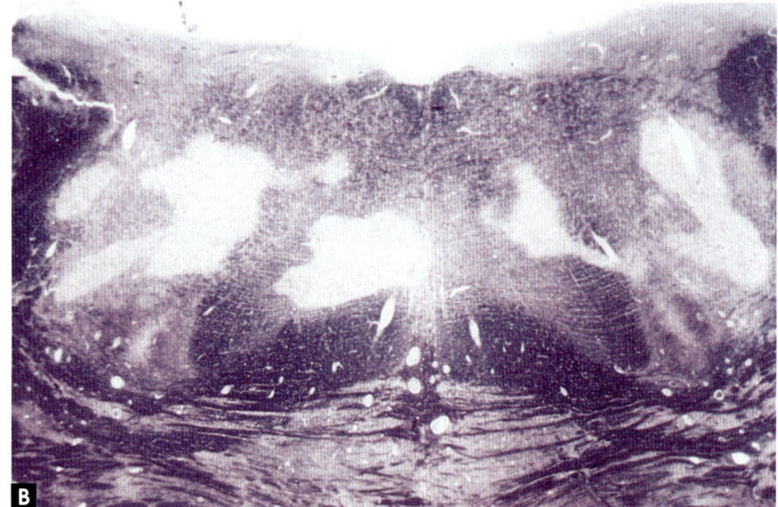

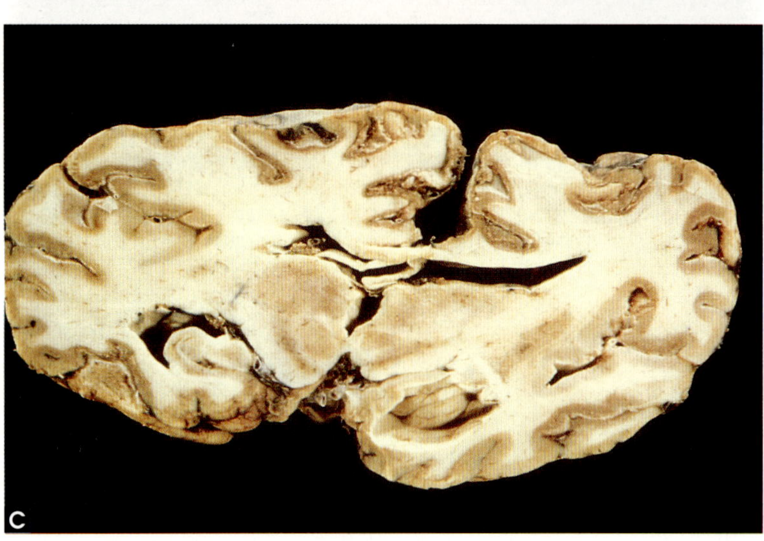

FIGURE 4.33

Neuropathology of ischemic brain lesions caused by generalized ischemia or hypoxia. **A**, Macroscopic aspect of hypotensive brain stem necrosis. **B**, Microscopic aspect of hypotensive brain stem necrosis at pontine tegmentum level (Luxol-Nissl stain). **C**, Macroscopic aspect of severe diffuse anoxic-ischemic encephalopathy (stage II).

REFERENCES

1. Fisher CM: Lacunar infarcts: a review. *Cerebrovasc Dis* 1991, 1:311–320.
2. Bogousslavsky J, Van Melle G, Regli F, for the Lausanne Stroke Registry Group: the Lausanne stroke Registry: Analysis of 1000 consecutive patients with first stroke. *Stroke* 1988, 19:1083–1092.
3. Bogousslavsky J, Regli F, Maeder P, Meuli R, Nader J: The etiology of posterior circulation infarcts: a prospective study using MRI and MR angiography. *Neurology* 1993, 43:1528-1533.
4. Bogousslavsky J, Van Melle G, Regli F: Middle cerebral artery–pial territory infarcts: a study of the Lausanne Stroke Registry. *Ann Neurol* 1989, 25:555–560.
5. Orgogozo JM, Bogousslavsky J: Lacunar syndromes. In *Handbook of Clinical Neurology: Vascular Diseases. Part 2.* Edited by Vinken PJ, Bruyn GW, Klawans HL, Toole JF. Amsterdam: Elsevier Science Publishers: 1989:235–269.
6. Donnan GA, Bladin PF, Berkovic SF, Langley WA, Saling MM: The stroke syndrome of striatocapsular infarction. *Brain* 1991, 114:51–70.
7. Caplan LR: Intracranial branch atheromatous disease: a neglected, understudied, and underused concept. *Neurology* 1989, 39:1246–1250.
8. Bogousslavsky J, Regli F, Maeder P: Intracranial large-artery disease and lacunar infarction. *Cerebrovasc Dis* 1991, 1:154–159.
9. Melo TP, Bogousslavsky J, Van Melle G, Regli F: Pure motor stroke: A reappraisal. *Neurology* 1992, 42:789–795.
10. Helgason CM: A new view of anterior choroidal artery territory infarction. *J Neurol* 1988, 235:387–391.
11. Bogousslavsky J, Regli F: Anterior cerebral artery territory infarction in the Lausanne stroke registry: clinical and etiologic patterns. *Arch Neurol* 1990, 47:144–150.
12. Bogousslavsky J, Regli F: Unilateral watershed cerebral infarcts. *Neurology* 1986, 36:373–377.
13. Sloan MA, Haley EC, Jr.: The syndrome of bilateral hemisphere border zone ischemia. *Stroke* 1990, 21:1668–1673.
14. Weiller C, Ringelstein EB, Reiche W, Buell U: Clinical and hemodynamic aspects of low-flow infarcts. *Stroke* 1991, 22:1117–1123.
15. Waterston JA, Brown MM, Butler P, Swash M: Small deep cerebral infarcts associated with occlusive internal carotid artery disease: a hemodynamic phenomenon? *Arch Neurol* 1990, 47:953–957.
16. Bogousslavsky J: The plurality of subcortical infarction. *Stroke* 1992, 23:629–631.
17. Bogousslavsky J, Regli F: Centrum ovale infarcts: subcortical infarction in the superficial territory in the middle cerebral artery. *Neurology* 1992, 42:1992–1998.
18. Donnan GA, Norrving B, Bamford JM, Bogousslavsky J: Subcortical infarction: classification and terminology. *Cerebrovasc Dis* 1993, 3:248–251.
19. Hebel N, Von Cramon DY: Der Posteriorinfarkt. *Fortschr Neurol Psychiatr* 1987, 55:37–53.
20. Pessin MP, Lathi ES, Cohen MB, Kwan ES, Hedges TR III, Caplan LR: Clinical features and mechanism of occipital infarction. *Ann Neurol* 1987, 21:290–299.
21. Amarenco P, Hauw JJ, Hénin D, *et al.*: Infarctus du territoire de l'artère cérébelleuse postéro-inférieure: etude clinico-pathologique de 28 cas. *Rev Neurol* 1989, 145:277–288.
22. Barth A, Bogousslavsky J, Regli F: The clinical and topographic spectrum of cerebellar infarcts: a clinical MRI correlation study. *Ann Neurol* 1993, 33:451–456.
23. Amarenco P, Hauw JJ: Cerebellar infarction in the territory of the anterior and inferior cerebellar artery: a clinico-pathological study of 20 cases. *Brain* 1990, 113:139–155.
24. Struck LK, Biller J, Bruno A, *et al.*: Superior cerebellar artery territory infarction. *Cerebrovasc Dis* 1991, 1:71–75.
25. Amarenco P, Caplan LR: Vertebrobasilar occlusive disease: Review of selected aspects, 3. Mechanism of cerebellar infarctions. *Cerebrovasc Dis* 1993, 3:66–73.
26. Caplan LR. "Top of the basilar" syndrome. *Neurology* 1980, 30:72–79.
27. Bogousslavsky J: Double infarction in one cerebral hemisphere. *Ann Neurol* 1991, 30:12–18.
28. Besson G, Bogousslavsky J, Regli F, Maeder P: Acute pseudo-bulbar and suprabulbar palsy. *Arch Neurol* 1991, 48:501–507.
29. Graham DI: Hypoxia and vascular disorders. In *Greenfield's Neuropathology*, 5th ed. Edited by Adams JH, Duchen LW. London: Edward Arnold; 1992:153–368.
30. Garcia JH: The evolution of brain infarcts: a review. *J Neuropathol Exp Neurol* 1992, 51:387–393.
31. Neurobiology of ischemic brain damage. In *Progress in Brain Research*, vol 96. Edited by Kogure K, Hossmann KA, Siesjö BK. Amsterdam: Elsevier Science Publishers; 1993.
32. Miklossy J, Van der Loos H: The long-distance effects of brain lesions: visualization of myelinated pathways in the human brain using polarising and fluorescence microscopy. *J Neuropathol Exp Neurol* 1991, 50:1–15.
33. Janzer RC, Friede RL: Hypotensive brain stem necrosis or cardiac arrest encephalopathy? *Acta Neuropathol (Berl)* 1980, 50:53–56.
34. Janzer RC, Friede RL: Perisulcal infarcts: lesions caused by hypotension during increased intracranial pressure. *Ann Neurol* 1979, 6:399–404.
35. Bogousslavsky J, Hommel M: Ischemic stroke syndromes: clinical features, anatomy, vascular territories. In *Handbook of Cerebrovascular Diseases.* Edited by Adams HP, Jr. New York: Marcel Dekker, Inc., 1993:51.
36. Bogousslavsky J, Meienberg O: Eye-movement disorders in brain-stem and cerebellar stroke. *Arch Neurol* 1987, 44:141–148.
37. Bogousslavsky J: Subcortical infarcts. In *Current Review of Cerebrovascular Disease.* Edited by Fisher M, Bogousslavsky J. Philadelphia: Current Medicine; 1993:31–40.

Chapter 5

Subarachnoid Hemorrhage

JEFFREY C. CURTIN
MICHAEL A. KELLY

Aneurysmal dilatation of intracranial blood vessels may arise from any of several etiologies. Berry aneurysms are the most common type and are responsible for the large majority of aneurysmal subarachnoid hemorrhages. Although sometimes referred to as congenital, they are rarely found in children. Some aneurysms may assume giant proportions (*ie*, greater than 25 mm in diameter) and cause symptoms on the basis of compression of neighboring brain structures. When such size is attained they are called giant aneurysms. Atherosclerosis may result in aneurysmal dilatation of intracranial vessels. Bleeding from these aneurysms is uncommon but may compress and distort surrounding brain structures. Thromboembolism and aneurysmal extension into penetrating arteries may result in symptoms of cerebral ischemia. Mycotic aneurysms are the result of septic emboli to more distal cerebral vessels and have the potential for rupture.

EPIDEMIOLOGY

Nontraumatic subarachnoid hemorrhage (SAH) comprises about 5% of all strokes with an incidence of 3.9 to 19.4 per 100,000 population [1–3]. Rupture of a berry aneurysm accounts for as many as 80% of cases [4]. Autopsy-based studies indicate that up to 2% to 5% of the population harbors an unruptured aneurysm. Thus, as many as 5 million North Americans may be at risk for rupture [1,4,5]. The peak incidence for rupture is between the ages of 55 and 60 [6]. Aneurysmal subarachnoid hemorrhage in children is rare, occurring most commonly in vascular trauma, infection, and metabolic connective tissue disease [7].

Berry Aneurysms

Berry aneurysms are found near the circle of Willis at the bifurcation of large arteries and rupture into the subarachnoid space. Although berry aneurysms are distributed throughout the circle of Willis, about 85% are found in the anterior circulation and the remainder in the posterior circulation (Figures 5.1 and 5.2). The pathologic process that results in the formation of a berry aneurysm is not clearly understood. The congenital theory advocates that the aneurysm develops due to a congenital defect in the media of the arterial wall [8]. This hypothesis was ultimately abandoned because much of the evidence was circumstantial and could not be supported scientifically. It has now been replaced by the degenerative theory that advocates that aneurysm formation occurs from degenerative changes induced by hemodynamic stress. Since berry aneurysms occur at the bifurcations of basal arteries, it is felt that this is an area of hemodynamic stress that could lead to mural atrophy and aneurysm formation [7]. Hypertension and atherosclerotic changes are the presumed stressors and have been substantiated as such in animal studies [9,10]. Berry aneurysms have been associated with coarctation of the aorta and polycystic kidney disease, both of which are congenital conditions. They are also associated with hemodynamic stress due to profound hypertension that may be sufficient to cause disruption of the elastic layers of the artery leading to aneurysm formation [7].

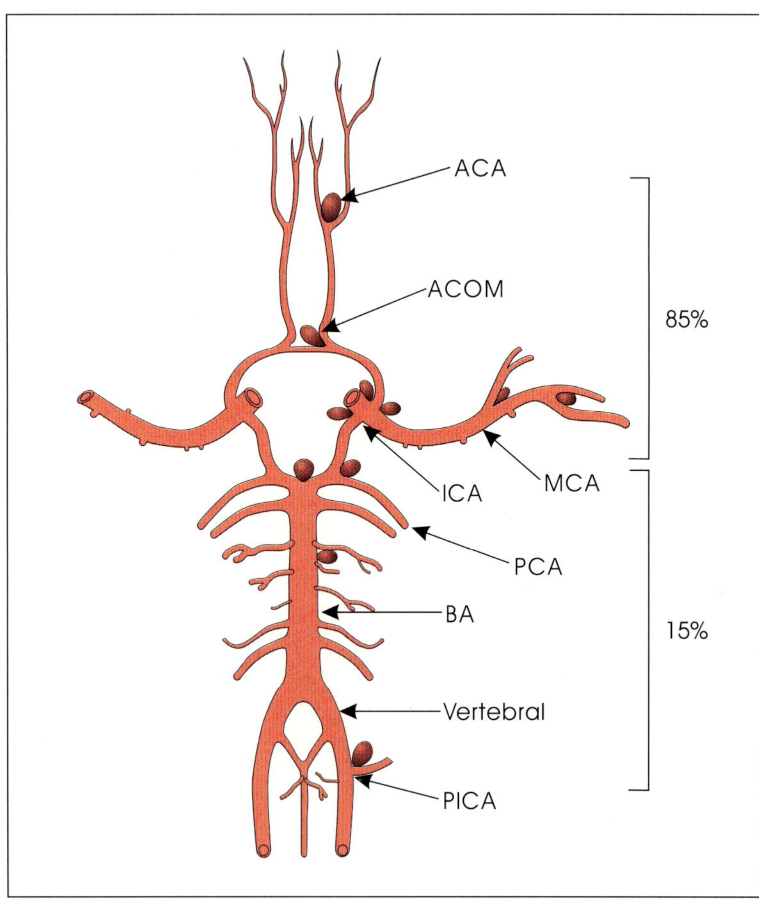

FIGURE 5.1

Circle of Willis and distribution of berry aneurysms. About 85% are located in the anterior circle (carotid territory) and about 15% are located in the posterior circle (vertebrobasilar territory). ACA—anterior cerebral artery; ACOM—anterior communicating artery; BA—basilar artery; ICA—internal carotid artery; MCA—middle cerebral artery; PCA—posterior cerebral artery; PICA—posterior inferior cerebellar artery.

Giant Aneurysms

The term *giant aneurysm* is reserved for those aneurysms with diameters greater than 25 mm [11]. They are three times as common in women than men and present most often between the ages of 30 and 60 years [12]. Giant aneurysms often present with symptoms of mass effect rather than subarachnoid hemorrhage (Figures 5.3 and 5.4). Ocular motor palsies, progressive hemiparesis, visual loss, and chronic headache are signs associated with anterior circulation giant aneurysm. Cranial nerve palsies and long tract signs are associated with posterior circulation aneurysm. Stagnation of blood flow within the aneurysm may induce formation of thrombus and subsequent embolism causing symptoms of cerebral ischemia distant from the site of the aneurysm. Although it is widely held that giant aneurysms bleed only rarely, studies have demonstrated subarachnoid hemorrhage in 30% to 80% of cases [11,13–16].

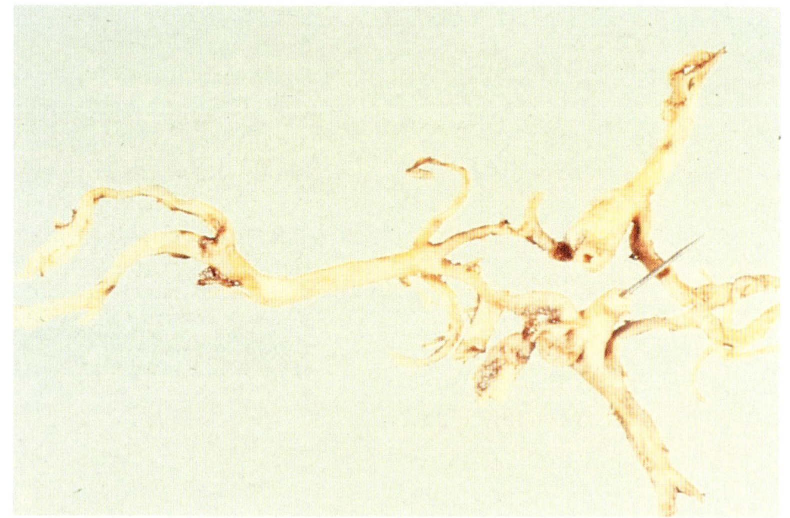

FIGURE 5.2

Autopsy specimen demonstrating a berry aneurysm of the right internal carotid artery.

MYCOTIC ANEURYSMS

Mycotic or infectious aneurysms are an uncommon cause of aneurysmal subarachnoid hemorrhage and account for about 5% of all intracranial aneurysms [17]. Since first described by Osler in 1881 [18], the term *mycotic* has been a source of confusion, as fungus is rarely if ever the infecting agent. Most cases of mycotic aneurysms are due to complications of infectious endocarditis with *Streptococcus* and *Staphylococcus* organisms being the most common agents. Mycotic aneurysms are located in cerebral artery branches distal from the circle of Willis as would be expected from their embolic origin.

The development of a mycotic aneurysm is a result of septic embolization. It is presumed that septic emboli become lodged in a distal segment of an artery or embolize into the vasovasorum. Exactly which mechanism is responsible is not clear, and certainly both may contribute. Once this process is established, the septic emboli cause degeneration of the vessel wall [19]. Molinari [19], who carried out sophisticated studies of mycotic aneurysm formation in rats, showed that injection of emboli infected with *Staphylococcus aureus* could result in aneurysm formation in as little as 24 hours with rapid progression to death if untreated.

ATHEROSCLEROTIC ANEURYSMS

Arteriosclerotic or dolichoectatic aneurysms are fusiform dilatations of intracerebral arteries attributed to long-standing hypertension resulting from breakdown of the elastic lamina and muscularis layer. The large basal arteries are most often involved, most commonly the basilar, but the internal carotid and anterior, and middle cerebral arteries may also be involved [20,21]. They rarely cause subarachnoid hemorrhage but may cause symptoms by compression of neighboring structures or by thromboembolism [22].

PATHOPHYSIOLOGY OF VASOSPASM

Since the first clinical description of vasospasm in 1951, the ischemic consequences have been recognized as a major source of delayed morbidity and mortality following aneurysmal subarachnoid hemorrhage [23,24]. Vasospasm can be defined by clinical, angiographic, or Doppler criteria. Angiographic studies have shown vasospasm in 30% to 70% of cases studied between 4 and 14 days [25]. The diagnosis of angiographic vasospasm has been made as early as 1 minute and as late as 3 weeks postrupture [26,27].

Several types of arteriographic vasospasm have been identified: diffuse, segmental, and local. In the diffuse form of vasospasm, all arteries are affected with essentially the same caliber of narrowing. The segmental form of vasospasm gives a sausage-like appearance to the artery. The local form of spasm is usually restricted to a vessel in close proximity to the site of aneurysm rupture [27]. Vasospasm can also be defined sonographically with the aid of transcranial Doppler (TCD) ultrasonography. TCD has become a valuable noninvasive technology for the assessment of vasospasm since its first clinical application in 1982 [28]. In the years since TCD was first used numerous reports have documented the correlation between angiographic vasospasm and increased flow velocities. Several studies have shown a correlation between increasing flow velocities in the middle cerebral artery and the degree of arterial narrowing [29,30]. In our blood flow laboratory we have found it useful to look at flow velocities in the basilar artery and the internal carotid artery at the siphon (Figure 5.5). Controversy exists, however, about its ability to predict delayed ischemic consequences [31].

Although the exact cause of vasospasm remains unknown, the presence of blood or one of its components in the subarachnoid space has long been implicated. In the past, vasospasm was attributed solely to arterial smooth muscle contraction. This

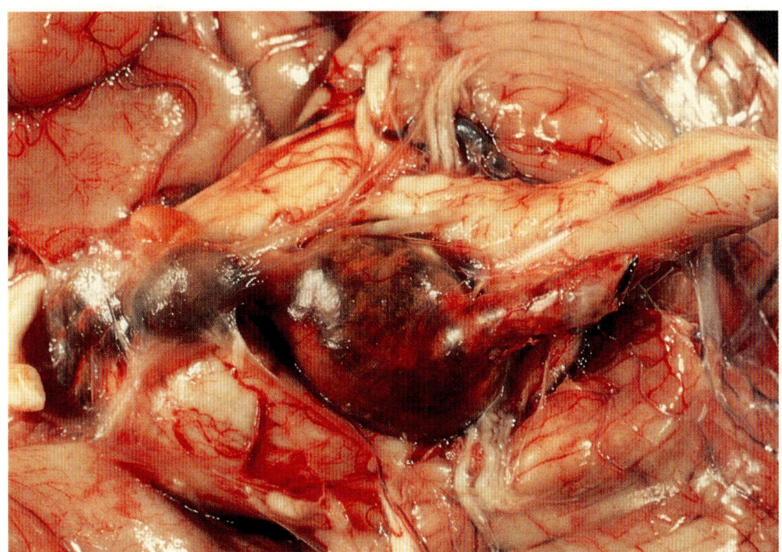

FIGURE 5.3

Autopsy specimen of a giant aneurysm of the basilar artery with associated compression of surrounding brain structures.

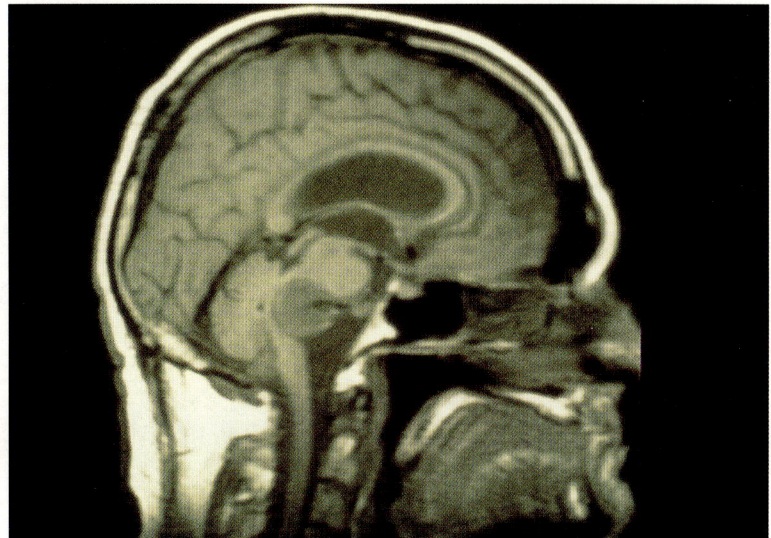

FIGURE 5.4

Antemortem magnetic resonance image of same case clearly demonstrates compression of the brain stem.

hypothesis led to numerous studies involving vasoactive amines, prostaglandins, and immunoreactive agents including complement C3 and IgG as potential causes. Vasospasm due to the production of red blood cell lysis was demonstrated in experimental animals as early as 1940 [32]. These substances need to be present in greater than physiologic amounts and are metabolized too rapidly to exert a sustained effect. One could argue that if these substances resided in a clot in high concentrations and were protected from metabolism, they could exert an effect. This seems reasonable as vasospasm tends to occur in vessels that are in close proximity to the clot. Nonetheless, numerous trials involving antispasmodic agents have been ineffective in treating vasospasm. This argues against smooth muscle contraction as being the sole cause, and one must look to other possibilities. Arteriopathy associated with subarachnoid hemorrhage has been described, and along with vasoconstriction, may contribute to vasospasm [33,34]. The triad of subintimal edema, myonecrosis, and leukocytic infiltration are found in the affected vessels and may explain why trials of antispasmodic agents are ineffective.

Contemporary studies have shown that injection of autologous red blood cells into the subarachnoid space does not result in vasospasm, but when the hemolysate of the red blood cells is injected, severe vasospasm occurs [35]. Several lines of evidence suggest that oxyhemoglobin, a potent vasoconstrictor, may be the offending agent. The presence of oxyhemoglobin could trigger a cascade involving phospholipid peroxidation in the vessel wall generating hydroperoxides and leukotrienes [36,37]. The subsequent free radical formation could lead to morphologic changes in the vessel wall [38]. Although this is an attractive hypothesis, it probably is only a small piece of the puzzle. The presence of blood in the subarachnoid space does not cause vasospasm by itself because most cases of nonaneurysmal subarachnoid hemorrhage do not lead to vasospasm, nor do operative procedures involving the brain that leave blood in the subarachnoid space. Thus, it seems that for vasospasm to occur there must be aneurysm rupture as well as subarachnoid blood [39].

LUMBAR PUNCTURE IN SUBARACHNOID HEMORRHAGE

Prior to the development of computed tomography (CT), lumbar puncture was the key to the diagnosis of subarachnoid hemorrhage. Because 10% of subarachnoid hemorrhage may be CT-negative, lumbar puncture remains important today [40]. CT may not demonstrate blood if the bleed is of small volume, severe anemia is present, or the time elapsed does not allow blood to settle into the spinal subarachnoid space.

Xanthochromia refers to the pigmentation of bloody cerebrospinal fluid (CSF), and it is usually yellow in color. Xanthochromia occurs when there is a release of pigments from lysed red blood cells. It is found in the supernatant of the sample and is highly suggestive of subarachnoid hemorrhage. Spectrophotometric studies have established oxyhemoglobin, bilirubin, and methemoglobin as the agents causing xanthochromia [41–45].

Traumatic Lumbar Puncture Versus Subarachnoid Hemorrhage

The traumatic or bloody tap is not an uncommon event when performing a lumbar puncture, and adds considerable confusion in the diagnosis of subarachnoid hemorrhage. When blood is encountered at the time of lumbar puncture the sample should be centrifuged and the supernatant compared to water. If the supernatant is clear the blood is probably due to a traumatic tap. If, on the other hand, the supernatant is xanthochromatic, subarachnoid hemorrhage is likely. However, this rule is not absolute as adequate time must pass to release red blood cell pigments through cell lysis. The supernatant may remain clear for 2 to 4 hours or as long as 12 hours after subarachnoid hemorrhage before cell lysis occurs [46,47]. Xanthochromia may persist for 3 weeks following SAH [46]. If the fluid is xanthochromic and the diagnosis of SAH is doubtful, one must rule out other causes including: 1) hyper-

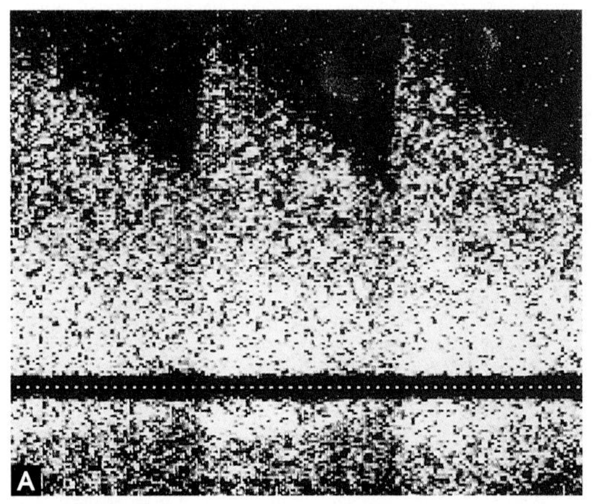

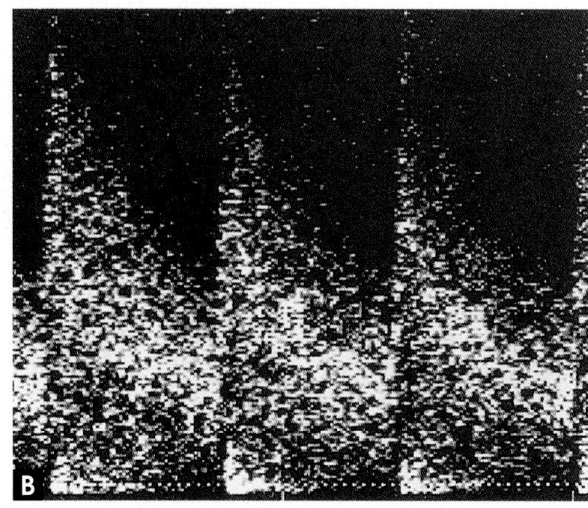

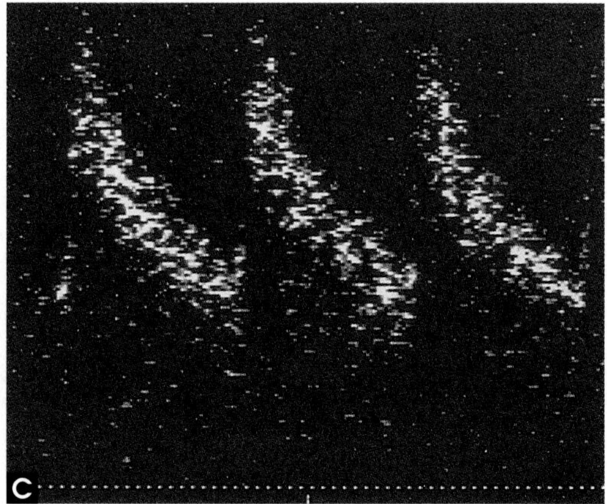

FIGURE 5.5

Transcranial Doppler of a patient in vasospasm demonstrates markedly increased flow velocities in the middle cerebral artery (**A**), internal carotid artery (**B**), and basilar artery (**C**).

carotenemia; 2) rifampin use; 3) malignant melanosis; and 4) CSF protein > 150 mg/dL.

The three-tube method is performed by collecting three consecutive tubes of CSF and obtaining a cell count on each tube. A declining trend in the number of red blood cells from tubes one to three suggests a traumatic tap (Figure 5.6). If there is remaining doubt, then four-vessel cerebral angiography should be considered to rule out aneurysm.

PATHOPHYSIOLOGY OF HYDROCEPHALUS

Hydrocephalus is a commonly encountered problem following subarachnoid hemorrhage and may be acute or delayed. Acute hydrocephalus occurs during the first 1 to 7 days following hemorrhage in 9% to 67% of cases [48]. This variability is in part due to differences in diagnostic criteria. Surprisingly, acute hydrocephalus as a complication of subarachnoid hemorrhage was rarely recognized prior to the CT era. The progressive ventricular dilation seems to arrest after the first few days after hemorrhage and remains static. Two factors that may contribute to this new equilibrium are transependymal reabsorption of CSF, and decreased production of CSF at the choroid plexus secondary to increased intracranial pressure [49,50]. The decision to divert the CSF is controversial. However, an increased bicaudate diameter by CT scan with a normal level of consciousness probably does not require diversion. A declining level of consciousness and impairment of upward gaze are signs of worsening hydrocephalus and CSF shunting may be indicated.

The presence of intraventricular blood correlates with the development of hydrocephalus [51]. Thus, it appears that most cases of acute hydrocephalus are communicating, but noncommunicating hydrocephalus may be seen. However, cases of hydrocephalus due to nonaneurysmal subarachnoid hemorrhage involving the perimesencephalic cistern and sparing the ventricles, suggest that clots at the tentorial hiatus may also lead to acute obstruction [52].

DELAYED HYDROCEPHALUS

Delayed hydrocephalus describes the condition in which hydrocephalus develops weeks or months after the initial hemorrhage. In general, hydrocephalus occurring beyond 10 to 14 days can be thought of as delayed. The main difference between the two lies in the pathology. Acute hydrocephalus is usually an obstructive or noncommunicating hydrocephalus, whereas delayed hydrocephalus is typically a communicating hydrocephalus. The probable site of obstruction is the arachnoid granulations (Figure 5.7), and pathologic studies have demonstrated the presence of hemosiderin-laden macrophages as well as adhesions involving the pia and arachnoid layers [53,54].

NEUROCARDIOLOGY

Cardiovascular abnormalities are a frequent occurrence following aneurysmal subarachnoid hemorrhage and were first reported in 1959 [55]. Electrocardiographic changes are paramount and include ischemic ST segment changes, prolonged Q-Tc interval, prominent U waves, and T wave alterations (Figure 5.8) [56]. In addition to these findings, disturbances of cardiac rhythm can be seen including malignant rhythms such as torsades de pointe, ventricular tachycardia, and ventricular fibrillation [57]. Other more benign conduction disturbances are frequent findings and include atrial fibrillation, premature ventricular complexes, and supraventricular tachycardia.

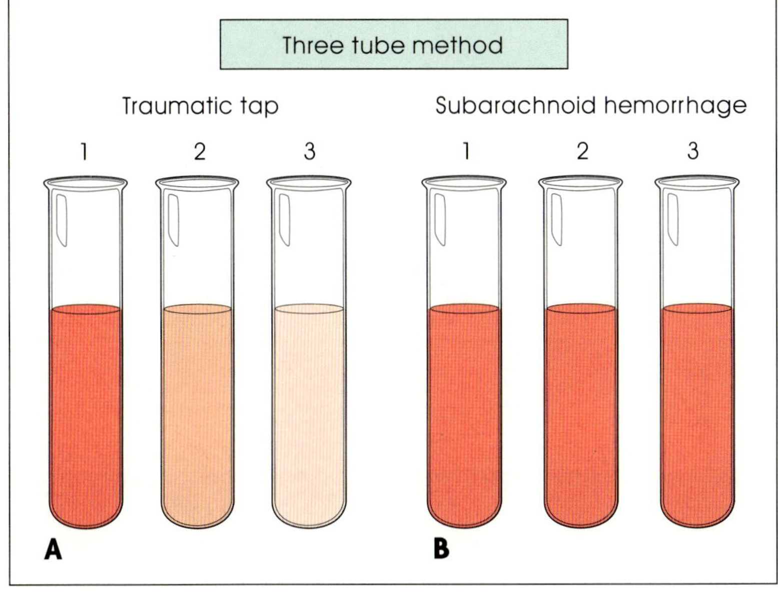

FIGURE 5.6

A, Traumatic tap. Gradual reduction in color and number of red blood cells from tubes one to three. **B**, Subarachnoid hemorrhage. No change in color and number of red blood cells from tubes one to three.

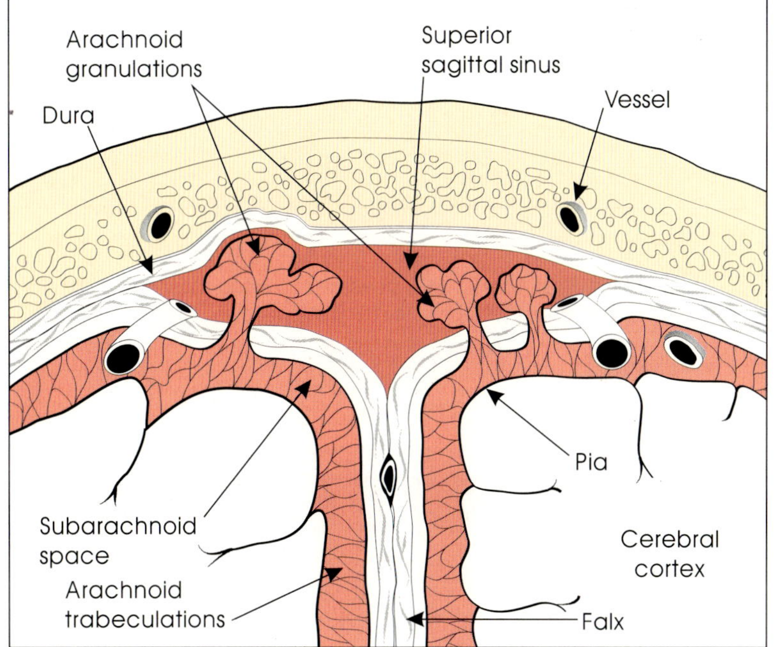

FIGURE 5.7

Coronal depiction of arachnoid granulations where cerebrospinal fluid is reabsorbed.

The presumed mechanism for the electrocardiographic changes is thought to be related to subendocardial ischemia of the left ventricle [58,59]. Animal studies have shown that lesions of the hypothalamus may result in comparable cardiac lesions. Stimulation of the posterior hypothalamus results in the release of enormous amounts of norepinephrine via the thoracolumbar sympathetic outflow tracts [60,61], which may be responsible for the observed responses. Considering the vascular anatomy of the hypothalamus, it is not difficult to imagine that a ruptured aneurysm of the circle of Willis could have adverse consequences. The hypothalamus receives its blood supply from the anteromedial perforators of the anterior cerebral and the anterior communicating arteries. Posteriorly, the hypothalamus is supplied by the posteromedial perforators of the posterior communicating and posterior cerebral arteries.

Thus, the frequently observed cardiovascular abnormalities following aneurysmal subarachnoid hemorrhage could be explained by a ruptured aneurysm involving the circle of Willis producing ischemia to the hypothalamus.

NEUROGENIC PULMONARY EDEMA

In one study [62], neurogenic pulmonary edema occurred in 11% of patients with subarachnoid hemorrhage. The presence of neurogenic pulmonary edema correlated with the severity of the hemorrhage [62]. Neurogenic pulmonary edema differs significantly in pathophysiology from that of cardiac origin. In pulmonary edema of cardiac origin, there is left ventricular dysfunction and elevated end diastolic pressures, leading to an increase in end diastolic volume. Neurogenic pulmonary edema occurs in the setting of a competent heart and therapeutic measures such as diuresis, preload reduction, and ionotropic agents are of no benefit.

As with cardiac disturbances associated with subarachnoid hemorrhage, a very high sympathetic output is probably the cause of neurogenic pulmonary edema. The underlying pathophysiology is the increased capillary permeability to solutes such as proteins resulting in increased oncotic pressure within the interstitial space. The result is an osmotic gradient favoring the transudation of water into the interstitial space and disruption of the normal Starling forces (Figure 5.9) [63]. This probably occurs because of sympathetic innervation to contractile proteins in the vascular endothelium [64,65]. There is also some evidence that sympathetic stimulation may cause lymphatic constriction leading to pulmonary edema [66].

ACKNOWLEDGMENTS

I would like to thank Drs. Raymond Clasen and Elizabeth Cochran for autopsy materials. I would also like to thank Laura Prezpiorka, RN, BSN, for the Doppler spectra and constructive criticism. I would also like to thank Jennifer Valasek for valuable comments and proofreading the manuscript.

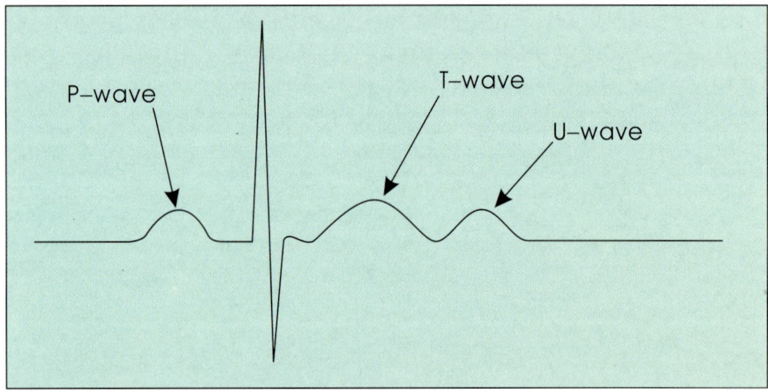

FIGURE 5.8

The U-wave is the deflection (usually positive) following the T-wave and may be prominent following subarachnoid hemorrhage.

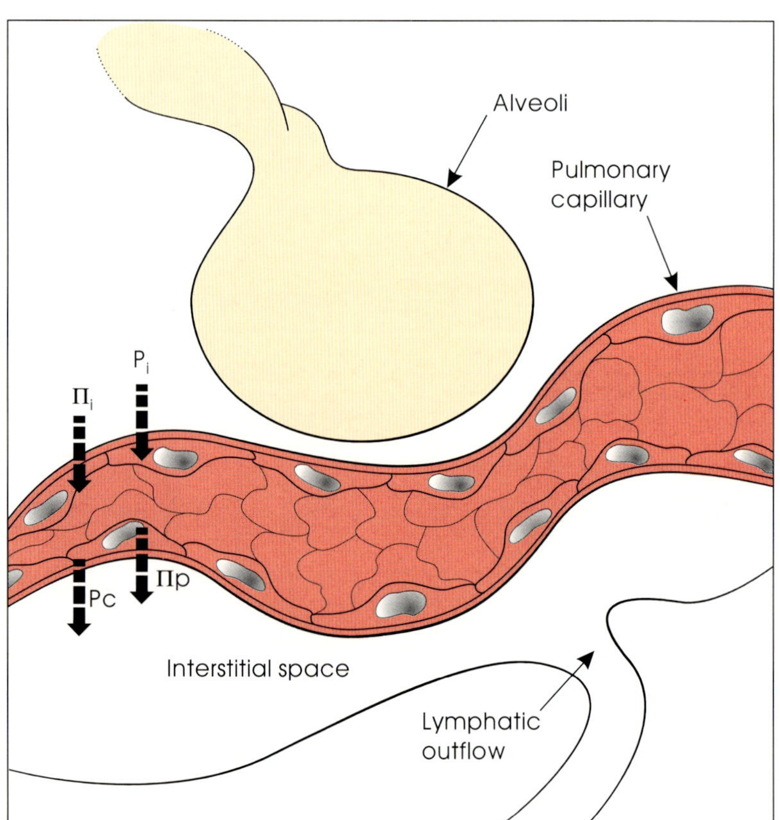

FIGURE 5.9

Starling relationship. P_C—capillary hydrostatic pressure; P_i—interstitial hydrostatic pressure; π_i interstitial oncotic pressure; π_p—capillary oncotic pressure.

REFERENCES

1. Sahs AL: Preface. In *Aneurysmal Subarachnoid Hemorrhage: Report of the Cooperative Study*. Edited by Sahs AL, Nibbelink DW. Baltimore: Urban and Schwarzenberg; 1981:xvii.
2. Peerless SJ, Yasargil MG: Adrenergic innervation of the cerebral blood vessels in the rabbit. *J Neurosurg* 1971, 35:158.
3. Fodstad H, Liliequist B, Schannog M, Thulin CA: Tranexamic acid in the preoperative management of ruptured intracranial aneurysms. *Surg Neurol* 1978, 10:9.
4. Stehbens WE: The pathology of intracranial artery aneurysms and their complications. In *Intracranial Aneurysms, Vol 1*. Edited by Fox JL. New York: Springer Verlag; 1983, 272–357.
5. Ingawa T, Hirano A: Autopsy study of unruptured incidental intracranial aneurysms. *Surg Neurol* 1990, 34:361.
6. Sahs AL, Nibbelink DW, Torner JC, eds.: *Aneurysmal Subarachnoid Hemorrhage: Report of the Cooperative Study*. Baltimore: Urban and Schwarzenberg; 1981.
7. Stehbens WE: Etiology of intracranial berry aneurysms. *J Neurosurg* 1989, 70:823.
8. Forbus WE: On the origin of miliary aneurysms of the superficial cerebral arteries. *Bull John's Hopkins Hos* 1930, 47:239.
9. Stehbens WE: Chronic changes in experimental saccular and fusiform aneurysms in rabbits. *Arch Pathol* 1981, 105:603.
10. Stehbens WE: Experimental arterial loops and arterial atrophy. *Exp Mol Pathol* 1986, 44:177.
11. Locksley HB: Report on the Cooperative Study of Intracranial Aneurysm and Subarachnoid Hemorrhage. Sect.V, Part I: Natural history of subarachnoid hemorrhage, intracranial aneurysms and arteriovenous malformations: based on 6368 cases in the cooperative study. *J Neurosurg* 1966, 25:219.
12. Morley TP, Barr HWK: Giant intracranial aneurysms: diagnosis, course and management. *Clin Neurosurg* 1969, 16:73.
13. Battaglia R, Pasqualin A, DaPian R: Italian Cooperative Study on Giant Intracranial Aneurysms. 1. Study design and clinical data. *Acta Neurochir (Wien)* 1988, 42(suppl):49.
14. Drake CG: Giant intracranial aneurysms: experience with surgical treatment in 174 patients. *Clin Neurosurg* 1979, 26:12.
15. Onuma T, Suzuki J: Surgical treatment of giant intracranial aneurysms. *J Neurosurg* 1979, 51:33.
16. Wittle IR, Dorsch NW, Besser M: Giant intracranial aneurysms diagnosis, management and outcome. *Surg Neurol* 1984, 21:218.
17. Krinsky LM, Merrit HH: Neurologic manifestations of SBE. *N Engl J Med* 1938, 218:563.
18. Osler W: Gulstonian lectures on malignant endocarditis. *Lancet* 1885, 1:393.
19. Molinari GF,*et al.*: Pathogenesis of cerebral mycotic aneurysms. *Neurology* 1973, 23:4, 325.
20. Yates PO: Vascular disease of the nervous system. In *Greenfields Textbook of Neuropathology*. Year Book Medical Publishers, Inc.; 1977:87.
21. Garcia CA, Dulcey S, Dulcey J: Ruptured aneurysm of the sinal artery of Adamkiewicz during pregnancy. *Neurology* 1977, 29:394.
22. Mohr JP, Kistler JP, Fink ME: Intracranial aneurysms. In *Stroke Pathophysiology, Diagnosis and Management, 2nd ed.* Edited by Barnett HJM, Mohr JP, Stein BM, Yatsu FM. New York: Churchill Livingstone; 1992:620.
23. Kassell NF, Sasaki T, Colohan ART, Nazar G: Cerebral vasospasm following aneurysmal subarachnoid hemorrhage. *Stroke* 1985, 16:562.
24. Ecker A, Reimenschneider PA: Arteriographic demonstration of spasm of the intracranial arteries with special reference to saccular arterial aneurysms. *J Neurosurg* 1951, 8:660.
25. Heros RC, Zervas NT, Varsos V: Cerebral vasospasm after subarachnoid hemorrhage: an update. *Ann Neurol* 1983, 14:599.
26. Weir B, Grace M, Hansen J, Rothberg C: Time course of vasospasm in man. *J Neurosurg* 1978, 48:173.
27. Taneda M, Otsuki H, Kumura E, Sakaguci T: Angiographic demonstration of acute phase of intracranial arterial spasm following aneurysm rupture. *J Neurosurg* 1990, 73:958.
28. Aaslid R, Markwalder TM, Nornes H: Noninvasive transcranial Doppler ultrasound recording of flow velocity in basal cerebral arteries. *J Neurosurg* 1982, 57:769.
29. Aaslid R, Huber P, Nornes H: Musical murmurs in human cerebral arteries after subarachnoid hemorrhage. *J Neurosurg* 1984, 60:32.
30. Sloan MA, *et al.*: Sensitivity and specificity of transcranial Doppler ultrasonography in the diagnosis of vasospasm following subarachnoid hemorrhage. *Neurology* 1989, 39:1514.
31. Laumer R, *et al.*: Cerebral hemodynamics in subarachnoid hemorrhage evaluated by transcranial Doppler sonography: Part 1. Reliability of flow velocities and clinical management. *Neurosurgery* 1993, 33:1.
32. Zucker MB: A study of the substances in blood serum and platelets which stimulate smooth muscle. *Am J Physiol* 1944, 142:12.
33. Crompton MR: Cerebral infarction following the rupture of cerebral berry aneurysms. *Brain* 1964, 87:491.
34. Connay LW, McDonald LW: Structural changes of the intradural arteries following subarachnoid hemorrhage. *J Neurosurg* 1972, 34:715.
35. Jackson IJ: Aseptic homogenic meningitis: an experimental study of aseptic meningeal reactions due to blood and its breakdown products. *Arch Neurol Psych* 1949, 62:572.
36. Paoletti P, Gaetani P, Grignani G, *et al.*: CSF leukotriene C4 following subarachnoid. *J Neurosurg* 1988, 69:488.
37. Saski T, Wakai S, Asano T, *et al.*: The effect of lipid hydroperoxide of arachidonic acid on the canine basilar artery: an experimental study on cerebral vasospasm. *J Neurosurg* 1981, 54:357.
38. Peterson JW, Roussos L, Kwun BD, *et al.*: Evidence of the role of hemolysis in experimental cerebral vasospasm. *J Neurosurg* 1990, 72:775.
39. Vermuelen M, Lindsay KW, Van Gijin J: Cerebral ischemia. In *Subarachnoid Hemorrhage*. Philadelphia: WB Saunders Co.; 1992:74–75.
40. Savoiardo M, Grisoli M; Computed tomography scanning. In *Stroke: Pathophysiology, Diagnosis and Management, 2nd ed.* Edited by Barnett HJM, Mohr JP, Stein BM. New York: Churchill Livingstone; 1992:174.
41. Barrows LJ, Hunter FT, Baker BQ: The nature and clinical significance of pigments in the cerebral spinal fluid. *Brain* 1955, 78:59.
42. Van Der Meulen JP: Cerebral spinal fluid xanthochromia: an objective index. *Neurology* 1966, 16:170.
43. Kreig AF: Cerebral spinal fluid and other body fluids. In *Clinical Diagnosis and Management by Laboratory Methods, 16th ed.* Edited by Henry JB. Philadelphia: WB Saunders; 1979:635–657.
44. Kjellin KG: Xanthochromic compounds in cerebral spinal fluid: quantitative spectrophotometry and electromigration. In *Neurobiology of Cerebral Spinal Fluid, Vol 2*. Edited by Wood J. New York: Plenum Press; 1980:559–570.
45. Britton M, Hultman E, Murray V, *et al.*: The diagnostic accuracy of CSF analysis in stroke. *Acta Med Scand* 1983, 214:3.
46. Fishman RA, ed.: *Cerebral Spinal Fluid in Diseases of the Nervous System*, ed. 2. Philadelphia: WB Saunders; 1992.
47. Walton JN, ed.: *Subarachnoid Hemorrhage*. Edinburgh: Livingstone; 1956.
48. Hasan D, Vermuelen M, Wijdicks EFM, *et al.*: Management problems in acute hydrocephalus after subarachnoid hemorrhage. *Stroke* 1989, 20:747.
49. Millhorat TH: Acute hydrocephalus. *N Engl J Med* 1970, 283:857.

50. Sahar A: The effects of pressure on the production of CSF by the choroid plexus. *J Neurolog Sci* 1972, 16:49.
51. Vermuelen M, Lindsay KW, Van Gijin J: Hydrocephalus. In *Subarachnoid Hemorrhage*. Philadelphia: WB Saunders Co.; 1992:87–99.
52. Rinkel GJE, Wijdicks EFM, Vermuelen M, *et al.*: Acute hydrocephalus in non aneurysmal perimesencephalic hemorrhage: evidence of CSF block at the tentorial hiatus. *Neurology* 1992, 242:623.
53. Kibler RF, Couch RSC, Crompton MR: Hydrocephalus in the adult following subarachnoid hemorrhage. *Brain* 1961, 84:45.
54. Ellington E, Margolis G: Block of the arachnoid villus by subarachnoid hemorrhage. *J Neurosurg* 1969, 30:305.
55. Beard EF, Robertson JW, Robertson RCL: Spontaneous subarachnoid hemorrhage simulating acute myocardial infarction. *Am Heart J* 1959, 58:755.
56. Vermeulen M, Lindsay KW, Van Gijn J: Medical complications. In *Subarachnoid Hemorrhage*. Philadelphia: WB Saunders Co.; 1992:103–106.
57. Marion DW, Segal RS, Thomson ME: Subarachnoid hemorrhage and the heart. *Neurosurgery* 1986, 18:101.
58. Smith RP, Tomlinson BE: Subendocardial hemorrhages associated with intracranial lesions. *J Pathol Bacteriol* 1954, 68:327.
59. Attar HJ, Gutierrez MR, Bellet S, Ravens JR: Effects of stimulation of the hypothalamus and reticular activating system on production of cardiac arrhythmias. *Circ Res* 1963, 12:14.
60. Melville KI, Blum B, Shister HE, Silver MD: Cardiac ischemic changes and arrhythmias induced by hypothalamic stimulation. *Am J Cardiol* 1963, 12:781.
61. Goldfien A, Ganong WF: Adrenal medullary and adrenal cortical response to stimulation of diencephalon. *Am J Physiol* 1962, 202:205.
62. Theordore J, Robin ED: Pathogenesis of neurogenic pulmonary oedema. *Lancet* 1975, ii:749.
63. Malik AB: Mechanisms of neurogenic pulmonary edema. *Circ Res* 1985, 57:1.
64. Simon RP, Bayne LL: Pulmonary lymphatic flow alterations during intracranial hypertension in sheep. *Ann Neurol* 1984, 15:188.
65. Rosell S: Neuronal control of microvessels. *Ann Rev Physiol* 1980, 42:359.
66. McHale NG, Roddie IC: Peripheral lymph flow during intravenous noradrenalin infusion in sheep [abstract]. *J Physiol* 1983, 50:334.

Chapter 6

Neuropathology and Pathophysiology of Intraparenchymal Hemorrhage

JANET L. WILTERDINK
EDWARD FELDMANN

Spontaneous, intraparenchymal hemorrhage (IPH) accounts for 10% to 15% of all strokes. Many etiologies of IPH are identified by their epidemiologic association, such as the high incidence of hypertension among patients with IPH. In most IPHs, there is very little direct evidence for the mechanism of hemorrhage. Prior to IPH, underlying causative conditions such as an arteriovenous malformation or amyloid angiopathy are often unsuspected. Putative precipitants, such as physical exertion, are also retrospectively identified. Finally, the brain parenchyma underlying the IPH is damaged by the hemorrhage, making its pathology difficult to define. Nonetheless, a wealth of indirect evidence, including epidemiologic data, pathologic examination of vessels remote from the hemorrhage in the same individual or in individuals without hemorrhage but with the same underlying condition, and studies in animal models have contributed to our understanding of the pathophysiology of IPH.

PATHOPHYSIOLOGY OF INTRAPARENCHYMAL HEMORRHAGE

The mechanisms underlying intraparenchymal hemorrhage (IPH) fall into three general categories (Figure 6.1). The first is an abnormality of the cerebral vessel wall. A variety of pathologic abnormalities of the cerebral vessel wall weaken its structure and make it susceptible to rupture. Some of these are congenital, such as arteriovenous malformations. Hypertensive arteropathy, amyloid angiopathy, and inflammatory vasculitides (Table 6.1) (Figure 6.2) are acquired conditions that damage and weaken cerebral vessel walls. Intracerebral neoplasms and Moyamoya disease produce new cerebral blood vessels that are structurally weak and prone to hemorrhage. Cerebral infarction and prolonged vasospasm in subarachnoid hemorrhage or migraine may cause ischemic injury of cerebral vessel walls leading to rupture and IPH in some patients [1].

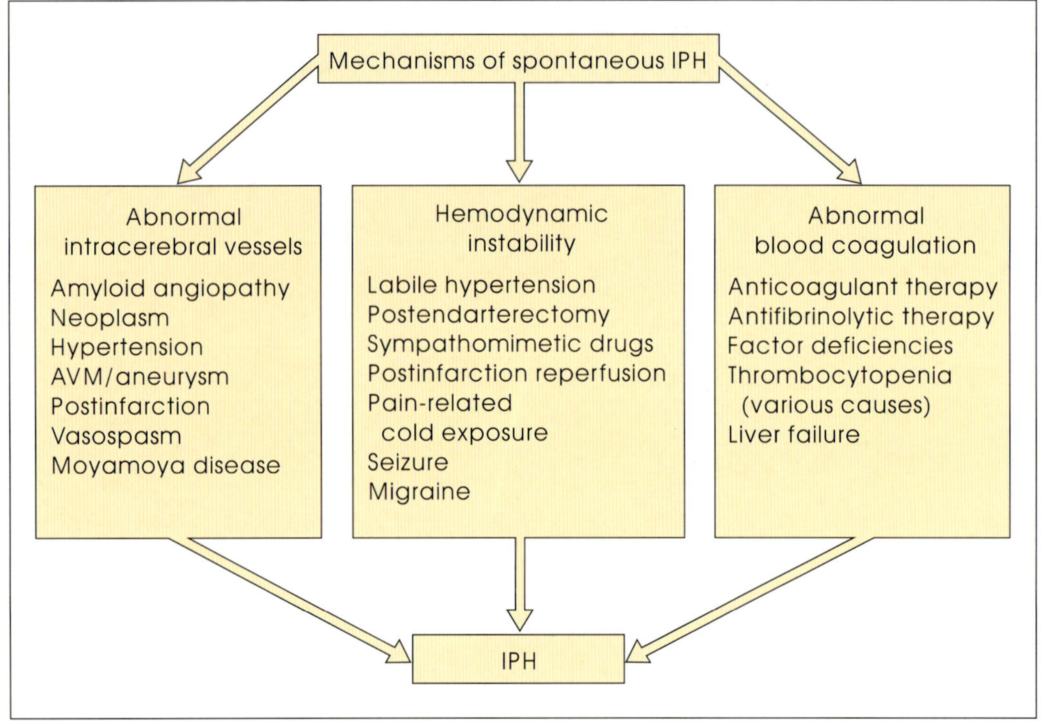

FIGURE 6.1

Mechanisms of intraparenchymal hemorrhage (IPH). AVM—arteriovenous malformation.

Table 6.1. Inflammatory vasculitides associated with intraparenchymal hemorrhage*

Polyarteritis nodosa
Churg-Strauss
Wegener's granulomatosis
Sarcoidosis
Systemic lupus erythematosus
Rheumatoid vasculitis†
Scleroderma
Polymyositis
Ulcerative colitis
Takayasu's arteritis
Varicella-zoster
Behcet's disease
Primary central nervous system vasculitis
Drug-related

**Data from* Cohen and Biller [138], and Petty and Mohr [139].

†*See* Fig. 6.2.

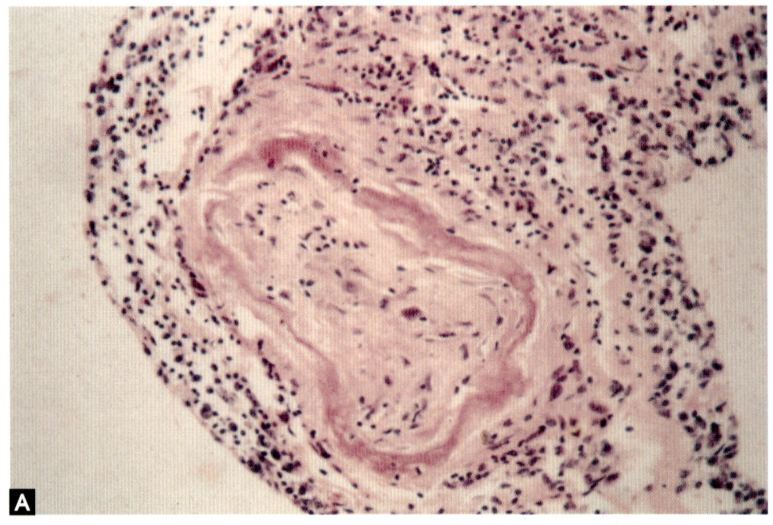

FIGURE 6.2

Cerebral vasculitis. **A**, Cerebral vasculitis in a patient with rheumatoid arthritis. There is a prominent perivascular inflammatory infiltrate. **B**, Higher power demonstrates plasma cells among the inflammatory infiltrate. (Hematoxylin-eosin stain.) (*Courtesy of* Dr. M. Ambler.)

Impaired blood clotting may also contribute to IPH. Potential causes are numerous (Table 6.2), including congenital factor deficiencies such as hemophilia, and acquired factor deficiencies such as disseminated intravascular coagulation. Conditions associated with decreased numbers of platelets (leukemia) or abnormal platelet function (uremia) are also associated with IPH [95]. Occasionally warfarin, heparin, or thrombolytic therapy is complicated by IPH. It is not clear that aspirin significantly increases the risk of IPH.

Abrupt changes in intracerebral hemodynamics are believed to play a role in many IPHs. Caplan [2] reviewed cases of IPH in unusual settings, such as after sympathomimetic drug use, cold exposure, and acute dental and other pain. He proposed that an acute rise in blood pressure and cerebral blood flow was a common and perhaps causative denominator [2]. Anecdotal reports show IPH in the setting of acute stress, both physical and emotional, such as running from a burning building or narrowly avoiding a motor vehicle accident [3,4]. Other authors have found a circadian rhythmicity of IPH onset that correlated with diurnal variation in blood pressure [5]. Reperfusion after carotid endarterectomy [6], hemodynamic changes in pregnancy [7], and increased blood flow before or during epileptic or electroconvulsive therapy-induced seizures [8] are also associated with IPH in rare circumstances.

These mechanisms are likely to coexist in most patients with IPH. Abnormal cerebral blood vessels are less effective in autoregulation and may provide inadequate protection against acute rises in systemic blood pressure. Similarly, a coagulopathy in a patient with an underlying vasculopathy may transform very limited subclinical bleeding into a catastrophic hemorrhage. The interactions of these various mechanisms in specific disorders are discussed in more detail below.

Table 6.2. Coagulopathies associated with intraparenchymal hemorrhage*

Congenital disorders of blood clotting
Factor VIII deficiency (hemophilia)
Factor VIII inhibitor
von Willebrand factor deficiency
Factor IX deficiency (hemophilia B, Christmas disease)
Factor VII deficiency
Factor XIII deficiency
Afibrinogenemia/dysfibrinogenemia
Acquired disorders of blood clotting
Diminished platelet number or function
Idiopathic thrombocytopenic purpura
Thrombotic thrombocytopenic purpura
Uremia
Antiplatelet agents
Leukemia
Other myeloproliferative/dysplastic disorders
Diminished or impaired clotting factors
Anticoagulants
Vitamin K deficiency
Impaired platelet and clotting function
Disseminated intravascular coagulation
Hepatic dysfunction
Fibrinolytic therapy

**Data from* del Zoppo and Mori [95]

GENERAL PATHOLOGY OF INTRAPARENCHYMAL HEMORRHAGE

When IPH occurs, the hemorrhage spreads along a path of least resistance, infiltrating between the fiber tracts of the white matter. The dense neuropil of gray matter is more resistant to the shearing forces of the growing hematoma and is more often compressed than infiltrated by the spreading hematoma [9–11]. Intraventricular and subarachnoid extension commonly occur when the hemorrhage is large. The size of the hematoma is quite variable and may correlate with the size of the ruptured artery [12] and the duration of bleeding. Coagulopathies tend to be associated with large hemorrhages [13]. Multifocal hemorrhages are uncommon, but do occur in severe coagulopathies, diffuse cerebral vasculitis, amyloid angiopathy, sympathomimetic drug abuse, or with multiple cerebral metastases. While IPH may occur anywhere within the brain substance, certain etiologies have predilections for specific sites.

Cytotoxic and vasogenic edema develop in the parenchyma surrounding the hematoma, becoming maximal in 3 to 5 days. After about 2 weeks, macrophages appear at the periphery of the hemorrhage. Resorption of blood takes place over weeks to months, depending on the hemorrhage size. Finally, a cavity is left behind, lined by hemosiderin-laden macrophages and surrounded by gliotic tissue [10,11].

There are several mechanisms by which IPH may injure brain tissue, such as the immediate destructive effect of the hemorrhage itself. Ischemic injury in brain parenchyma surrounding the hemorrhage appears to be the most important mechanism of tissue damage. The sudden introduction of the clot into a closed intracranial space produces mass effect that compresses and interrupts the local microcirculation. In animal models, stereotactic injection of blood or inert material into brain parenchyma is accompanied by a decrease in regional cerebral blood flow in the immediate clot penumbra within minutes after clot formation [11,14–16]. The development of edema may exacerbate this process and worsen the resulting ischemia [11,14,15,17]. Pathologic studies demonstrate an area of ischemic necrosis around the hemorrhage, proportional in severity and extent to the size of the hemorrhage [14,16]. Injection of blood affects regional cerebral blood flow differently than the injection of inert material, suggesting that chemical as well as mechanical effects of the clot may be important [16,17]. Pretreatment with the calcium channel blocker nimodipine partially reduces secondary perilesional ischemia and final lesion size in experimental models of IPH [15].

SPECIFIC DISORDERS

While the number of causes of IPH are enormous, the majority of IPHs are caused by a relatively small number of common conditions. A discussion of all causes of IPH is beyond the scope of this chapter, which will concentrate on the more common causes (Table 6.3).

Hypertension

Hypertension is the single most common risk factor for spontaneous IPH, which can occur in individuals with hypertension of all causes, including essential hypertension, renal vascular hypertension, and pregnancy-induced hypertension [18]. Improved treatment of hypertension is credited with the overall decline of IPH in the past 20 years [19].

Cerebrovascular pathology in hypertensive individuals has been extensively described. Small arteries and arterioles in chronically hypertensive individuals with and without IPH show a spectrum of pathologic change, referred to as lipohyalinosis and fibrinoid degeneration (Figure 6.3). Medial smooth muscle cells become necrotic and ultimately replaced by collagen. The elastic lamina becomes fragmented and the intima thickened. Granular and vesicular debris accumulate due to insudation of plasma contents in the vessel wall [12,20–24]. Microaneurysms may arise from small arterioles (Figure 6.3). These are 200- to 300-µm diameter saccular or fusiform disruptions of the vessel wall. The aneurysm wall lacks medial smooth muscle and an internal elastic lamina. Microaneurysms may originate from diseased or otherwise normal appearing arterioles [12,20,25–28]. Both severely damaged arterial walls and microaneurysms likely represent sufficient structural weakening to cause arterial rupture. The actual source of bleeding in any individual with hypertensive IPH is difficult to identify.

The mechanism by which hypertension produces these pathologic changes is unclear. Age, chronicity, and severity of hypertension may contribute independently [20,22,25,26]. Medial smooth muscle, hypertrophied in response to increased hemodynamic stress, may become ischemic because oxygen and nutrient supply is insufficient for its metabolic requirements. Muscle cells may then become necrotic, releasing lysosomal enzymes that are destructive to other vessel wall constituents [9,20,24]. Alternatively, hypertension-induced mechanical and shear forces may disrupt endothelial integrity, allowing insudation of plasma contents, damaging the intima and media [20,23,24]. The former may result from chronic hypertension, the latter from repeated acute elevations in blood pressure.

The most common sites of IPH in hypertensive individuals are the basal ganglia, thalamus, cerebellum, and pons (Table 6.4) (Figure 6.4) [13]. These sites are supplied by small penetrating arteries that are more frequent and more severely affected by hypertensive arteropathy than cortical vessels of similar size. Unlike the small cortical vessels, these arteries originate directly from large caliber parent arteries and lack anastomoses with other end arteries. They are therefore less protected from the effects of systemic hypertension [9,26]. The small vessel arteropathy of hypertension is also believed to cause small lacunar infarcts and subcortical encephalomalacia, both frequently found in patients with hypertensive IPH [29].

An acute rise in blood pressure may precede many hypertensive IPHs. In one series of 393 patients with hypertensive IPH, 10 occurred during some form of emotional excitement, and only 14.5% occurred during sleep when blood pressure was relatively low [30]. Chronic and acute elevations in blood pressure in patients with essential hypertension may play a role in IPH associated with other etiologies, such as aneurysm rupture, cerebral amyloid angiopathy, and cerebral infarction.

Amyloid Angiopathy

The prevalence of sporadic cerebral amyloid angiopathy (CAA) in the general population increases dramatically with age, from 8% in patients aged in their 60s to 60% in patients aged over 90 years. Two autosomal dominantly inherited forms have also been described in Dutch and Icelandic families [31]. Defining the incidence of CAA-related IPH is difficult because its diagnosis requires pathologic examination.

Pathologically, deposition of amyloid material in the media and adventitia results in an acellular mural thickening of affected vessels. The material is eosinophilic on routine hematoxylin and eosin staining, stains with thioflavin S or T, and with Congo red,

Table 6.3. Relative frequency of the more common causes of intraparenchymal hemorrhage*

Cause	Frequency, %
Hypertension	40–60
Amyloid angiopathy	5–10
Neoplasm	2–10
Vascular malformation, aneurysm	10–20
Alcohol and drug abuse	1–5
Anticoagulants and thrombolytic therapy	5
Other	5

*Hemorrhagic infarctions are excluded from most series of intraparenchymal hemorrhage.

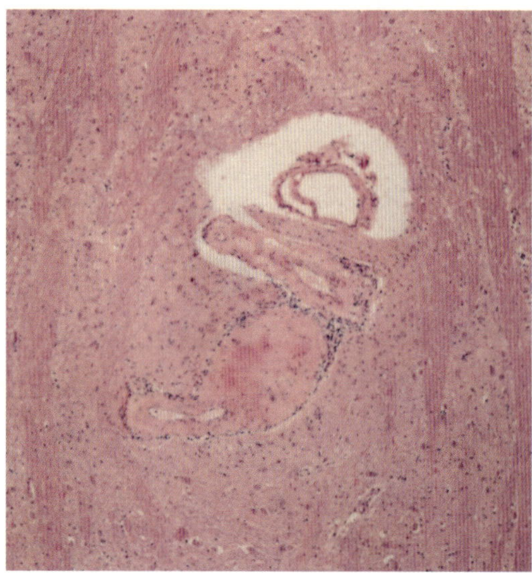

FIGURE 6.3 Saccular microaneurysm arising from a penetrating vessel in a 64-year-old hypertensive patient. The vessel wall of the parent artery demonstrates lipohyalinotic change and mural necrosis. (Hematoxylin-eosin stain.) (*Courtesy of* Dr. M. Ambler.)

and shows birefringence under polarized light (Figure 6.5). Ultrastructural analysis demonstrates 7- to 9-nm amyloid fibrils. Medial smooth muscle cells are split apart by the deposition of amyloid material, and the elastic lamina is fragmented, split, or destroyed. In severely affected arteries, all three wall layers are affected. The arterial walls may also develop segmental fibrinoid necrosis similar to that seen in hypertensive arteropathy. The lumen may be narrowed by this process, or develop segmental dilatation with microaneurysm formation. The development of mural clefts leads to a double-barrel lumen appearance [31–34]. Occasionally, some affected vessels demonstrate an inflammatory response similar in appearance to the arteritis of rheumatoid arthritis or granulomatous angiitis. This may represent a giant cell foreign body response to the amyloid protein [31,35,36]. Severe arteropathy with fibrinoid necrosis or microaneurysms may increase the risk of IPH in CAA [35,37].

The origin of the amyloid protein in CAA and the mechanism of its deposition in cerebral vessels is not clear. While circulating factors have been proposed in its genesis, the fact that CAA is not associated with systemic amyloidosis, but is associated with other cerebral amyloidoses, suggests that local factors may be more important. Forty percent of patients with CAA have the pathologic changes associated with Alzheimer's disease and a similar number have clinical dementia. The protein deposited in the arteries of CAA is biochemically similar to that of the amyloid plaques of Alzheimer's disease [31,34].

The pathogenesis of fibrinoid necrosis in CAA is unclear. Some but not all patients have hypertension as well as CAA [32]. Severe CAA may distort the vessel wall, causing disruption in the endothelium and leakage of plasma contents into the vessel wall. Whether this plays a primary or secondary role in the pathogenesis of CAA is unclear [31].

In contrast to the vasculopathy of hypertensive disease, CAA affects veins and capillaries as well as small- and medium-sized arteries and arterioles. Vascular involvement is patchy and asymmetric with striking involvement of superficial cortical and leptomeningeal vessels. While some authors have noted that CAA occurs primarily in the parietal and occipital lobes [31], others have noted a frontal predominance [32,35]. The temporal cortex is often involved, the cerebellum and the deep hemispheric structures less commonly, and the brainstem almost never [32,35,38,39]. The location of IPH in CAA mirrors the distribution of the arteropathy (Table 6.5).

The hematomas are usually superficial and often quite large. They may recur over months to years, and are rarely multiple simultaneously [33,35,38]. Subdural, subarachnoid, and intraven-

Table 6.4. Most frequent anatomic sites of hypertensive intraparenchymal hemorrhage*

Site	Incidence, %
Putamen	53
Thalamus	13
Pons	5
Cerebellum	10
Other (including lobar)	19

**Data from* Ojemann and Mohr [13]

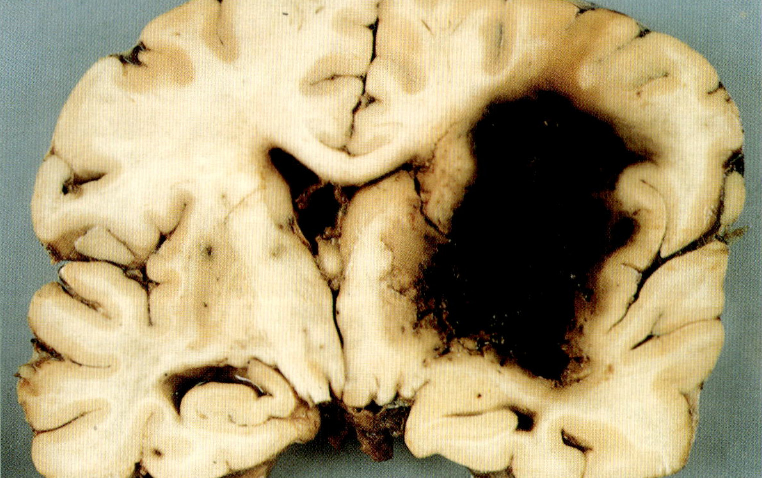

FIGURE 6.4

Large intraparenchymal hemorrhage originating from the basal ganglia in a hypertensive patient. (*Courtesy of* Dr. M. Ambler.)

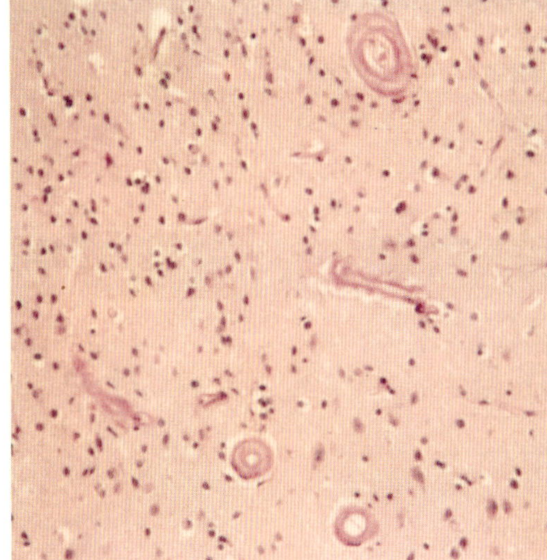

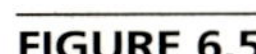

FIGURE 6.5

Cerebral amyloid angiopathy in an elderly patient. There is an acellular, eosinophilic thickening of the cerebral vessel walls. (Hematoxylin-eosin stain.) (*Courtesy of* Dr. M. Ambler.)

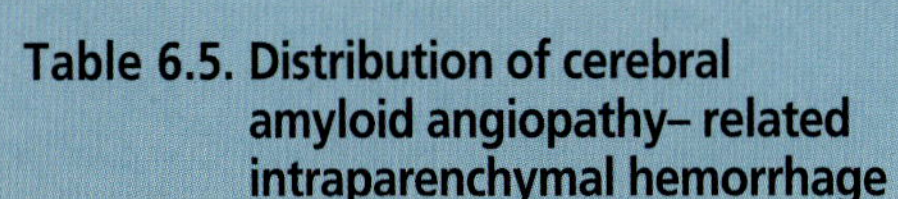

Table 6.5. Distribution of cerebral amyloid angiopathy– related intraparenchymal hemorrhage

Site	Incidence, %
Frontal	35
Temporal	14
Parietal	26
Occipital	19
Deep gray matter	4
Cerebellum	2
Corpus callosum	<1

tricular hemorrhages are not uncommon [31–33,38]. As in hypertensive vasculopathy, vascular occlusion and small infarcts may be seen. CAA is also associated with myelin loss in the deep periventricular white matter [31,35,40].

Intraparenchymal hemorrhage in CAA is usually a spontaneous event, but may also occur after minor head trauma, neurosurgical procedures, and thrombolytic therapy [32,35, 41,42]. Rapid changes in blood pressure may also be a risk factor for IPH in some but not all patients with CAA, and anticoagulant and antiplatelet therapy may play a role in others [32]. The high incidence of CAA in elderly patients may explain why IPH is a more frequent complication of anticoagulant therapy in the elderly.

Vascular Malformations

Vascular malformations are congenital lesions resulting from abnormal fetal development. They are of four major subtypes with different anatomic and clinical features (Table 6.6). All have been associated with IPH and subarachnoid hemorrhage, but with different frequencies. Ten percent of vascular malformations are multiple [43]. Most occur sporadically. There are a number of familial disorders with intracranial vascular malformations in which there is an increased incidence of either single or multiple subtypes of vascular malformations, including the Sturge-Weber and Osler Weber Rendu syndromes and others [44].

Arteriovenous malformations (AVM) are the most frequent source of malformation-associated bleeding. The defining anatomic feature of an AVM is a direct artery to vein anastomosis without intervening capillaries. An AVM may be a single fistula between artery and vein, but usually there is a tangle of vessels with intervening neural tissue (Figure 6.6). AVM size is variable, from less than 1 cm in diameter to enormous, multilobar lesions. They may be located anywhere in the central nervous system, with no predilection for any particular site. Eighty percent of AVMs are supratentorial. Of these, 20% are located deep in the hemispheres [43,45].

The vessels forming the malformation nidus are tortuous, with abnormal vessel wall architecture, making it difficult to distinguish arterial and venous components. The elastica and muscularis are markedly attenuated or absent, and the wall is often thickened, sclerotic, and mineralized. Intervening neural tissue is usually highly gliotic with evidence of prior hemorrhage. Intranidal aneurysms are formed by segmental dilatation of these abnormal arteries [43].

Arteries feeding the AVM may be single or multiple, and usually arise from one or more of the main arterial trunks. These feeding arteries are abnormally large and ectatic, with abnormal vessel wall structure characterized by either medial hypertrophy, or attenuated muscular components with hyalin change. These arteries have decreased responsivity to autoregulatory stimuli and to changes in CO_2 tension. Saccular aneurysms are associated with 10% of AVMs. These may be multiple and are usually found on the feeding arteries, rarely elsewhere. Veins draining the AVM may also be single or multiple, draining into deep central venous structures, superficial cortical veins, or directly into the sinuses. They are often abnormally distended and carry an increased blood volume [43,46].

Cavernous hemangiomas are closely related to AVMs. These consist of sinusoidal, dilated, endothelial-lined vascular channels without intervening neural tissue (Figure 6.7). The hyalinized vessel walls lack elastic and smooth muscle tissue. Calcification, sclerosis, and thrombosis are quite common. The tissue surrounding the malformation may show gliosis and hemosiderin deposition. They have an anatomic distribution similar to AVMs but are more often angiographically occult. While classically thought to have a low bleeding potential, their increased diagnosis by magnetic resonance imaging has shown that they are not as benign as once believed and may infrequently produce serious and recurrent hemorrhages [44,47–49].

Venous angiomas are also increasingly recognized to be a rare source of serious IPH. The malformation is composed of anomalous venous structures that are hyalinized, with diminished or absent elastic and smooth muscle tissue, converging on a single draining vein. These may arise anywhere in the brain. While the risk of hemorrhage is lower than with other malformations, serious and recurrent IPHs from venous angiomas do occur [50,51].

Capillary telangiectasis are the most benign vascular malformation. Angiographically occult, they are commonly an incidental finding on pathologic examination. They are most often located in the pontine base, cerebellum, or cerebral white matter. They are made up of capillary-like vessels with a single endothelial layer. Clinically significant bleeding is very rare [43].

Table 6.6. Cerebral vascular malformations

Type	Anatomic characteristic	Bleeding potential
AVM	Direct artery to vein connections with intervening neural tissue	Moderate, higher if AVM small, or if associated with aneurysm
Cavernous angioma	Abnormal arteriovenous structures without intervening neural tissue	Small
Venous malformation	Large abnormal draining veins	Small
Capillary telangiectasia	Capillary-like vessels	Very small

AVM—arteriovenous malformation.

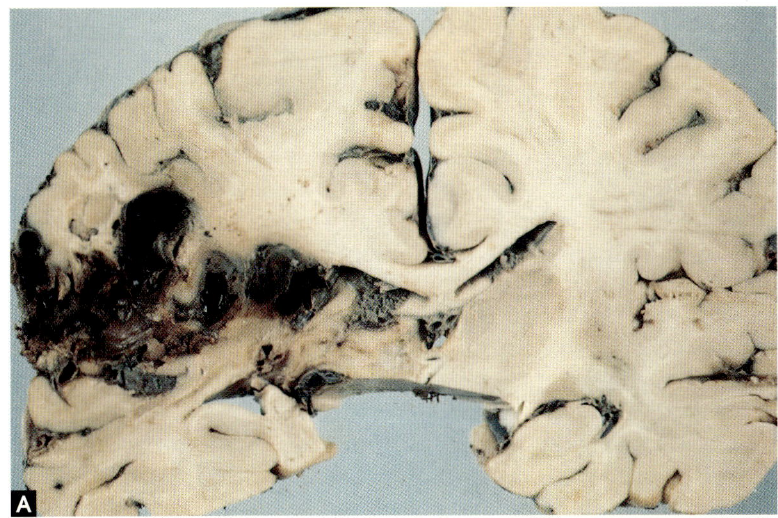

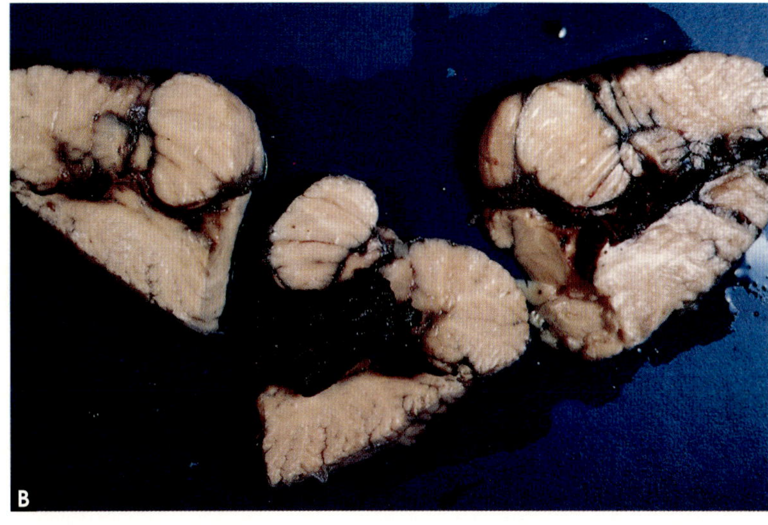

FIGURE 6.6

Arteriovenous malformations (AVMs). **A**, An AVM with intraparenchymal hemorrhage involving the inferior parietal cortex, the subinsular region, and the lateral basal ganglia. **B**, Cerebellar hemorrhage associated with amphetamine abuse in an 18-year-old with a previously unsuspected cerebellar AVM. The hemorrhage extends to the subarachnoid space. **C**, Microscopic evaluation shows abnormal vessel wall structure with adventitial connective tissue and varying thickness of smooth muscle, elastic, and subintimal tissue. Some vessels are occluded by thrombus with recanalization. The intervening neural tissue is highly gliotic. (*Courtesy of* Dr. M. Ambler.)

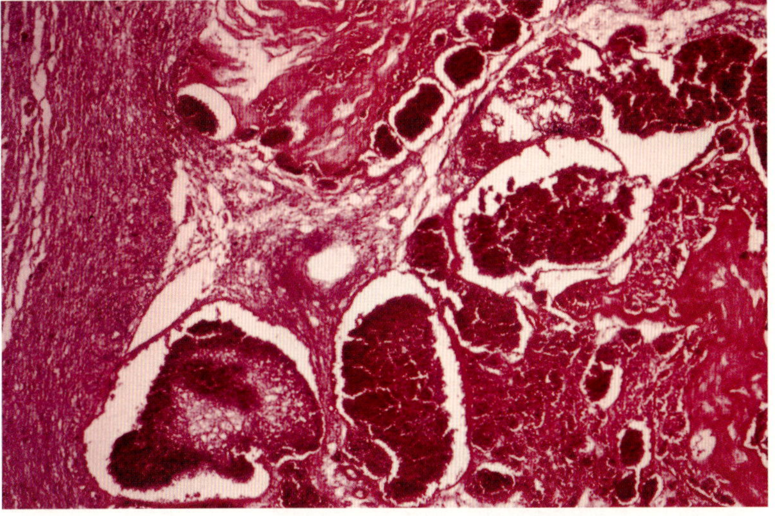

FIGURE 6.7

Cavernous angioma. The vessel walls are thinned with attenuated components. Many of the dilated vascular channels are occluded by thrombus. There is no intervening neural tissue between the vascular channels. (Phosphotungshi acid hematoxylin [PTAH].) (*Courtesy of* Dr. M. Ambler.)

Hemorrhage occurs in approximately one half of AVMs. Like the vascular anomalies, IPH occurs anywhere within the substance of the brain as well as in the subarachnoid and intraventricular space [43]. Specific characteristics of an AVM that correlate with bleeding risk vary among studies (Table 6.7) [45,46,52,53]. The role of hemodynamic factors in producing IPH in these patients is undefined. Circadian blood pressure variation and acute changes in blood pressure do not seem to have the same importance as in other etiologies of IPH [54,55], however, hemorrhage has been associated with sympathomimetic drug use [56,57] and physical exertion in a few patients. Venous pressure may be more important than arterial pressure in producing IPH. Short, central, and single draining veins, venous stenosis, and venous thrombosis are associated with both increased venous pressure and an increased risk of hemorrhage, while multiple, superficial draining veins are associated with decreased venous pressure and a decreased risk of hemorrhage [52,58]. Also, the increased risk of hemorrhage from AVMs late in pregnancy correlates with an increase in blood volume and venous pressure that peaks in the third trimester, resolving a few weeks after delivery [59–61].

Aneurysm

Saccular aneurysms are acquired vascular abnormalities, but may arise on the basis of congenital vessel wall weakening. They most commonly arise from the arterial bifurcations in, or just proximal to, the circle of Willis. The aneurysm wall varies in structure but is often thinned, fibrosed, and lacks complete wall constituents such as a muscularis and internal elastic lamina, making it susceptible to rupture [62].

The subarachnoid space is the most common site of bleeding following aneurysm rupture, but 30% to 40% of aneurysmal hemorrhages are associated with significant or even predominant IPH [63,64]. The anatomic site of the aneurysm is important in determining whether there is predominant IPH. Aneurysms embedded in or compressed against the parenchyma are most likely to produce IPH. Aneurysms having a relatively high association with IPH include those arising from the middle cerebral artery bifurcation (into the temporal lobe), the anterior communicating artery and distal anterior cerebral artery (into the medial frontal lobe), and the internal carotid artery bifurcation (into the basal ganglia) (Figure 6.8) [63].

Intraparenchymal hemorrhage is believed to be associated with rehemorrhage from an aneurysm rather than with its initial rupture [63,65]. Prior hemorrhage produces fibrosis and adhesions in the aneurysm wall and surrounding arachnoid that may limit hemorrhage into the subarachnoid space and direct the trajectory of recurrent bleeding intraparenchymally [62]. Another contributing factor in this setting is cerebral infarction from vasospasm, which decreases the intraparenchymal resistance to hemorrhage [62].

Rupture from saccular aneurysms has been associated with acute increase in systemic blood pressure, with a classic onset during physical exertion, straining, or during coitus. It has also occurred in temporal relation to cocaine use [66]. However, spontaneous rupture during normal activity and even during sleep does occur. Other risk factors for hemorrhage are usually absent.

Mycotic aneurysms are associated with bacterial and fungal infections, most commonly with bacterial endocarditis, but also with contiguous infections such as meningitis, abscess, osteomyelitis, and sinusitis. A pyogenic arteritis is believed to result from bacterial invasion of the artery wall, whether blood borne as a septic embolus from infected cardiac valves or from local infection. Pathologic studies reveal a brisk inflammatory response in the adventitia, spreading to involve other wall structures (Figure 6.9). Within 48 hours, this may produce sufficient structural weakening of the vessel wall to produce mycotic aneurysm, intracerebral hemorrhage, or both. Subcortical arterial branches are the most common site of embolism. Therefore, IPH is typically lobar in this setting [67–70].

Staphyloccal endocarditis has the highest risk of complicating mycotic aneurysms and IPH, accounting for almost one half of all mycotic aneurysms. Many other bacteria have been associated with mycotic aneurysm formation including *Streptococcus* species, *Escherichia coli*, and other enterococci, as well as a number of fungi, especially *Aspergillus* species and *Candida albicans* [68–71]. Anticoagulant therapy and other coagulopathies may play a role in many IPHs associated with bacterial endocarditis [67,69].

Table 6.7. Risk factors for arteriovenous malformation hemorrhage

Small size (< 3 cm)
Associated aneurysm
Short, central draining vein
Venous thrombosis or stenosis

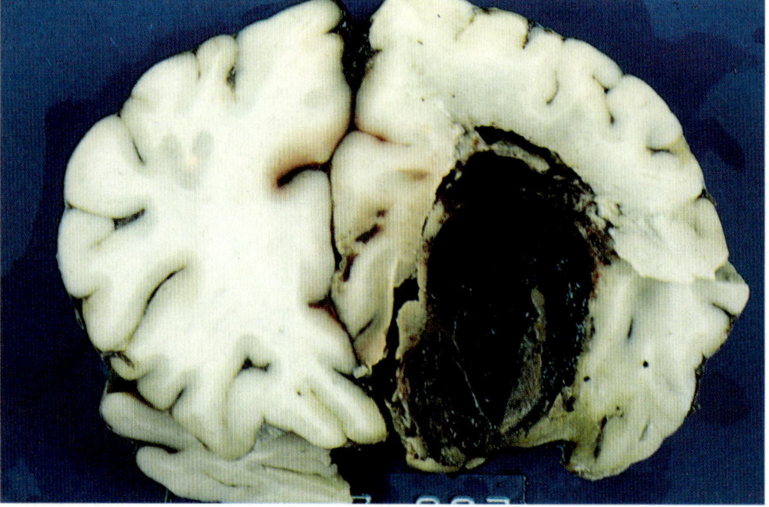

FIGURE 6.8
Intraparenchymal hemorrhage following rerupture of a saccular aneurysm that originated from the bifurcation of the right internal carotid artery into the anterior and middle cerebral arteries. The hemorrhage involved the inferior frontal lobe and basal ganglia. (*Courtesy of* Dr. M. Ambler.)

Hemorrhagic Infarction

The management of cerebral infarction is complicated by the significant incidence of hemorrhagic transformation, which varies among studies from 5% to 70%. Hemorrhagic transformation (HT) is highly associated with embolic, particularly cardioembolic, sources of infarction. In recent studies, the incidence of HT is 25% to 45% in nonanticoagulated patients with cardioembolic stroke [72–74]. The spectrum of IPH varies in these patients from patchy, petechial areas of hemorrhage within the infarction to frank hematoma, and has a corresponding range of clinical significance (Figure 6.10). The location of hemorrhage corresponds to the site of infarction. Cardioembolic strokes are usually cortical and often large [72–74].

The mechanism of HT is believed to be related to "migrating embolism." With prolonged arterial occlusion, the distal parenchyma and the arterial wall become ischemic, structurally weakened, and cannot withstand the pressure of sudden reperfusion that occurs after spontaneous or medical fibrinolysis of the embolus. This mechanism is consistent with the observed timing of hemorrhagic transformation, which is rare in the first few hours, and most common within the first few days after infarction [72,73]. Others have shown that HT may occur despite persistent arterial occlusion and suggest that it may be related in some cases to an arterial tear produced by the embolus, sudden reperfusion from collateral flow, or acute surges in blood pressure [74,75].

While less common, venous occlusion has a higher association with HT than does arterial occlusion. Most venous thromboses occur in the superior sagittal sinus and adjacent cortical veins, producing hemorrhagic infarction in the cortex of the convexities (Figure 6.11). Venous thrombosis occurs in the setting of hypercoagulable states, as a complication of meningitis (thrombophlebitis), and in pregnancy (Table 6.8) [76–78].

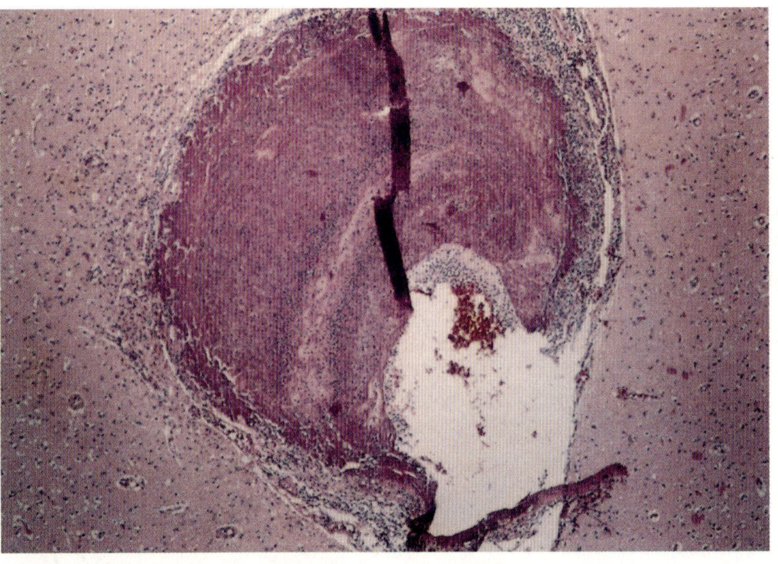

FIGURE 6.9

Mycotic aneurysms. The vessel walls and surrounding parenchyma are infiltrated by bacteria and polymorphonuclear cells. (Hematoxylin-eosin stain.) (*Courtesy of* Dr. M. Ambler.)

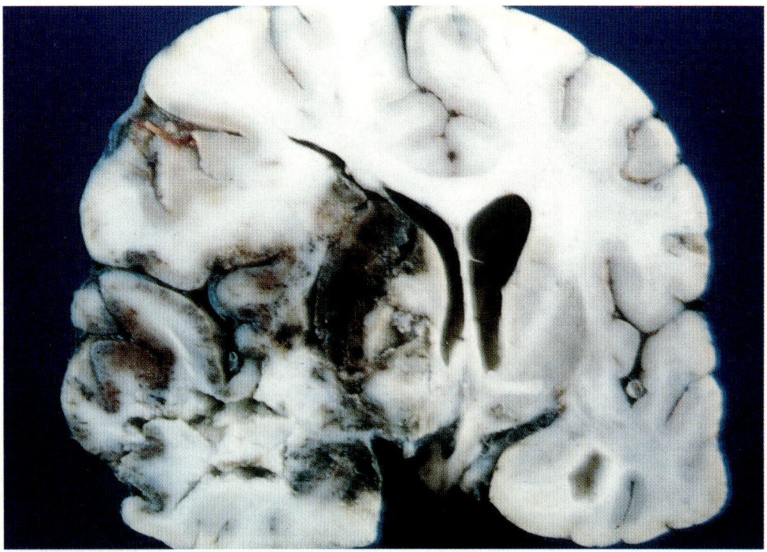

FIGURE 6.10

Hemorrhagic infarction in the left middle cerebral artery distribution in a 78-year-old patient with a dilated cardiomyopathy. There is marked swelling and softening of the left hemisphere in the distribution of the middle cerebral artery, with patchy hemorrhage involving the cortex and basal ganglia. (*Courtesy of* Dr. M. Ambler.)

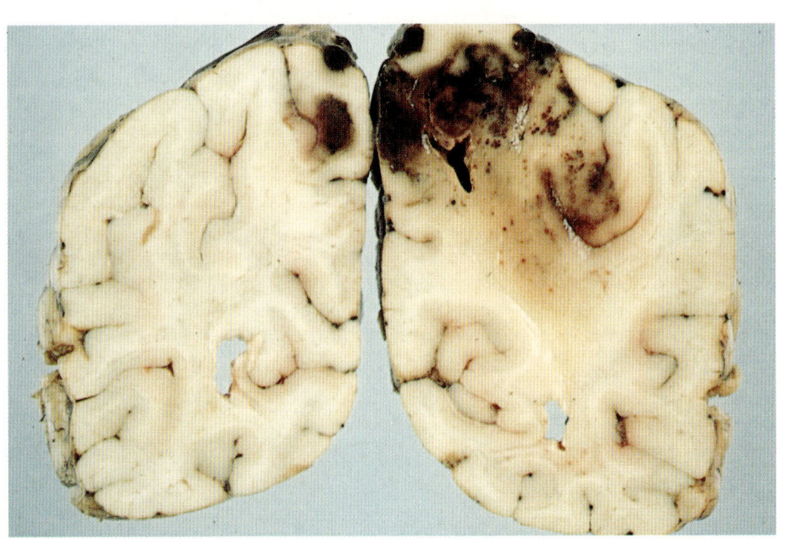

FIGURE 6.11

Hemorrhagic infarction in parasaggital convexities in a 14-year-old patient with superior sagittal sinus thrombosis secondary to an underlying hypercoagulable state. (*Courtesy of* Dr. M. Ambler.)

Other stroke mechanisms also may be associated with HT. HT has been observed late (20–30 days) after subarachnoid hemorrhage, corresponding to resolution of vasospasm [79]. IPH also rarely occurs after a migraine attack, perhaps also related to sudden reperfusion of blood flow after resolution of vasospasm in an ischemic artery [1]. Early carotid endarterectomy after acute cerebral infarction may also be a risk factor for hemorrhagic transformation [6,80].

The role of anticoagulant therapy in HT is disputed. Some believe that anticoagulation increases the risk of HT, while others believe that heparin may increase the size and morbidity of HT but not its overall incidence. Age, concomitant hypertension, and size of the infarction are also believed to be risk factors for HT [72–74,81].

Tumor

While an underlying intracerebral tumor is a relatively infrequent cause of IPH, occurring in 2% to 10%, it has important implications for prognosis and treatment [82–84]. IPH may occur in almost every tumor type (Table 6.9), and in one third to one half of tumor-related IPH, it is the presenting feature of the tumor. Primary brain tumors bleed rarely, less than 1% of the time [85]. Among astrocytomas, the risk of hemorrhage correlates with the grade of malignancy, with the highest rate of bleeding in glioblastoma multiforme, and malignant astrocytomas. Oligodendrogliomas are an exception to this, being relatively benign tumors that have a higher incidence of bleeding [86]. Pilocystic astrocytomas also bleed somewhat more frequently than other low-grade astrocytomas [87]. Meningiomas bleed rarely and almost never into the brain parenchyma [86]. Hemorrhage occurs more frequently (16%) in pituitary adenomas than in other primary intracranial tumors (<1%) [88].

Metastatic tumors bleed more frequently than primary brain tumors, about 10% to 14% of the time [85]. IPH may be presenting symptom of a brain metastasis. While brain metastases from almost every known primary may bleed, IPH is overwhelmingly associated with a few, namely bronchogenic and renal carcinomas, melanoma, and choriocarcinoma. Melanomas and choriocarcinomas are relatively uncommon causes of intracerebral metastases, but have a high, 40% to 60%, risk of intraparenchymal bleeding [85,86]. Bronchogenic carcinoma bleeds relatively infrequently, but its high prevalence makes it the most common cause of hemorrhagic metastases. One half of metastatic hemorrhages are multiple, an important clue to their diagnosis [89].

Tumor-related IPH may occur in any location in the deep and superficial cerebral hemispheres, cerebellum, and brainstem (Figure 6.12) [85]. Glioblastomas often bleed into deep hemispheric structures, such as the basal ganglia, and, uniquely, into the corpus callosum. Metastatic tumors often bleed into the subcortical white matter at the gray white junction where many metastatic lesions are located, or into the cerebellum [83–85]. Hemorrhages may be small and clinically silent or massive and clinically devastating [82]. Both small microscopic and large tumors may produce IPH [85].

The propensity of brain tumors to produce hemorrhage is multifactorial, in part related to their neovascularity. The abundant vessels of primary and secondary brain tumors may be large and often appear "immature" with poorly formed wall elements, lacking tight endothelial junctions [82,85,90]. Calcification of the vessel walls in some tumors, such as oligodendrogliomas, weaken their structure and may increase bleeding risk. Necrosis, produced by rapid growth of the tumor beyond its blood supply, decreases the central support of blood vessels and increases the risk of IPH [85]. Certain malignancies, especially choriocarcinoma and rarely astrocytoma, invade

Table 6.8. Conditions associated with cerebral venous thrombosis*

Condition
Pregnancy
Malignancy
Local infections (thrombophlebitis)
Systemic infections
Dehydration
Hypercoagulable states
Thrombocythemia
Erythrocyte disorders
Sickle cell anemia
Paroxysmal nocturnal hemoglobinuria
Polycythemia
Leukemia
Connective tissue disorders

**Data from* Bousser and Barnett [76]

Table 6.9. Intracerebral tumors associated with intraparenchymal hemorrhage

Tumor
Primary
Glioblastoma multiforme
Anaplastic astrocytoma
Oligodendroglioma
Pilocytic astrocytoma
Pituitary adenoma
Metastatic
Choriocarcinoma
Melanoma
Lung
Renal
Leukemia
Rare (chordoma [140], colon, breast, teratoma [141], adrenal carcinoma, hemangiopericytoma [84], laryngeal carcinoma, testicular carcinoma, carcinoid [85], lymphoma [86])

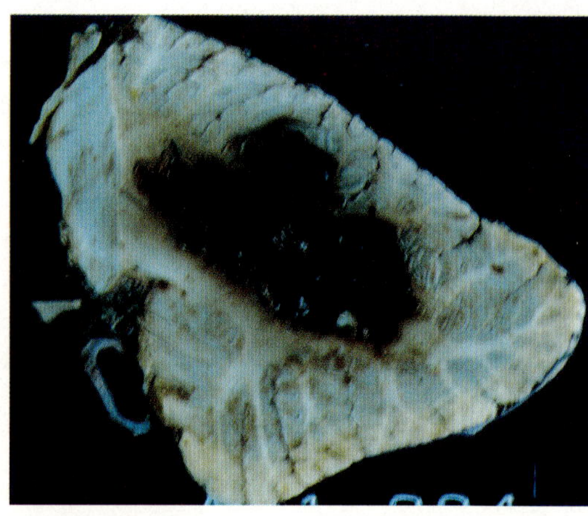

FIGURE 6.12

Cerebellar hemorrhage arising from metastatic carcinoma. This 54-year-old patient was subsequently found to have underlying squamous cell lung cancer. (*Courtesy of* Dr. M. Ambler.)

the walls of normal blood vessels and produce massive IPH [85,91,92]. Some tumors are associatd with aneurysms. These have been found in choriocarcinoma, bronchogenic tumors, atrial myxomas, and gliomas [85,91,93,94]. IPH associated with small microscopic tumors have been postulated to occur as a result of hemorrhagic infarction after tumor embolism [85].

Leukemias may produce IPH by several mechanisms. Very high leukocyte counts may produce sludging of blood flow with associated hemorrhagic venous infarction. Associated thrombocytopenia and disseminated intravascular coagulation in leukemia may also play a role in producing or extending the hemorrhage [95].

Disseminated intravascular coagulation with bleeding is associated with systemic neoplasms. While theoretically a risk for tumor-related IPH, it does not appear to play a large role [85]. Other coagulopathies, such as thrombocytopenia appear to play a role in some series [86]. Anticoagulant therapy, however, is believed to be relatively safe in most patients with brain tumors [96].

Most tumor-related IPHs arise spontaneously. However, some have been associated with head trauma or with shunting procedures [85,86,88]. Some authors believe hypertension increases the risk of IPH in patients with tumors [82], while others have found no association [86].

Substance Abuse

A number of abused substances have been implicated in the pathogenesis of IPH (Table 6.10). Although IPH most often occurs with drug abuse, it may also occur after nonillicit use of prescribed or over the counter medication. The drug is believed to be responsible for IPH when IPH occurs in a young person using the drug, in the absence of other identifiable risk factors, or in close temporal proximity to its administration. IPH often occurs immediately after drug use but may be delayed by hours or days. Oral, intranasal, and intravenous routes of administration are all associated with IPH. IPH may follow a single administration of the drug or may occur after chronic use [57,97,98].

The mechanism of IPH in this setting is obscured by several issues. There is very little pathologic data in these patients. Multisubstance abuse is common, making it difficult to attribute IPH to a single drug. The notorious unreliability of drug abusers makes historical information questionable and obscures possible temporal and dose relationships [99]. Nonetheless, a variety of pathophysiologic mechanisms both proven and speculative are believed to play a role in drug-related IPH (Table 6.11).

The vasculitis of substance abuse has received much attention, but has been proven to underlie IPH in only a minority of patients. A drug-related vasculitis has been best documented in association with amphetamine and amphetamine-like substances, particularly phenylpropanolamine, but has also been described in cocaine, heroin, and other substance abusers. The vasculitis may produce cerebral infarction as well as hemorrhage [2,100]. This is a necrotizing angiitis, similar in appearance to polyarteritis nodosa, which involves the vessel walls of arteries and arterioles with fibrinoid necrosis of the media and intima, and destruction of muscle and elastic components that are replaced by collagen. A cellular infiltrate of neutrophils, eosinophils, lymphocytes, and histiocytes surrounds the vessel and extends to the surrounding parenchyma. This may represent a direct toxic effect of the drug on the vessel wall or a hypersensitivity reaction to the drug or an adulterant [100–103]. Drug-related vasculitis may involve other organs including peripheral nerves, kidney, liver, and skin [104].

In drug-related and other vasculitides, angiography may be normal or demonstrate "beading." This is a nonspecific pattern that by itself is not proof of vasculitis that requires pathologic data [105]. In some instances, angiographic "beading" does not represent vasculitis but may represent vasospasm or another form of arteropathy. These pathologies may be responsible for some drug-related IPH [66,105–107].

Cocaine, phencyclidine, and the amphetamine-like drugs have sympathomimetic actions and may produce an acute rise in blood pressure by direct cardiostimulation and vasoconstriction [57,108]. Because many IPHs occur soon after drug administration, this is

Table 6.10. Drugs associated with intraparenchymal hemorrhage

Drug	Most common pathogenesis
Amphetamine-like drugs	Vasculitis, acute rise in blood pressure
Amphetamine	
Phenylpropanolamine	
Ephedrine	
Pseudephedrine	
Dextroamphetamine	
Cocaine	Underlying vascular lesion, acute rise in blood pressure
Heroin and other opiates	Subacute bacterial endocarditis
Pentazocine and tripelennamine	Mechanism unclear, arteropathy [107]
Phencyclidine	Acute rise in blood pressure [108]
Alcohol	Coagulopathy, hypertension

Table 6.11. Possible mechanisms in intraparenchymal hemorrhage related to substance abuse

Vasculitis
Bacterial endocarditis and septic embolism
Hypertensive arteropathy
Underlying vascular malformation
Foreign body embolism with hemorrhagic transformation
Thrombocytopenia
Liver failure
Acute hypertension

believed to be important in their pathogenesis [109]. Nearly 50% of cocaine-related IPHs occur soon after drug use in patients who have an underlying vascular lesion, such as a vascular malformation, aneurysm, or tumor [57,66,106,110]. The effects of repeated acute increases in blood pressure from sympathomimetic drug use on the cerebrovasculature is not known but may produce a vasculopathy similar to that seen in essential hypertension. The use of heroin and other opiates may produce a nephropathy with associated hypertension. A hypertensive vasculopathy may underlie deep IPH in substance abusers when no other underlying vascular lesion is discovered [66,106].

Intravenous drug abuse carries the risk of subacute bacterial endocarditis, with complicating pyogenic arteritis, mycotic aneurysm, and IPH. *Staphylococcus aureus* is both the most common organism involved in subacute bacterial endocarditis associated with intravenous drug abuse and carries the highest risk of mycotic aneurysm and IPH [69].

A variety of coagulopathies may occur with substance abuse. An autoimmune thrombocytopenia occurs in heroin and cocaine abusers, sometimes related to concomitant HIV infection [111–113]. Hepatitis B with complicating liver failure and coagulopathy may also complicate intravenous drug abuse.

Most (70%) IPHs occurring in relation to drug abuse are lobar [97]. Many are deep in the cerebral hemispheres, but cerebellar and brainstem locations are very uncommon. Multiple simultaneous hemorrhages occur infrequently [106,109].

Alcohol abuse appears to be associated with IPH [114]. Age, concomitant hypertension, and black race appear to increase the risk of IPH in alcoholics [115]. Chronic alcohol abuse may produce or exacerbate systemic hypertension, but this mechanism is not believed to account for most alcohol-related IPHs, which are usually large, lobar hemorrhages [116]. Many of these hemorrhages occur in the setting of chronic hepatic cirrhosis, with dysfibrinogenemia, decreased vitamin K–dependent clotting factors, thrombocytopenia, and occasionally disseminated intravascular coagulation [117,118]. Alcohol is also directly toxic to bone marrow causing thrombocytopenia and impaired platelet aggregability [119]. Head trauma occurs with high frequency in this population and may play a role in many IPHs. Alcohol may potentiate the effects of illicit drugs by reducing hepatic metabolism, prolonging their action, and perhaps increasing the risk of associated IPH [106].

Fibrinolytic and Anticoagulant Therapies

Intraparenchymal hemorrhage is a dreaded complication of fibrinolytic therapy. All types of fibrinolytic therapy (urokinase, streptokinase, and tissue plasminogen activator) have been associated with this complication. There is no clear, consistent, dose-response relationship. When thrombolysis is given for acute myocardial infarction, the overall risk of IPH is 0.4% to 2.2% [120]. IPH may occur during administration or up to 24 hours later, but is quite uncommon after this. Most IPHs (70%) are lobar, and 15% to 33% are multiple. Risk factors variably include age, hypertension, use of other drugs (heparin, aspirin, and warfarin), prolonged cardiopulmonary resuscitation, and a history of neurologic disease (Table 6.12). Other less well established risk factors include female sex, dose and type of fibrinolytic agent, low body weight, and prior invasive cardiovascular procedures [120–124].

Preexisting cerebral or cerebrovascular disease provides a substrate for hemorrhage in a number of patients. Often the diagnosis of prior brain disease is not known until IPH has occurred. Such conditions include CAA, AVM, hypertensive vascular disease, aneurysm, cerebral infarction, and brain tumor [41,125,126]. Some IPHs after thrombolytic therapy may represent hemorrhagic infarction [122]. It is believed that fibrinolytic therapy leads to lysis of a recently formed hemostatic plug at sites of cerebrovascular injury, either microvascular or due to major underlying vascular pathology. Thrombolytic therapy often produces hypofibrinogenemia and fibrin degradation products that have anticoagulant properties, deplete factors V and VIII, and impair platelet function. These effects may further increase the risk and potential size of IPH [41,125,127,128]. Concomitant anticoagulant therapy may exacerbate this risk [124]. The poor correlation between the risk of IPH and laboratory measures of the fibrinolytic state may simply reflect the differences between local and systemic fibrinolysis [127].

There is less experience with thrombolysis given for acute cerebral infarction. The major risk is of hemorrhagic transformation of the infarction for which the drug is administered. The incidence of HT varies between 8% and 53% in recent clinical trials [129,130]. Similar risk factors to those considered above may be important. The timing of drug administration is clearly important, with the risk of major HT increasing if the drug is given more than 6 hours after stroke onset [129]. Larger infarctions have a higher risk of HT with thrombolytic therapy [131].

The risk of IPH in patients treated with chronic anticoagulant therapy is low (1.5%–2%) [132,133]. Similar risk factors apply, including age and concomitant hypertension. Supratherapeutic prothrombin time seems to increase the risk, but IPH also occurs in patients who have normal or subtherapeutic levels. IPH may occur at any time after the onset of therapy [133–136]. In many series there seems to be a high prevalence of patients anticoagulated for cerebrovascular disease [135]. This may represent selection bias or may suggest a role for underlying structural vascular pathology, ischemic or hypertensive, in the pathogenesis of anticoagulant-related IPH. Hemorrhages are often large and may occur anywhere in the brain, but seem to have a predilection for the subcortical white matter and the cerebellum [135–137].

Table 6.12. Risk factors for thrombolytic or anticoagulant-related intraparenchymal hemorrhage

Age
Hypertension
Dose of bolus infusion
Supratherapeutic prothrombin time or partial thromboplastin time
Cardiac embolism
Septic embolism
Other underlying structural brain disease
Anticoagulant/thrombolytic/antiplatelet drug combinations

REFERENCES

1. Cole AJ, Aube M: Migraine with vasospasm and delayed intracerebral hemorrhage. *Arch Neurol* 1990, 47:53–56.
2. Caplan L: Intracerebral hemorrhage revisited. *Neurology* 1988, 38:624–627.
3. Freytag E: Fatal hypertensive intracerebral haematomas: a survey of the pathological anatomy of 393 cases. *J Neurol Neurosurg Psychiatry* 1968, 31:616–620.
4. Dinsdale HB: Spontaneous hemorrhage in the posterior fossa. *Arch Neurol* 1964, 10:200–217.
5. Sloan MA, Price TR, Foulkes MA, *et al.*: Circadian rhythmicity of stroke onset: intracerebral and subarachnoid hemorrhage. *Stroke* 1992, 23:1420–1426.
6. Caplan LR, Skillman J, Ogemann R, Fields WS: Intracerebral hemorrhage following carotid endarterectomy: a hypertensive complication. *Stroke* 1978, 9:457–460.
7. Wilterdink JL, Feldmann E: Cerebral hemorrhage. In *Neurologic Complications of Pregnancy.* Edited by Devinsky O, Feldmann E, Hainline B. New York: Raven Press; 1994:13–23.
8. Weisberg LA, Elliott D, Mielke D: Intracerebral hemorrhage following electroconvulsive therapy. *Neurology* 1991, 41:1849.
9. Huckman MS, Weinberg PE, Kim KS, Davis DO: Angiographic and clinico-pathologic correlates in basal ganglionic hemorrhage. *Radiology* 1970, 95:79–92.
10. Kaufman HH, Schochet SS: Pathology, pathophysiology, and modeling. In *Intracerebral Hematomas.* Edited by Kaufman HH. New York: Raven Press; 1992:13–22.
11. Bullock R, Brock-Utne J, van Dellen J, Blake G: Intracerebral hemorrhage in a primate model: effect on regional cerebral blood flow. *Surg Neurol* 1988, 29:101–107.
12. Takebayashi S, Kaneko MK: Electron microscopic studies of ruptured arteries in hypertensive intracerebral hemorrhage. *Stroke* 1984, 14:28–36.
13. Ojemann RG, Mohr JP: Hypertensive brain hemorrhage. *Clin Neurosurg* 1975, 23:220–244.
14. Kingman TA, Mendelow AD, Graham DI, Teasdale GM: Experimental intracerebral mass: description of model, intracranial pressure changes and neuropathology. *J Neuropathol Exp Neurol* 1988, 47:128–137.
15. Nath FP, Jenkins A, Mendelow AD, *et al.*: Early hemodynamic changes in experimental intracerebral hemorrhage. *J Neurosurg* 1986, 65:697–703.
16. Nehls DG, Mendelow AD, Graham DI, *et al.*: Experimental intracerebral hemorrhage: progression of hemodynamic changes after production of a spontaneous mass lesion. *J Neurosurg* 1988, 23:439–444.
17. Mendelow AD: Spontaneous intracerebral hemorrhage. *J Neurol Neurosurg Psychiatry* 1991, 54:193–195.
18. Richards A, Graham D, Bullock R: Clinicopathological study of neurologic complications due to hypertensive disorders of pregnancy. *J Neurol Neurosurg Psychiatry* 1988, 51:416–421.
19. Furlan AJ, Whisnant JP, Elveback LR: The decreasing incidence of primary intracerebral hemorrhage: a population study. *Ann Neurol* 1979, 5:367–373.
20. Yoshida Y, Shinkai H, Ooneda G: Morphogenesis of microaneurysm and plasmatic anterionecrosis in hypertensive cerebral hemorrhage. In *Hypertensive Intracerebral Hemorrhage.* Edited by Mizukami M, Kogure K, Kanaya H, Yamori Y. New York: Raven Press; 1983:181–190.
21. Rosenblum WI: Miliary aneurysms and "fibrinoid" degeneration of cerebral blood vessels. *Hum Pathol* 1977, 8:133–139.
22. Takebayashi S: Ultrastructural morphometry of hypertensive medial damage in lenticulostriate and other arteries. *Stroke* 1985, 16:449–453.
23. Fredriksson K, Nordborg C, Kalimo H, *et al.*: Cerebral microangiopathy in stroke-prone spontaneously hypertensive rats: an immunohistochemical and ultrastructural study. *Acta Neuropathol* 1988, 75:241–252.
24. Tagami M, Nara Y, Kubota A, *et al.*: Ultrastructural characteristics of occluded perforating arteries in stroke-prone spontaneously hypertensive rats. *Stroke* 1987, 18:733–740.
25. Cole FM, Yates P: Intracerebral microaneurysms and small cerebrovascular lesions. *Brain* 1967, 90:759–767.
26. Russell RWR: Observations on intracerebral aneurysms. *Brain* 1963, 86:425–441.
27. Fisher CM: Cerebral miliary aneurysms in hypertension. *Am J Pathol* 1972, 66:313–330.
28. Fisher CM: Pathological observations in hypertensive cerebral hemorrhage. *J Neuropathol Exp Neurol* 1971, 30:536–550.
29. Inzitari D, Giordano GP, Ancona AL, *et al.*: Leukoaraiosis, intracerebral hemorrhage, and arterial hypertension. *Stroke* 1990 , 21:1419–1423.
30. Douglas MD, Haerer AF: Long-term prognosis of hypertensive intracerebral hemorrhage. *Stroke* 1982, 13:488–491.
31. Vinters HV: Cerebral amyloid angiopathy: a critical review. *Stroke* 1987, 18:311–324.
32. Cosgrove GR, Leblanc R, Meagher-Villemure K, Ethier R: Cerebral amyloid angiopathy. *Neurology* 1985, 35:625–631.
33. Kalyan-Raman UP, Kalyan-Raman K: Cerebral amyloid angiopathy causing intracranial hemorrhage. *Ann Neurol* 1984, 16:321–329.
34. Okazaki H, Reagan TJ, Campbell RJ: Clinicopathologic studies of primary cerebral amyloid angiopathy. *Mayo Clin Proc* 1979, 54:22–31.
35. Vonsattel JPG, Myers RH, Hedley-Whyte ET, *et al.*: Cerebral amyloid angiopathy without and with cerebral hemorrhages: a comparative histological study. *Ann Neurol* 1991, 30:637–649.
36. Powers JM, Stein MB, Torres RAA: Sporadic cerebral amyloid angiopathy with giant cell reaction. *Acta Neuropathol* 1990, 81:95–98.
37. Case records of the Massachusetts General Hospital. 10-1988. *N Engl J Med* 1988, 318:623–631.
38. Itoh Y, Yamada M, Hayakawa M, *et al.*: Cerebral amyloid angiopathy: a significant cause of cerebellar as well as lobar cerebral hemorrhage in the elderly. *J Neurol Sci* 1993, 116:135–141.
39. Duchen LW: Current status review: cerebral amyloid. *Int J Exp Pathol* 1992, 73:535–550.
40. Gray F, Dubas F, Foullet E, Escourolle R: Leukoencephalopathy in diffuse haemorrhagic cerebral amyloid angiopathy. *Ann Neurol* 1985, 18:54–59.
41. Leblanc R, Haddad G, Robitaille Y: Cerebral hemorrhage from amyloid angiopathy and coronary thrombolysis. *Neurosurgery* 1992, 31:586–590.
42. Torack RM: Congophilic angiopathy complicated by surgery and massive hemorrhage. *Am J Pathol* 1975, 81:349–366.
43. Stein BM, Wolpert SM: Arteriovenous malformations of the brain. I. Current concepts and treatment. *Arch Neurol* 1980, 37:1–5.
44. Rigamonti D, Hadley MN, Drayer BP, *et al.*: Cerebral cavernous malformations: incidence and familial occurrence. *N Engl J Med* 1988, 319:343–347.
45. Spetzler RF, Hargraves RW, McCormick PW, *et al.*: Relationship of perfusion pressure and size to risk of hemorrhage from arteriovenous malformations. *J Neurosurg* 1992, 76:918–923.
46. Brown RD, Wiebers DO, Forbes GS: Unruptured intracranial aneurysms and arteriovenous malformations: frequency of intracranial hemorrhage and relationship of lesions. *Neurosurg* 1990, 73:859–863.
47. Requena I, Arias M, Lopez-Ibor L, *et al.*: Cavernomas of the central nervous system: clinical and neuroimaging manifestations in 47 patients. *J Neurol Neurosurg Psychiatry* 1991, 54:590–594.
48. Robinson JR, Awad IA, Little JR: Natural history of the cavernous angioma. *J Neurosurg* 1991, 75:709–714.
49. Tung H, Giannotta SL, Chandrasoma PT, Zee CS: Recurrent intraparenchymal hemorrhages from angiographically occult vascular malformations. *J Neurosurg* 1990, 73:174–180.

50. Malik GM, Morgan JK, Boulos RS, Ausman JI: Venous angiomas: an underestimated cause of intracranial hemorrhage. *Surg Neurol* 1988, 30:350–358.

51. Garner TB, Curling OD, Kelly DL, Laster DW: The natural history of intracranial venous angiomas. *J Neurosurg* 1991, 75:715–722.

52. Marks MP, Lane B, Steinberg GK, Chang PJ: Hemorrhage in intracerebral arteriovenous malformations: angiographic determinants. *Radiology* 1990, 176:807–813.

53. Graf CJ, Perret GE, Torner JC: Bleeding from cerebral arteriovenous malformations as part of their natural history. *J Neurosurg* 1983, 58:331–337.

54. Szabo MD, Crosby G, Sundaram P, *et al.*: Hypertension does not cause spontaneous hemorrhage of intracranial arteriovenous malformations. *Anesthesiology* 1989, 70:761–763.

55. Brown RD, Wiebers DO, Forbes G, *et al.*: The natural history of unruptured intracranial arteriovenous malformations. *J Neurosurg* 1988, 68:352–357.

56. Lukes SA: Intracerebral hemorrhage from an arteriovenous malformation after amphetamine injection. *Arch Neurol* 1983, 40:60–61.

57. Klonoff DC, Andrews BT, Obana WG: Stroke associated with cocaine use. *Arch Neurol* 1989, 46:989–993.

58. Miyasaka Y, Yada K, Kurata A, *et al.*: Correlation between intravascular pressure and risk of hemorrhage due to arteriovenous malformations. *Surg Neurol* 1993, 29:370–373.

59. Metcalfe J, McAnulty J, Ueland K: Cardiovascular physiology. *Clin Obstet Gynecol* 1981, 24:693–709.

60. Robinson J, Hall C, Seczimir C: Arteriovenous malformations, aneurysms and pregnancy. *J Neurosurg* 1974, 41:63–70.

61. Sadasivan B, Malik G, Lee C, Ausman J: Vascular malformations and pregnancy. *Surg Neurol* 1990, 33:305–313.

62. Masson RL, Day AL: Aneurysmal intracerebral hemorrhage. *Neurosurg Clin* 1992, 3:539–550.

63. Pasqualin A, Bazzan A, Cavazzani P, *et al.*: Intracranial hematomas following aneurysmal rupture: experience with 309 cases. *Surg Neurol* 1986, 25:6–17.

64. Inagawa T, Hirano A: Ruptured intracranial aneurysms: an autopsy study of 133 patients. *Surg Neurol* 1990, 33:117–123.

65. Hijdra A, Vermeulen M, van Gijn J, van Crevel H: Rerupture of intracranial aneurysms: a clinicoanatomic study. *J Neurosurg* 1987, 67:29–33.

66. Brown E, Prager J, Lee HY, Ramsey RG: CNS complications of cocaine abuse: prevalence, pathophysiology and neuroradiology. *Am J Radiol* 1992, 159:137–147.

67. Masuda J, Yutani C, Waki R, *et al.*: Histopathological analysis of the mechanisms of intracranial hemorrhage complicating infective endocarditis. *Stroke* 1992, 23:843–850.

68. Brust JCM, Dickinson PCT, Hughes JEO, Holtzman RNN: The diagnosis and treatment of cerebral mycotic aneurysms. *Ann Neurol* 1990, 27:238–246.

69. Hart RG, Kagan-Hallet K, Joerns SE: Mechanisms of intracranial hemorrhage in infective endocarditis. *Stroke* 1987, 18:1048–1056.

70. Clare CE: Infectious intracranial aneurysms. *Neurosurg Clin* 1992, 3:551–566.

71. Salgado AV: Central nervous system complications of infective endocarditis. *Stroke* 1991, 22:1461–1463.

72. Babikian VL, Kase CS, Pessin MS, *et al.*: Intracerebral hemorrhage in stroke patients anticoagulated with heparin. *Stroke* 1989, 20:1500–1503.

73. Cerebral Embolism Study Group: Immediate anticoagulation of embolic stroke: brain hemorrhage and management options. *Stroke* 1984, 15:779–789.

74. Okada Y, Yamaguchi T, Minematsu K, *et al.*: Hemorrhagic transformation in cerebral embolism. *Stroke* 1989, 20:598–603.

75. Bougousslavsky J, Regli F, Uske A, Maeder P: Early spontaneous hematoma in cerebral infarct: is primary cerebral hemorrhage overdiagnosed? *Neurology* 1991, 41:837–840.

76. Bousser MG, Barnett HJM: Cerebral venous thrombosis. In *Stroke. Pathophysiology, Diagnosis, and Management.* 2nd ed. Edited by Barnett HJM, Mohr JP, Stein BM, Yatsu FM. New York: Churchill Livingstone; 1992:517–537.

77. Beal MF, Wechsler LR, Davis K: Cerebral vein thrombosis and multiple intracranial hemorrhages by computed tomography. *Arch Neurol* 1982, 39:437–438.

78. Bousser MG, Chiras J, Bories J, Castaigne P: Cerebral venous thrombosis: a review of 38 cases. *Stroke* 1985, 16:199–213.

79. Terada T, Komai N, Hayashi S, *et al.*: Hemorrhagic infarction after vasospasm due to ruptured cerebral aneurysm. *Neurosurgery* 1986, 18:415–418.

80. Reith HB, Edelmann M, Reith C: Spontaneous intracerebral hemorrhage following carotid endarterectomy: experience of 328 operations from 1983-1988. *Int Surg* 1992, 77:224–225.

81. Shields RW Jr, Laureno R, Lachman T, Victor M: Anticoagulant-related hemorrhage in acute cerebral embolism. *Stroke* 1984, 15:426–437.

82. Bitoh S, Hasegawa H, Ohtsuki H, *et al.*: Cerebral neoplasms initially presenting with massive intracerebral hemorrhage. *Surg Neurol* 1982, 22:57–62.

83. Scott M: Spontaneous intracerebral hematoma caused by cerebral neoplasms. *J Neurosurg* 1975, 42:338–342.

84. Little JR, Dial B, Belanger G, Carpenter S: Brain hemorrhage from intracranial tumor. *Stroke* 1979, 10:283–288.

85. Mandybur TI: Intracranial hemorrhage caused by metastatic tumors. *Neurology* 1977, 27:650–655.

86. Kondziolka D, Bernstein M, Resch L, *et al.*: Significance of hemorrhage into brain tumors: clinicopathological study. *J Neurosurg* 1987, 67:852–857.

87. Lones MA, Verity MA: Fatal hemorrhage in a cerebral pilocytic astrocytoma-adult type. *Acta Neuropathol* 1991, 81:688–690.

88. Wakai S, Yamakawa K, Manaka S, Takakura K: Spontaneous intracranial hemorrhage caused by brain tumor: its incidence and clinical significance. *Neurosurgery* 1982, 10:437–444.

89. Gildersleeve N, Koo AH, McDonald CJ: Metastatic tumor presenting as intracerebral hemorrhage. *Radiology* 1977, 124:109–112.

90. Hirano A, Matsui T: Vascular structures in brain tumors. *Hum Pathol* 1975, 6:611–621.

91. Giannakopoulos G, Nair S, Snider C, Amenta PS: Implications for the pathogenesis of aneurysm formation: metastatic choriocarcinoma with spontaneous splenic rupture: case report and a review. *Surg Neurol* 1992, 38:236–240.

92. Hart MN, Byer JA: Rupture of middle cerebral artery branches by invasive astrocytoma. *Neurology* 1974, 24:1171–1174.

93. Ho KL: Neoplastic aneurysm and intracranial hemorrhage. *Cancer* 1982, 50:2935–2940.

94. New PFJ, Price DL, Carter B: Cerebral angiography in cardiac myxoma. *Radiology* 1970, 96:335–345.

95. del Zoppo GJ, Mori E: Hematologic causes of intracerebral hemorrhage and their treatment. *Neurosurg Clin* 1992, 3:637–658.

96. Ruff RL, Posner JB: Incidence and treatment of peripheral venous thrombosis in patients with glioma. *Ann Neurol* 1983, 13:334–336.

97. Kaku DA, Lowenstein DH: Emergence of recreational drug abuse as a major risk factor for stroke in young adults. *Ann Intern Med* 1990, 113:821–827.

98. Harrington H, Heller HA, Dawson D, *et al.*: Intracerebral hemorrhage and oral amphetamine. *Arch Neurol* 1983, 40:503–507.

99. Sloan MA, Kittner SJ, Rigamonti D, Price TR: Occurrence of stroke associated with use/abuse of drugs. *Neurology* 1991, 41:1358–1364.

100. Fredericks RK, Lefkowitz DS, Challa VR, Troost BT: Cerebral vasculitis associated with cocaine abuse. *Stroke* 1991, 22:1437–1439.

101. Yin PA: Ephedrine-induced intracerebral hemorrhage and central nervous system vasculitis. *Stroke* 1984, 15:1641.
102. Yu YJ, Cooper LR, Wellenstein DE, Block B: Cerebral angiitis and intracerebral hemorrhage associated with amphetamine abuse. *J Neurosurg* 1983, 58:108–111.
103. Wooten MR, Khangure MS, Murphy MJ: Intracerebral hemorrhage and vasculitis related to ephedrine abuse. *Ann Neurol* 1983, 13:337–340.
104. Citron BP, Jhalpern M, McCarron M, *et al.*: Necrotizing angiitis associated with drug abuse. *N Engl J Med* 1970, 19:1003–1011.
105. Stoessl AJ, Young GB, Feasby TE: Intracerebral hemorrhage and angiographic beading following ingestion of catecholaminergics. *Stroke* 1985, 16:734–736.
106. Green RM, Kelly KM, Gabrielsen T, *et al.*: Multiple intracerebral hemorrhages after smoking "crack" cocaine. *Stroke* 1990, 21:957–962.
107. Caplan LR, Thomas C, Banks G: Central nervous system complications of addiction to "T's and Blues." *Neurology* 1982, 32:623–628.
108. Bessen HA: Intracranial hemorrhage associated with phencyclidine abuse. *JAMA* 1982, 248:585–586.
109. Kitka DG, Devereaux MW, Chandar K: Intracranial hemorrhages due to phenylpropanolamine. *Stroke* 1985, 16:510–512.
110. Yapor WY, Gutierrez FA: Cocaine-induced intratumoral hemorrhage: case report and review of the literature. *Neurosurgery* 1992, 30:288–291.
111. Adams WH, Rufo RA, Talarico L, *et al.*: Thrombocytopenia and intravenous heroin use. *Ann Intern Med* 1978, 89:207–211.
112. Karpatkin S: Immunologic thrombocytopenic purpura in HIV-seropositive homosexuals, narcotic addicts and hemophiliacs. *Sem Hematol* 1988, 25:219–229.
113. Leissinger CA: Severe thrombocytopenia associated with cocaine use. *Ann Intern Med* 1990, 112:708–710.
114. Gorelick PB: The status of alcohol as a risk factor for stroke. *Stroke* 1989, 20:1607–1610.
115. Klatsky AL, Armstrong MA, Friedman GD: Alcohol use and subsequent cerebrovascular disease hospitalizations. *Stroke* 1989, 20:741–746.
116. Gill JS, Shipley MJ, Tsementzis SA, *et al.*: Alcohol consumption: a risk factor for hemorrhagic and non-hemorrhagic stroke. *Am J Med* 1991, 90:489–497.
117. Weisberg LA: Alcoholic intracerebral hemorrhage. *Stroke* 1988, 19:1565–1569.
118. Niizuma H, Suzuki J, Yonemitsu T, Otsuki T: Spontaneous intracerebral hemorrhage and liver dysfunction. *Stroke* 1988, 19:852–856.
119. Cowan DH: Effect of alcoholism on hemostasis. *Sem Hematol* 1980, 17:137–147.
120. DeJaegere PP, Arnold AA, Balk AH, Simoons ML: Intracranial hemorrhage in association with thrombolytic therapy: incidence and clinical predictive factors. *J Am Coll Cardiol* 1992, 19:289–294.
121. Alpert JS: Intracranial hemorrhage after thrombolytic therapy: a therapeutic conflict. *J Am Coll Cardiol* 1992, 19:295–296.
122. Gore JM, Sloan M, Price TR, *et al.*: Intracerebral hemorrhage, cerebral infarction, and subdural hematoma after acute myocardial infarction and thrombolytic therapy in the thrombolysis in myocardial infarction study. *Circulation* 1991, 83:448–459.
123. Anderson JL, Karagounis L, Allen A, *et al.*: Older age and elevated blood pressure are risk factors for intracerebral hemorrhage after thrombolysis. *Am J Cardiol* 1991, 68:166–170.
124. Kase CS, O'Neal AM, Fisher M, *et al.*: Intracranial hemorrhage after use of tissue plasminogen activator for coronary thrombolysis. *Ann Intern Med* 1990, 112:17–21.
125. Pendlebury WW, Iole ED, Tracy RP, Dill BA: Intracerebral hemorrhage related to cerebral amyloid angiopathy and t-PA treatment. *Ann Neurol* 1991, 29:210–213.
126. Ramsay DA, Penswick JL, Robertson DM: Fatal streptokinase-induced intracerebral haemorrhage in cerebral amyloid angiopathy. *Can J Neurol Sci* 1990, 17:336–341.
127. Sane DC, Califf RM, Ropol EG, *et al.*: Bleeding during thrombolytic therapy for acute myocardial infarction: mechanisms and management. *Ann Intern Med* 1989, 111:1010–1022.
128. DaSilva VF, Bormanis J: Intracerebral hemorrhage after combined anticoagulant-thrombolytic therapy for myocardial infarction: two case reports and a short review. *Neurosurgery* 1992, 30:943–945.
129. Teal PA, Pessin MS: Hemorrhagic transformation: the spectrum of ischemia-related brain hemorrhage. *Neurosurg Clin* 1992, 3:601–610.
130. del Zoppo GJ, Poeck K, Pessin MS, *et al.*: Recombinant tissue plasminogen activator in acute thrombotic and embolic stroke. *Ann Neurol* 1992, 32:78–86.
131. Wolpert SM, Bruckmann H, Greenlee R, *et al.*: Neuroradiological evaluation of patients with acute stroke treated with recombinant tissue plasminogen activator. *Am J Neuroradiol* 1993, 14:3–13.
132. Landefeld CS, Goldman L: Major bleeding in outpatients with warfarin: incidence and prediction by factors known at the start of outpatient therapy. *Am J Med* 1989, 87:144–152.
133. Fogelholm R, Eskola K, Kiminkinen T, Kunnamo I: Anticoagulant treatment as a risk factor for primary intracerebral haemorrhage. *J Neurol Neurosurg Psych* 1992, 55:1121–1124.
134. Wintzen AR, de Jonge H, Loeliger EA, Bots GTAM: The risk of intracerebral hemorrhage during oral anticoagulant treatment: a population study. *Ann Neurol* 1984, 16:553–558.
135. Kase CS, Robinson RK, Stein RW, *et al.*: Anticoagulant-related intracerebral hemorrhage. *Neurology* 1985, 35:943–948.
136. Franke CL, de Jonge J, van Swieten JC, *et al.*: Intracerebral hematomas during anticoagulant treatment. *Stroke* 1990, 21:726–730.
137. Radberg JA: Prognostic parameters in spontaneous intracerebral hematomas with special reference to anticoagulant treatment. *Stroke* 1991, 22:571–576.
138. Cohen BA, Biller J: Hemorrhagic stroke due to cerebral vasculitis and the role of immunosuppressive therapy. *Neurosurg Clin* 1992, 3:611–624.
139. Petty GW, Mohr JP: Stroke in the setting of collagen vascular disease. In *Stroke: Pathophysiology, Diagnosis, Management.* Edited by Barnett HJM, Mohr JP, Stein BM, Yatsu FM. New York: Churchill Livingstone Inc.; 1992:691–720.
140. Levi ADO, Kucharczyk W, Lang AP, Schutz H: Clival chordoma presenting with acute brain stem hemorrhage. *Can J Neurol Sci* 1991, 18:515–518.
141. Sze G, Krol G, Olsen WL, *et al.*: Hemorrhagic neoplasms: MR mimics of occult vascular malformations. *AJR* 1987, 149:1223–1230.

Chapter 7

Nonatherosclerotic Stroke

NABIH M. RAMADAN
PANAYIOTIS MITSIAS

Cerebral atherosclerosis is implicated in over one half of ischemic strokes (IS) [1]. Cerebral cardioembolism is the cause of IS in 6% to 36% of cases [1–3]. Occasionally, hematologic abnormalities, nonatherosclerotic arteriopathies, illicit drug use, oral contraceptive use, migraine, or cerebral venous thrombosis are presumed causes of cerebral infarction, particularly when the patient is younger than 50 years of age. In such instances where atherosclerotic and common cerebral cardioembolic mechanisms of cerebral ischemia are unlikely, a thoughtful, exhaustive, and frequently expensive search for these unusual nonatherosclerotic causes of IS is indicated because the treatment of some of the underlying conditions may substantially reduce the risk of recurrent cerebral ischemic events. The focus of this chapter is on nonatherosclerotic causes of ischemic stroke that can be classified as cardiac, vascular, hematologic, and miscellaneous (Table 7.1).

CARDIAC CAUSES OF CEREBRAL INFARCTION

Approximately 15% of all IS patients have a presumed cardiac mechanism [2]. In young patients (*ie,* less than 45 years old), the frequency of cardioembolic stroke may be higher, reaching 36% in one study [3]. Commonly, young patients undergo more extensive evaluation (*eg,* transesophageal echocardiography with contrast, such as color-flow imaging or agitated intravenous saline) than the older stroke victims and, thus, the reported lower incidence of cardioembolism in the older age group could be due to underdiagnosis of this condition.

Typically, cardioembolic strokes are seen as wedge-shaped hypodensities on cranial computed tomography (CT) scan (Figure 7.1), involving both cortical gray and white matter. Arterial territories commonly involved in cerebral cardioembolism include the main subdivisions of the middle cerebral artery or the tip of the basilar artery. Small deep cerebral infarcts (lacune if <1.5 cm and involving the territory of a single arterial perforator, "lagoone" if the infarct is larger than 1.5 cm or if the ischemia is in the territory of multiple arterial perforators) have been seen with cardioembolic strokes, albeit infrequently.

Cardiac emboli are caused by abnormalities of the following: 1) cardiac rhythm; 2) cardiac valves; and 3) cardiac chamber or wall (Table 7.2).

Abnormalities of Cardiac Rhythm

Nonvalvular atrial fibrillation (NVAF) accounts for 45% of all cardioembolic strokes in elderly patients [4]. In the Framingham study [5], the age-specific incidence rate of atrial fibrillation exponentially increased from 0.2 per 1000 for patients aged 30 to 39 years to 39 per 1000 for those aged 80 to 89 years. The rate of stroke in patients older than 70 years of age who have atrial fibrillation exceeds 5% per year [2,4,5]. Recent (within 3 months) congestive heart failure, a history of hypertension, previous thromboembolic events, global left ventricular dysfunction, and increased left atrial diameter by echocardiography are strong predictors of IS in patients with NVAF [6,7]. Both paroxysmal and chronic atrial fibrillation are associated with an increased risk of IS [2,6,8]. Lone atrial fibrillation, defined as atrial fibrillation in patients less than 60 years of age who have no valvular or ischemic heart disease (*ie,* no risk factors), does not increase the risk of IS substantially [2,8]. The risk of IS with NVAF is maximal in the first year following the diagnosis of the arrhythmia [2,4,8,9] or after a transition from paroxysmal to chronic atrial fibrillation [10]. Wolf and coworkers [9] reported that nearly 25% of IS occurred when NVAF was initially diagnosed; an additional 14% occurred in the first year of the onset of atrial fibrillation. In addition to clinically manifested IS, "silent" cerebral infarction occurs in about 15% of patients with chronic atrial fibrillation [2]. In atrial fibrillation, thrombi are usually attached to the left atrium or the left atrial appendage [11]. Histopathologically, these thrombi are composed of alternating layers of fibrin and platelets mixed with coagulated erythrocytes [11]. Fresh thrombi tend to be poorly organized and fragment readily resulting in systemic and cerebral embolization, the latter more frequently.

Sick sinus syndrome is a rare cause of cerebral cardioembolism [12–14]. Fairfax and coworkers [15] reported 16 embolic events in 100 patients with sick sinus syndrome; 13 were cerebral. They also reported more embolic events in patients with prolonged atrial systole. Bathen and coworkers [13] found that

Table 7.1. Nonatherosclerotic causes of ischemic stroke

Cardiac	Arteriopathic	Hematologic	Toxic	Other
Abnormal rhythm Valve disease Abnormal chamber and wall	Idiopathic Infectious Inflammatory Hereditary Substance-related Traumatic Postradiation	Natural anticoagulant defect* Clotting factor increased Fibrinolytic defect Platelet hyperactivity Hyperviscosity syndromes Immune-mediated prothrombotic states	Illicit substance Oral contraceptives Anabolic steroids "Diet pills" Anticancer therapy Alcohol	Migraine Cerebral venous/sinus thrombosis

*Anticoagulant defect could be a decrease in absolute concentration or reduced activity.

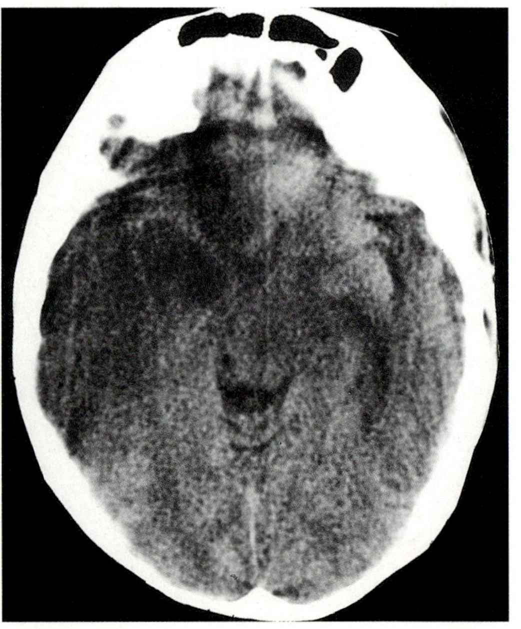

FIGURE 7.1

Cardioembolic stroke. Cranial computed tomography showing a large hypodense area compatible with ischemic stroke in the frontotemporal region. Note the dense middle cerebral artery sign.

patients with the brady-tachycardia syndrome have the highest risk of embolism formation.

Abnormalities of Cardiac Valves

Rheumatic heart disease frequently causes IS in patients not treated with anticoagulants [16,17]. Rheumatic mitral stenosis carries the highest risk of systemic and cerebral emboli [18], followed by aortic valve disease (stenosis or insufficiency) and mitral insufficiency [16–18]. Dervall and coworkers [19] reported that systemic embolization occurred at a rate of 1.5% to 4.7% per year in patients with rheumatic mitral stenosis prior to valve surgery. It is believed that a patient with mitral stenosis will have a one chance in five of developing systemic embolization during the course of the disease [17]. Low cardiac output, atrial fibrillation, and age increase the risk of embolization in patients with rheumatic mitral stenosis [16–18]. Left atrial size, mitral calcification, mitral valve surface area, and clinical classification (*ie*, cardiac class) correlate poorly with the risk of systemic embolism. In noninfected, rheumatic mitral stenosis, platelet-fibrin clots form on the left atrium or the left atrial appendage. Recurrent embolism occurs in 30% to 75% of patients with rheumatic mitral stenosis who do not receive anticoagulants [20].

Mitral annular calcification is often discovered in predominantly elderly women with generalized atherosclerosis [2,17]. Mitral annular calcification is associated with increased risk of IS and is often associated with other factors such as mitral stenosis or regurgitation, endocarditis, and arrhythmias including atrial fibrillation [2,17]. Fibrin clots and calcified material from a heavily calcified and ulcerated annulus embolize to the brain and systemically [21–23].

Infective endocarditis (Figure 7.2) is another well-recognized cause of cerebral embolism. Garvey and Neu [24] reported that 33% of patients with infective endocarditis of the natural valves and 50% of those with infection of prosthetic valves developed IS. In the postantibiotic era, the prevalence of embolism in infective endocarditis ranges from 12% to 40% [17]. IS occurs predominantly upon presentation or within 48 hours of the diagnosis of infective endocarditis [25]. In Garvey's series, Group D *Streptococcus* and *Staphylococcus aureus* were the most common pathogens in infective endocarditis of the natural valves, while *Aspergillus* species and *Streptococcus viridans* were the most likely organisms in infections of the prosthetic valves [24]. The risk of embolism seems particularly high with *S. aureus* [25]. IS in patients with infective endocarditis is caused by embolization of infected or sterile vegetations and, perhaps, embolization from mycotic aneurysms or vasculitis. Mycotic aneurysms are formed when material from infected cardiac valves embolize to the adventitia of the cerebral arteries [26]. Unlike berry aneurysms, mycotic aneurysms are detected on the distal branches of the main intracranial cerebral vessels (*eg*, distal branches of the middle cerebral artery).

Table 7.2. Causes of cerebral cardioembolism

Abnormal rhythm	Abnormal valve	Abnormal chamber/wall
Atrial fibrillation	Rheumatic heart disease	Myocardial infarction
Sick sinus syndrome	Prosthetic valve	Patent foramen ovale/atrial septal defect
Atrioventricular block*	Mitral annular calcification	Atrial/ventricular aneurysm
Supraventricular tachycardia	Infective endocarditis	Atrial septal aneurysm
	Noninfective endocarditis	Ventricular aneurysm
	Mitral valve prolapse*	Cardiomyopathy
	Calcific aortic stenosis	Cardiac tumors: atrial myxoma, metastatic melanoma, rhabdomyosarcoma
	Bicuspid aortic valve	

*With myxomatous changes or significant mitral insufficiency.

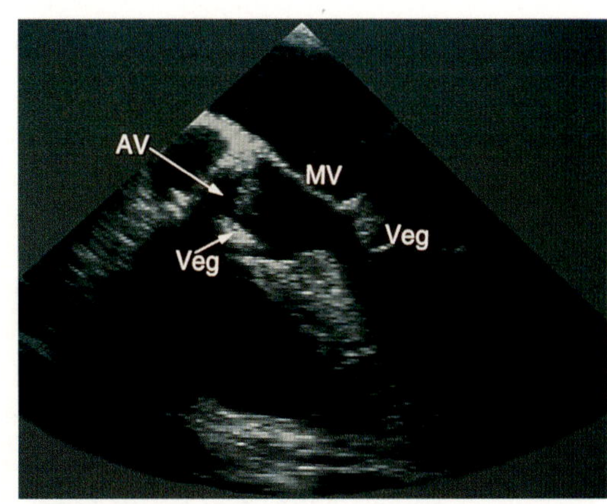

FIGURE 7.2

Infective endocarditis. Transesophageal echocardiogram showing vegetations (Veg) on aortic (AV) and mitral (MV) valves.

Table 7.3. Conditions associated with nonbacterial thrombotic endocarditis

Systemic lupus erythematosus
Antiphospholipid antibody syndrome
Peripartum
Malignant melanoma
Mucinous cancer
Adenocarcinoma

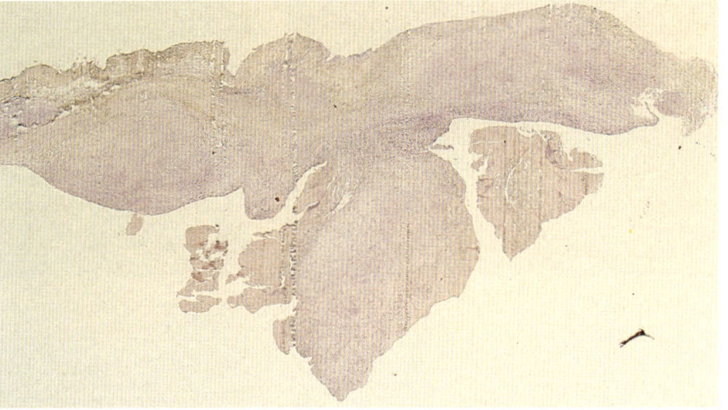

FIGURE 7.3

Libman-Sacks endocarditis. Vegetation on the aortic valve in a patient with positive anticardiolipins and multiple strokes (magnification × 5).

Nonbacterial thrombotic ("marantic") endocarditis (NBTE) develops in patients with chronic illnesses [27], as listed in Table 7.3 and accounts for up to 27% of strokes in patients with known cancer [2,27]. Patients with malignant melanoma and mucinous cancer are particularly vulnerable [26–28]. Systemic emboli occur in about 42% of patients with NBTE [27] and can be the initial manifestation of malignancy [29,30]. NBTE affects patients with normal cardiac valves, particularly the mitral and aortic valves. Vegetations in NBTE consist of bland fibrin-platelet thrombi sometimes mixed with valvular collagen debris [17,26]. Unlike the vegetations of infective endocarditis, they are sterile and tend to be small. Libman-Sacks vegetations (Figure 7.3) develop in patients with systemic lupus erythematosus (SLE) and the antiphospholipid antibody syndrome [31], and they consist of fibrin, necrotic debris of fibroblasts, and inflammatory cells. Thrombi in NBTE form on the atrial surface in mitral or tricuspid valve disease and on the ventricular surface in patients with aortic or pulmonic valve involvement [27]. Both small and large cerebral vessel occlusions occur in NBTE [26,28]. Evidence of multiple small-vessel occlusion, coexisting disseminated intravascular coagulopathy, and the presence of Trousseau's syndrome in some patients suggest that NBTE represents a prothrombotic state [2,26–30,32].

Both mitral valve prolapse (MVP) and patent foramen ovale are thought to account for a large number of IS in patients younger than 45 years of age [3]. The Cerebral Embolism Task Force [2] has estimated that the risk of IS in young adults with MVP is one per 11,000 per year. In a case-control study, Barnett and coworkers [33] found MVP in 40% of patients younger than 45 years of age who developed cerebral ischemic events. Six percent of older patients with cerebral ischemic events had evidence of MVP, whereas 7% of the control group did not. There is a general consensus in the literature that most subjects with MVP will not develop stroke. At risk are those with myxomatous degeneration of the valve, significant mitral insufficiency, and men. The use of oral contraceptives and protein S deficiency may increase the risk of stroke in patients with MVP [34,35]. A prothrombotic state is suspected in a patient with IS and MVP who also has protein S deficiency or who is taking oral contraceptives [34,35]. Fibrinous endocarditis, endothelial denudation of the mitral valve with fibrin deposition, and mural thrombus at the junction of a prolapsed leaflet and the atrial wall are the histopathologic substrates of cerebral cardioembolism in patients with MVP [17].

Calcific aortic stenosis (CAS) is a common finding in elderly patients, yet embolic strokes from CAS are believed to be rare [2,17]. Calcium emboli have been found in the retinas of patients with CAS [36]. Bicuspid aortic valve, another relatively common abnormality of the aortic valve, is rarely reported to cause IS [37].

Abnormalities of the Cardiac Chambers or the Myocardium

Acute myocardial infarctions (AMI) may be complicated by IS [2,38]. In a recent placebo-controlled, double-blind, randomized trial of warfarin following AMI, stroke occurred in 44 of 607 (7%) patients who received placebo and in 3% (18) of those treated with warfarin [39]. The risk of stroke in patients with anterior AMI is 2% to 6% [38], and 1% with inferior AMI [2]. Most strokes following AMI occur in the first 2 weeks of the cardiac event [2,38]. Mural thrombus formation, large cardiac size, poorly functioning dilated left ventricle, atrial fibrillation, heart failure, and acute left ventricular aneurysm increase the risk of IS in patients with AMI [2,38]. Cerebral cardioembolism following AMI is believed to be secondary to the formation of left ventricular thrombi (Figure 7.4), which are detected echocardiographically in about 40% of patients with anterior AMI [2,38]. Echocardiography is sensitive in detecting large ventricular thrombi [40], however, its value in detecting small (<5 mm), yet potentially devastating, mural thrombi is still doubtful [2]. The majority of ventricular thrombi are formed between days 1 and

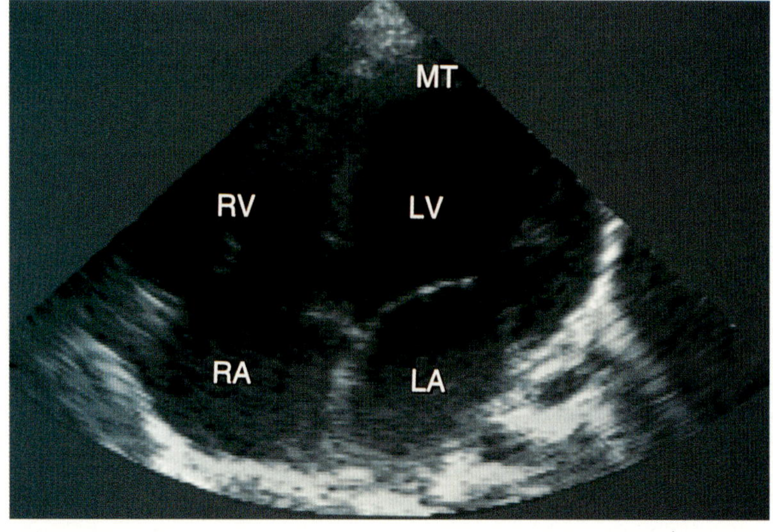

FIGURE 7.4

Mural thrombus (MT). Transesophageal electrocardiogram showing left ventricular (LV) thrombus. LA—left atrium; RA—right atrium; RV—right ventricle.

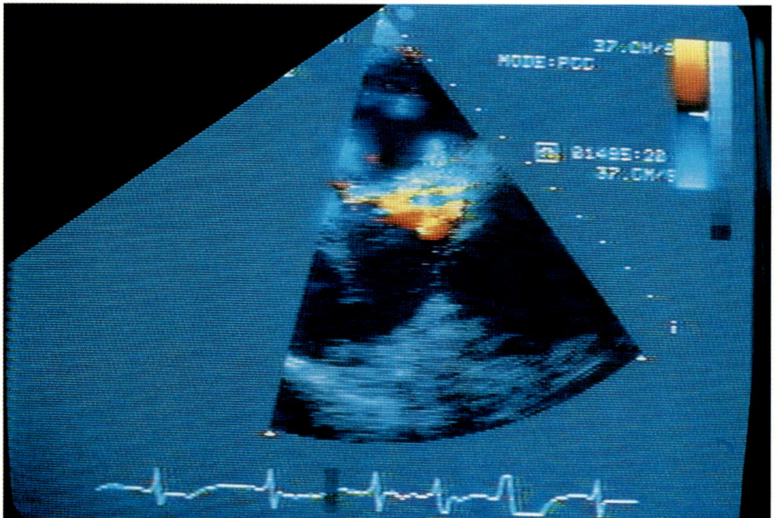

FIGURE 7.5

Right-to-left shunt. Color-flow transesophageal electrocardiogram showing interatrial blood flow in yellow and orange colors.

14 following AMI; most strokes occur during this critical period. These thrombi form over damaged akinetic myocardium or ventricular aneurysms. In such instances, activated clotting factors combined with locally abnormal hemorrheology promote the formation of thrombi that can embolize, especially when they protrude into the ventricular cavity [41].

Ventricular aneurysms develop in 7% to 10% of patients following AMI. They are typically apical or anterior and the risk of associated cerebral embolism is 5% [42].

Patent foramen ovale (Figure 7.5) is an increasingly recognized cause of cerebral cardioembolism [43]. Lechat and coworkers [43] found that 40% of 60 IS patients younger than 55 years of age had patent foramen ovale on contrast echocardiography. Patent foramen ovale was detected in 10% of their control non-IS group. This value is significantly lower than the percentage of patent foramen ovale detected at autopsy [44]. The mechanism of stroke in patients with patent foramen ovale and the related congenital atrial septal defect (Figure 7.6) is believed to be due to embolization from the venous side through the interatrial defect to the arterial circulation (paradoxical embolism). Left atrial pressure is normally higher than the right atrial pressure and, therefore, blood would flow from right to left only in such conditions as pulmonary hypertension. Hagen and coworkers [44] demonstrated, however, that spontaneous reversal of the usual direction of intra-arterial blood flow occurs, especially in early cardiac systole. In fact, in the majority of their patients with patent foramen ovale, right-to-left shunt was demonstrated spontaneously without Valsalva maneuvers. Bogousslavsky and Pierre [3] argue that an isolated patent foramen ovale in a young patient with stroke may be incidental. It is only in patients with documented peripheral venous thrombosis and in those whose stroke is temporally linked to Valsalva maneuvers that patent foramen ovale with paradoxical embolism can be the likely mechanism of cerebral ischemia.

Atrial septal aneurysm (Figure 7.7) is rare and has been reported to cause cerebral cardioembolism in a few cases [45].

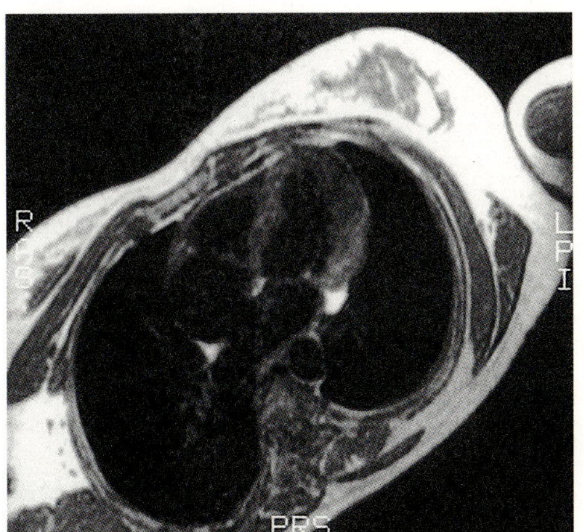

FIGURE 7.6

Atrial septal defect (ASD). Gated cardiac magnetic resonance image showing ASD in a patient with ischemic stroke and antiphospholipid antibodies.

Neurologic signs and symptoms of atrial myxoma (Figure 7.8), the most common cardiac tumor, occur in 45% of patients and are chiefly related to cerebral embolization [46]. Multiple cerebral infarctions, usually in the territory of the middle cerebral artery, are shown on cranial CT in the majority of patients and are thought to be due to degenerated myxomatous material that embolizes to the cerebral circulation. Cerebral aneurysms have been described as well in patients with atrial myxoma [47].

NONATHEROSCLEROTIC ARTERIOPATHIES

In addition to atherosclerosis, the cerebral blood vessels can be injured by systemic, or central nervous system inflammatory conditions, infections, trauma, or radiation. Vessel wall damage also occurs in hereditary disorders such as Fabry's disease [48].

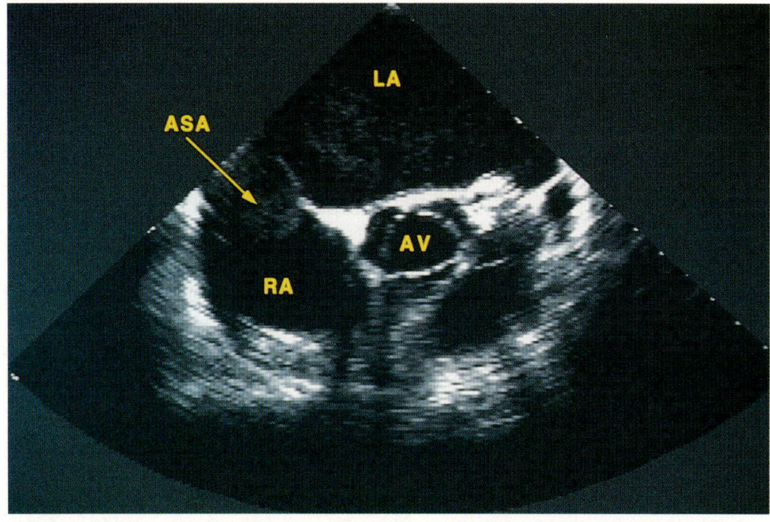

FIGURE 7.7

Atrial septal aneurysm (ASA) shown on transesophageal electrocardiogram. AV—aortic valve; LA—left atrium; RA—right atrium.

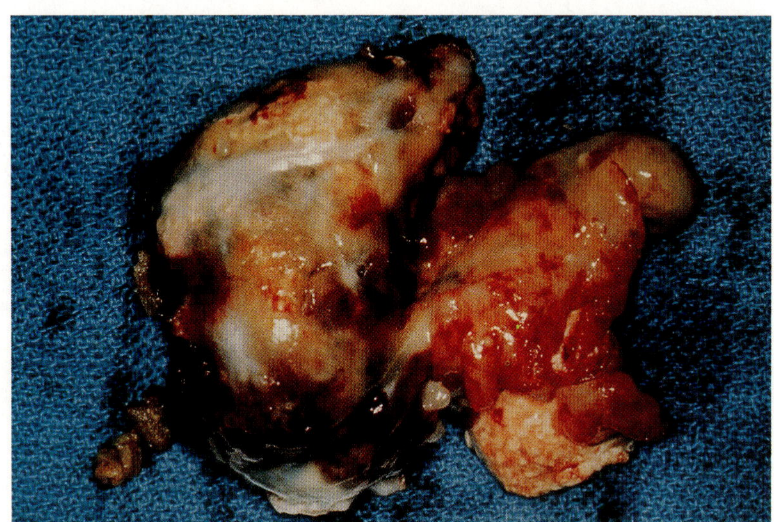

FIGURE 7.8

Atrial myxoma. Gross pathologic specimen.

The causes of cerebral ischemia in nonatherosclerotic arteriopathies are similar to those related to atherosclerosis and they include in situ thrombosis, artery-to-artery embolism, perfusion failure (watershed infarction), and vasospasm. Nonatherosclerotic arteriopathies can occur at any age, however, they are most prevalent in patients younger than 50 years of age. Nonatherosclerotic arteriopathies can be idiopathic, hereditary, inflammatory, infectious, or drug or substance induced as delineated in Table 7.4. The description of every reported nonatherosclerotic arteriopathy linked to IS is beyond the scope of this chapter. Only select conditions will be discussed.

Idiopathic Arteriopathies

Spontaneous dissection of the cervicocephalic arteries (Figure 7.9) is a rare cause of cerebral infarction in elderly patients but

Table 7.4. Nonatherosclerotic arteriopathies

Idiopathic	Infectious	Inflammatory	Hereditary	Toxic
Nontraumatic dissection Fibromuscular dysplasia Moyamoya disease Vanishing vasculopathy	Bacterial: Acute meningitis, syphilis, Lyme disease, tuberculosis Viral: Varicella-zoster virus, cytomegalovirus Fungal: Mucormycosis, aspergillosis Parasitic: Cysticerosis Rickettsial: Rocky mountain spotted fever	Granulomatous central nervous system angiitis Takayasu's disease Central nervous system angiitis Polyarteritis nodosa Churg-Strauss syndrome Systemic lupus erythematosus Sneddon's syndrome Wegener's granulomatosis Rheumatoid arthritis Scleroderma Behçet's disease Inflammatory bowel disease Sarcoidosis Malignant atrophic papulosis Lymphomatoid granulomatosis	Down's syndrome Fabry's disease Homocystinuria Sickle cell disease Amyloid angiopathy α-Glucosidase deficiency Mitochondrial disease (*eg*, MELAS)	Oral contraceptives Sympathomimetics Cocaine Alcohol Heroin Phencyclidine LSD Antineoplastic agents Pentazocine Marijuana

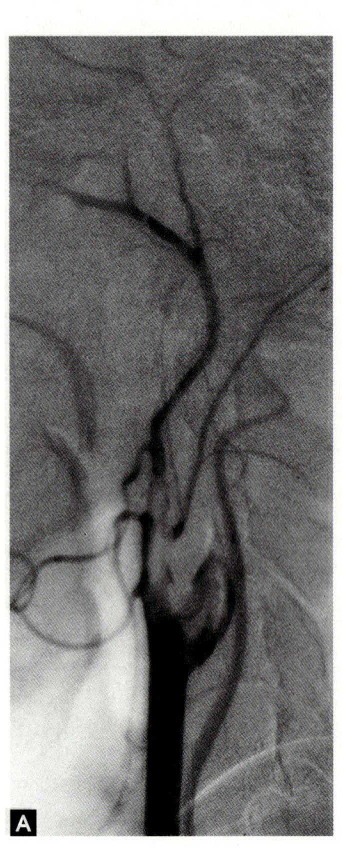

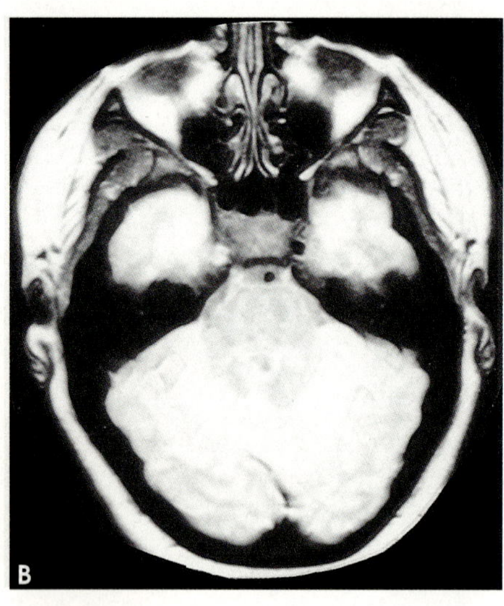

FIGURE 7.9

Cervicocephalic arterial dissection. **A**, Selective carotid angiogram showing tapered occlusion of the right internal carotid artery (ICA). **B**, T2-weighted cranial magnetic resonance image (MRI) demonstrating absence of flow void signal in the ICA. Patient is a migraine suffer and the suspected dissection on MRI was demonstrated on angiography.

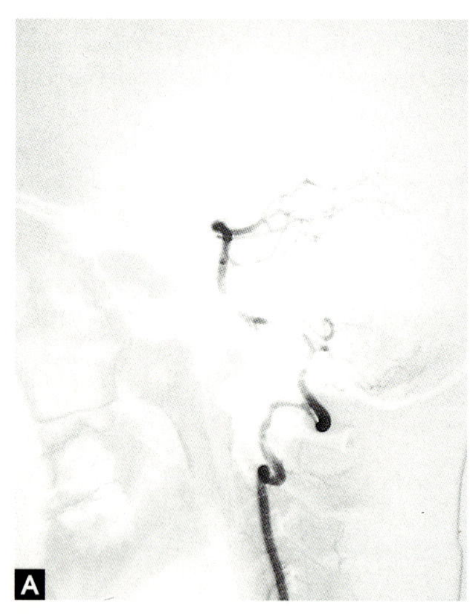

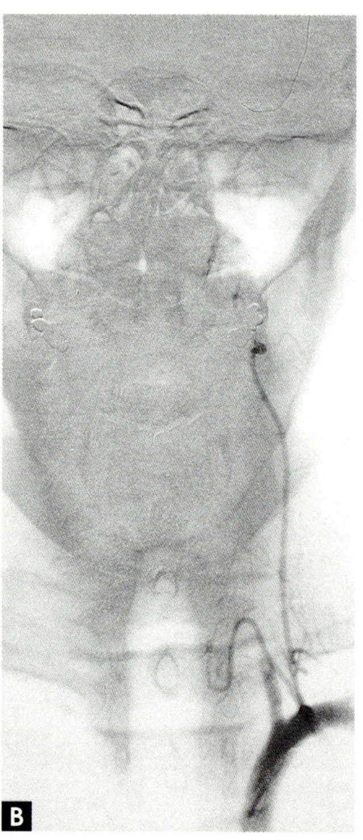

FIGURE 7.10

Bilateral vertebral artery (VA) dissection. Cerebral angiogram showing severe narrowing of the right vertebral artery (**A**) (*lateral view*) and tapered occlusion of the left VA (**B**) (*antereoposterior view*).

has been recognized as an important etiology of IS in young adults [3]. Biller and coworkers [49] reported that the incidence of dissection of the cerebral arteries was 0.4% when cerebral angiography was performed to evaluate patients with stroke. Among 1200 patients with acute stroke, Bogousslavsky and coworkers [50] found carotid dissection in 2.5%. The mean age of patients with carotid dissection was 41 years. Dissection of the carotid arteries is significantly more common than dissection of the vertebral arteries (Figure 7.10); involvement of the extracranial segment of the carotid artery 2- to 3-cm distal to the carotid bifurcation is distinctly more common than involvement of the intracranial portions of the vessel [51,52]. Multiple arterial dissections (Figure 7.11) are found in 10% to 30% of patients [51,52]. Dissection of the cervicocephalic arteries is frequently associated with minor trauma or physical stress [51,52]. A variety of physical activities as listed in Table 7.5 are believed to result in arterial dissection [51–53]. Fibromuscular dysplasia (FMD), hypertension, Marfan's syndrome, or migraine headache may predispose to or are associated with cervicocephalic arterial dissection [51,52,54,55]. Cerebral ischemia occurs in over two thirds of patients with cervicocephalic arterial dissection and can be the initial manifestation of the dissection in one third of patients [51,52]. Patients with distal internal carotid artery or distal vertebral artery dissection can present with subarachnoid hemorrhage [51,52]. Pathologically, extracranial arterial dissections are associated with the formation of hematomas in the media, intimal tears, pseudoaneurysms (Figure 7.12), and luminal stenosis or obstruction [51,52]. An overlying thrombus may be observed occasionally. In contrast, intracranial dissections develop in the plane between the internal elastic lamina and the media [52], suggesting that the dissection is the result of an intimal tear [51,52].

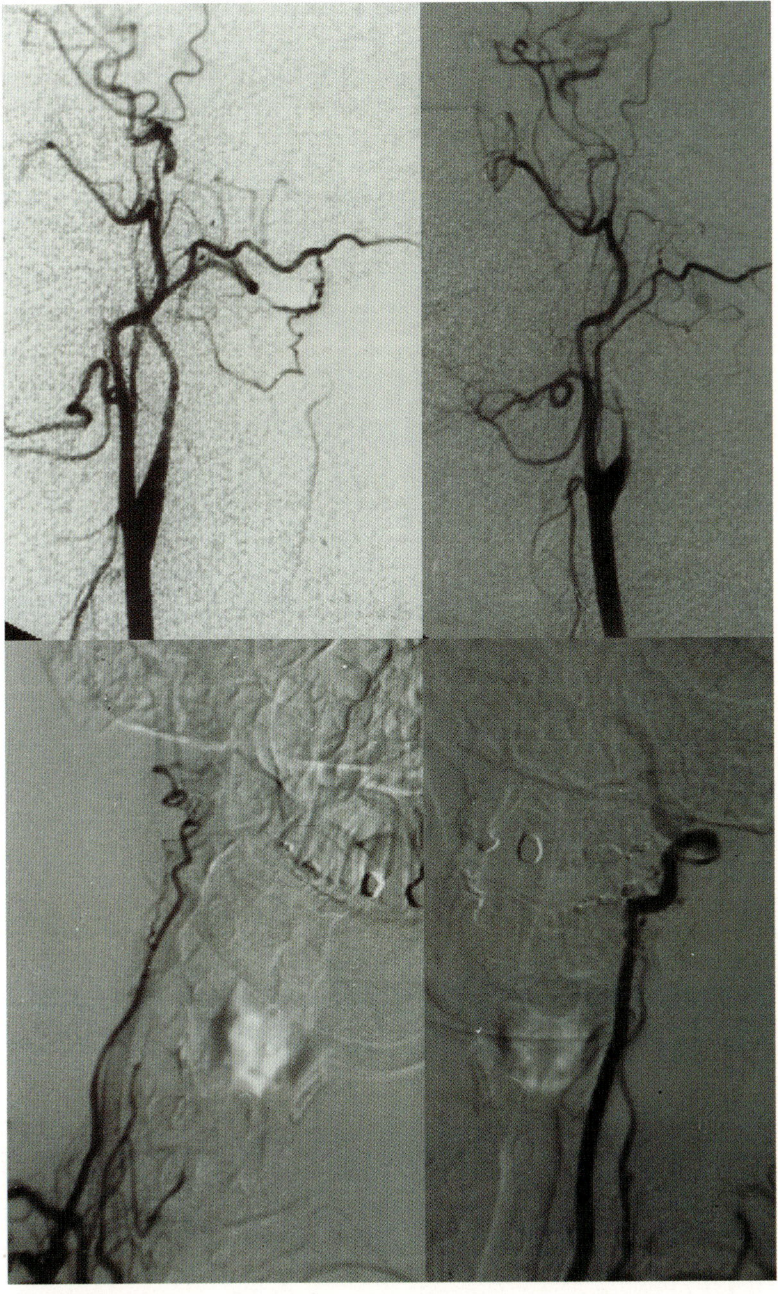

FIGURE 7.11

Four-vessel dissection. Cerebral angiogram showing tapered occlusion of left and right internal carotid artery (*top row, lateral views*), and of distal left vertebral artery (VA) (*bottom right, antereoposterior [AP] view*), and elongated severely narrowed right VA (*bottom left, AP view*).

Fibromuscular dysplasia is a nonatherosclerotic arteriopathy of the medium-sized arteries, affecting the renal, visceral, peripheral, and cerebral vessels [56]. FMD is a disease of unknown etiology predominantly affecting women in the sixth and seventh decades. FMD is usually asymptomatic; however, it can present as hypertension, peripheral vascular occlusive disease, or stroke. IS from FMD is related to thromboembolic occlusion or hemodynamic compromise of the distal cerebral arterial fields (*ie*, watershed zones). Cervicocephalic arterial dissection, aneurysmal formation, and carotid-cavernous fistulae are other complications of FMD [51,52,56]. The pathologic changes described in patients with FMD are the same in the cerebral and peripheral arteries. Segments of fibromuscular hypertrophy causing luminal stenosis alternate with dilated areas resulting from a thinning of the media

Table 7.5. Activities reported to be associated with arterial dissection

Coughing
Eating
Nose blowing
Shaving
Tooth brushing
Sexual intercourse
"Bottoms-up" drinking
Shampooing in beauty parlor
Childbirth
Turning head while leading a parade
Whiplash
Chiropractic manipulation
"Head banging" during punk-rock dancing
Heavy lifting
Straightening up after bending
Neck flexing with child scolding
Sports: basketball, bowling, diving, football, hockey, polo, skiing, tennis, trampoline exercise, volleyball

and loss of the elastic membrane [56]. This most common form of FMD, referred to as the medial type, produces the characteristic appearance of a string of beads on cerebral angiography (Figure 7.13). Occasionally, intraluminal thrombi are detected. The pathogenesis of FMD remains largely unknown. A viral infection, local trauma, hormonal mechanisms, and heredity are suggested etiologies or associated conditions.

Moyamoya disease (Figure 7.14) is an angiographically diagnosed entity of unknown etiology [57]. Reports from Japan show that about 60% of patients are women [57]. The age of onset of the disease is usually the first and fourth decades, regardless of sex [57]. Cerebral infarction tends to occur more frequently in men with moyamoya disease. Cerebral hemorrhage is more common in women. The pathologic hallmarks of definite moyamoya disease are: 1) intimal thickening of the terminal segment of both internal carotid arteries with subsequent stenosis or occlusion; 2) fibrous intimal proliferation, tortuosity of the elastic lamina, and thinning of the media; 3) the presence of perforating and anastomosing tributaries arising from the circle of Willis; and 4) a small pial vascular network [57]. Inflammatory changes are not present. The angiographic moyamoya pattern has been described in various disorders as shown in Table 7.6.

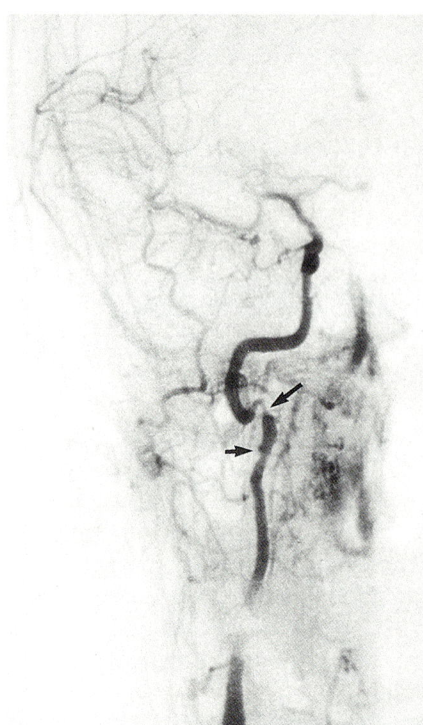

FIGURE 7.12

Pseudoaneurysm (*short arrow*). Selective carotid angiogram (*lateral view*) demonstrating a pseudoaneurysm. Patient suffered a stroke secondary to internal carotid artery (ICA) dissection following orgasm. Note ICA siphon stenosis (*long arrow*).

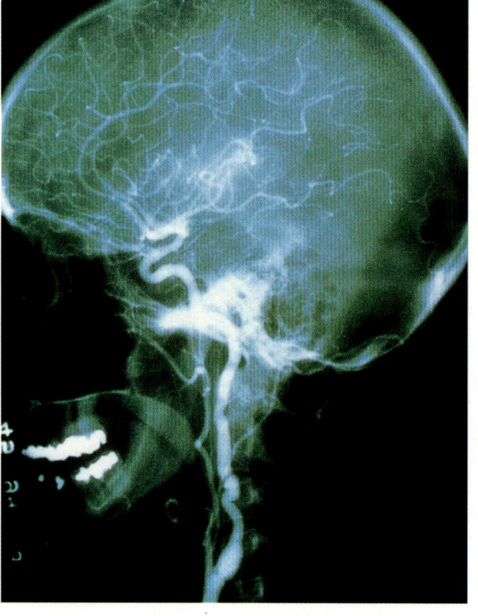

FIGURE 7.13

Fibromuscular dysplasia. "String of beads" sign of the internal carotid artery demonstrated on selective carotid angiogram (*lateral view*).

Infectious Arteriopathies

Ischemic stroke can complicate a whole host of bacterial, fungal, or viral infections [58]. In a recent study, Pfister and coworkers [59] reported that 24 of 86 patients with bacterial meningitis developed focal neurologic signs during the acute phase of the infection. Cerebrovascular arterial complications of bacterial meningitis include a narrowing of the supraclinoid internal carotid artery; wall irregularity, focal dilatation, and

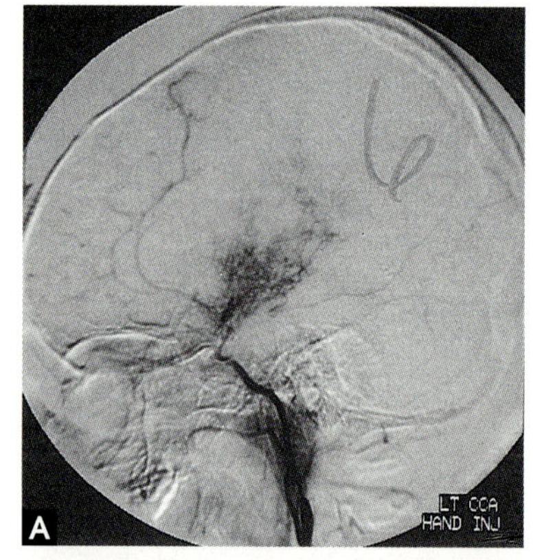

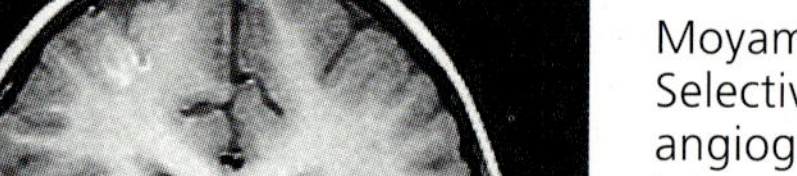

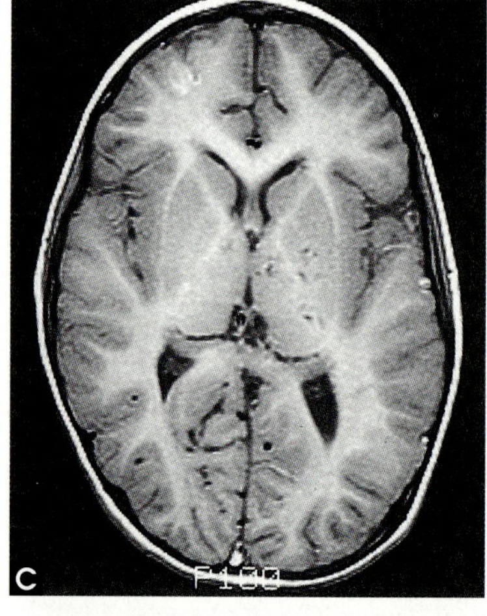

FIGURE 7.14

Moyamoya disease. **A** and **B**, Selective right and left carotid angiogram demonstrating distal internal carotid artery stenosis with abnormal collateral channels. The angiographic patterns of the basal collateral channels have been referred to as the *puff of smoke*. **C**, Proton density cranial magnetic resonance image showing multiple flow void areas corresponding to the collateral channels seen on angiography.

Table 7.6. Conditions associated with angiographic moyamoya

Idiopathic	Leptospirosis
Fibromuscular dysplasia	Postradiation
Neurofibromatosis	Arteriosclerosis
Down's syndrome	Severe vasospasm
Tuberculous meningitis	Oral contraceptives

occlusion of the distal branches of the middle cerebral artery; and focal parenchymatous blush [59,60]. Most arterial complications of bacterial meningitis occur in the first 2 weeks of the infection [59]. Histopathologically, infiltration of the small and medium-sized arteries by acute inflammatory cells results in vessel wall edema and necrosis, proliferation of subintimal tissue, endothelial damage, platelet aggregation, and luminal thrombosis [58]. Occasionally, extramural compression of the arteries from brain edema leads to perfusion failure and watershed infarction [58,59].

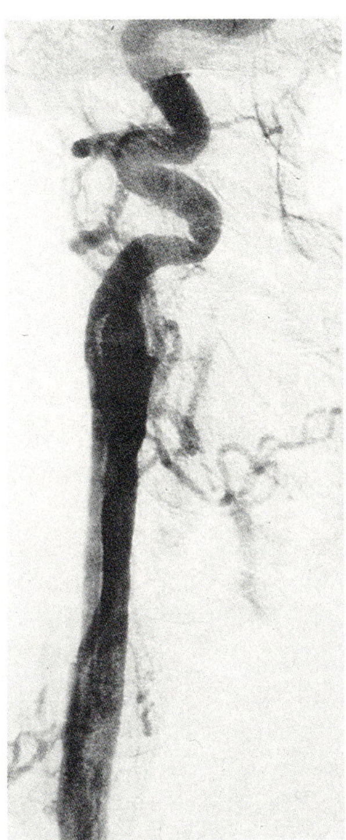

FIGURE 7.15

Common carotid artery dissection. Patient had giant cell arteritis. Note the false lumen.

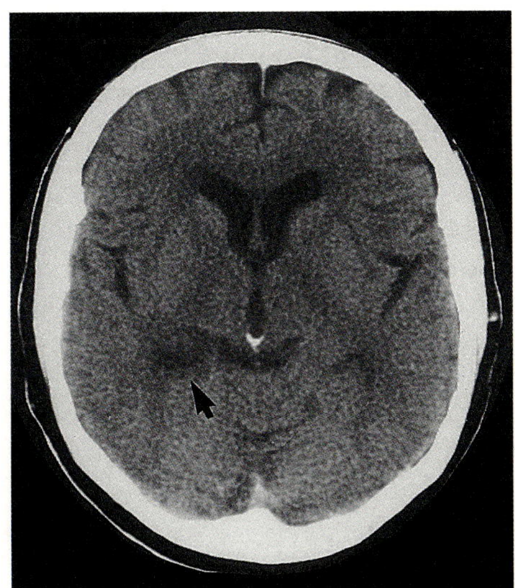

FIGURE 7.16

Systemic lupus rythematosus–associated ischemic stroke. Cranial computed tomography scan showing an area of hypodensity in the right parietooccipital area (*arrow*).

Reports of cerebrovascular neurosyphilis have increased with the epidemic of AIDS [61]. Burke and Schaberg [62] report that meningovascular syphilis was found in 19% of 2019 patients with symptomatic neurosyphilis. Cerebral infarction in neurosyphilis is the result of either Nissl-Alzheimer's arteritis, characterized by intimal proliferation without inflammation of the small cerebral vessels, or Heubner's arteritis, characterized by lymphocytic and plasma cell perivascular cuffing of the adventitia of the medium and large-sized arteries [58]. Fibrosis of the subintimal zone and thinning of the media of these vessels are also observed.

Ischemic stroke has been reported rarely in association with Lyme borreliosis [63], neurotuberculosis [58], and varicella-zoster virus infection [58,64]. Herpes zoster infection has been linked to granulomatous angiitis of the central nervous system [58,64].

In a recent case-control study [65], evidence of cerebral infarction was pathologically demonstrated in 10 of 181 patients who died with AIDS. The frequency was not significantly different from the control patients who died of chronic illness but not AIDS. Higher frequency of IS (29%), however, was reported in another pathologic study [66]. Cerebral vasculopathy, cardioembolism, and alteration in coagulation factors are some suggested mechanisms of IS in these patients.

Mucormycosis is most common in diabetic and immunocompromised patients, and can rarely result in IS from extension of the infection into the cavernous sinus and occlusion of the internal carotid artery [58]. Aspergillosis is encountered in immunocompromised patients and in AIDS patients. Invasion of the cerebral blood vessel walls by the hyphae results in strokes, usually hemorrhagic, and in subarachnoid hemorrhage [67].

Inflammatory Arteriopathies

Ischemic stroke complicates several arteritides (systemic and primary nervous system) as shown in Tables 7.4 and 7.7 (Figures 7.15–7.20). One cause of IS in these conditions is the

Table 7.7. Inflammatory arteropathies

Condition	Vessels involved	Pathology	Study
Giant cell arteritis	Temporal artery, middle cerebral artery, main aortic branches	Infiltration of arterial wall by monocytes, occassionally eosinophils and neutrophils	Mumenthaler [68]
Takayasu's disease	Aorta and its branches	Granulomatous arteritis	Schwartzman and Parker [69]
Granulomatous central nervous system angiitis	Precapillary arterioles	Granulomatous arteritis	Younger and coworkers [64], Moore [70]
Polyarteritis nodosa	Small- and medium-sized arteries	Segmental necrotizing vasculitis (cerebral hemorrhage also occurs)	Brown and Swash [71]
Systemic lupus erythematosus	Cartoid artery	Cervicocephalic dissection	Futrell and Millikan [72], Devinsky and coworkers [73], Mitsias and Levine [74]
Wegener's granulomatosis	Branches of large intracranial arteries and small-sized perforating arteries	Necrotizing granulomatous vasculitis; fibrinoid necrosis	Lucas and coworkers [75]
Neurosarcoidosis	Cerebral arterial and venous perforators	Granulomatous vasculitis involving the media and elastic lamina	Younger and coworkers [64], Brown and Swash [71]
Inflammatory bowel disease	No vessel involvement	Platelet-fibrin thrombi; no vessel wall inflammation	Brown and Swash [71], Talbot and coworkers [76]

invasion of the vessel wall by inflammatory cells, mural necrosis, thrombus formation, luminal stenosis, or occlusion with resultant perfusion failure. Often, however, cardiac embolization from Libman-Sacks vegetations and a prothrombotic state coexit with the inflammatory arteriopathy and therefore add to the risk of cerebral ischemia. The target vessel in these vasculitides is variable and multiple arterial, and sometimes venous beds are involved as indicated in Table 7.7.

FIGURE 7.17

Systemic lupus erythematosus–associated internal carotid artery (ICA) dissection. Selective carotid angiogram (*lateral view*) showing severe narrowing of the ICA (*arrow*) and a pseudoaneurysm (*arrowheads*).

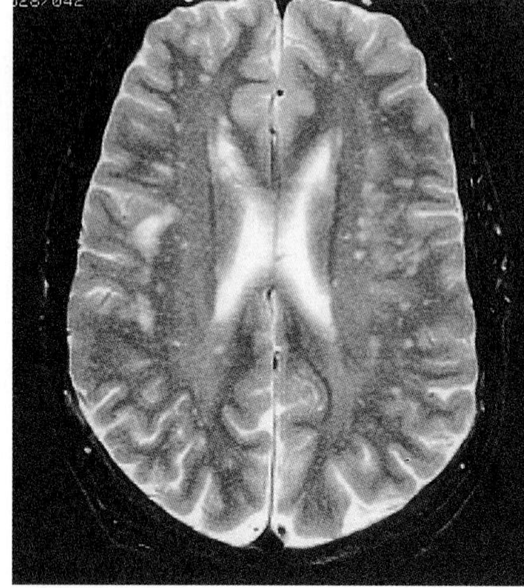

FIGURE 7.18

Inflammatory bowel disease (Crohn's disease). T2-weighted cranial magnetic resonance image showing multiple hyperintense signals compatible with ischemic strokes. Infectious, inflammatory, and demyelinating conditions were ruled out.

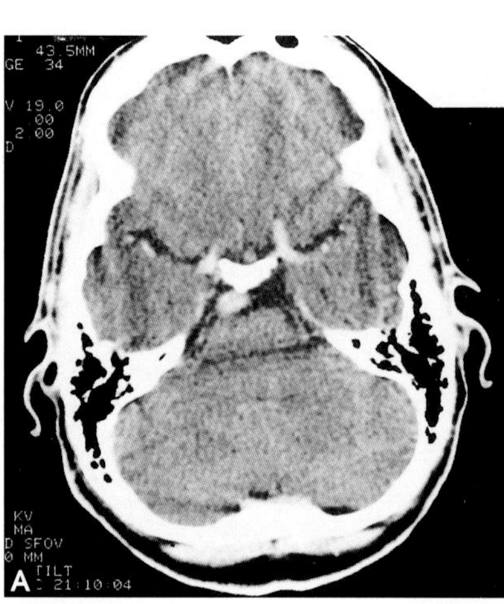

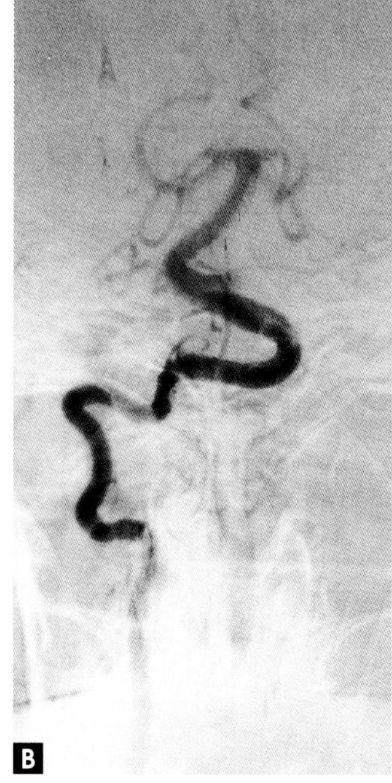

FIGURE 7.19

Fabry's disease. Cranial computed tomography scan (**A**) and selective right vertebral angiogram (**B**) demonstrating fusiform dilatation of the basilar artery (BA). Note compression of the brain stem by the BA (**A**).

Hereditary and Congenital Causes of Ischemic Stroke

Nonacquired, congenital, and hereditary causes of ischemic stroke [77] as shown in Tables 7.4 and 7.8 can be cardiac (*eg*, familial myxoma, MVP), vasculopathic (*eg*, Fabry's disease), hematologic (*eg*, familial dysfibrinogenemia, hereditary protein C or S deficiency), indeterminate (*eg*, mitochondriopathy), or mixed (*eg*, homocystinuria and sickle cell disease wherein a vasculopathy and a prothrombotic state coexist). Both hemorrhagic and ischemic strokes are encountered in these conditions. The genetic defect and the pathology observed in some of the hereditary arteriopathies are outlined in Table 7.8.

Arteriopathies Related to Drugs

In recent years, licit and illicit drug use and abuse (Table 7.4) have been implicated in both hemorrhagic and ischemic strokes, especially in young and otherwise healthy individuals. Drug- or substance-related strokes occur as the result of cerebral vasculitis, cerebral vasospasm, infective endocarditis, foreign body embolism, or a prothrombotic or procoagulant state [84,85].

Oral contraceptive use has been linked to ischemic and hemorrhagic strokes in some epidemiologic studies [84,85]. Cerebral venous and sinus occlusive disease has also been described in oral contraceptive users. The risk of ischemic stroke with oral contraceptive use may increase with advancing age and in cigarette smokers, hypertensives, and migraine sufferers [84–86]. Pathologically, cerebrovascular changes associated with oral contraceptive use resemble the ones observed in moyamoya disease, intimal hyperplasia, and subendothelial fibrosis [85]. Levine and coworkers [86] suggest that oral contraceptive arteriopathy is induced by ethinyl estradiol antibodies that cross react with endothelial tissue. IS related to oral contraceptive use can also result from hematologic alterations [84,85] discussed later in this chapter.

Sympathomimetics including amphetamines and amphetamine-like compounds such as phenylpropanolamine (PPA),

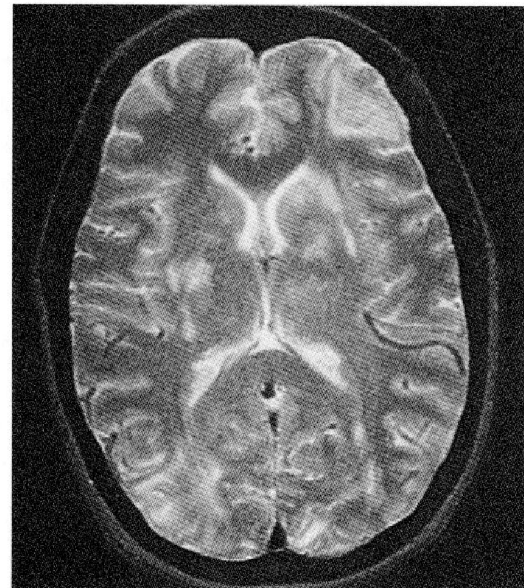

FIGURE 7.20

Sickle cell disease. T2-weighted cranial magnetic resonance image showing multiple hyperintense signals compatible with ischemic strokes.

found in "diet pills," have been linked to IS (Figure 7.21) in various reports [84,85]. Even occasional use, and not necessarily abuse, of PPA has been associated with stroke, especially hemorrhagic stroke [87]. Necrotizing vasculitis with involvement of the arterioles and medium- and small-sized arteries is the pathologic substrate of amphetamine-induced arteriopathy [84,85,87]. Autopsy specimens of the brains of monkeys given amphetamines have revealed areas of cerebral infarction, subarachnoid and intraparenchymal hemorrhage, microaneurysms, and perivascular cuffing by inflammatory cells [84,85].

On the streets of the United States, cocaine exists most commonly as the hydrochloride (cocaine-HCl) or the alkaloid freebase form known as *crack* [84,85,88]. Cerebral infarction, transient ischemic attacks, parenchymatous, and subarachnoid hemorrhage have been reported with the use of either form of cocaine [84,85,88]. Cerebral hemorrhage tends to be more frequent in cocaine-HCl users than in patients who have smoked crack [88]. Cerebral vasculitis following cocaine use has been described angiographically (Figure 7.22) without pathologic confirmation. Levine and coworkers [88] believe that several pathogenetic mechanisms (*eg*, cerebral vasospasm, arteriopathy, cardioembolism, or hypercoagulability) can account for cocaine-related stroke and that vasculitis is rare.

Table 7.8. Hereditary arteriopathies

Conditions	Mode of inheritance	Genetic defect	Pathology	Study
Fabry's disease	X-linked recessive	α-Galactosidase deficiency	Premature ischemic stroke and intracerebellar hemorrhage in the vertebrobasiliar system; aneurysm formation; sphingolipid deposition in large and small cerebral vessels	Kaye and coworkers [48], Natowicz and Kelley [77]
Homocystinuria*	Autosomal recessive	Cystathione β-synthase deficiency	Accumulation of homocystine causing endothelial injury and promoting atherogenicity	Natowicz and Kelley [77], Vonsattel and Hedley-Whyte [78], Schaffer and Kroll [79], Rodgers and Conn [80]
Sickle cell disease†	Autosomal recessive	Formation of hemoglobin S and hemoglobin C hemoglobin molecules	Stroke in 6%–17% (ischemic [cortical and subcortical] in 75%, hemorrhagic in 25%); fibrous proliferation of the intima of the distal internal caroid artery, proximal middle cerebral artery, and anterior cerebral artery leading to progressive luminal occlusion	Powars and coworkers [81], Hart and Kanter [82], Coull and Goodnight [83]

*Ischemic stroke occurs in homozygotes and heterozygotes for homocystinuria. Homocysteine accumulation promotes thrombogenicity by inhibiting the activation of protein C.
†Ischemic stroke occurs in hemoglobin SS, hemoglobin SC, and hemoglobin SA variants of sickle cell disease.

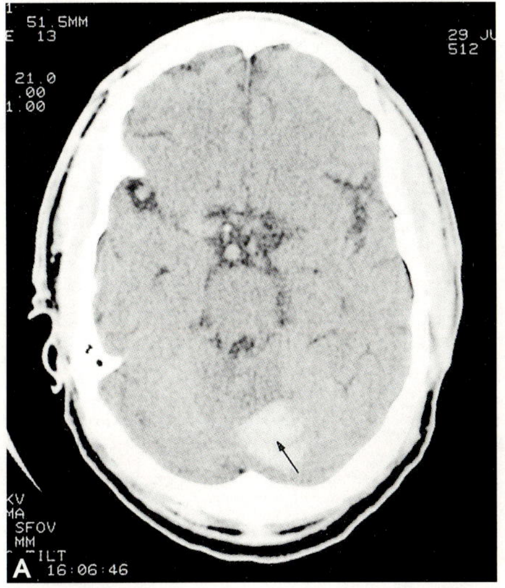

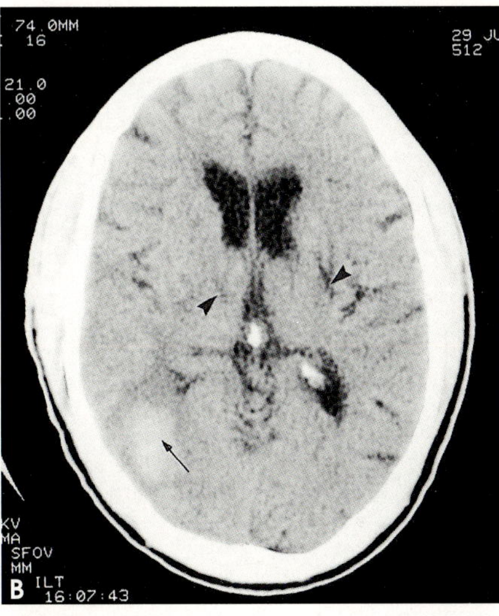

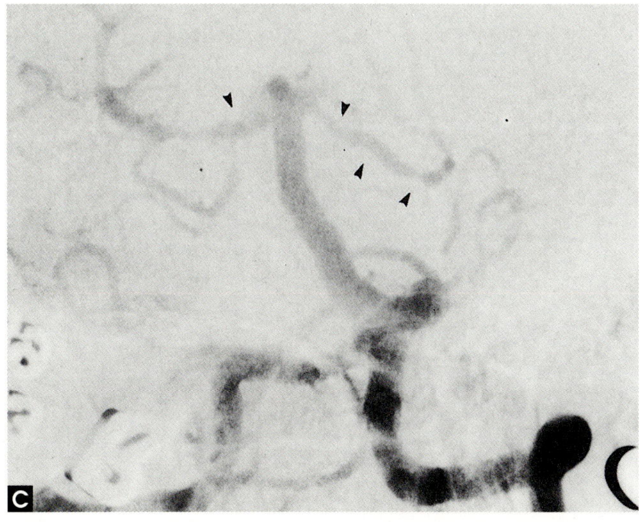

FIGURE 7.21

Suspected sympathomimetic-related stroke. Cranial computed tomography (**A**) showing areas of increased photon density (*arrows*) compatible with multiple hemorrhages, and areas of hypodensities (*arrowheads*) (**B**) compatible with multiple ischemic strokes. Selective left vertebral angiogram (**C**) showing areas of segmental narrowing (*arrowheads*) in both posterior cerebral arteries.

HEMATOLOGIC CAUSES OF ISCHEMIC STROKE

Less than 5% of ischemic strokes in patients of all ages are related to hematologic abnormalities [82]. The frequency of these abnormalities in young (<40 years of age) patients with IS is 9% [89]. A delicate balance between the clotting system, the naturally occurring anticoagulants (*eg*, protein C, protein S, antithrombin III), and the fibrinolytic system, and tightly regulated concentrations of blood cellular elements, platelets, and erythrocytes, are essential for the maintenance of normal homeostasis. Activation of the coagulation cascade, increased concentration of clotting factors, deficiency of an anticoagulant protein, limited activity of the fibrinolytic system, abnormally high concentrations of erythrocytes or platelets, platelet cell activation, or increased adhesiveness of blood cellular elements can result in arterial thrombosis [79]. When endothelial damage coexists with abnormalities of the blood cellular elements, as in heparin-associated thrombocytopenia and thrombosis or in the antiphospholipid antibody syndrome, the risk of arterial thrombosis increases [79]. Table 7.9 lists some of the hematologic causes of IS.

Hypercoagulable States

Protein C deficiency can be inherited as an autosomal dominant trait with incomplete penetrance or can be acquired [90]. In type I heterozygous protein C deficiency, there is an absolute reduction of the protein concentration, whereas in type II deficiency, protein C anticoagulant activity is reduced but its concentration is normal [90]. Venous thromboembolism is the most common manifestation of protein C deficiency; however, cerebral arterial infarction has also been reported [91]. In a more recent study, Camerlingo and coworkers [92] found protein C deficiency in three of 50 patients with IS who were younger than 45 years of age. Two patients had no history of thromboembolic events. Other causes of IS were ruled out in all three patients. Occlusion of branches of the middle cerebral artery was demonstrated angiographically in two patients, and occlusion of the carotid siphon was seen in the third. Large case-control and epidemiologic studies are needed to determine the true prevalence of protein C deficiency in stroke. Until then, stroke related to protein C deficiency should be considered rare.

Protein S is another vitamin K–dependent anticoagulant protein which, unlike protein C, circulates in the blood in both active and inactive forms [90]. Protein S potentiates the inactivation of factors V_a and VIII_a by protein C. Protein S deficiency is inherited or acquired in conditions such as consumptive coagulopathy, hepatic or renal failure, and inflammatory bowel disease [76]. Similar to protein C deficiency, most thromboembolic events associated with protein S deficiency are venous, and arterial strokes (Figure 7.23) are very rare [90]. A recent case-control study has shown that 21% of hospitalized patients with acute IS and 20% of hospitalized controls had free–protein S deficiency, defined as less than 20% of total protein S [93]. The authors concluded that free–protein S deficiency is common in hospitalized patients and is not a risk factor for IS.

Inherited deficiency of antithrombin III is less frequent than deficiency of either protein S or protein C. Deep vein thrombosis and pulmonary embolism are the more common manifestations of antithrombin III deficiency, and IS is distinctly rare [89,94].

Clotting Factor Excess

Activation of factor X and prothrombin by surgery, tissue necrosis, malignancy, inflammatory, or infectious disorders results in the release and activation of interleukin-1 or tumor necrosis factor, thus enhancing thrombogenicity [83]. The role of these clotting factors in stroke is unknown. High concentrations of factors V and VIII may increase the risk for stroke in patients with inflammatory bowel disease or AIDS and during preg-

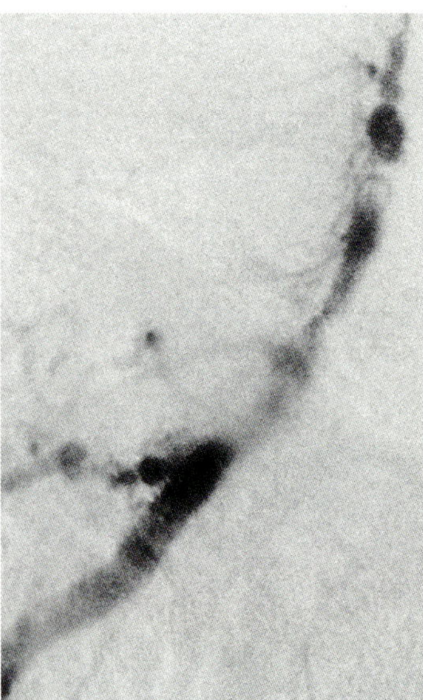

FIGURE 7.22
Cocaine-related stroke. Cerebral angiogram (*lateral view*) demonstrating irregular, beaded basilar artery with distal occlusion.

Table 7.9. Hematologic causes of ischemic stroke

Natural anticoagulant deficiency	Clotting factor excess	Fibrinolytic factor deficiency	Immune-mediated prothrombotic state	Others
Protein C Protein S Antithrombin III	Factor V Factor VIII Factor X Fibrinogen	Plasminogen Plasminogen activator Factor XII Dysfibrinogenemia	TTP aPL	Increased platelet activity aggregability HATT ET Hyperviscosity syndrome Hemoglobinopathies

aPL—antiphospholipid antibody syndrome; ET—essential thrombocytosis; HATT—heparin-associated thrombocytopenia and thrombosis; TTP—thrombotic thrombocytopenic purpura.

nancy. Fibrinogen excess (hyperfibrinogenemia) and fibrin monomer polymerization defect (dysfibrinogenemia) have been linked to ischemic strokes [95]. High levels of fibrinogen increase blood viscosity and activate platelets, thus predisposing patients to thrombosis [95].

Immune-mediated Prothrombotic States

Thrombotic thrombocytopenic purpura is a syndrome characterized by hemolytic anemia, thrombocytopenia, fever, and renal dysfunction. The majority of patients with TTP develop neurologic signs and symptoms, and strokes (Figure 7.24) are common [79,83,96]. IS tends to become hemorrhagic in TTP. Terminal arterioles and capillaries are occluded by fibrin-platelet thrombi and the vascular endothelium is hyperplastic [83,97]. Endothelial injury, resulting in decreased production of PGI_2, and reduced fibrinolysis are suggested mechanisms of thrombosis in TTP [83,97].

Antiphospholipid antibodies are a heterogenous group of autoantibodies, including the lupus anticoagulant and anticardiolipins, which have been associated with fetal loss, thrombocytopenia, and recurrent thromboembolic venous and arterial occlusive events [79,98]. Neurologic manifestations of antiphospholipid antibodies include transient ischemic attacks, cerebral and retinal infarction (Figure 7.25), dementia, chorea, cranial neuropathies, and migraine-like headache [79,83,98,99]. In a recent case-control study [100], anticardiolipin positivity was detected in about 10% of 255 patients with their first ischemic stroke and 4% of 255 age- and sex-matched hospitalized controls (odds ratio = 2.3). Antiphospholipid antibodies are found in 40% of patients with SLE [83,99] and have been detected in several other autoimmune conditions, such as rheumatoid arthritis and TTP [83]. These antibodies may cause a hypercoagulable state as the result of the following: 1) a deficiency of protein S; 2) inhibition of the protein C–protein S complex binding; 3) increased levels of thromboxane A_2; 4) defective release of prostacyclin; 5) increased expression of procoagulant tissue factor; or 6) increased von Willebrand's factor [79,83]. Cardioembolism is another potential mechanism of stroke in patients with antiphospholipid antibodies [31,79,83,99].

Miscellaneous Hematologic Causes of Ischemic Stroke

Hyperviscosity syndromes [101] include diseases of erythrocyte deformability, such as sickle cell disease, and disorders of plasma proteins, such as multiple myeloma (Figure 7.26). As a result of increased cell-protein-cell bridging, a phenomenon encountered in the paraproteinemias, erythrocytes tend to form rouleaux and thereby block small vascular channels such as capillaries and terminal arterioles [101]. Rouleaux formation is also seen in conditions of increased erythrocyte production (Figure 7.27), especially when these cells are immature as in polycythemia rubra vera. In sickle cell disease and related hemoglobinopathies, on the other hand, erythrocytes do not readily cross the capillary lumen, particularly in hypoxic conditions where the erythrocyte membranes are very rigid, resulting in thrombosis and perfusion failure [81,101]. Table 7.10 lists some of the hyperviscosity syndromes that have been reported to cause stroke. Of note is that in most of these conditions, the mechanism of ischemic stroke could be an endothelial injury, intracardiac thrombi, a hypercoagulable state, or

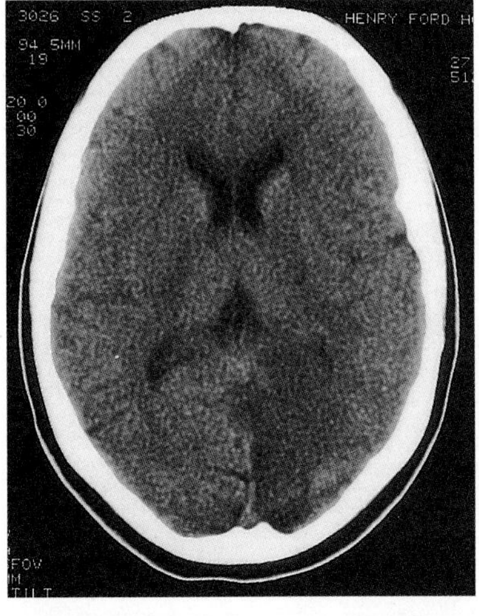

FIGURE 7.23

Protein S deficiency and stroke. Cranial computed tomography scan showing an area of decreased photon density in the left occipital lobe compatible with ischemic stroke. Aside from protein S deficiency, the workup for causes of stroke was otherwise negative.

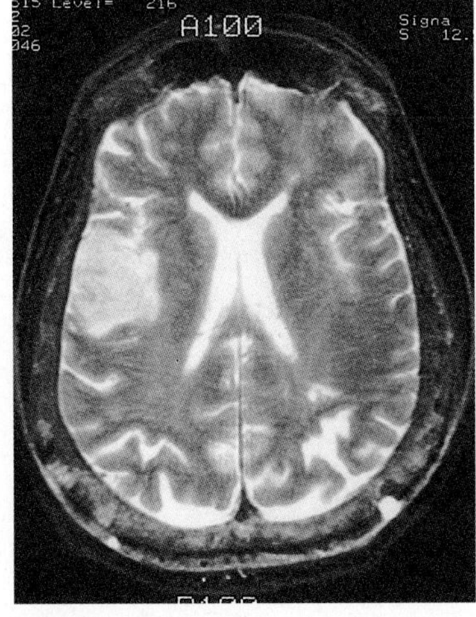

FIGURE 7.24

Thombotic thrombocytopenic purpura and stroke. T2-weighted cranial magnetic resonance image showing a large hyperintense signal in the right frontotemporal region compatible with ischemic stroke.

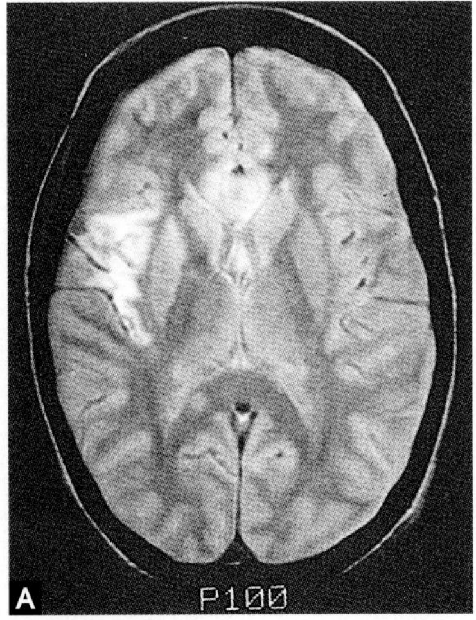

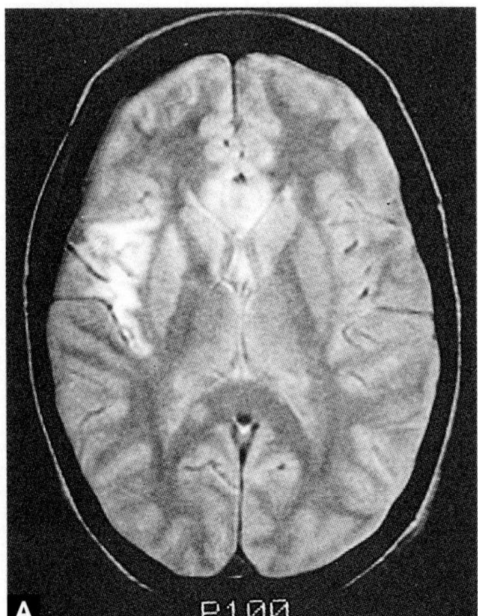

FIGURE 7.25

Antiphospholipid antibodies and stroke. Proton density cranial magnetic resonance image showing areas of increased signal intensity in the left lateral (**A**) and medial (**B**) frontal lobe compatible with cerebral infarction in multiple arterial territories.

disseminated intravascular coagulopathy, in addition to increased blood viscosity.

MISCELLANEOUS CAUSES OF ISCHEMIC STROKE

Migraine may be a risk factor for stroke [102], however, the mechanism of migrainous infarction remains unknown [102,103]. Chatillon and coworkers [54] found that migraine predisposes the patient to cervicocephalic dissection. Migrainous infarction (Figure 7.28) should be diagnosed only in patients with history of migraine, and after more common mechanisms of IS are ruled out [102].

Cerebral venous and sinus thrombosis is a rare cause of IS in the United States, although it is the most common cause of peripartum stroke in India [104]. Typically, there is extensive thrombosis of cerebral venous structures, most commonly the superior sagittal sinus, causing infarction in multiple cerebral territories [103]. Cerebral venous– and sinus thrombosis–related infarctions tend to be hemorrhagic (Figure 7.29) and poorly circumscribed, unlike arterial strokes. Cerebral venous and sinus thrombosis occurs as the result of 1) vessel wall damage as seen in central nervous system infections, sarcoidosis, or lymphoma; 2) venous stasis as in dehydration; or 3) hypercoagulability [104].

ACKNOWLEDGMENTS

Drs. M. Gorman, S.R. Levine, N. Samuel, and G.E. Tietjen have provided some of the figures.

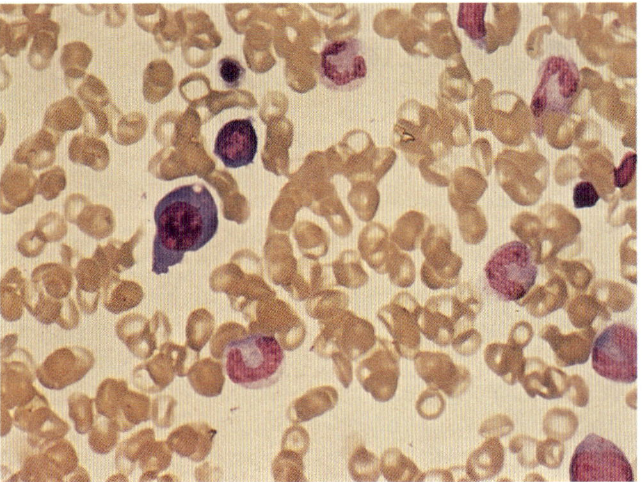

FIGURE 7.26

Multiple myeloma. Bone marrow biopsy showing increased number of plasma cells in a patient with stroke and smoldering myeloma.

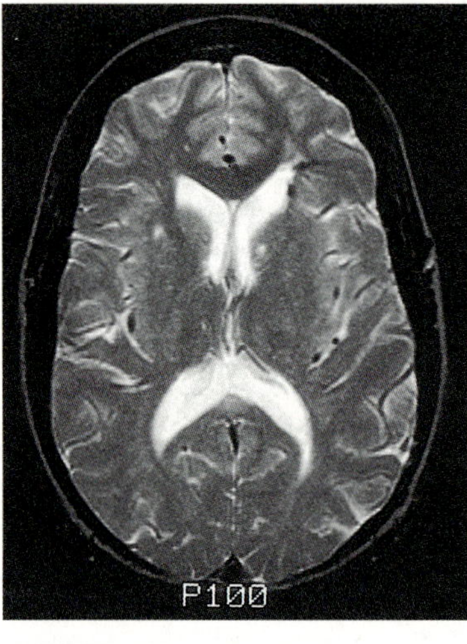

FIGURE 7.27

Secondary polycythemia. T2-weighted cranial magnetic resonance image showing two foci of ischemic infarction in a patient with cyanotic heart disease.

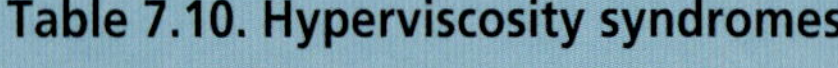

Table 7.10. Hyperviscosity syndromes

- Paraproteinemias
  - Multiple myeloma
  - Waldenström's macroglobulinemia
  - Lymphoma
- Cryoglobulinemia
- Hyperfibrinogenemia
- Heavy chain diseases
- Polycythemia
  - Polycythemia rubra vera
  - Erythrocytosis
  - Leukemia
  - Relative polycythemia
- Hemoglobinopathies
- Spherocytosis

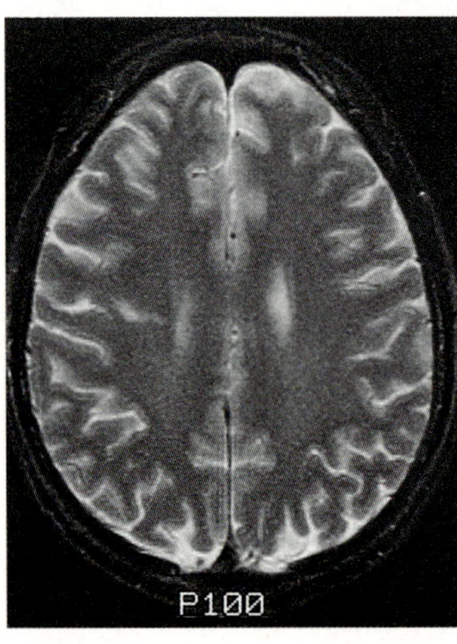

FIGURE 7.28

Migrainous infarction. T2-weighted cranial magnetic resonance image showing an area of increased signal intensity in the deep right frontal region compatible with cerebral infarction.

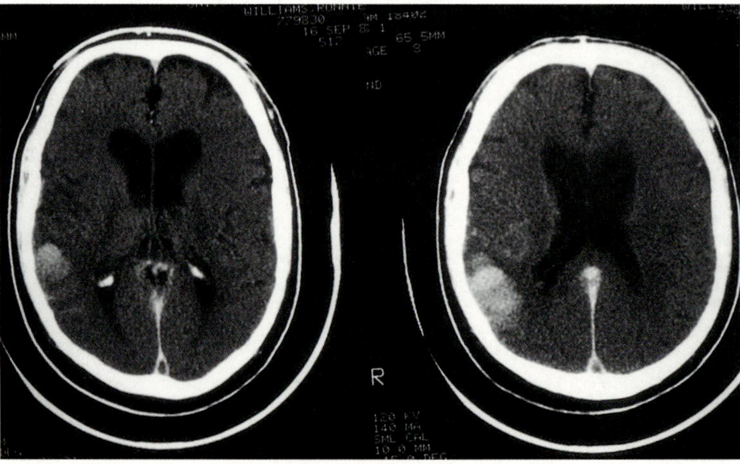

FIGURE 7.29

Cerebral venous thrombosis. Cranial computed tomography scan showing an area of hemorrhage in the right parietal lobe and the *empty delta* sign. Patient was dehydrated and had severe congestive heart failure.

REFERENCES

1. Foulkes MA, Wolf PA, Price TR, *et al.*: The stroke data bank: design, methods, and baseline characteristics. *Stroke* 1988, 19:547–554.
2. Cerebral Embolism Task Force: Cardiogenic brain embolism: the second report of the Cerebral Embolism Task Force. *Arch Neurol* 1989, 46:727–743.
3. Bogousslavsky J, Pierre P: Ischemic stroke in patients under age 45. *Neurol Clin* 1992, 10:113–124.
4. Cerebral Embolism Task Force: Cardiogenic brain embolism. *Arch Neurol* 1986, 43:71–84.
5. Wolf PA, Abbott RD, Kannel WB: Atrial fibrillation: a major contributor to stroke in the elderly. *Arch Intern Med* 1987, 147:1561–1564.
6. The Stroke Prevention in Atrial Fibrillation Investigators: Predictors of thromboembolism in atrial fibrillation (I): clinical features of patients at risk. *Ann Intern Med* 1992, 116:1–5.
7. The Stroke Prevention in Atrial Fibrillation Investigators: Predictors of thromboembolism in atrial fibrillation, part II: echocardiographic features of patients at risk. *Ann Intern Med* 1992, 116:6–12.
8. Laupacis A, Albers G, Dunn M, Feinberg W: Antithrombotic therapy in atrial fibrillation. *Chest* 1992, 102(suppl):426–433.
9. Wolf PA, Kannel WB, McGee DL, *et al.*: Duration of atrial fibrillation and imminence of stroke: the Framingham study. *Stroke* 1983, 14:664–667.
10. Peterson P, Godtfredsen J: Embolic complications in paroxysmal atrial fibrillation. *Stroke* 1986, 17:622–626.
11. Hinton RC, Kistler JP, Fallon JT, *et al.*: Influence of etiology of atrial fibrillation on incidence of systemic embolism. *Am J Cardiol* 1977, 40:509–515.
12. Rubenstein JJ, Schulman LL, Yurchak PM, *et al.*: Clinical spectrum of sick sinus syndrome. *Circulation* 1972, 46:5–13.
13. Bathen J, Sparr S, Rokseth R: Embolism in sinoatrial disease. *Acta Med Scand* 1978, 203:7–11.
14. Norris JW, Frogatt GM, Hachinski VC: Cardiac arrhythmia in acute stroke. *Stroke* 1978, 9:392–396.
15. Fairfax AJ, Lambert CD, Leatham A: Systemic emboli in chronic sinoatrial disorder. *N Engl J Med* 1976, 295:190–193.
16. Levine HJ, Pauker SG, Salzman EW: Antithrombotic therapy in valvular heart disease. *Chest* 1989, 95(suppl):107–117.
17. Levine HJ, Pauker SG, Salzman EW, Eckman MH: Antithrombotic therapy in valvular heart disease. *Chest* 1992, 102(suppl):434–444.
18. Easton JD, Sherman DG: Management of cerebral embolism of cardiac source. *Stroke* 1980, 11:433–442.
19. Dervall PB, Olley PM, Smith DR, *et al.*: Incidence of stenosis embolism before and after mitral valvotomy. *Thorax* 1968, 23:530–540.
20. Sherman DG: Prevention of cardioembolic stroke. In *Prevention of Stroke.* Edited by Hachinski VC, Norris JW. New York: Springer-Verlag; 1991:149–159.
21. Korn D, DeSanctis RW, Sell S: Massive calcification of the mitral valve. *N Engl J Med* 1962, 269:900–909.
22. Fulkerson PK, Beaver BM, Auseon J, *et al.*: Calcification of the mitral annulus: etiology, clinical associations, complications, and therapy. *Am J Med* 1979, 66:967–977.
23. Ridolfi RL, Hutchins GM: Spontaneous calcific emboli from calcific mitral annular fibrosis. *Arch Pathol Lab Med* 1976, 100:117–120.
24. Garvey GT, Neu HC: Infective endocarditis: an evolving disease. *Medicine* 1978, 57:105–127.
25. Salgado AV, Furlan AJ, Keys TF, *et al.*: Neurologic complications of native and prosthetic valve endocarditis. *Neurology* 1989, 30:173–178.
26. Caplan LR, Stein RW, eds: Cerebral embolism. In *Stroke: A Clinical Approach.* Boston: Butterworth Publishers; 1986:197–218.
27. Lopez JA, Ross RS, Fishbein MC, *et al.*: Nonbacterial thrombotic endocarditis: a review. *Am Heart J* 1987, 113:773–784.
28. Amico L, Caplan LR, Thomas C: Cerebrovascular complications of mucinous cancer. *Neurology* 1989, 39:522–526.
29. Kooiker JC, McLean JM, Sumi SM: Cerebral embolism, marantic endocarditis and cancer. *Arch Neurol* 1976, 33:260–264.
30. Rogers LR, Cho ES, Kempin S, Posner JB: Cerebral infarction from nonbacterial thrombotic endocarditis: clinical and pathological study including the effects of anticoagulation. *Am J Med* 1987, 83:746–756.
31. Hess DC: Stroke associated with antiphospholipid antibodies. *Stroke* 1992, 23 (suppl 1):23–28.
32. Reagan TJ, Okasaki H: The thrombotic syndrome associated with carcinoma. *Arch Neurol* 1974, 31:390–395.
33. Barnett HJM, Boughner DR, Taylow DW, *et al.*: Further evidence relating mitral valve prolapse to cerebral ischemic events. *N Engl J Med* 1980, 302:139–144.
34. Busch EH, Snyder DW, Burron RE: Embolic stroke in a woman with mitral valve prolapse who used oral contraceptives. *Chest* 1986, 90:454–455.
35. Wallis DE, Godwin J: Mitral valve prolapse, cerebral ischemia and protein S deficiency. *Am J Med* 1988, 84:974.
36. Brockmeier LP, Adolph RJ, Gustin BW, *et al.*: Calcium emboli to the retinal artery in calcific aortic stenosis. *Am Heart J* 1981, 101:32–37.
37. Pleet A, Massey E, Vengrowe M: TIA, stroke, and the bicuspid aortic valve. *Neurology* 1981, 31:1540–1542.
38. Cairns JA, Hirsh J, Daniel Lewis H, *et al.*: Antithrombotic agents in coronary artery disease. *Chest* 1992, 102(suppl):456–481.
39. Smith P, Arnesen H, Holme I: The effect of warfarin on mortality and reinfarction after myocardial infarction. *N Engl J Med* 1990, 323:147–152.
40. Starling MR, Crawford MH, Sorensen SG, Groven FL: Comparative value of invasive and noninvasive techniques for identifying left ventricular mural thrombi. *Am Heart J* 1983, 106:1143–1149.
41. Visser CA, Kan G, Meltzer RS, *et al.*: Embolic potential of left ventricular thrombus after myocardial infarction: a two-dimensional echocardiographic study of 119 patients. *J Am Coll Cardiol* 1985, 5:1276–1280.
42. Reeder GS, Lengyel M, Tajik AJ, *et al.*: Mural thrombus in left ventricular aneurysm: incidence, role of angiography, and relation between anticoagulation and embolization. *Mayo Clin Proc* 1981, 56:77–81.
43. Lechat PH, Mas JL, Lascault G, *et al.*: Prevalence of patent foramen ovale in patients with stroke. *N Engl J Med* 1988, 318:1148–1152.
44. Hagen PT, Scholz DG, Edwards WD: Incidence and size of patent foramen ovale during the first 10 decades of life: an autopsy study of 965 normal hearts. *Mayo Clin Proc* 1984, 59:17–20.
45. Pasquale G, Andreoli A, Grazi P, *et al.*: Cardioembolic stroke from atrial septal aneurysm. *Stroke* 1988, 19:640–643.
46. Knepper LE, Biller J, Adams HP, Bruno A: Neurologic manifestations of atrial myxoma: a 12-year experience and review. *Stroke* 1988, 19:1435–1440.
47. Damasio H, Seabra-Gomes R, da Silva JP, *et al.*: Multiple cerebral aneurysms and cardiac myxoma. *Arch Neurol* 1975, 32:269–270.
48. Kaye EM, Kolodny EH, Logigian EL, Ullman MD: Nervous system involvement in Fabry's disease. *Ann Neurol* 1988, 23:505–509.
49. Biller J, Hingtgen WL, Adams HP, *et al.*: Cervicocephalic arterial dissections: a ten-year experience. *Arch Neurol* 1986, 43:1234–1238.
50. Bogousslavsky J, Despland PA, Regli F: Spontaneous carotid dissection with acute stroke. *Arch Neurol* 1987, 44:137–140.
51. Hart RG, Easton JD: Dissection of cervical and cerebral arteries. *Neurol Clin* 1983, 1:155–182.
52. Culebras A, Hodge CJ, Petro GR: Carotid and vertebral dissecting hematomas. In *Handbook of Clinical Neurology: Vascular Diseases.* Part II. Edited by Vinken PJ, Bruyn GW, Klawans HL; co-edited by Toole JF. Amsterdam: Elsevier Science Publishers; 1989:271–285.
53. Trosch RM, Hasbani M, Brass LM: "Bottoms up" dissection. *N Engl J Med* 1989, 320:1564–1565.
54. Chatillon JD, Ribiero V, Mas JL, *et al.*: Migraine—a risk factor for dissection of cervical arteries. *Headache* 1989, 29:560–561.
55. Ramadan NM, Tietgen GE, Levine SR, Welch KMA: Scintillating scotoma associated with internal carotid artery dissection: report of three cases. *Neurology* 1991, 41:1084–1087.

56. Sandok BA: Fibromuscular dysplasia of the cephalic arterial system. In *Handbook of Clinical Neurology: Vascular Diseases.* Part 3. Edited by Vinken PJ, Bruyn GW, Klawans HL; co-edited by Toole JF. Amsterdam: Elsevier Science Publishers; 1989:283–292.
57. Kitamura K, Fukui M, Oka K, *et al.*: Moyamoya disease. In *Handbook of Clinical Neurology: Vascular Diseases.* Part 2. Edited by Vinken PJ, Bruyn GW, Klawans HL; co-edited by Toole JF. Amsterdam: Elsevier Science Publishers; 1989:293–306.
58. Dalal PM, Dalal KP: Cerebrovascular manifestations of infectious disease. In *Handbook of Clinical Neurology: Vascular Diseases.* Part 3. Edited by Vinken PJ, Bruyn GW, Klawans HL; co-edited by Toole JF. Amsterdam: Elsevier Science Publishers; 1989:411–441.
59. Pfister HW, Feiden W, Einhäupl KM: Spectrum of complications during bacterial meningitis in adults: results of a prospective clinical study. *Arch Neurol* 1993, 50:575–581.
60. Pfister HW, Borasio GD, Dirnagl U, *et al.*: Cerebrovascular complications of bacterial meningitis in adults. *Neurology* 1992, 42:1497–1504.
61. Katz DA, Berger JR, Duncan RC: Neurosyphilis: a comparative study of the effects of infection with human immunodeficiency virus. *Arch Neurol* 1993, 50:243–249.
62. Burke JM, Schaberg DR: Neurosyphilis in the antibiotic era. *Neurology* 1985, 35:1368–1371.
63. May EF, Jabbari B: Stroke in neuroborreliosis. *Stroke* 1990, 21:1232–1235.
64. Younger DS, Hays AP, Brust JCM, Rowland LP: Granulomatous angiitis of the brain: an inflammatory reaction of diverse etiology. *Arch Neurol* 1988, 45:514–518.
65. Berger JR, Harris JO, Gregoris J, Norenberg M: Cerebrovascular disease in AIDS: a case-control study. *AIDS* 1990, 4:239–244.
66. Mizusawa H, Hirano A, Llena JF, Shintaku M: Cerebrovascular lesions in acquired immune deficiency syndrome (AIDS). *Acta Neuropathol* 1988, 76:451–457.
67. Walsh TJ, Hier DB, Caplan LR: Aspergillus of the CNS: clinicopathological analysis of 17 patients. *Ann Neurol* 1985, 18:574–582.
68. Mumenthaler M: Cranial arteritis. In *Handbook of Clinical Neurology: Vascular Diseases.* Part 3. Edited by Vinken PJ, Bruyn GW, Klawans HL; co-edited by Toole JF. Amsterdam: Elsevier Science Publishers; 1989:341–351.
69. Schwartzman RJ, Parker JC: The aortic arch syndrome. In *Handbook of Clinical Neurology: Neurological Manifestations of Systemic Diseases.* Part 3. Edited by Vinken PJ, Bruyn GW, Klawans HL. Amsterdam: North Holland Publishing Co.; 1980:213–238.
70. Moore PM: Diagnosis and management of isolated angiitis of the central nervous system. *Neurology* 1989, 39:167–173.
71. Brown MM, Swash M: Polyarteritis nodosa and other systemic vasculitides. In *Handbook of Clinical Neurology: Vascular Diseases.* Part 3. Edited by Vinken PJ, Bruyn GW, Klawans HL; co-edited by Toole JF. Amsterdam: Elsevier Science Publishers; 1989:353–368.
72. Futrell N, Millikan C: Frequency, etiology, and prevention of stroke in patients with systemic lupus erythematosus. *Stroke* 1989, 20:583–591.
73. Devinsky O, Petito CK, Alonso DR: Clinical and neuropathological findings in systemic lupus erythematosus: the role of vasculitis, heart emboli, and thrombotic thrombocytopenic purpura. *Ann Neurol* 1988, 23:380–384.
74. Mitsias P, Levine SR: Large cerebral vessel occlusive disease in systemic lupus erythematosus. *Neurology* 1994, 44:385–393.
75. Lucas FV, Benjamin SP, Steinberg MC: Cerebral vasculitis in Wegener's granulomatosis. *Cleve Clin Q* 1976, 43:275–281.
76. Talbot RW, Heppell J, Dozois RR, Beart RW: Vascular complications of inflammatory bowel disease. *Mayo Clin Proc* 1986, 61:140–145.
77. Natowicz M, Kelley RI: Mendelian etiologies of stroke. *Ann Neurol* 1987, 22:175–192.
78. Vonsattel JPG, Hedley-Whyte ET: Homocystinuria. In *Handbook of Clinical Neurology: Vascular Diseases.* Part 3. Edited by Vinken PJ, Bruyn GW, Klawans HL; co-edited by Toole JF. Amsterdam: Elsevier Science Publishers; 1989:325–334.
79. Schaffer AI, Kroll MH: Nonatheromatous arterial thrombosis. *Ann Rev Med* 1993, 44:155–170.
80. Rodgers GM, Conn MT: Homocysteine, an atherogenic stimulus, reduces protein C activation by arterial and venous endothelial cells. *Blood* 1990, 4:895–901.
81. Powars DR, Wilson B, Imbus C, *et al.*: The natural history of stroke in sickle cell disease. *Am J Med* 1978, 65:461–471.
82. Hart RG, Kanter MC: Hematologic disorders and ischemic stroke. *Stroke* 1990, 21:1111–1121.
83. Coull BM, Goodnight SH: Hematological abnormalities in stroke. In *Handbook of Cerebrovascular Diseases.* Edited by Adams HP. New York: Marcel Dekker; 1993:191–220.
84. Brust JCM: Stroke and drugs. In *Handbook of Clinical Neurology: Vascular Diseases.* Part 3. Edited by Vinken PJ, Bruyn GW, Klawans HL; co-edited by Toole JF. Amsterdam: Elsevier Science Publishers; 1989:517–531.
85. Kelly MA, Gorelick PB, Mirza D: The role of drugs in the etiology of stroke. *Clin Neuropharmacol* 1992, 15:249–275.
86. Levine SR, Fagan SC, Pessin MS, *et al.*: Accelerated intracranial occlusive disease, oral contraceptives, and cigarette smoking. *Neurology* 1991, 41:1893–1901.
87. Forman HP, Levin S, Stewart B, *et al.*: Cerebral vasculitis and hemorrhage in an adolescent taking diet pills containing phenylpropanolamine: case report and review of the literature. *Pediatrics* 1989, 83:737–741.
88. Levine SR, Brust JCM, Futrell N, *et al.*: A comparative study of the cerebrovascular complications of cocaine: alkaloid versus hydrochloride: a review. *Neurology* 1991, 41:1173–1177.
89. Hart RG, Miller VT: Cerebral infarction in young adults: a practical approach. *Stroke* 1983, 14:110–114.
90. High KA: Antithrombin III, protein C, and protein S: naturally occurring anticoagulant proteins. *Arch Pathol Lab Med* 1988, 112:28–36.
91. D'Angelo A, Landi G, Orazio EN, *et al.*: Protein C in acute stroke. *Stroke* 1988, 19:579–583.
92. Camerlingo M, Finazzi G, Casto L, *et al.*: Inherited protein C deficiency and nonhemorrhagic arterial stroke in young adults. *Neurology* 1991, 41:1371–1373.
93. Mayer SA, Sacco RL, Hurlet-Jensen A, *et al.*: Free protein S deficiency in acute ischemic stroke: a case-control study. *Stroke* 1993, 24:224–227.
94. Arima T, Motomura M, Nishiata Y: Cerebral infarction in a heterozygote with variant antithrombin III. *Stroke* 1992, 23:1822–1825.
95. Dang CV, Bell WR, Shuman M: The normal and morbid biology of fibrinogen. *Am J Med* 1989, 87:567–576.
96. Kay AC, Solberg LA, Nichols DA, Petitt RM: Prognostic significance of computed tomography of the brain in thrombotic thrombocytopenic purpura. *Mayo Clin Proc* 1991, 66:602–607.
97. Ross Russell RW, Wade JPH: Haematological causes of cerebrovascular disease. In *Handbook of Clinical Neurology: Vascular Diseases.* Part 3. Edited by Vinken PJ, Bruyn GW, Klawans HL; co-edited by Toole JF. Amsterdam: Elsevier Science Publishers; 1989:463–481.
98. Harris EN, Asherson RA, Hughes GRV: Antiphospholipid antibodies: autoantibodies with a difference. *Ann Rev Med* 1988, 39:261–271.
99. Levine SR, Deegan MJ, Futrell N, Welch KMA: Cerebrovascular and neurologic disease associated with antiphospholipid antibodies: 48 cases. *Neurology* 1990, 40:1181–1189.
100. The Antiphospholipid Antibody in Stroke Study (APASS) Group: Anticardiolipin antibodies are an independent risk factor for first ischemic stroke. *Neurology* 1993, 43:2069–2073.
101. Ott E: Hyperviscosity syndromes. In *Handbook of Clinical Neurology: Vascular Diseases.* Part 3. Edited by Vinken PJ, Bruyn GW, Klawans HL; co-edited by Toole JF. Amsterdam: Elsevier Science Publishers; 1989:483–492.
102. Levine SR, Ramadan NM: The relationship of stroke and migraine. In *Handbook of Cerebrovascular Diseases.* Edited by Adams HP. New York: Marcel Dekker; 1993:221–231.
103. Ramadan NM: Migrainous infarction: the Charcot-Féré syndrome? *Cephalalgia* 1993, 13:249–251.
104. Tietjen GE, Mitsias P: Cerebral venous thrombosis. *Heart Dis Stroke* 1993, 2:19–25.

Chapter 8

Cranial Computed Tomography and Magnetic Resonance Imaging of Cerebrovascular Disorders

GLEN GEREMIA
WILLIAM M. GREENLEE

Cerebral ischemia is a significant decrease in blood flow to regions of the brain. Major causes of cerebral ischemia are hypoperfusion, artery-to-artery embolism, cardiac embolism, thrombosis, vasospasm, and venous thrombosis. Cerebral infarction is the progression of ischemia to irreversible changes characterized by coagulation necrosis. Coagulation necrosis is the result of cell death. Brain infarcts are often classified as bland (anemic) or hemorrhagic, depending on the presence of extravasated blood within the parenchyma. Hemorrhagic infarcts are generally due to cardiac embolism or venous occlusion.

PATHOPHYSIOLOGY OF CEREBRAL ISCHEMIA AND INFARCTION

Neurons subjected to ischemia for 30 to 60 minutes (in experimental models of ischemia) reveal swelling of cytoplasm due to cytotoxic edema as a result of ionic pump dysfunction caused by ATP depletion to ≤ 40% of normal [1,2]. Water accumulates in the cytoplasm because the ATP levels are not sufficient to fuel the membrane-based ionic pumps. The influx of sodium and potassium into the cell and the build-up of lactic acid from anaerobic glycolysis increases the osmotic gradient resulting in water diffusion into the cytoplasm, worsening the cytotoxic edema. Ischemic changes in astrocytes and oligodendrocytes occur at about the same time as they occur in neurons. However, of the three cell types, neurons are the least tolerant of ischemic change.

Reperfusion and hemorrhage into an ischemic area are sometimes observed in arterial occlusion caused by an embolus. This is seen following lysis of the embolus when flow is reestablished. Reperfusion before endothelial cell damage, 3 to 6 hours postictus, can prevent cytotoxic edema. However, reperfusion after endothelial cell injury can add vasogenic edema to a brain region already swollen from cytotoxic edema. Endothelial cell injury will effect the integrity of the blood-brain barrier. Water and plasma protein will deposit into the extracellular space from leaky capillaries. The volume of edema reaches maximum at between 1 to 5 days postictus and resolution occurs over the next 1 to 2 weeks.

Anatomic safeguards are present that may prevent an ischemic process from progressing to infarction. There exists a continuous capillary network between adjacent arterial territories that may obviate progression to infarction following proximal arteriolar occlusion. For example, the vascular territory of the subcortical "u" fibers is supplied by both terminal branches of cortical arteries and by the proximal branches of long medullary arteries [2]. This dual blood supply is also seen in the external capsule, claustrum, and extreme capsule. Regions of the brain without these protective collateral vascular beds are present in the basal ganglia, thalamus, and centrum semiovale, which receive their blood supply from long penetrating arteries that do not interdigitate and that arise adjacent to each other from the same vessel.

Evaluation of patients suspected of having intracranial vascular disease relies heavily on diagnostic radiology techniques. Imaging modalities such as computed tomography (CT) and magnetic resonance (MR) imaging are the tools used to visibly observe otherwise imperceptible underlying pathophysiologic changes *in vivo*. The predominant goals of use of these diagnostic techniques include definition of the location and extent of a disease process along with the delineation of the underlying pathogenesis. Also, the response to therapy can be monitored by serial interval radiologic studies in some instances.

VASCULAR TERRITORIES

Familiarization of vascular territories (Figures 8.1, 8.2) as they appear in the axial or coronal planes can help distinguish infarction from other pathologic lesions on CT and MR scans. A focal brain lesion that does not respect a vascular distribution pattern would be unlikely to be a thromboembolic infarction. There are three major vascular territories of the cerebrum, the anterior, middle, and posterior cerebral arteries. These are further divided into two major groups, the superficial cortical branches and deep penetrating branches [3,4].

Anterior Cerebral Artery

The anterior cerebral artery supplies the medial portion of the cerebral hemisphere. The anterior cerebral artery has been further divided into three major groups, the medial lenticulostriate, deep pericallosal, and cortical branches [5]. The medial lenticulostriate arteries supply the anterior regions of the putamen, caudate nucleus, and internal capsule. The deep pericallosal branches supply the anterior two thirds of the corpus callosum. The cortical branches supply the medial and inferior frontal lobe.

Middle Cerebral Artery

The middle cerebral artery supplies the lateral portion of the cerebral hemisphere. The middle cerebral artery is further divided into the deep system of lateral lenticulostriate arteries and the peripheral cortical branches. Lateral lenticulostriate branches supply the head and body of the caudate nucleus, putamen, lateral aspect of the globus pallidus, and the anterior fiber tracts of the internal capsule [4]. The cortical branches supply the anterolateral aspects of the temporal lobes and the lateral convexity surface of the frontal, temporal, and parietal lobes [6].

Posterior Cerebral Artery

The posterior cerebral arteries supply the inferomedial portion of the cerebral hemisphere. The posterior cerebral artery is divided into two major groups, deep penetrating arteries to the thalamus, brain stem, and posterior choroidal arteries, and peripheral branches that supply the medial cortical surface of the temporal, parietal, and occipital lobes.

The posterior fossa is supplied predominantly from the superior cerebellar artery (superior cerebellum, vermis, and quadrigeminal plate), anterior inferior cerebellar artery (anterior cerebellum and dorsal medulla), and the posterior inferior cerebellar artery (inferolateral cerebellum, inferior vermis, cerebellar tonsil, and the medulla). The vertebral and basilar arteries give rise to the aforementioned cerebellar arteries. The vertebral and basilar arteries supply blood circulation to vital areas of the brain stem.

Watershed Zones

Watershed zones (Figure 8.3) are regions located at the junctions between the anterior, middle, and posterior cerebral arteries. Infarctions in these zones are usually caused by arterial hypoperfusion. The parietal-occipital zone is the region most vulnerable to a watershed infarct since this is the point of termination of the distal branches of the anterior, middle, and posterior cerebral arteries.

ROLE OF COMPUTED TOMOGRAPHY AND MAGNETIC RESONANCE IMAGING

The clinical role of neuroimaging in cerebral infarction has been primarily to evaluate for other causes of neurologic dysfunction that may mimic the stroke syndrome (*eg*, tumor, subdural hematoma), provide radiologic evidence of tissue infarction and determine the vascular territories involved, and rule out the presence of hemorrhage in anticipation of anticoagulation administration or experimental hyperacute ischemic stroke therapy.

Computed Tomography

The role of CT in the diagnosis of cerebral infarction is well established [7]. CT can distinguish between an ischemic bland (nonhemorrhagic) stroke, hemorrhagic infarction, and primary intracerebral hemorrhage [8].

In the clinical setting of a transient ischemic attack (TIA) the CT scan is usually normal, however, the detection of white matter or capsular hypodensity (chronic ischemic change) establishes the presence of underlying vascular disease [9]. It has been reported that 18% to 34% of patients evaluated for TIAs may have lacunar infarcts in the basal ganglia and internal capsule detected by CT [9–11].

The classic neuropathologic processes that occur during the evolution of an infarction are well reflected by the CT scan. An understanding of the classic evolutionary changes of infarction

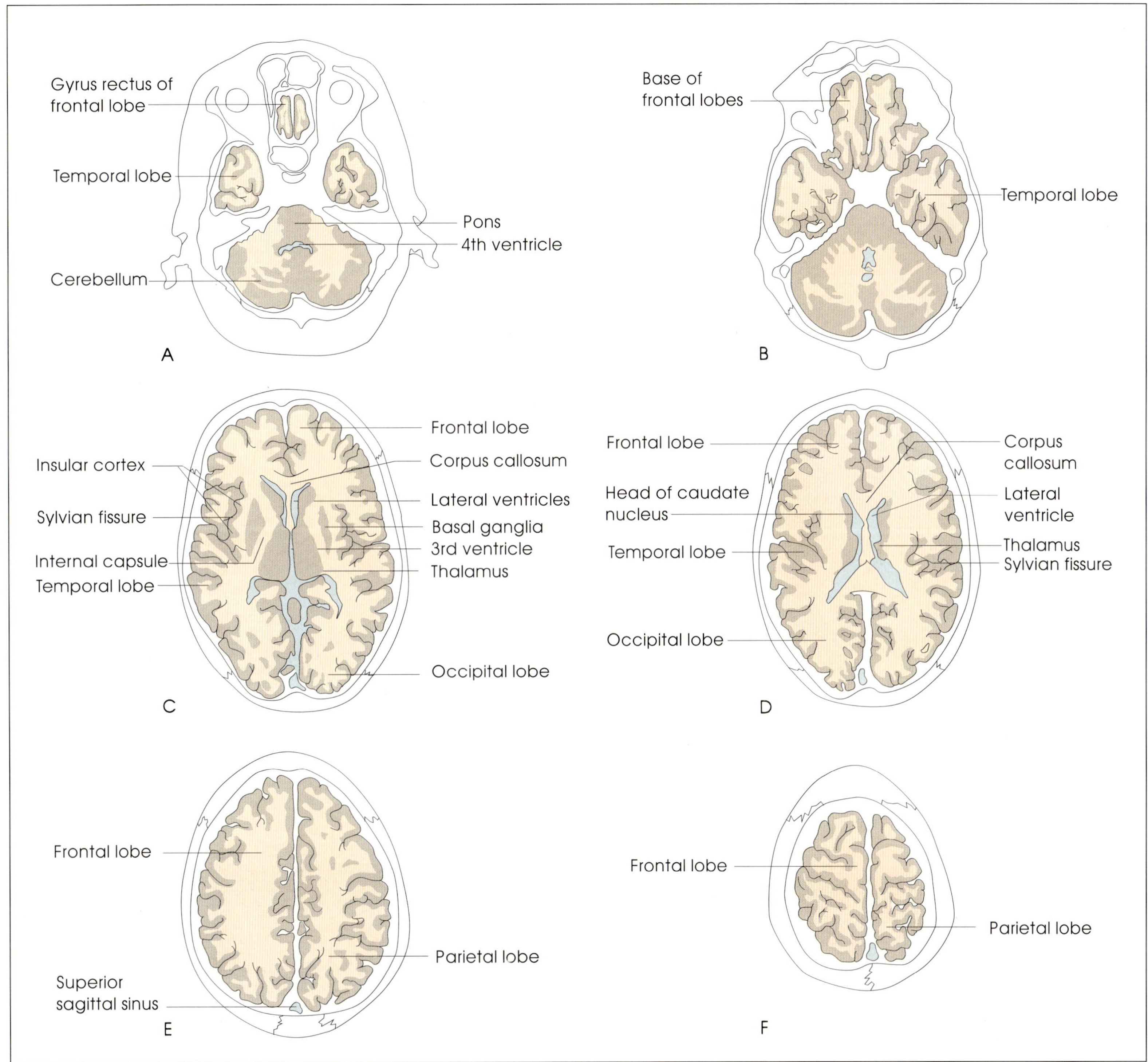

FIGURE 8.1

Illustrative drawings of normal brain anatomy in the axial plane (**A**–**F**) from base of brain (**A**) to top (**F**).

on serial CT imaging is necessary in distinguishing infarction from other intracerebral processes such as primary or secondary brain neoplasm. The radiologic imaging characteristics are divided into four stages and are dependent on the time from the onset of the ictus. These stages are divided into 1) hyperacute (less than 24 hours); 2) acute (24 hours to 7 days); 3) subacute (8–21 days); and 4) chronic (greater than 21 days) (Figure 8.4) (Table 8.1).

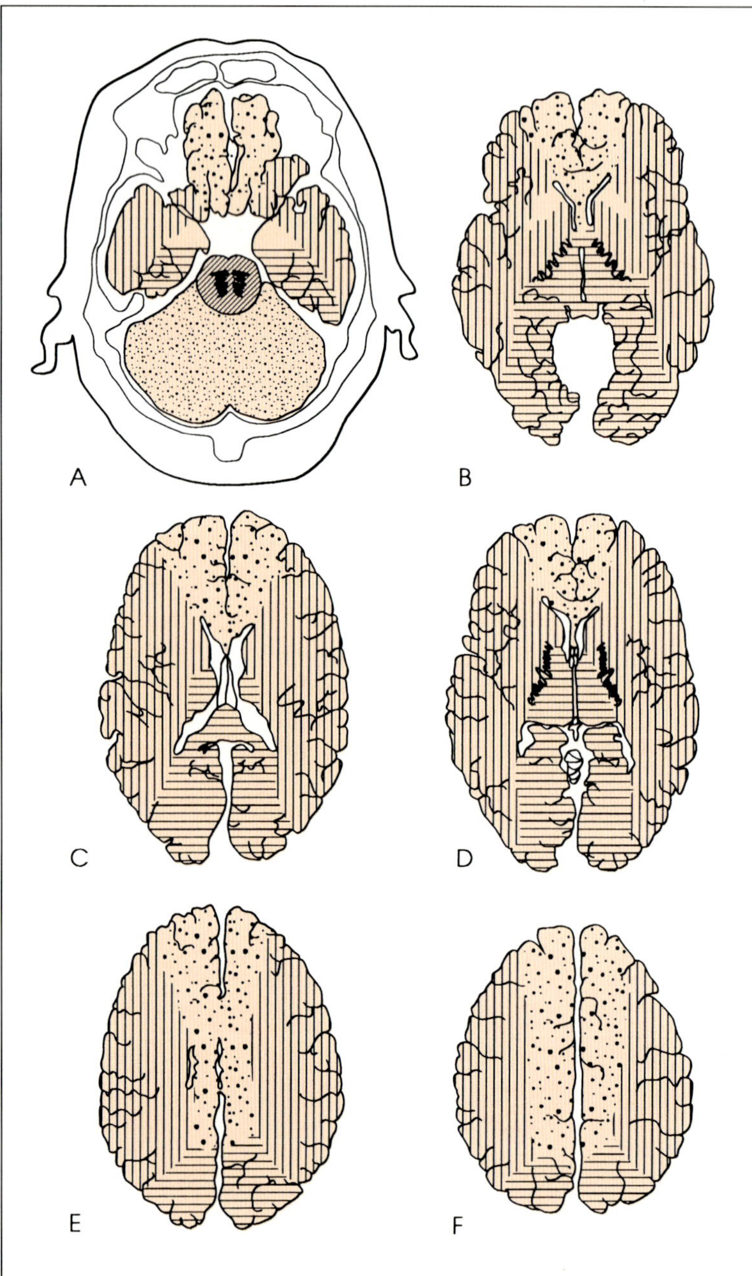

FIGURE 8.2

A–F, Schematic drawings of brain in the axial plane vascular territories defined. *Lightly stippled* areas represent anterior cerebral artery; *vertically lined* areas represent middle cerebral artery; *horizontally lined* areas represent posterior cerebral artery; *diagonally lined* areas represent basilar perforations; and *heavily stippled* areas represent cerebellar arteries.

Hyperacute Infarction

The ability to detect an infarction during the first 24 hours is dependent on the size and degree of the ischemic insult [12]. Most scans will demonstrate little or no mass effect (Figure 8.5A). When detected, the changes of an infarct during this stage include a poorly marginated region with subtle decrease in the density of the gray matter causing it to become isodense with white matter, and thus the gray-white differentiation is obscured [8,12–14]. This hypodense region will become more distinct after several days and assumes a wedge shape with its broad base along the cortical brain surface. This initial low-density appearance represents intracellular (cytotoxic) edema [15]. The cytotoxic edema is caused by the redistribution of sodium and water within the brain. The sensitivity of CT in the detection of an early infarction, however, remains limited and only about half of all infarcts are seen in the first 24 hours [16].

Acute Infarction

Hypodensity and mass effect increase within the first week of the infarction (Figure 8.5B). Tissue necrosis and intracellular edema

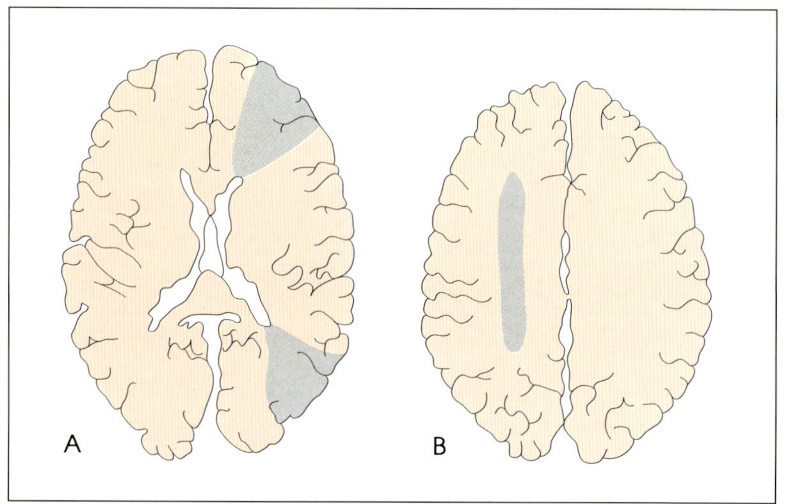

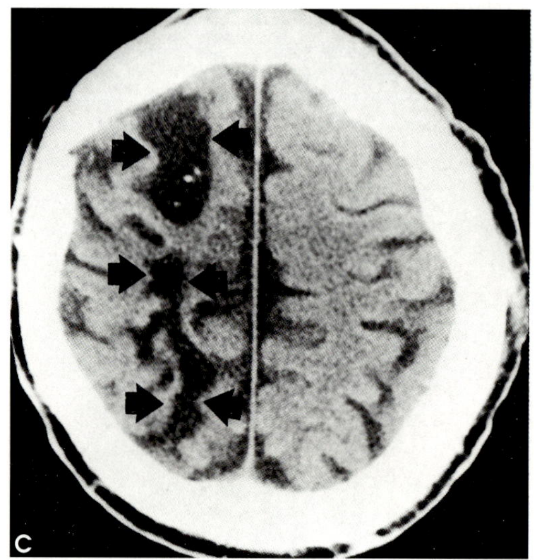

FIGURE 8.3

Watershed zones represented as shaded areas (**A** and **B**). Watershed infarction seen on computed tomography between anterior and middle cerebral artery territories (**C**) (*arrows*).

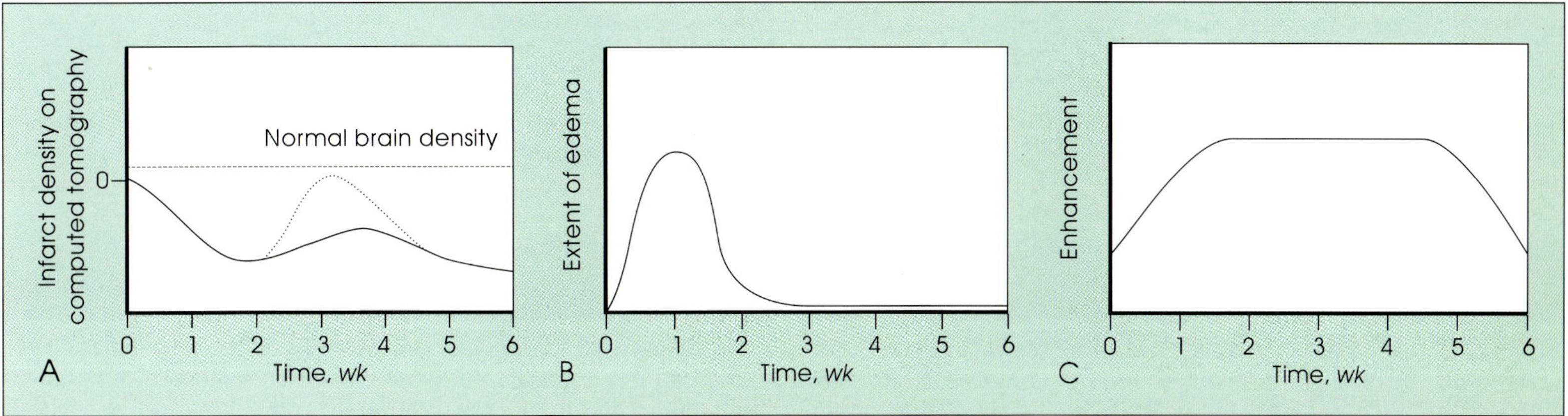

FIGURE 8.4

Summary of computed tomography (CT) findings in cerebral infarction. **A**, CT hypodensity following infarction; *dotted line* indicates the "paradoxical" or "fogging" effect that may obscure the area of infarction in the subacute phase, occurring when resolution of edema is superimposed on coagulative necrosis. **B**, Mass effect and edema typically peak between 3 and 10 days after infarction. **C**, Blood-brain barrier breakdown as reflected by contrast enhancement following intravenous contrast administration. (*Adapted from* Djang and coworkers [9]; with permission.)

Table 8.1. Imaging findings in cerebral infarction: computed tomography and magnetic resonance imaging

		MR signal intensity		
Infarction (stage)	**CT density**	**T1WI**	**T2WI**	**CT/MR gyral enhancement**
Hyperacute (< 24 hrs)	Iso-hypodense	Iso-hypointense	Iso-hyperintense	NE
Acute (> 24 hrs–7 days)	Hypodense	Hypointense	Hyperintense	NE to E*
Subacute (8–21 days)	Hypodense	Hypointense	Hyperintense	E
Chronic (> 21 days)	Hypodense	Hypointense	Hyperintense	NE

*In the acute stage there may or may not be enhancement.
CT—computed tomography; E—enhancement; MR—magnetic resonance; NE—no enhancement; T1WI—T1-weighted; T2WI—T2-weighted.

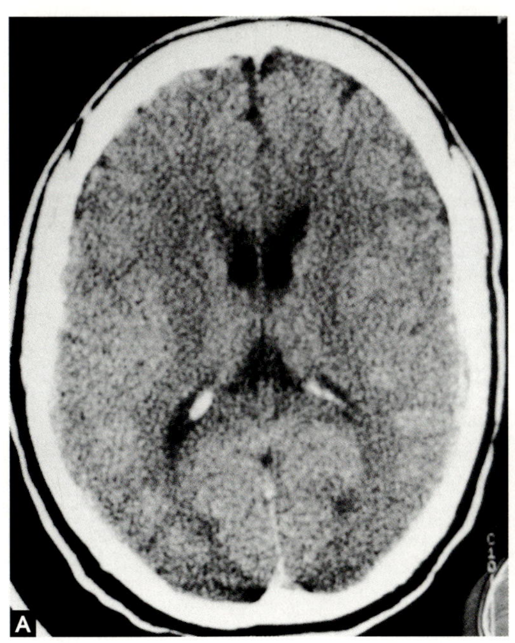

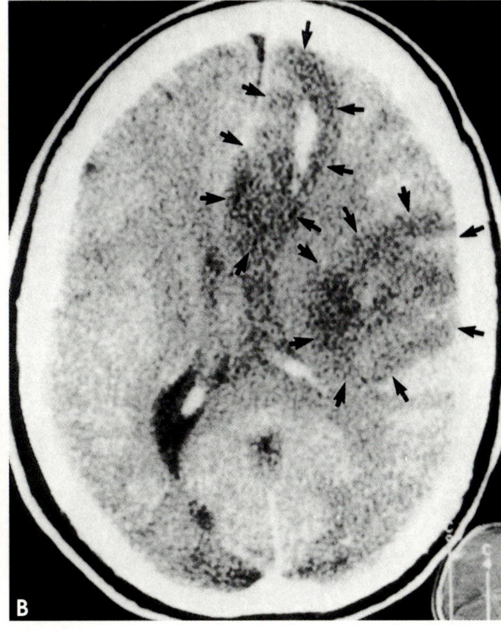

FIGURE 8.5

Sequential changes of an infarct on computed tomography (CT) in the distribution of the anterior and middle cerebral arteries. **A**, Hyperacute stage. CT scan performed 8 hours postictus is normal. **B**, Acute stage. CT performed several days later reveals cytotoxic edema and mass effect (*arrows*).

reach maximum at this time. The greatest degree of mass effect is reportedly between the third and fifth days and is seen in 21% to 70% of infarcts [16–18]. The swelling begins to subside after the first week and usually resolves completely in 12 to 21 days [12]. Extreme mass effect may cause midline shift and transtentorial temporal lobe herniation with resultant occipital lobe infarction from posterior cerebral artery occlusion. Infarcts in multiple vascular territories and of the same age are usually caused by emboli (Figure 8.6). With embolic infarction, greater brain swelling may occur due to vasogenic edema when clot lysis results in reestablished circulation. This results in leakage of intravascular fluids and protein through ischemically damaged capillary endothelium into the extracellular spaces [19]. In severe global hypoperfusion infarction may occur in "watershed" or border zones between major arterial distal distributions of the anterior, middle, and posterior cerebral artery circulation (Figure 8.3).

Subacute Infarction

Mass effect begins to subside during this period (8–21 days postictus). Resolution of edema and mass effect may make the area isodense relative to brain and therefore less conspicuous. This phenomenon has been called the "fogging effect."

Contrast enhancement occurs during this period and follows maximum mass effect [20–22] (Figure 8.7). The intensity of enhancement begins to decline by the third week and usually persists for 6 weeks following the acute event. Several pathophysiologic mechanisms are responsible for enhancement, the major factor being extravasation of contrast into extracellular space caused by breakdown in the capillary endothelium blood-brain barrier [23]. Neovascular capillary proliferation also occurs, and these blood vessels have an incompetent blood-brain barrier. The pattern of enhancement with cortical infarction is gyral. Infarction in the deep basal ganglia demonstrates a ringlike appearance of enhancement.

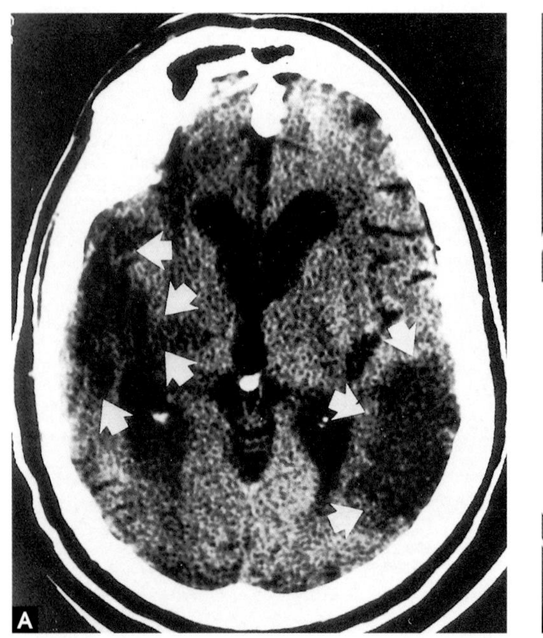

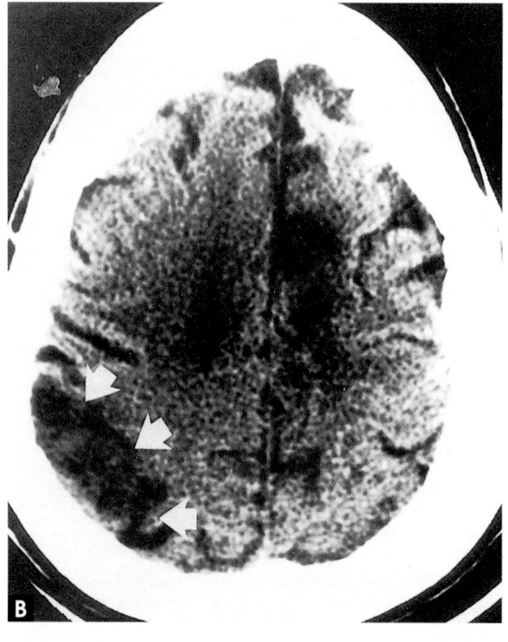

FIGURE 8.6

A and **B**, Computed tomography scan without contrast. Bilateral scattered areas of infarction (*arrows*) consistent with multiple emboli.

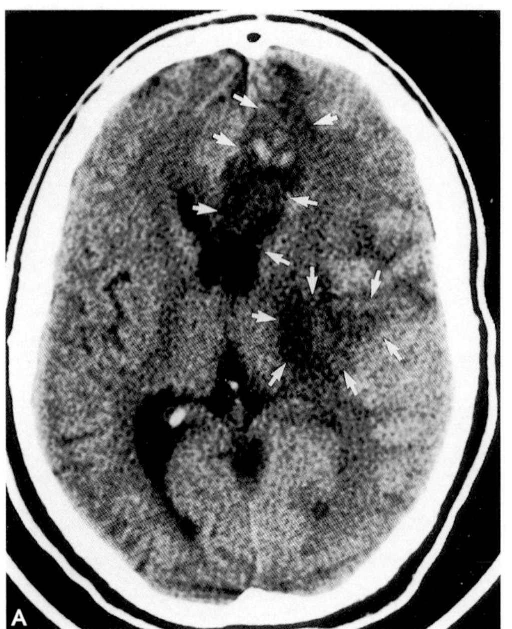

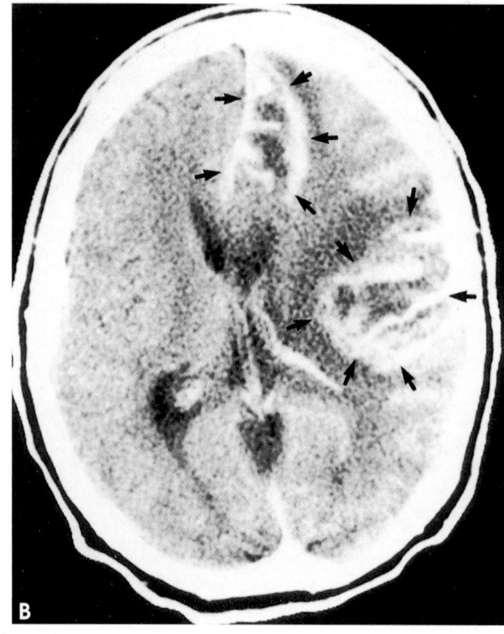

FIGURE 8.7

Same patient as seen in Figure 8.5. Subacute stage. Computed tomography obtained 10 days postictus reveals slightly less mass effect (*white arrows*) (**A**) and contrast enhancement (*black arrows*) (**B**).

Chronic Infarction

The area that previously demonstrated low-density edema and mass effect is now seen as a well-marginated zone of cystic encephalomalacia whose density is similar to cerebral spinal fluid (Figure 8.8). There may also be a surrounding zone of gliosis or calcification (Figure 8.9). The edema at this stage has resorbed, thus making the margins of the infarcted region more distinct. An overall loss of tissue volume with prominent cortical sulci and compensatory dilatation of the ipsilateral ventricle are seen on CT in a region of infarction. Contrast enhancement may be seen as long as 6 to 8 weeks following the acute stroke. At this time the blood-brain barrier has undergone the reparative process and has regained its integrity.

MAGNETIC RESONANCE IMAGING

Image contrast with MR imaging is dependent on three tissue variables: T1 relaxation time; T2 relaxation time; and proton density. These variables are inherent properties of the tissue to be scanned and are not operator controlled. However, there are several time variables that are controlled by the operator. These are the pulse repetition time (TR) and the echo delay time (TE). By varying the TR and TE an image can be obtained that will predominantly favor either the T1 or T2 properties of the tissue. In disease states, T1 and T2 characteristics will be altered relative to those of normal tissue. The image changes seen in disease tissue predominantly reflect an increase in the free water content of the ischemic brain. The superiority of MR imaging over CT in the detection of cerebral infarcts has been reported [24] (Figure 8.10). Experimental models have suggested detection of ischemia 1 hour after the event by MR imaging [25].

ISCHEMIC STROKE

Acute Stage

The earliest changes seen with MR imaging of an acute infarct are low signal in the infarcted region of the T1-weighted images and high (bright) signal on the T2-weighted images. These changes represent prolongation of the T1 and T2 relaxation times consistent with an increase in the free water content

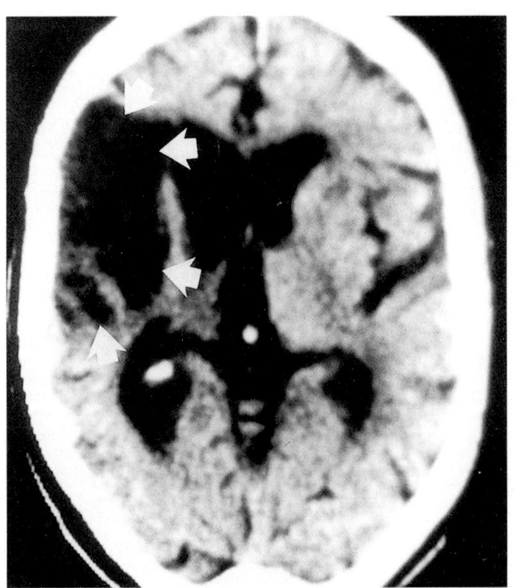

FIGURE 8.8

Chronic infarction. Area of low density consistent with cystic encephalomalacia in the temporal lobe (*arrows*). Note compensatory dilatation of the ipsilateral lateral ventricle due to the loss of brain parenchyma.

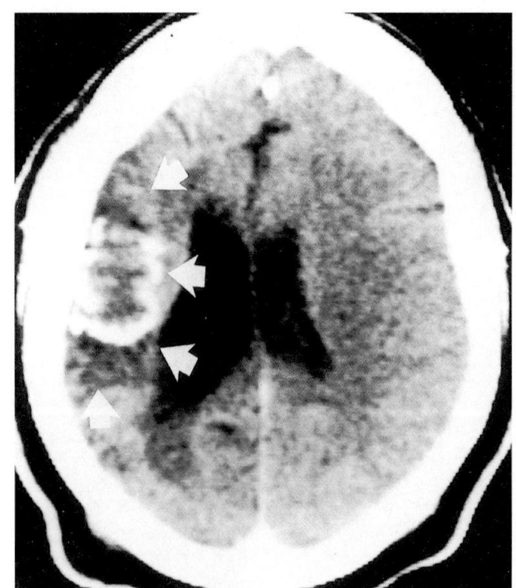

FIGURE 8.9

Chronic infarction with area of calcification (*arrows*).

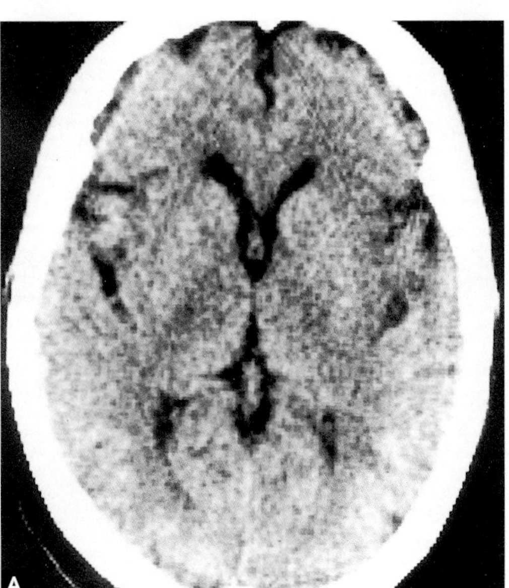

FIGURE 8.10

Acute infarct not detected on computed tomography (**A**) but demonstrated on magnetic resonance image (**B**) as an area of hyperintensity (*arrows*).

within the zone of infarction. The signal intensity changes are not reliably present until 8 hours after the ictus with signal changes being greatest at 24 to 48 hours [26,27].

As with CT, the area of involvement is in a vascular distribution. In some series mass effect was seen 2 hours after the onset of symptoms but was usually seen within 8 hours [28]. Peak mass effect is not generally seen in the acute stage but is present about 3 to 10 days after infarction. Contrast enhancement with gadolinium is not usually a feature in early acute stroke. However, early enhancement of arterioles and leptomeninges has recently been reported and may be seen before parenchymal signal changes (Figure 8.11) [29].

Subacute Stage

The subacute period is between 7 and 21 days. Signal changes here are similar to those seen in the acute phase. The region of infarction is hypointense on the T1-weighted images and hyperintense (bright) on the T2-weighted images. Contrast enhancement with gadolinium is similar in pattern to that seen with CT

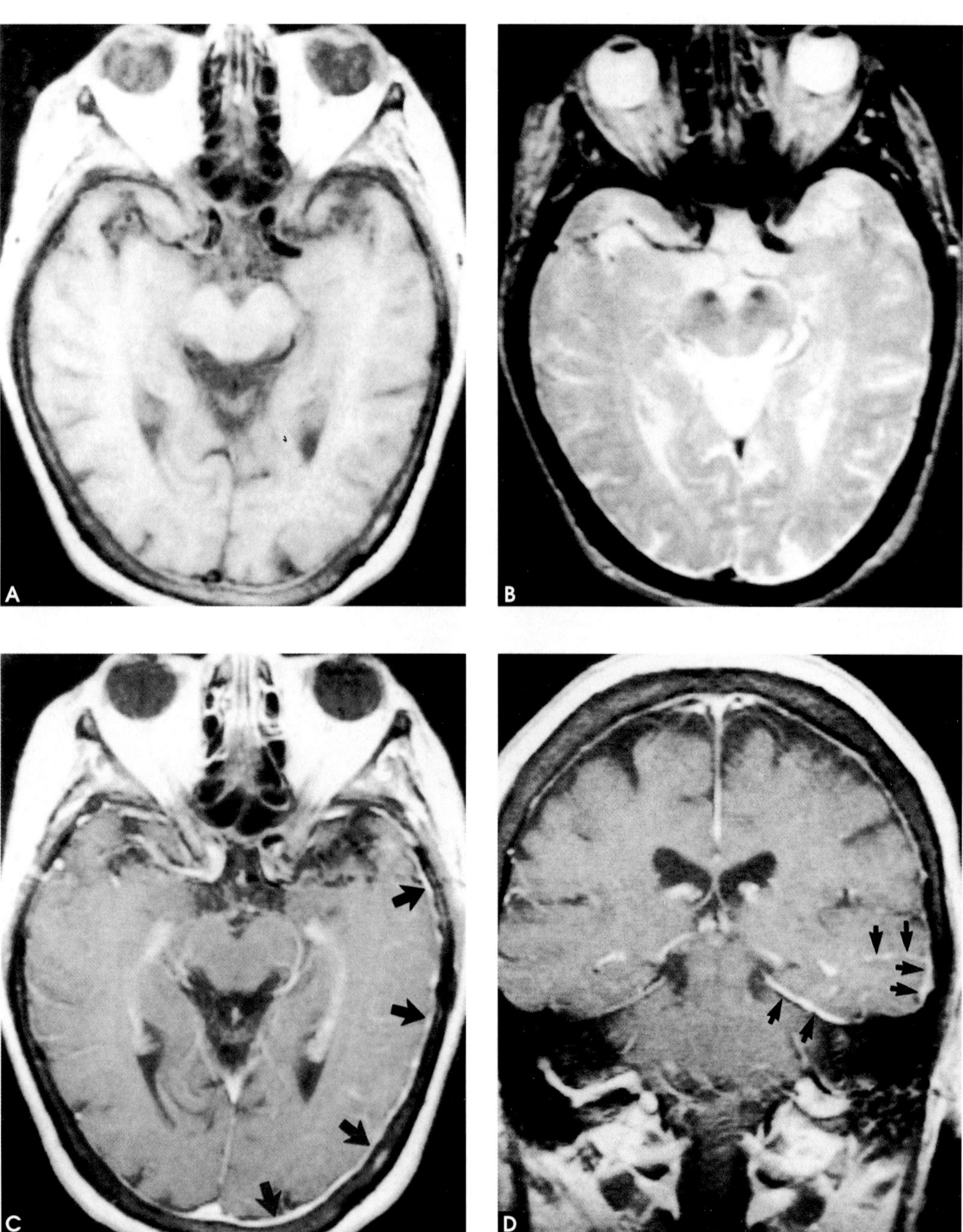

FIGURE 8.11

Acute infarct. T1-weighted (**A**) and T2-weighted (**B**) images are unremarkable. Contrast infused T1-weighted images (**C** and **D**) reveal meningeal and arterial enhancement (*arrows*).

(Figure 8.12). Also, the mechanism for enhancement, contrast extravasation due to breakdown of the blood-brain barrier, is also the same as with CT. Contrast enhancement is best appreciated on the T1-weighted images. Subtle enhancement in infarcted regions has been reported to be more conspicuous on MR images than CT [30].

Chronic Infarction

This stage is generally considered to begin about 3 weeks postictus. As in CT, the major findings are loss of mass effect and characteristics consistent with encephalomalacia and gliosis. The cystic areas demonstrate hypointensity and hyperintensity similar to that of cerebral spinal fluid on the T1- and T2-weighted images, respectively (Figure 8.13). Contrast enhancement may persist as a uniform pattern until several months after the infarct. The parenchymal enhancement eventually subsides following repair of the capillary endothelium blood-brain barrier.

LACUNAR INFARCTS

Lacunar infarcts are focal lesions within the basal ganglia and thalami and are often seen in patients with a clinical history of hypertension [9]. These are caused by ischemia to or occlusion of small penetrating end arteries. CT and MR images reveal

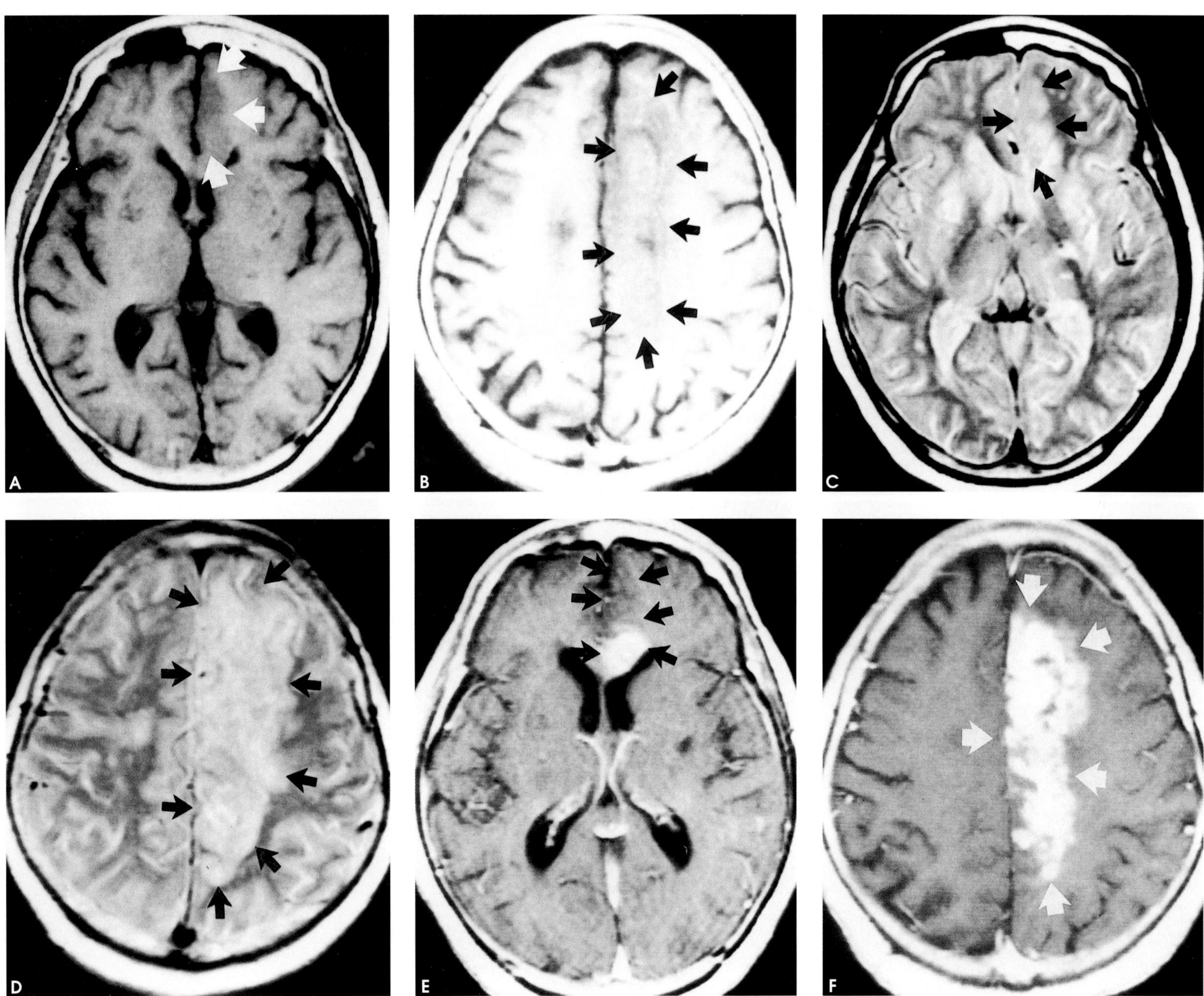

FIGURE 8.12

Subacute infarction in distribution of anterior cerebral artery (*arrows*). The area of infarction is hypointense on the T1-weighted images (**A** and **B**) and hyperintense (bright) on the T2-weighted images (**C** and **D**). There is parenchymal enhancement following contrast infusion (**E** and **F**).

punctate focal areas of abnormal density or signal intensity within these deep structures (Figure 8.14).

White Matter Lesions

Deep white matter focal and confluent lesions are often seen in the elderly with underlying small vessel disease. MR imaging is far superior in detecting these lesions over CT. The MR appearance is of bilaterally symmetric patchy deep white matter lesions that are hyperintense on the T2-weighted images (Figure 8.15) and slightly hypointense on the T1-weighted images [31]. CT reveals hypodensity in these regions (Figure 8.16). The white matter involvement is primarily located adjacent to the body and atrium of the lateral ventricles. This region is a deep border zone (watershed area) between the penetrating transmedullary white matter arteries originating from the cortical surface and short arterial branches extending out from the ependymal surface of the lateral ventricles. The abnormal appearance is most commonly caused by atrophic perivascular ischemic demyelination that is a degenerative process caused by arteriolar wall thickening and may or may not be associated with symptoms [32]. Another less common cause for this appearance is subcortical arteriosclerotic encephalopathy (Binswanger's disease) [33,34]. Binswanger's disease is associated with dementia, and is caused by arteriosclerotic and hypertensive vasculopathy that results in multiple deep infarctions [32] (Figure 8.17). These two entities look similar and are indistinguishable by imaging techniques.

SPECIFIC SIGNS

Obscuration of the Lentiform Nucleus

Tomura and coworkers [35] described obscuration of the lentiform nucleus (Figure 8.18) as a sign of acute infarction. The CT scans of

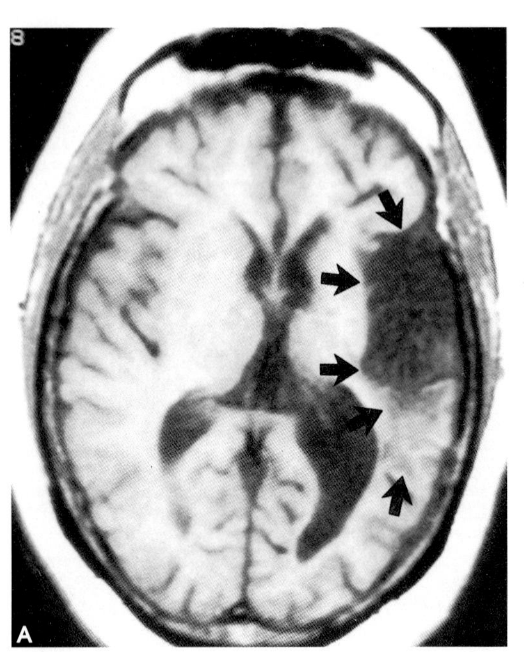

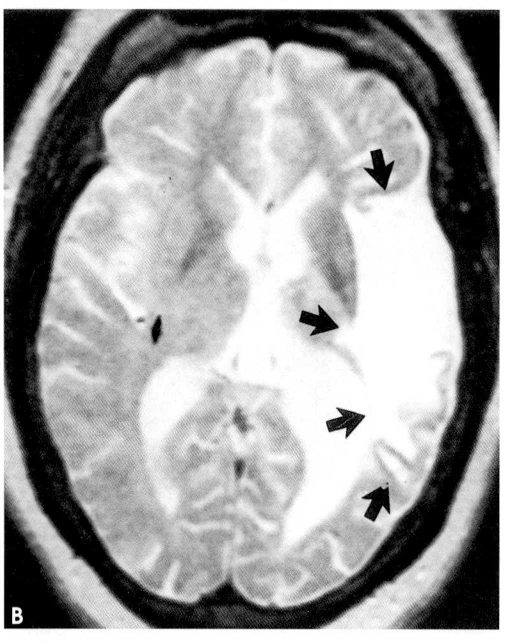

FIGURE 8.13

Chronic infarction. Areas of cystic encephalomalacia (*arrows*) reveal signal intensity similar to that of cerebrospinal fluid on T1-weighted (**A**) and T2-weighted (**B**) images. There is compensatory dilatation of the ipsilateral lateral ventricle due to parenchymal loss.

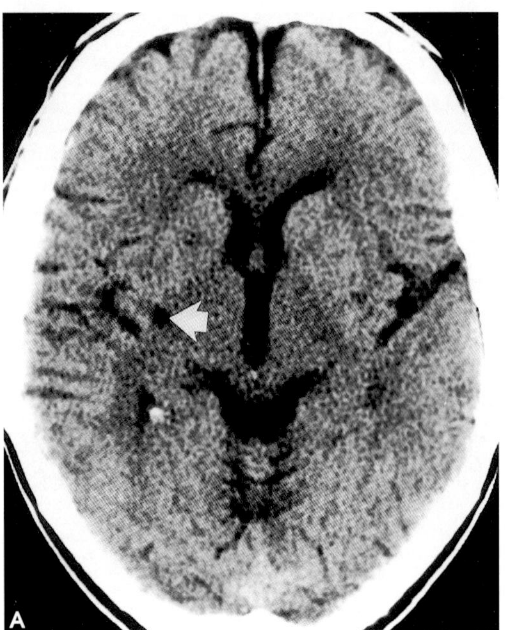

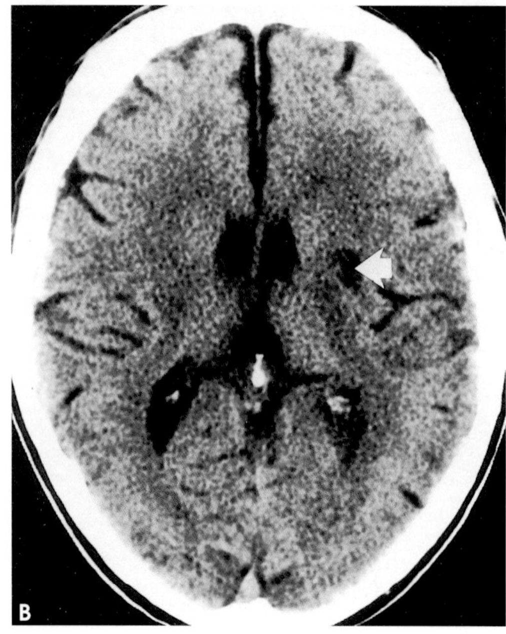

FIGURE 8.14

A and **B**, Lacunar infarcts. Low-density, well-defined lacunar infarcts (*arrows*) are seen within the basal ganglia in a hypertensive patient.

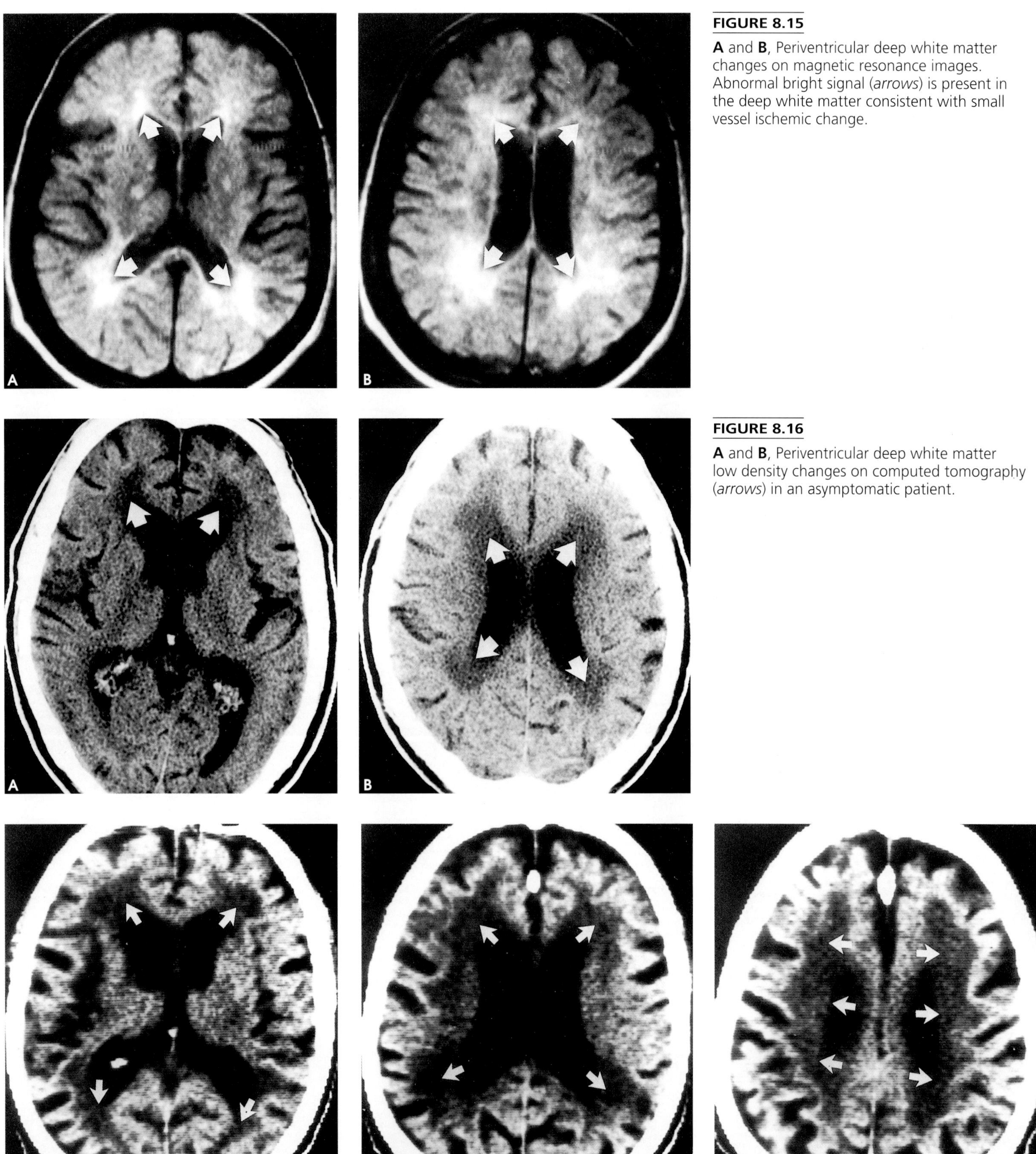

FIGURE 8.15

A and **B**, Periventricular deep white matter changes on magnetic resonance images. Abnormal bright signal (*arrows*) is present in the deep white matter consistent with small vessel ischemic change.

FIGURE 8.16

A and **B**, Periventricular deep white matter low density changes on computed tomography (*arrows*) in an asymptomatic patient.

FIGURE 8.17

A–C, Deep white matter low density changes on computed tomography (*arrows*) seen in a patient with Binswanger's disease.

25 patients with acute (less than 6 hours) embolic cerebral infarction of the middle cerebral artery territory were retrospectively analyzed. The most common finding was of an obscured outline or partial disappearance of the lentiform nucleus, which was found in 23 patients (92%). In several cases this finding was seen 1 hour after the onset of stroke. Follow-up CT scans obtained 1 to 4 days after stroke onset demonstrated areas with markedly decreased density and mass effect in all patients.

Fogging Effect

Several authors have described a phenomenon called the *fogging effect* (Figure 8.19) whereby an initially hypodense acute infarct can become isodense during the second or third week after the onset of infarction. Skriver and Olsen [36] prospectively studied the sequential CT changes 3 days, 18 days, and 6 months after stroke that were performed on 50 consecutive patients. The fogging effect was found in 54% of these cases. In 1978, Becker and coworkers [37] studied 10 selected patients with cerebral infarction by serial CT. In this series the fogging effect was reported to be a constant finding during the second and third weeks after stroke. No definitive pathophysiologic explanation for this sign has been evaluated. One theory is that the diminution of edema and mass effect along with proliferation of capillaries and extravasation of macrophages causes a previous hypodense area of acute infarction to return to isodensity. If a CT study is performed 2 to 3 weeks after an acute stroke (when the fogging effect is maximal) an area of infarction

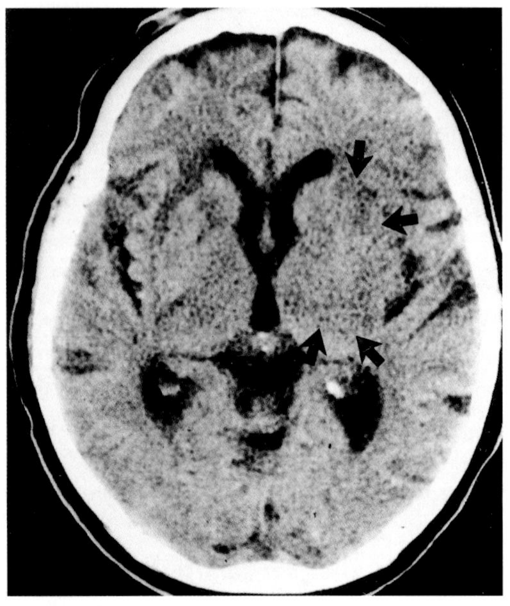

FIGURE 8.18

Obscuration of the lentiform nucleus. The margins of the infarcted basal ganglia are not identifiable (*arrows*) compared with the opposite uninvolved basal ganglia.

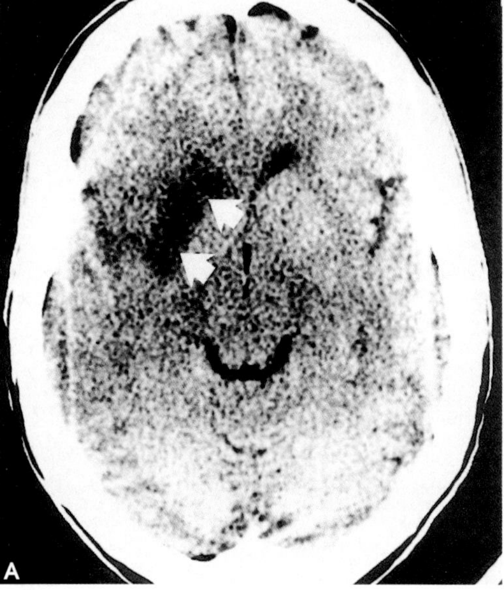

FIGURE 8.19

Fogging effect. **A**, Initial computed tomography (CT) scan performed several days postictus demonstrates low density changes in the basal ganglia (*arrows*). **B**, Follow-up CT performed 16 days later is unremarkable.

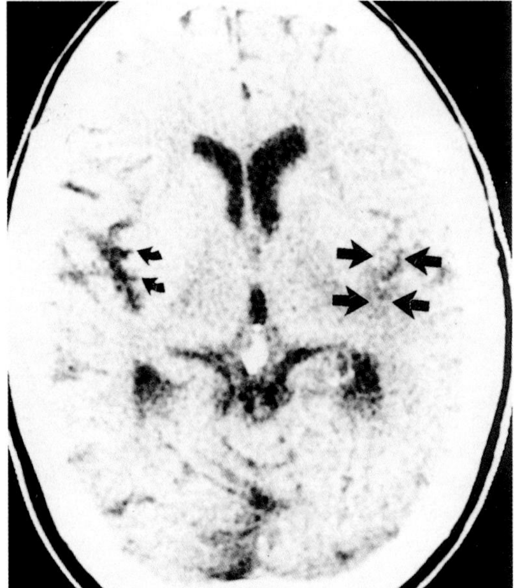

FIGURE 8.20

Loss of the insular ribbon. Effacement of the sylvian fissure and insular ribbon (*straight arrows*) is seen on the infarcted side of brain compared with the normal insular ribbon (*curved arrows*).

may be missed. Thus, a "normal" CT during this period does not rule out cerebral infarction and must be performed with contrast administration or repeated at a later date in order to exclude or confirm the diagnosis.

Loss of Insular Ribbon

Truwit and coworkers [38] identified loss of definition of the gray-white interface in the lateral margins of the insula ("insular ribbon") (Figure 8.20) in acute middle cerebral artery strokes less than 6 hours old. Loss of the insular ribbon was seen in 12 of 16 patients studied prospectively and in 11 of 11 patients reviewed retrospectively. The insular ribbon is supplied by the insular segments of the middle cerebral artery and its claustral branches. With occlusion or hypoperfusion of the middle cerebral artery the insular ribbon becomes the region most distal from the anterior and posterior cerebral collateral circulations and thus acts as a watershed arterial zone. Loss of the insular ribbon is a reflection of acute edema due to infarction. The authors concluded that loss of the insular ribbon is a reliable finding in acute middle cerebral artery stroke.

Hyperdense Middle Cerebral Artery Sign on Computed Tomography

Several authors have described the appearance of a hyperdense middle cerebral artery on CT (Figure 8.21) in patients presenting with acute stroke [39–43]. There was positive correlation between the angiographic findings of middle cerebral artery occlusion and the hyperdense middle cerebral artery on CT. The authors conclude that in the clinical setting of acute stroke, an artery visualized on noncontrast CT as diffuse high density and higher density than other visualized vessels should be suspected as acutely occluded by clot.

Wallerian Degeneration

A large hemispheric infarction may result in antegrade degeneration of axons and their myelin sheaths (Wallerian degeneration) (Figure 8.22). This is secondary to injury of the axon proximally or after death of its neuronal cell body. MR imaging reveals atrophic change in the ipsilateral mesencephalon and pons [44]. Abnormal intensity changes are seen in the corticospinal tracts.

OTHER VASCULAR LESIONS AND CONDITIONS

Hemorrhagic Lesions

Hemorrhagic lesions include reperfusion into an infarcted region of brain, hypertensive hemorrhage, and venous infarction with secondary hemorrhage. Hemorrhage occurs in about 10% of stroke patients in North America. Hypertension is present in 70% of these patients. The detection of cerebral hemorrhage has important therapeutic implications. One type of hemorrhage is associated with reperfusion in an area of ischemia following lysis of an embolus (Figure 8.23). The embolus lodges in a proximal vessel producing ischemic damage to the underlying brain and endothelial damage of the capillaries. Lysis of the embolus restores the circulation to the ischemic area that results in extravasation of erythrocytes through the capillary wall and into the parenchyma.

Hypertensive hemorrhages are most commonly located in the basal ganglia, thalami, deep cerebellum, and pons (Figure 8.24). Mass effect may be present and there may be hemorrhagic

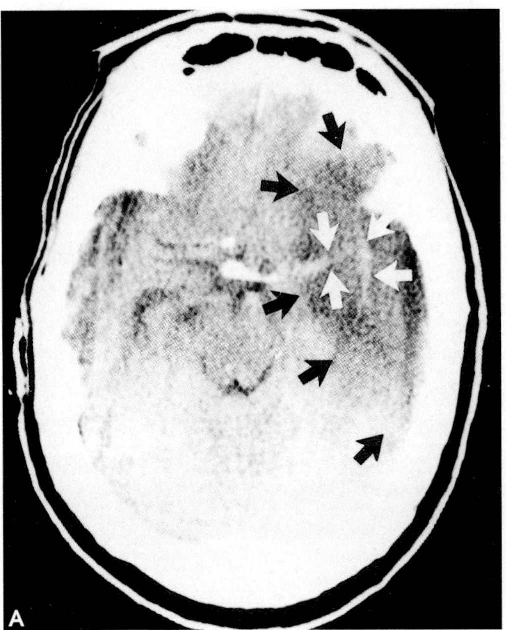

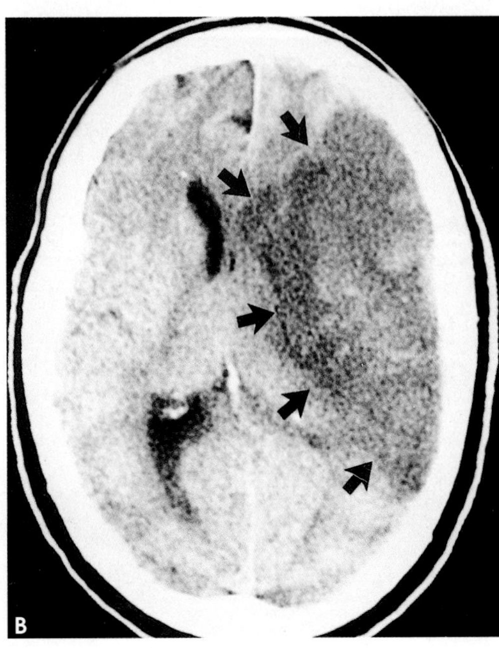

FIGURE 8.21

A and **B**, Hyperdense middle cerebral artery (*white arrows*) consistent with acute clot is seen surrounded by low density parenchymal edema (*black arrows*).

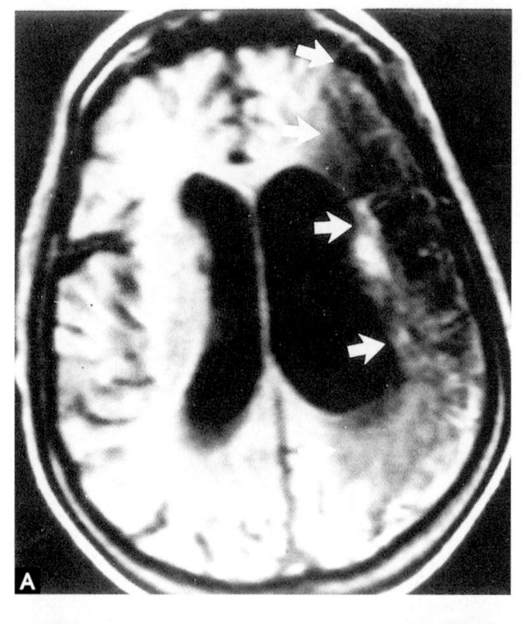

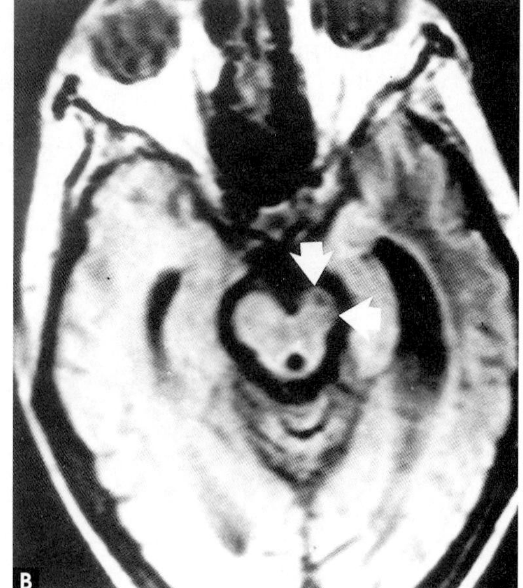

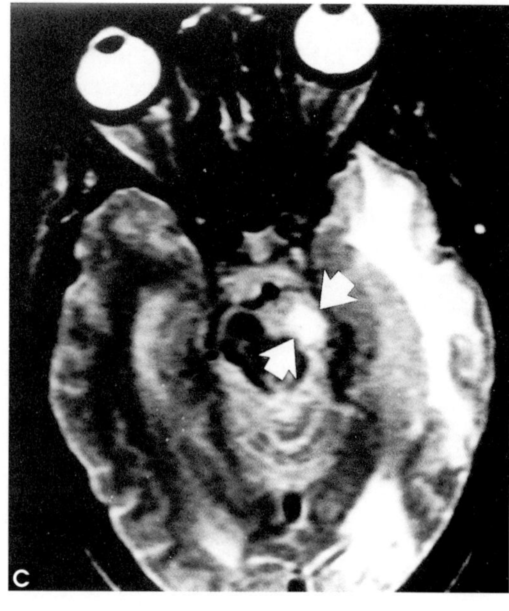

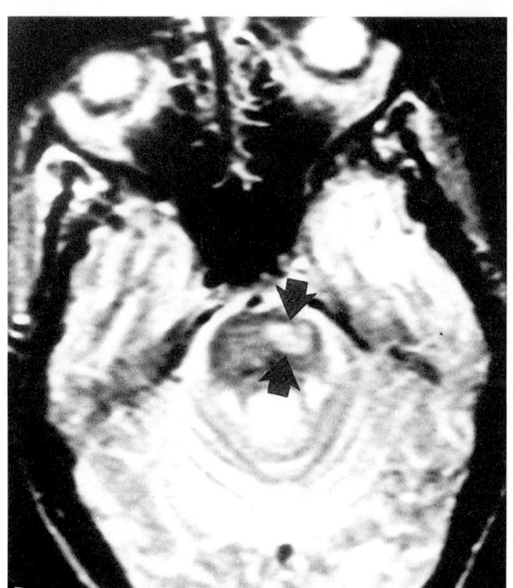

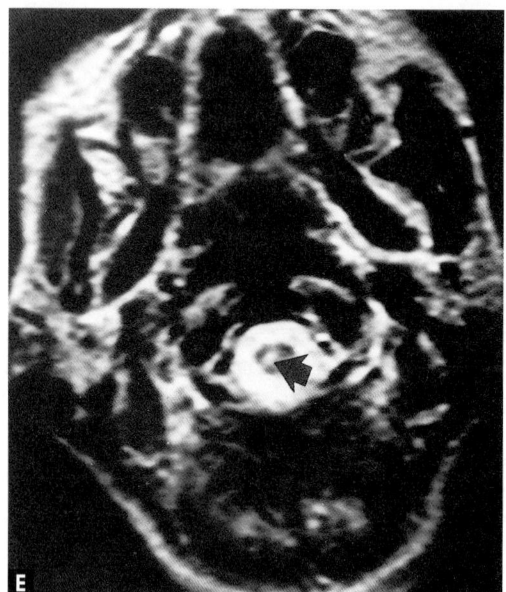

FIGURE 8.22

Wallerian degeneration. Low-signal changes (*arrows*) consistent with cystic encephalomalacia (**A**) are seen along with atrophy of the ipsilateral cerebral peduncle (*arrows*) (**B**) on the T1-weighted images. Abnormal high signal on the T2-weighted images is present in the ipsilateral cerebral peduncle (*arrows*) (**C**) and pons (*arrows*) (**D**) due to antegrade axonal degeneration. T2-weighted axial image (**E**) reveals abnormal signal in the contralateral lower medulla (*arrow*) caused by Wallerian degeneration of the corticospinal tract below its decussation.

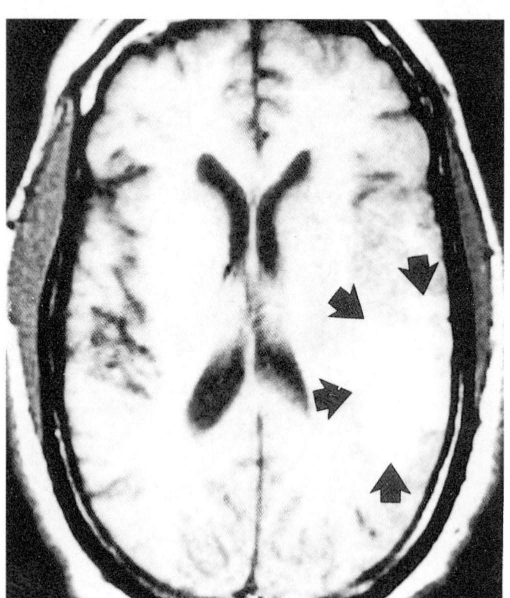

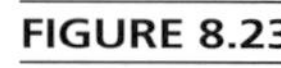

FIGURE 8.23

T1-weighted image reveals hemorrhage in the posterior temporal lobe (*arrows*) due to reperfusion into an area of infarction.

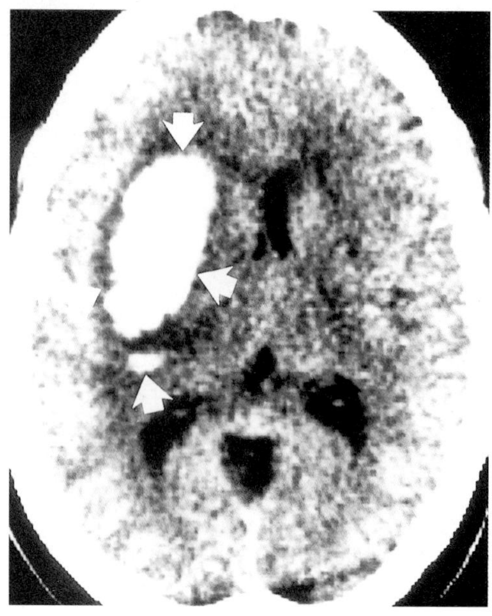

FIGURE 8.24

Computed tomography scan demonstrates typical hypertensive hemorrhage (*arrows*) into the basal ganglia.

rupture into an adjacent ventricle. Acute hemorrhage is best detected with CT. Acute blood appears bright white on noncontrast CT. Detectability of acute hemorrhage on MR images is variable. The MR characteristics of hemorrhage depend on the age of the hemorrhage, state of oxidation, and magnetic field strength [45] (Table 8.2). Acute hemorrhage (< 1 week) is iso- to hypointense on the T1-weighted images, and is iso- to markedly hypointense on the T2-weighted images [45,46]. The appearance is due to the presence of deoxygenated hemoglobin. Subacute hematomas (> 1 week) develop a hyperintense peripheral ring of bright signal on the T1- and T2-weighted images. This is due to lysis of erythrocytes and the presence of oxidized methemoglobin. The central aspect of the lesion eventually becomes bright as progressive lysis and oxidation affects the central components of the hematoma. Thus, the bright signal fills in the hematoma in the late subacute and chronic stage. In the chronic stage, phagocytes have ingested hemosiderin that causes local field inhomogeneities. This appears as a dark peripheral ring of hypointensity especially conspicuous on the T2-weighted images.

Venous Infarction

Cerebral infarction may be caused by occlusion of cerebral veins and dural sinuses and may result in intracerebral hemorrhage. Venous outflow obstruction causes venous congestion, which results in cerebral edema and eventual extravasation of erythrocytes into the parenchyma due to blood-brain barrier damage. Causes of venous thrombosis and occlusion include hypercoagulable states, pregnancy, sepsis, and tumor involvement of the venous sinus [46]. Features that differentiate venous from arterial infarction include bilaterality, lack of correspondence with a specific arterial territory, involvement of more than one vascular territory, and involvement of dural venous sinus [47]. CT or MR imaging may reveal acute clot in a venous sinus and underlying brain parenchyma (Figure 8.25) [48].

Computed tomography or MR images in patients with the acute onset of sustained elevated arterial blood pressure (hypertensive encephalopathy) may reveal findings of cerebral edema in the white matter of posterior parietal and occipital lobes bilaterally (Figure 8.26). The edematous changes usually resolve

Table 8.2. Appearance of intracranial hemorrhage on magnetic resonance images*

Stage	Biochemical type	Time of appearance	Appearance on T1WI (short) TR sequence	Appearance on T2W1 (long) TR sequence
Acute	Deoxyhemoglobin	Hours to several days	Hypointense (dark)	Hypointense
Subacute	Intracellular methemoglobin	Several days	Hyperintense (bright)	Hypointense
	Extracellular methemoglobin	Days to several weeks	Hyperintense	Hyperintense
Chronic	Hemosiderin	Several weeks to months	Hypointense	Very hypointense

*Signal intensities are relative to gray matter. TR—time to repetition; T1WI—T1-weighted; T2WI—T2-weighted.

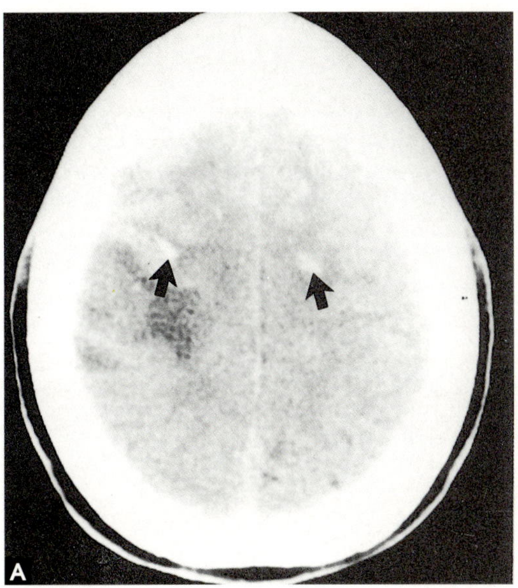

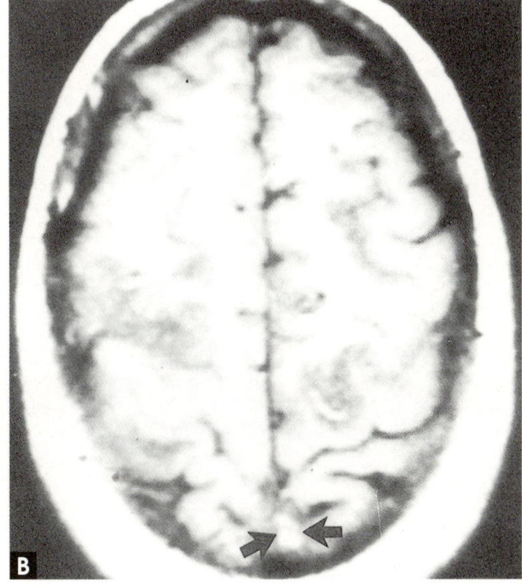

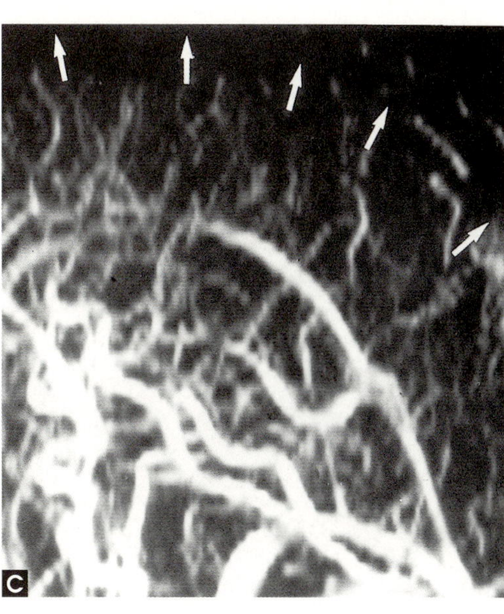

FIGURE 8.25

Superior sagittal sinus thrombosis and associated venous hemorrhage. **A**, Computed tomography scan reveals acute blood bilaterally (*arrows*). **B**, Magnetic resonance (MR) image demonstrates acute clot within the superior sagittal sinus (*arrows*). **C**, MR angiography documents no flowing blood (absence of white signal) in the superior sagittal sinus (*arrows*) consistent with occlusion.

following therapy (Figure 8.27). Other symptoms include severe headache, nausea, vomiting, and altered consciousness. Pathologic evaluation may reveal small petechial hemorrhages that may be undetected by CT and MR imaging.

Subarachnoid Hemorrhage

Subarachnoid hemorrhage is the usual initial clinical presentation of berry aneurysms. Most berry aneurysms occur at the origins of branching intracranial arteries of the Circle of Willis and are less than 1 cm in diameter. Noncontrast CT is the diagnostic radiologic procedure of choice in the initial work-up of subarachnoid hemorrhage [31]. High-density acute blood is identified in the subarachnoid cisterns on noncontrast CT following rupture of an aneurysm into the subarachnoid space (Figure 8.28). Contrast-infused CT may identify the aneurysm if it's larger than 5 mm in diameter. CT is superior to MR imaging in the detection of acute subarachnoid hemorrhage. Subarachnoid blood tends to be isointense to normal brain parenchyma, thus causing it to be inconspicuous in the acute stage of MR images. Subarachnoid hemorrhage develops MR hyperintensity about 1 week following an acute aneurysm rupture [31].

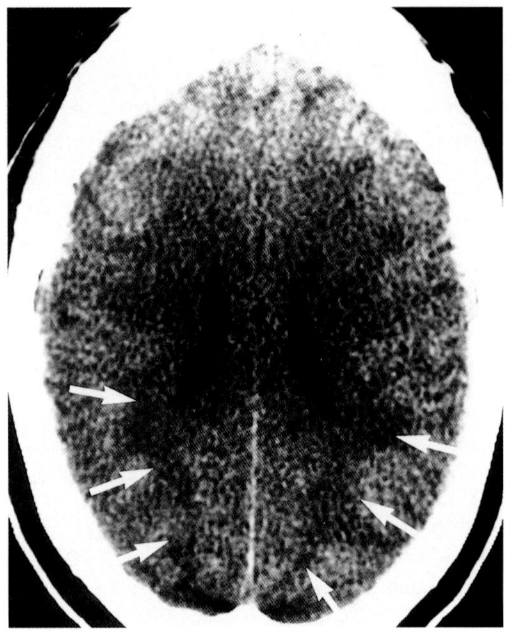

FIGURE 8.26

Computed tomography scan in acutely hypertensive young woman. Low-density changes are seen in the deep white matter of posterior parietal lobes bilateral (*arrows*).

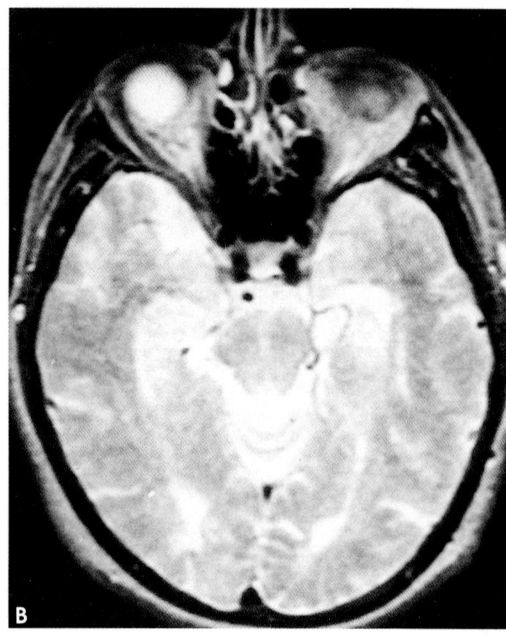

FIGURE 8.27

T2-weighted images on an acutely hypertensive patient before therapy (**A**) and several days after therapy (**B**). The previously identified region of abnormal signal (*arrows*) is no longer seen on the follow-up study.

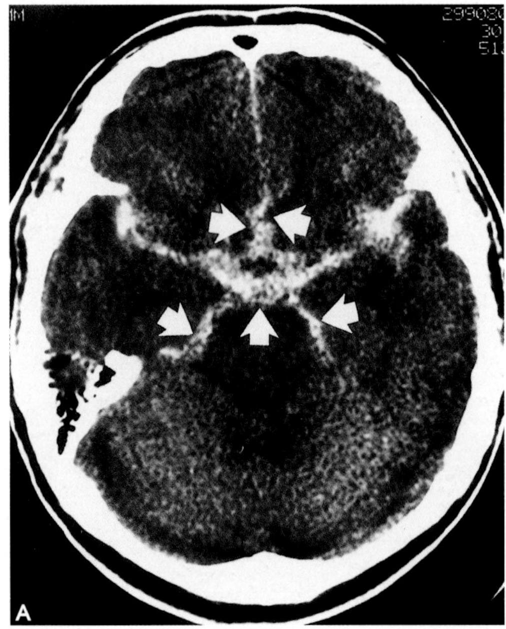

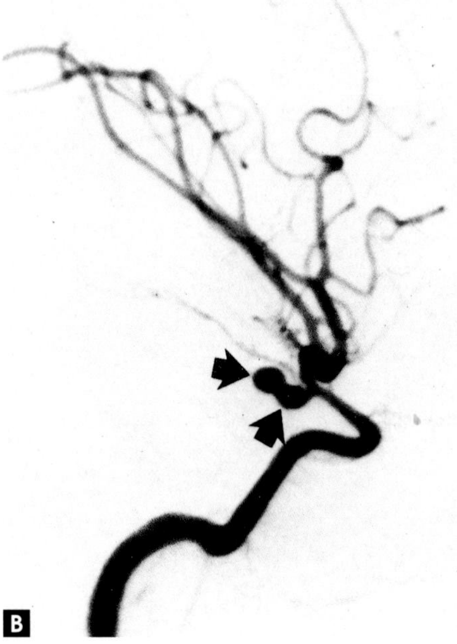

FIGURE 8.28

A, Acute subarachnoid blood fills the suprasellar cistern (*arrows*). **B**, Angiography identifies the posterior cerebral artery aneurysm (*arrows*) responsible for the subarachnoid hemorrhage.

REFERENCES

1. Garcia JH, Lossiasky AS, Kauffman FC, *et al.*: Neuronal ischemic injury: light microscopy, ultrastructure and biochemistry. *Acta Neuropathologica* 1978, 43:85–95.
2. terPenning B: Pathophysiology of stroke. In *Neuroimaging Clinics of North America.* Edited by Weingarten K, Zimmerman RD. Philadelphia: WB Saunders and Co.; 1992:389–408.
3. Hayman LA, Berman SA, Hinck VC: Correlation of CT cerebral vascular territories with function: II. Posterior cerebral artery. *AJNR* 1981, 2:219–225.
4. Berman SA, Hayman LA, Hinck VC: Cerebrovascular territories. In *Clinical Brain Imaging.* Edited by Hayman LA, Hinck VC. St. Louis: Mosby-Year Book, Inc.; 1992:402–416.
5. Berman SA, Hayman LA, Hinck VC: Correlation of CT cerebral vascular territories with function. In *Anterior Cerebral Artery. Am J Roentgenol* 1980, 135:253–257.
6. Bryan RN, Whitlow WD, Levy LM: Cerebral infarction and ischemic disease. In *Magnetic Resonance Imaging of the Brain and Spine.* Edited by Atlas SW. New York: Raven Press; 1991:411–437.
7. Monajati A, Heggeness L: Patterns of edema in tumor vs. infarcts: visualization of white matter pathways. *AJNR* 1982, 3:251–255.
8. Weingarten K: Computed tomography of cerebral infarction. In *Neuroimaging Clinics of North America.* Edited by Weingarten K, Zimmerman RD. Philadelphia: WB Saunders and Co.; 1992:409–419.
9. Djang WT, Gray L, Drayer B: Intracranial occlusive vascular disease. In *Radiology.* Edited by Taveras JM, Ferrucci JT. Philadelphia: J.B. Lippincott Co.; 1991:1–23.
10. Ladurner G, Sager WD, Iliff LD, *et al.*: A correlation of clinical findings and CT in ischemia cerebrovascular disease. *Eur J Neurol* 1979, 18:281.
11. Perrone P, Candelise L, Scotti G: CT evaluation in patients with transient ischemic attack: correlation between clinical and angiographic findings. *Eur J Neurol* 1979, 18:217.
12. Goldberg HI: Stroke. In *Cranial Computed Tomography and MRI.* Edited by Lee SH, Raok C. New York: McGraw-Hill Book Co.; 1987:643–716.
13. Inoue Y, Takemoto K, Miyamoto T, *et al.*: Sequential computed tomography scans in acute cerebral infarction. *Radiology* 1980, 135:655–662.
14. Wall SD, Zawadzki MB, Jeffrey RB, *et al.*: High frequency CT findings within 24 hours after cerebral infarction. *AJNR* 1981, 2:553–557.
15. Alcala H, Gado M, Torack RM: The effect of size, histologic elements, and water content on the visualization of cerebral infarcts. *Arch Neurol* 1978, 35:1–7.
16. Houser OW, Campbell JK, Baker HL, *et al.*: Radiologic evaluation of ischemic cerebrovascular syndromes with emphasis on computed tomography. *Radiol Clin North Am* 1982, 20:123–142.
17. Masdeu JC, Berhooz A-K, Rubina FA: Evaluation of recent cerebral infarction by computerized tomography. *Arch Neurol* 1977, 34:417–424.
18. Yock DH, Marshall WH: Recent ischemic brain infarcts at computed tomography: appearance pre and post contrast infusion. *Radiology* 1975, 117:599–600.
19. Millikan CH, McDowell F, Easton JD: General pathology and neuropathology of stroke. In *Stroke.* Edited by Millkan CH, McDowell F, Easton JD. Philadelphia: Lea and Febiger; 1987:33–44.
20. Pullicino P, Kendall BE: Contrast enhancement in ischemic lesions. *J Neuroradiol* 1980, 19:235–239.
21. Crain MR, Yuh WT, Greene GM: Cerebral ischemia: evaluation with contrast-enhanced MR imaging. *AJNR* 1991, 12:631–639.
22. Weisberg LA: Computerized tomographic enhancement patterns in cerebral infarction. *Arch Neurol* 1980, 37:21–24.
23. Gado MH, Phelps ME, Coleman RE: An extravascular component of contrast enhancement in cranial computed tomography. *Radiology* 1975, 117:595–597.
24. Bryan RN, Levy LM, Whitlow WD, *et al.*: Diagnosis of acute cerebral infarction: comparison of CT and MR imaging. *AJNR* 1991, 12:611–620.
25. Brant-Zawadski M, Pereira B, Weinstein P, *et al.*: MRI of acute experimental ischemia in rats. *AJNR* 1986, 7:7–11.
26. Yuh WT, Crain MR: Reply: acute cerebral ischemia: CT and MR findings [letter]. *AJNR* 1992, 13:829–830.
27. Yuh WT, Crain MR: Magnetic resonance imaging of acute cerebral ischemia. In *Neuroimaging Clinics of North America.* Edited by Weingarten K, Zimmerman RD. Philadelphia: WB Saunders and Co.; 1992:421–439.
28. Yuh WT, Crain MR, Loes DJ: MR imaging of cerebral ischemia: findings in the first 24 hours. *AJNR* 1991, 12:621–629.
29. Elster AD, Moody DM: Early cerebral infarction. gadopentetate dimeglumine enhancement. *Radiology* 1990, 177:627–632.
30. Sato A, Takahashis S, Soma Y, *et al.*: Cerebral infarction: early detection by means of contrast-enhanced cerebral arteries CT MR imaging. *Radiology* 1991, 178:433–439.
31. Grossman CB: Cerebrovascular disorders. In *Magnetic Resonance Imaging and Computed Tomography of the Head and Spine.* Edited by Grossman CB. Baltimore: Williams and Wilkins; 1990:145–183.
32. Kirkpatrick JB, Haymon LA: White matter lesions in MR imaging of clinically healthy brains of elderly subjects: possible pathological basis. *Radiology* 1987, 162:509–511.
33. Kinkel WR, Jacobs L, Polachini I, *et al.*: Subaortical arteriosclerotic encephalopathy (Binswanger's disease) computed tomographic, nuclear magnetic resonance, and clinical correlations. *Arch Neurol* 1985, 42:951–959.
34. Lotz PR, Ballinger WE, Quisling RG: Subcortical arteriosclerotic encephalopathy: CT spectrum and pathological correlation. *AJNR* 1986, 7:817–822.
35. Tomura N, Nemura K, Inngram A, *et al.*: Early CT finding in cerebral infarction: obscuration of the lentiform nucleus. *Radiology* 1988, 168:463–467.
36. Skriver EB, Olsen TS: Transient disappearance of cerebral infarctions on CT scan, the so-called fogging effect. *Neuroradiology* 1981, 22:61–65.
37. Becker H, Desch H, Hacker H, *et al.*: CT fogging effect with ischemic cerebral infarcts. *J Neuroradiol* 1979, 18:185–192.
38. Truwit CL, Barkovich AJ, Gean-Martin A, *et al.*: Loss of the insular ribbon: another early CT sign of acute middle cerebral artery infarction. *Radiology* 1990, 176:801–806.
39. Tomsick TA, Brott TG, Chambers AA, *et al.*: Hyperdense middle cerebral artery sign on CT. *AJNR* 1990, 11:473–477.
40. Schuknecht B, Ratzkam, Hoffman E: The "dense artery sign" - major cerebral artery thromboembolism demonstrated by computed tomography. *J Neuroradiol* 1990, 32:98–103.
41. Bastianello S, Pierallini A, Colonnese C, *et al.*: Hyperdense middle cerebral artery CT sign. *Neuroradiology* 1991, 33:207–211.
42. Gacs G, Fox AJ, Barnett HJ, *et al.*: CT visualization of intracranial arterial thromboembolism. *Stroke* 1983, 14:756–762.
43. Pressman BD, Tourje EJ, Thompson JR: An early CT sign of ischemic infarction: increased density in a cerebral artery. *AJNR* 1987, 8:645–648.
44. Kuhn MJ, Johnson KA, Davis KR: Wallerian degeneration: evaluation with MR imaging, *Radiology* 1988, 168:199–202.
45. Seidenwurm D, Meng TK, Kowalski H, *et al.*: Intracranial hemorrhagic lesions: evaluation with spin-echo and gradients refocused MR imaging at 0.5 and 1.5 T. *Radiology* 1989, 172:189–194.
46. Gomori JM, Grossman RI, Goldberg HI: Intracranial hematomas: imaging by high field MR. *Radiology* 1985, 157:87–93.
47. Zawadzki MB, Kucharczyk W: Vascular disease: ischemia. In *Magnetic Resonance Imaging of the Central Nervous System.* Edited by Brant-Zawadzki M, Norman O. New York: Raven Press; 1987:221–234.
48. Secrist RD, Traynelis V, Schochett S: MR imaging of acute cortical venous infarction: preliminary experience with an animal model. *Magnetic Reson Imag* 1989, 7:149–153.

Chapter 9

Diagnosing Cerebrovascular Disease Using Magnetic Resonance Angiography and Conventional Cerebral Angiography

ANN MARIE RITTER
L. ANNE HAYMAN
DALE CHARLETTA

Conventional cerebral angiography (CCA) has traditionally been the standard diagnostic modality for the evaluation of cerebrovascular ischemic disease. However, it is expensive and not without complications. Therefore, less invasive methods for examination of the cerebral vessels have been investigated. Magnetic resonance angiography (MRA) has recently become a powerful tool in the assessment of intra- and extracranial vascular lesions. This chapter summarizes the usefulness and limitations of CCA and MRA. Digital subtraction angiography (DSA) is discussed briefly as a subset of CCA. The first section of this chapter describes the techniques used in CCA and MRA. The next describes the general clinical applications for each, and the third outlines their use in specific clinical situations.

TECHNICAL CONSIDERATIONS

Conventional Angiography

The cerebral vessels are identified by CCA when contrast medium is injected into the cerebral or vertebral arteries via a fluoroscopically placed catheter. Sequential standard radiographic images demonstrate the flow of contrast through the vessels [1,2]. CCA may be supplemented by DSA. In this method, the image is digitized and stored in a computer. The precontrast bony image is used to subtract the soft tissue detail from all subsequent postcontrast images. The resultant "subtracted" DSA image displays only the contrast within the vessels [2,3]. Compared with CCA, DSA uses less contrast medium, and is quicker and less expensive [4]. These are distinct advantages for patients with symptoms caused by vascular disease.

Magnetic Resonance Angiography

The goals of MRA are to noninvasively detect the intensity of flowing protons in blood and to maximally suppress the background stationary protons. This is currently achieved by two methods: time-of-flight (TOF) and phase-contrast (PC) imaging.

In a TOF acquisition, radiofrequency pulses are applied repeatedly to a preselected volume (slab) of the head or neck. This "saturates" the signal from the stationary tissues, causing them to appear *hypo*intense on MRA. When the "unsaturated" flowing blood enters this slab, it absorbs the pulse and generates an intense signal, causing it to appear *hyper*intense on MRA. This is termed *flow-related enhancement* (Figure 9.1) [5–7]. Addition of a moving saturation band can eliminate arterial or venous vessels from the TOF images (Figure 9.2). However, techniques that elimi-

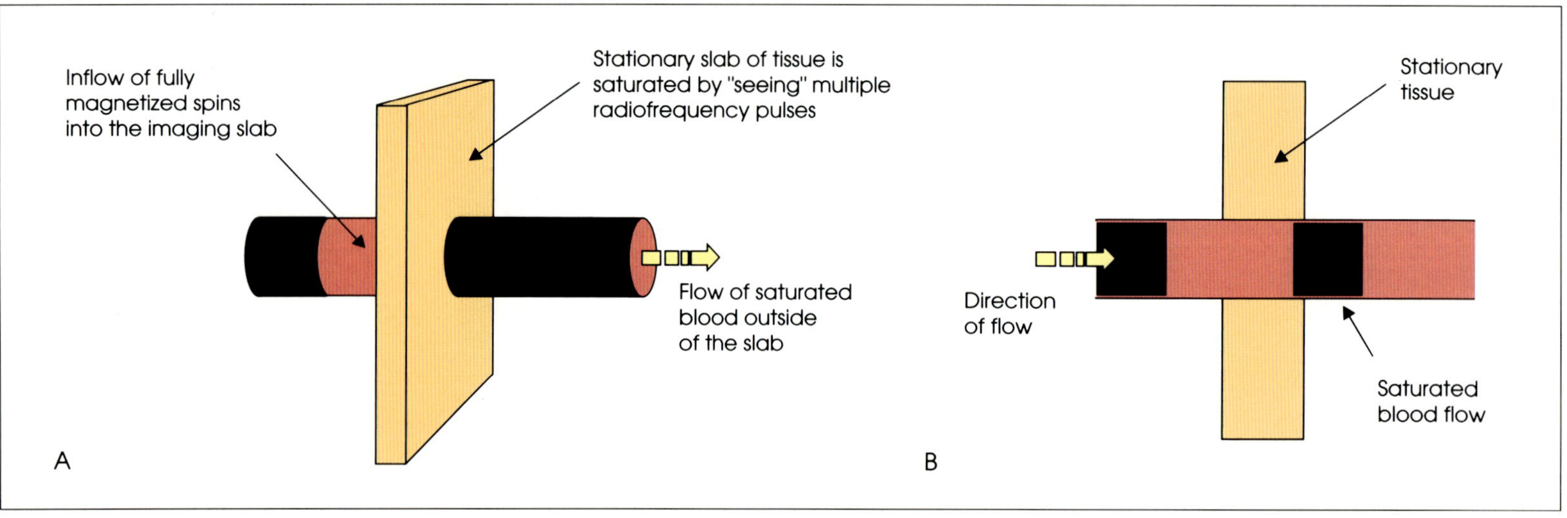

FIGURE 9.1

The "flow enhancement phenomenon" used to generate time-of-flight magnetic resonance angiography. The inflow of blood into the slab of tissue (*light areas*) introduces unsaturated protons that have a hyperintense signal compared with the saturated protons of stationary tissue and blood (*dark areas*) that exit the slab. (*From* Turski [25]; with permission.)

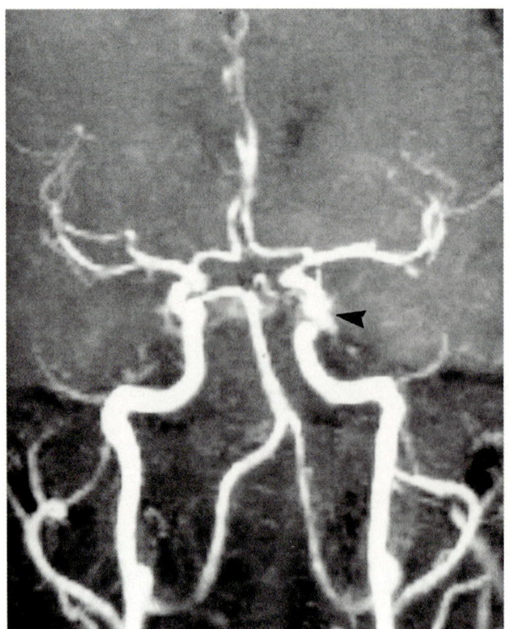

FIGURE 9.2

Two-dimensional time-of-flight magnetic resonance angiography of the normal extracranial and intracranial vasculature. A saturation pulse at the top of the head renders venous flow invisible. Note an area of interrupted signal at a site of turbulent flow (*arrowhead*).

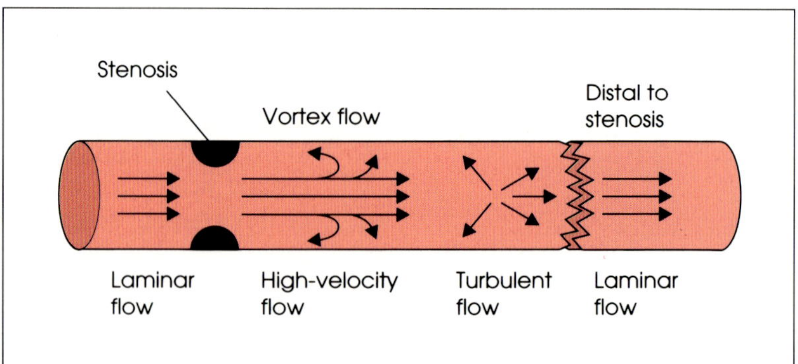

FIGURE 9.3

Laminar vascular flow distortions at sites of narrowing. Note that laminar blood flow exists prior to a stenotic site. Past this point, patterns of complex flow are produced. Turbulence is the chaotic flow of blood distal to a narrowing, caused by the increased velocity that occurs when the blood travels through the narrower lumen. Proton dephasing in these distal areas of complex flow leads to overestimation of the degree of stenosis in the narrowed region on phase-contrast magnetic resonance angiography. (*From* Turski [25]; with permission.)

nate the veins will eliminate retrograde flow in the vertebral artery, which has clinical significance in cases of subclavian steal. The TOF technique is degraded by air-bone artifacts caused by susceptibility gradients.

The second type of MRA is PC angiography. PC angiography is visually more attractive because there is better background noise suppression than on TOF MRA. The images are based on the position of the proton's intrinsic angular motion. Two gradient pulses of equal but opposite polarity are applied to a tissue volume. Stationary protons are unstimulated by these gradient pulses. Flowing protons that move into the gradient plane exhibit phase shifts. The laminar blood flow that occurs in normal vessels is composed of protons in similar phases. These protons react to the magnetic field with equal but opposite polarity, resulting in a net zero phase shift, which generates a strongly hyperintense signal on PC MRA. Vascular stenosis, tortuosity, or ulceration creates protons that are not at the same phase. This results in a net non-zero (uneven) phase shift that diminishes the signal creating a hypointense zone on PC MRA (Figures 9.3 and 9.4) [5–8]. A unique aspect of PC MRA is its sensitivity to flow velocities. Gradient pulses may be selected to show areas of slow or fast flow (Figure 9.5). PC MRA also provides information on direction of flow, and cine-phase MRA evaluates quantitation flow with the cardiac cycle [9,10].

Time-of-flight and PC MRA can be imaged as two- or three-dimensional blocks, called *slabs* or *source images*. The thinner

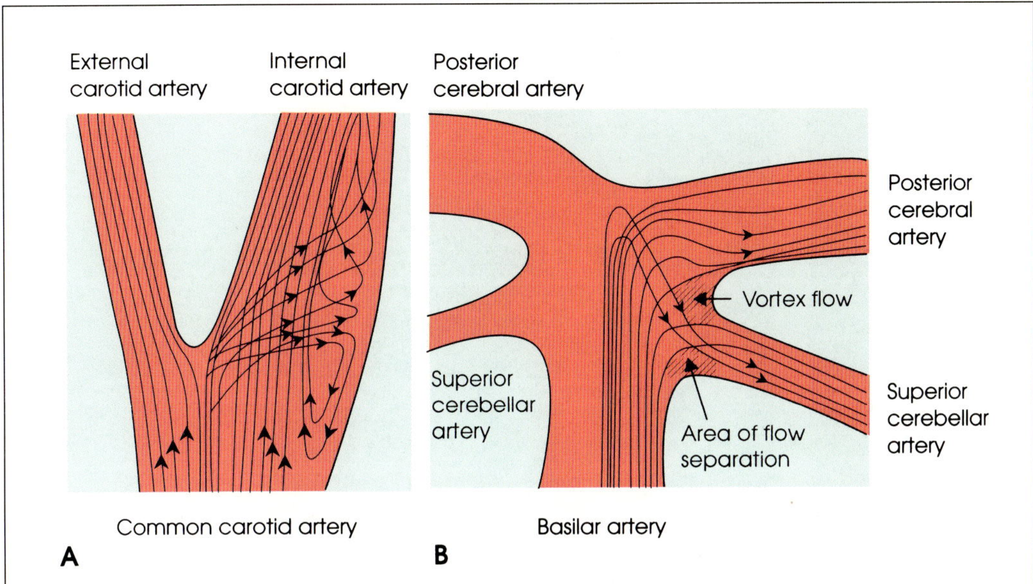

FIGURE 9.4

Laminar flow distortions at sites of vessel bifurcation (**A**) and branching (**B**). Vortex flow is the slow swirling motion of blood in a dilated vessel distal to a stenosis or at a bifurcation. It is demonstrated at sharp angles of vessel division. Proton dephasing in these areas leads to erroneous loss of signal on phase-contrast magnetic resonance angiography. (*From* Turski [25]; with permission.)

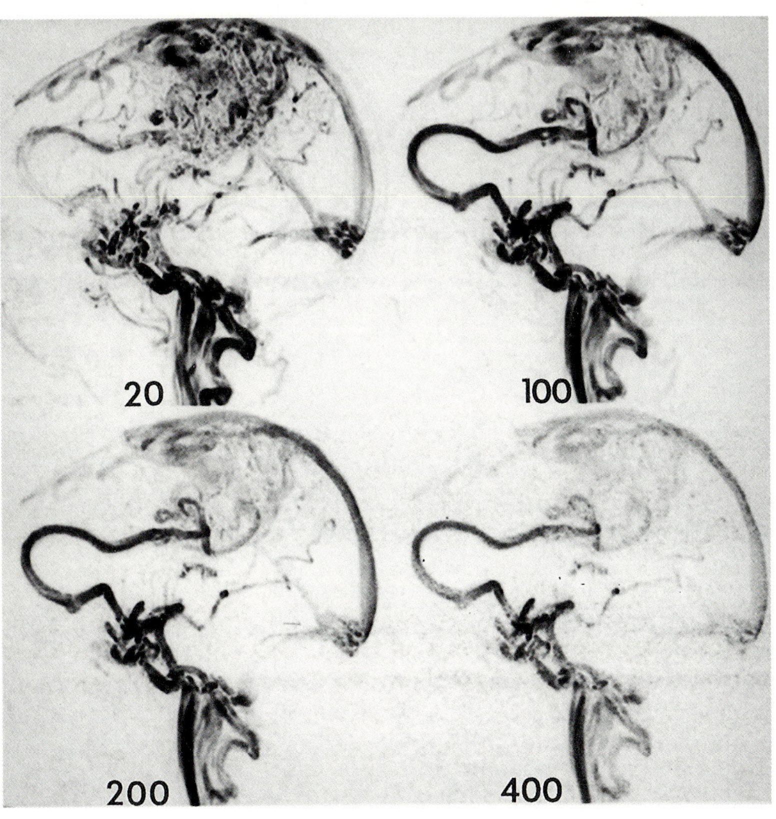

FIGURE 9.5

Multiple two-dimensional phase-contrast magnetic resonance angiographic images with increasing velocity encodings of 20, 100, 200, and 400 cm/s offer a rapid method to evaluate velocity information in a right frontoparietal arteriovenous malformation. The nidus and arterialized flow in the veins draining this huge malformation are best seen on the 20 cm/s image. Increasing the velocity encoding increases visualization of the arteries and diminishes the visualization of the nidus and venous drainage. (*From* Huston and Ehman [9]; with permission.)

sections of the three-dimensional technique make it better suited for imaging small intracranial vessels and the thicker two-dimensional slices appear satisfactory for imaging the neck vessels [5,6]. Slabs of two- or three-dimensional information are processed by the "maximal intensity pixel" (MIP) projection computer algorithm, which automatically locates the brightest signals and connects them together to form the MRA image. The resultant radiographic picture is similar to the projections used for CCA (Figure 9.2) [5–7]. Software is available to rotate these images in space, thus allowing the physician to untangle overlapped vascular images (Figure 9.6) [11]. Information can be lost when the MR arteriogram is constructed. The "source," or raw, MR images are needed to correctly assess vessel caliber, which may appear artifactually narrowed on the MRA reconstruction. The use of intravenous gadolinium contrast medium improves the visualization of vascular components using either PC or TOF techniques (Figure 9.7).

CLINICAL APPLICATIONS AND LIMITATIONS

Conventional Angiography

Conventional cerebral angiography is still the gold standard for diagnosing and delineating most cerebrovascular pathology because it accurately evaluates the extra- and intracranial vessels. It is the only study available for patients with ferromagnetic implants or foreign bodies, and is the only technique that measures arteriovenous circulation time and arterial stump pressures (Figure 9.8).

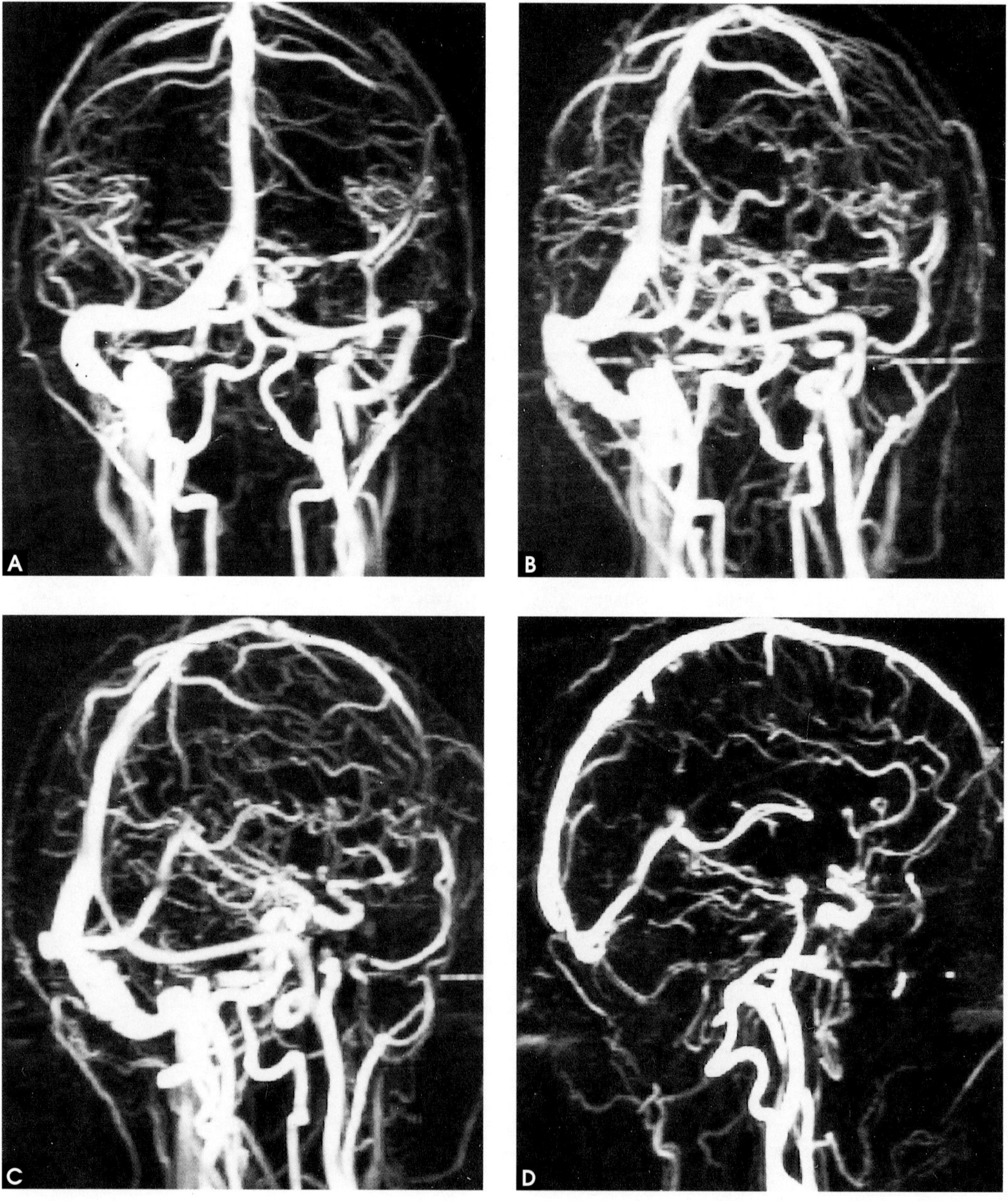

FIGURE 9.6

Three-dimensional data rotated at 0° (**A**), 30° (**B**), 60° (**C**), and in the sagittal plane (**D**) by the maximum intensity algorithm. As the images rotate, the deeper arterial and venous structures can be visualized. *Arrows* and *arrowheads* indicate signal loss as the vertebral arteries pass through bony structures. (*From* Pernicone and coworkers [11]; with permission.)

The limitations of CCA relate to its invasiveness and the use of contrast material. There is a 1% risk of permanent neurologic sequelae and a less than 0.1% risk of death from CCA [12]. In approximately 4% of patients, a puncture site hematoma, arterial dissection, hypotension, nausea, vomiting, urticara, or cardiac arrhythmias may occur [13,14]. The risk of CCA complications is greater if the patient has frequent transient ischemic attacks, diabetes, renal failure, a history of cerebrovascular disease, or is dehydrated [12–15].

The complications of arterial DSA are generally inconsequential. There was a 0.45% incidence of transient neurologic deficit, a 0.09% incidence of permanent deficits, and no deaths in a recent study of 1095 patients. The overall complication rate was 0.9%, which included local hematoma and urticara [16]. Compared with CCA, the only disadvantage is the limited spatial resolution of vascular structures; arterial DSA cannot accurately image vessels less than 1 mm in diameter [17,18]. This is clinically significant because the difference between a 75% stenosis and a 60% stenosis of a 5-mm carotid artery is less than 1 mm. Arterial DSA may not accurately separate these *clinically* significant degrees of stenosis [18].

Although the risks of CCA and DSA are minimal in a given patient, they become significant because large numbers of patients who do not ultimately require surgical intervention are studied. In one survey, although 78% of CCA patients did not require vascular surgery, they were still subjected to the risk of conventional arteriography [19].

Magnetic Resonance Angiography

Magnetic resonance angiography is used in the evaluation of cerebrovascular disease in patients *without* acute intracranial hemorrhage. A concurrent MR imaging study can add valuable information concerning ischemia, infarct, hemorrhage, gliosis, and encephalomalacia [20,21]. Table 9.1 lists the types of MRA

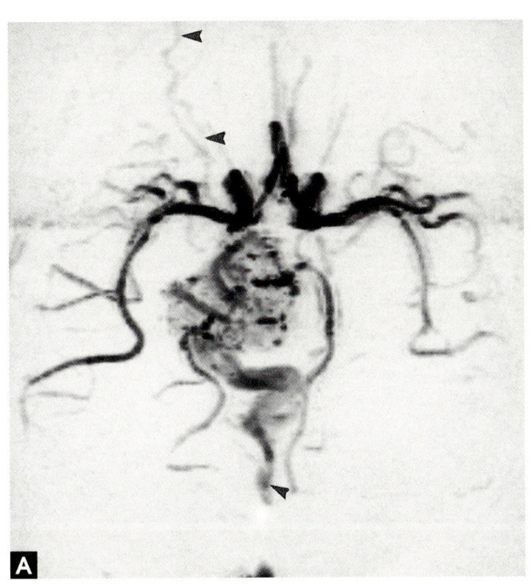

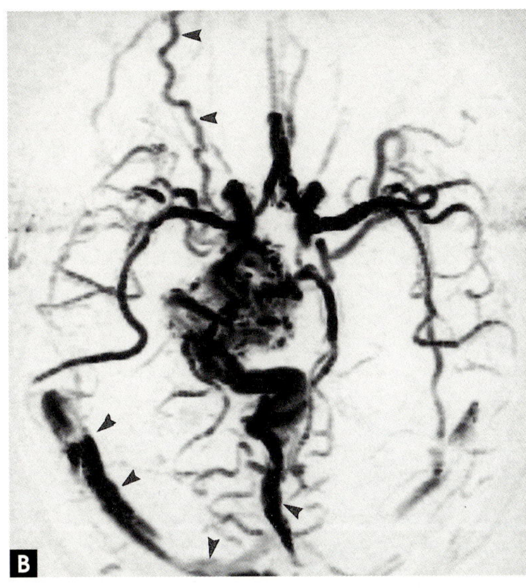

FIGURE 9.7

Axial three-dimensional phase-contrast magnetic resonance angiographic images of thalamic arteriovenous malformations before (**A**) and after (**B**) administration of contrast material show that gadopentetate dimeglumine increases the visualization of vascular structures. Note draining veins (*arrowheads*) on both images. (*From* Huston and Ehman [9]; with permission.)

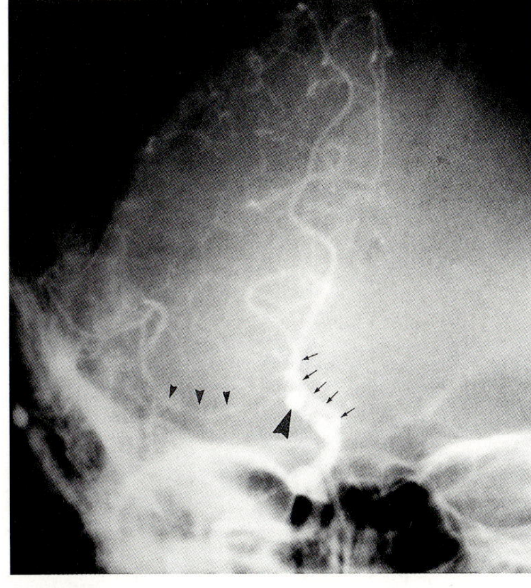

FIGURE 9.8

Conventional cerebral angiography (frontal view) in a patient with numerous shotgun pellets to the head and neck. Note a pellet (*large arrowhead*) lodged in the right internal carotid artery, which prevents filling of the middle and anterior cerebral arteries. The fetal posterior cerebral artery (*arrows*) and retrograde filling of the middle cerebral artery (*small arrowheads*) are visualized.

Table 9.1. Preferred magnetic resonance angiography technique for specific causes of ischemic cerebrovascular disease

MRA technique	Cerebrovenous thrombosis	Extracranial occlusive vascular disease	Intracranial occlusive vascular disease	Collateral blood flow	Cerebral aneurysm	Arteriovenous malformations
Two-dimensional TOF	X	X*				X (venous phase)
Three-dimensional TOF		X	X		X	X (arterial phase)
Three-dimensional PC			X	X	X*	X*
Two-dimensional PC			X	X	X	

*Velocity encoding can differentiate the arterial from the venous anatomy.
PC—phase-contrast; TOF—time-of-flight.

used to image specific cranial vascular lesions and Table 9.2 describes its benefits and limitations. The major limitations included erroneous signal loss and MIP processing losses; however, refinements in acquiring and processing MRA data that may eliminate these drawbacks in the future are being investigated [22].

Figures 9.3 and 9.4 depict the signal loss at areas of complex flow and proton dephasing. These occur at vessel bifurcations, tortuosities, and distal to stenoses (Figure 9.9), and can lead to dampening or loss of the MRA signal and erroneous appearance of stenosis or increased length of the stenosis. These are also

Table 9.2. Advantages and disadvantages of various imaging techniques for magnetic resonance angiography*

Technique	Advantages	Disadvantages
Two-dimensional TOF	Sensitivity to slow flow; relatively short scan times; lack of saturation effects; multiple projections, including subvolumes	Thrombus or other short T_1 substance may simulate flow; patient motion artifact; insensitivity to in-plane flow; relatively long echo time
Three-dimensional TOF	Short scan times; high spatial resolution; very short echo times; reprojection and subvolume images possible	Thrombus or other short T_1 substance may simulate flow; insensitivity to slow flow; saturation effects; field distortion artifacts such as air-bone susceptibility gradients
Two-dimensional PC	Short acquisition time; variable velocity encoding, allowing imaging of slow or fast flow; directional flow images; excellent background suppression	No reprojection images; large voxel size; relatively long echo times
Three-dimensional PC	Variable velocity encoding, allowing imaging of slow or fast flow; excellent background suppression; minimized saturation effects; small voxel size; directional flow information; reprojection and subvolume images possible	Long acquisition time; relatively long echo times
Cine-phase contrast	Variable velocity encoding, allowing imaging of cerebrospinal fluid, venous, or arterial flow; quantitative flow measurement; time-resolved information; hemodynamic flow information	Loss of signal intensity with overlapping vessels; large voxel size

**From* Huston and Ehman [9]; with permission.
PC—phase-contrast; TOF—time-of-flight.

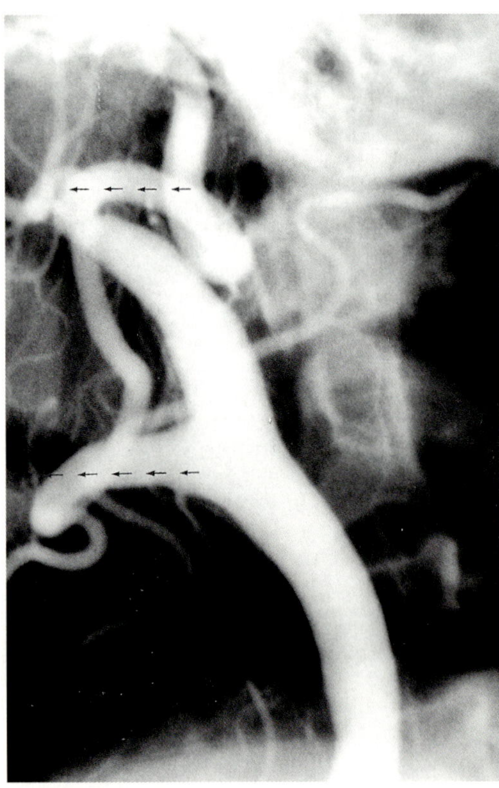
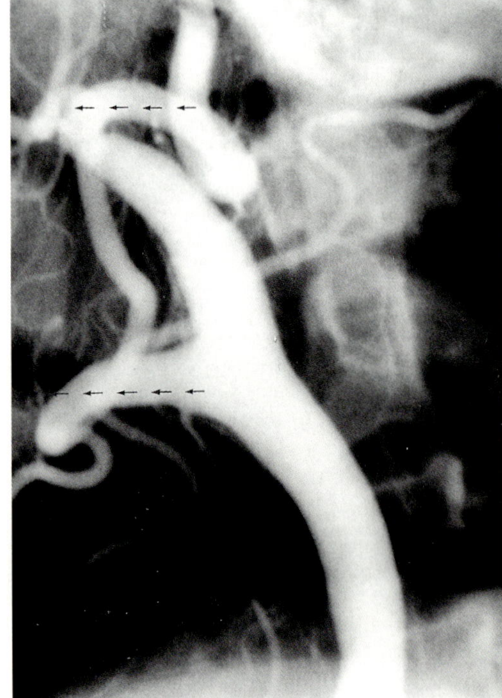
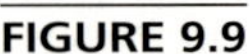

FIGURE 9.9

Conventional cerebral angiogram showing an extremely tortuous internal and external carotid artery. The horizontal flow within the slab will not be visualized on time-of-flight (TOF) magnetic resonance angiography (MRA) and the segments (*arrows*) will be absent on the TOF image. They would be seen if phase-contrast MRA was used.

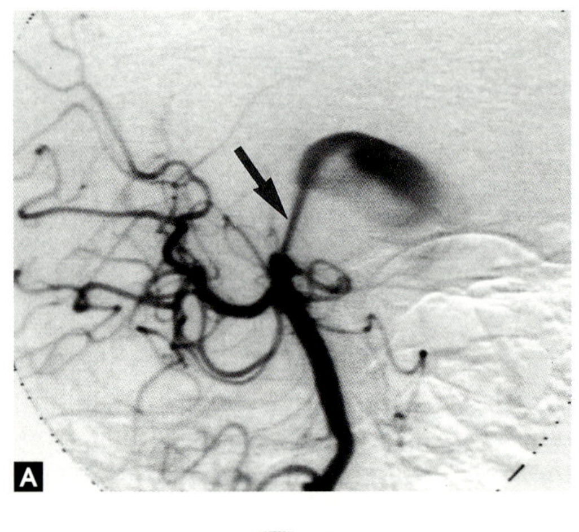

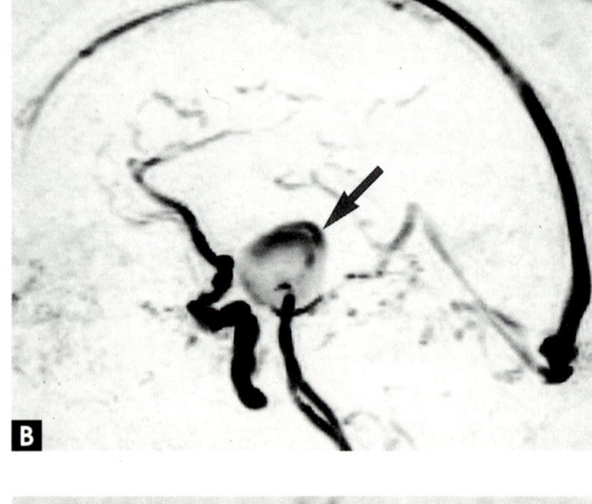

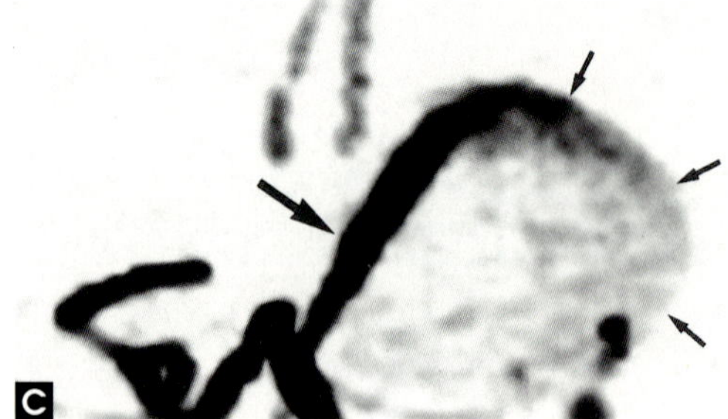
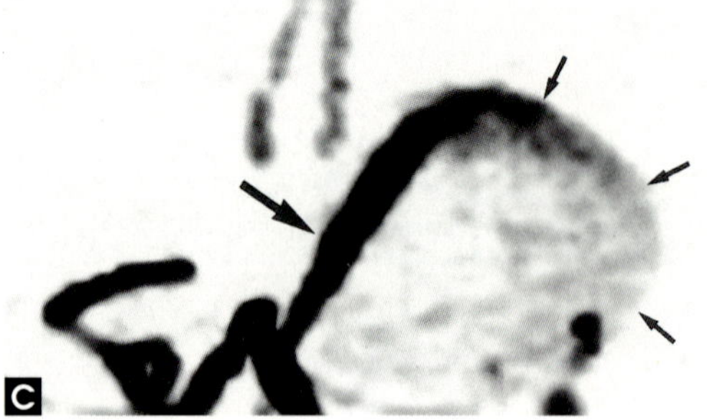
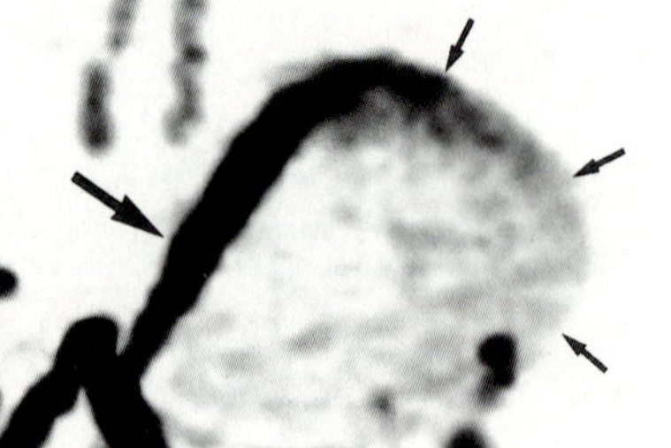

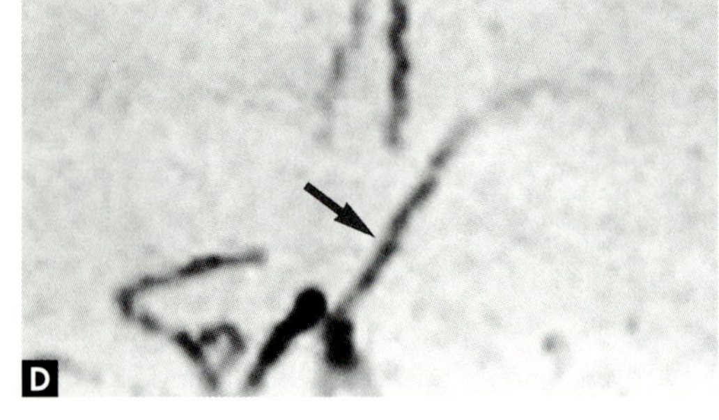

FIGURE 9.10

A, Digital subtraction angiography of a large aneurysm of the left posterior cerebral artery. The flow jet is depicted (*arrow*) and the dome is visualized. **B,** Two-dimensional phase-contrast (PC) image obtained with 30 cm/s velocity encoding depicts only the aneurysm dome (*arrow*). **C,** Three-dimensional PC image illustrates the flow jet (*long arrow*) and the aneurysm dome (*small arrows*). **D,** Three-dimensional time-of-flight image demonstrates the flow jet (*arrow*), but because of slow blood flow saturating the large aneurysm, the dome is not visualized (*From* Huston and Ehman [9]; with permission.)

precise areas of atheroma formation, which can lead to a diagnostic dilemma [5–8]. Signal loss may also occur if the blood remains in the pulsed field, becoming saturated and exhibiting diminished or absent flow [5–7, 23–25] (Figure 9.10).

Magnetic resonance angiography is also hindered by a problem inherent in the MIP algorithm. The computer program is not yet sensitive enough to distinguish the slight difference between the signal of stationary tissue and small vessels, or the difference between the hyperintense signal of subacute thrombus and blood flow (Figure 9.11) [5–7,23–25]. In addition, if a vessel is outside the excited slab, it will not be visualized on the MIP image.

Table 9.3 lists other factors that preclude the use of MRA to evaluate cerebrovascular disease [26]. Of particular concern is the patient with ferromagnetic implants, such as intracranial clips, hemostatic clips, and ferromagnetic foreign bodies. The hazards associated with these products are related to their deflection in the magnetic field, which causes disruption of vascular structures and neural tissues. Research has demonstrated that they do not produce heat or electrical current [26]. Table 9.4 lists common intracranial devices and their deflection in the magnetic field, as well as their propensity to distort the final image [27–29]. Table 9.5 describes similar data for ballistic objects [27,30]. Figures 9.12 and 9.13 depict these distortions.

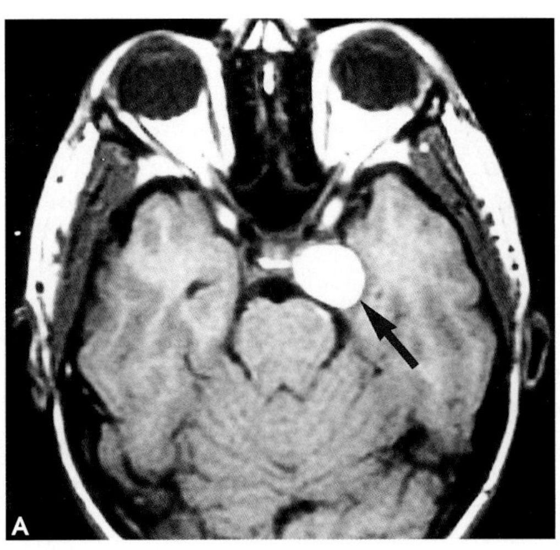

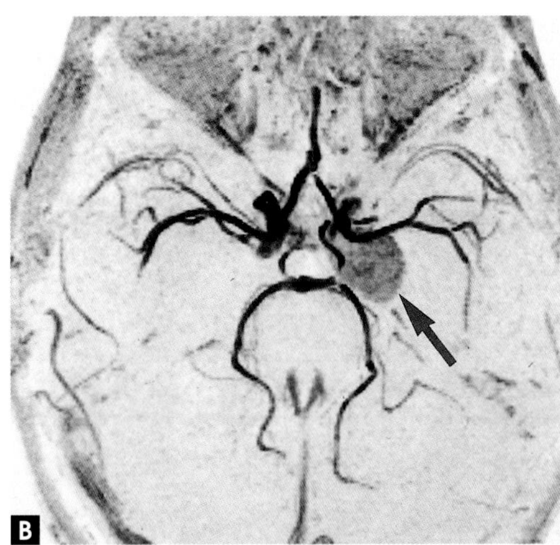

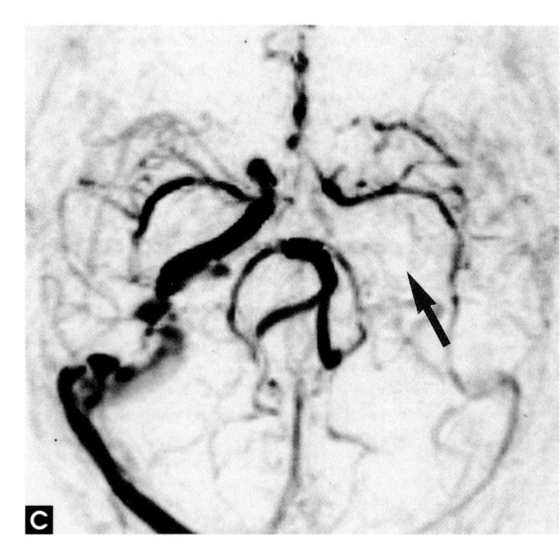

FIGURE 9.11

A 14-year-old boy underwent balloon occlusion of the left carotid artery to thrombose a cavernous sinus aneurysm. **A,** T1-weighted magnetic resonance image demonstrates a high-intensity thrombosis (*arrow*) in the cavernous sinus. **B,** Three-dimensional time-of-flight (TOF) image shows the aneurysm with what appears to be flow (*arrow*). **C,** Two-dimensional phase-contrast (PC) image, which is more sensitive to actual flow, shows no flow within the aneurysm (*arrow*). Notice the air-bone and soft tissue artifact in the TOF image (**B**) compared with the excellent background suppression in the PC image (**C**). (*From* Huston and Ehman [9]; with permission.)

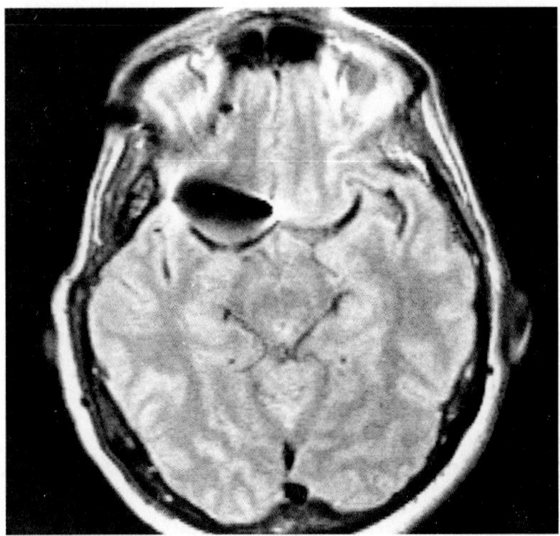

FIGURE 9.12

Mild artifact at the level of the clip in a 58-year-old woman who had a 2.5-cm aneurysm of the right internal carotid artery near the right ophthalmic artery clipped using a Yasargil 316LVM aneurysm clip. Higher level axial cut demonstrated no artifact. No deflection was noted when the clip was pretested in the magnet. (*From* Becker and coworkers [29]; with permission.)

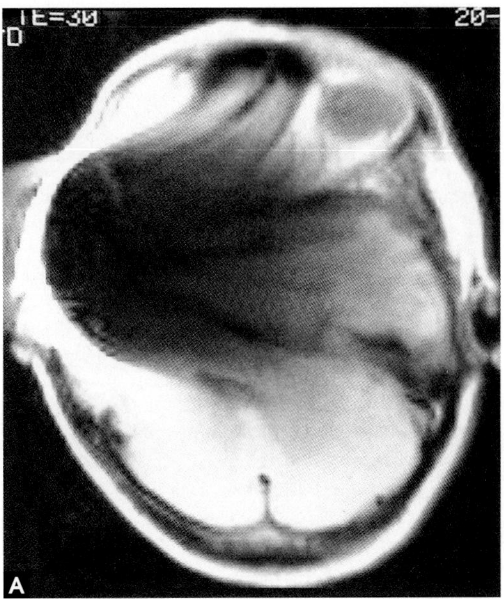

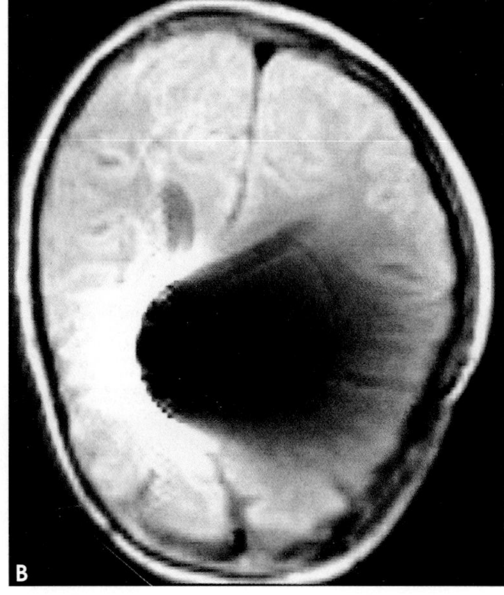

FIGURE 9.13

A 74-year-old woman had a right internal carotid aneurysm clipped with a Heifetz 17-7PH clip. **A,** Extensive artifact at the level of the clip, which persisted at a higher axial cut (**B**). No deflection was observed when pretesting the clip in the magnetic field. (*From* Becker and coworkers [29]; with permission.)

CLINICAL SITUATIONS

Intracranial Venous and Dural Sinus Occlusive Disease

The venous sinuses are formed between the dura mater and internal table of the cranial vault. Smaller cerebral veins drain into these sinuses, which empty into the internal jugular veins. The channels most commonly affected by thrombosis are the superior sagittal sinus (75%), the lateral sinus (72%), and the cavernous sinus (2.7%). Most occlusions involve more than one sinus [31,32].

In the past, the venous phase of CCA was the investigative modality of choice to define venous occlusions. CCA findings consistent with thrombosis include complete loss or partial filling of venous channels and retrograde blood flow through these vessels. Indirect signs include an increase in collateral circulation, a delay in the arterial to venous circulation time, an abnormal drainage pattern, tortuous dilated veins, and a prolonged brain blush [32,33]. Cortical vein thrombosis is difficult to discern unless a visualized vein ends abruptly [31]. Flow defects on angiography must be differentiated from an inadequate injection of contrast, a decrease in cerebral perfusion pressure, or arterial occlusion [32,33]. Such defects may also be due to the high variability in normal dural sinus anatomy [34].

Recently, two-dimensional TOF MRA has been advocated as the gold standard for diagnosing intracranial venous and dural thrombosis (Figure 9.14) [35–37]. The reduction or absence of flow within the venous channels is consistent with thrombosis [35–39]. Normal venous channels may appear thrombosed secondary to saturation effects of diminished cerebral flow. Methemoglobin in a subacute clot may erroneously mimic blood flow. Current MRA techniques do not adequately define small cortical vessel thrombosis [35].

Extracranial Occlusive Cerebrovascular Disease

The most prevalent cause of ischemic stroke is atherosclerosis of the carotid arteries [40,41]. Thirty-four percent of patients have involvement of the posterior wall of the proximal 1 to 2 cm of the internal and external carotid arteries, and over half have narrowing of multiple arteries. Tandem lesions involving the internal carotid artery and the carotid siphon are prevalent (Figure 9.15) [41,42].

Table 9.3. Other factors precluding the use of magnetic resonance angiography*

Contraindications
- Large body habitus
- Cardiac pacemakers
- Implantable cardiac defibrillators
- Cochlear implants
- Nerve and bone stimulators
- Drug infusion pumps
- Pregnancy†

Patient considerations‡
- Claustrophobia
- Anxiety
- Movement disorders

*From Shellock and Kanal [26]; with permission.
†No studies have evaluated the use of magnetic resonance angiography in pregnant women. Therefore, caution is advised due to legal considerations.
‡Short-acting sedation may be helpful in these situations.

Table 9.5. Common ballistic projectiles in the urban setting

Projectile	Deflection?	Magnetic field, *T*	Distortion
BBs [27]			
(Daisy)	Yes	1.5	Unknown
(Crosman)	Yes	1.5	Unknown
0.357-inch lead bullet [30]			
(Cascade)	No	1.5	Slight
(Remington)	No	1.5	Slight
(Winchester)	No	1.5	Yes
(Hornady)	No	1.5	Yes
9-mm lead bullet [30]			
(Norma)	Yes	1.5	Strong
(Remington)	No	1.5	Slight
Lead shot [30]			
7.5	No	1.5	Slight
4	No	1.5	Slight
00	No	1.5	Slight

Table 9.4. Common intracranial implants, their reaction to a magnetic field, and distortion of magnetic resonance imaging

Implant	Deflection?	Magnetic field, *T*	Distortion
Aneurysm clips			
Heifetz (Edward Weck)			
Elgiloy [27]	No	1.89	Evident
17-7PH [27,29]	No	1.89	Strong
Mayfield (Codman and Shurtleff) [27]			
301SS	Yes	1.5	Unknown
304SS	Yes	1.89	Unknown
McFadden (Codman and Shurtleff) [27]	No	1.5	Unknown
301SS	Yes	1.5	Unknown
Scoville (Downs) [28]			
Large	Yes	1.5	Strong
Small	Yes	1.5	Evident
Sugita (Downs) [27,28]	No	1.89	Slight
Vari-angle (Codman and Shurtleff) [27]			
17-7PH	Yes	1.89	Unknown
McFadden MP35N	No	1.89	Unknown
Micro 17-7PM SS	Yes	0.15	Unknown
Spring 17-7PM SS	Yes	0.15	Unknown
Yasargil (Aesculap)			
316 SS [27,29]	No	1.89	Unknown
Phynox [27,29]	No	1.89	Unknown
316 LVM [29]	No	0.35	Slight
Intravascular coils [28]			
Gianturco (Cook)	Yes	1.5	Unknown
Ventricular shunts			
Tube connectors			
(Ethicon) [28]	Yes	1.5	Slight
Accuflow (Codman and Shurtleff) [27]	No	1.5	Unknown
Shunt valves [28]			
Holter (Holter)	Slight	1.5	Evident
Holter-Hanson (Holter-Hanson)	No	1.5	Slight
Hakim (Cordis)	Slight	1.5	Evident
Other			
Tantalum hemoclips [27,28]	No	1.5	Unknown
Stainless steel wire [28]	No	1.5	Evident

Duplex Doppler studies are the established screening tool for the evaluation of occlusive disease of the carotid and vertebral arteries [43,44]. However, MRA is becoming a more attractive screening tool for the following reasons. First, the sensitivity and specificity of MRA is not dependent on operator skill. Second, it offers a complete view of the aortic arch, proximal carotid system, and distal carotid siphon. Authors have found more perioperative strokes in patients with tandem lesions involving these locations. Lastly, MRA does not have difficulty distinguishing severe stenosis from occlusion; the latter is a contraindication to surgery [43–47].

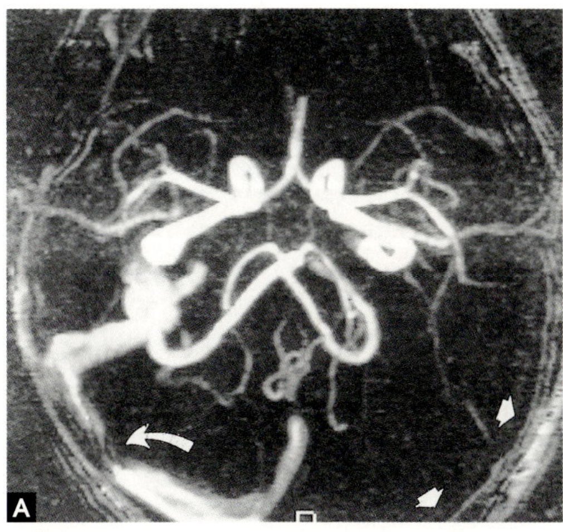

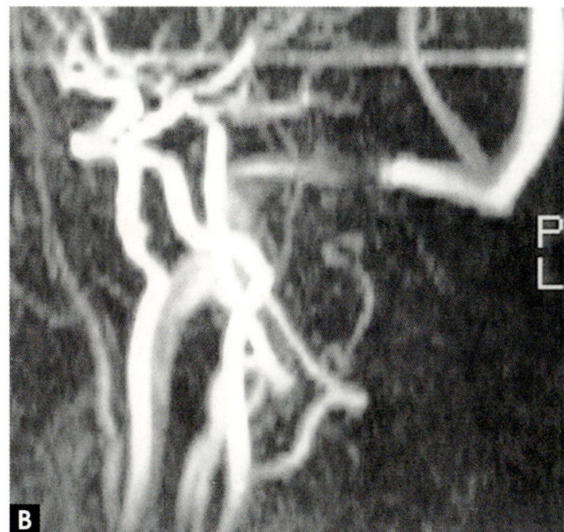

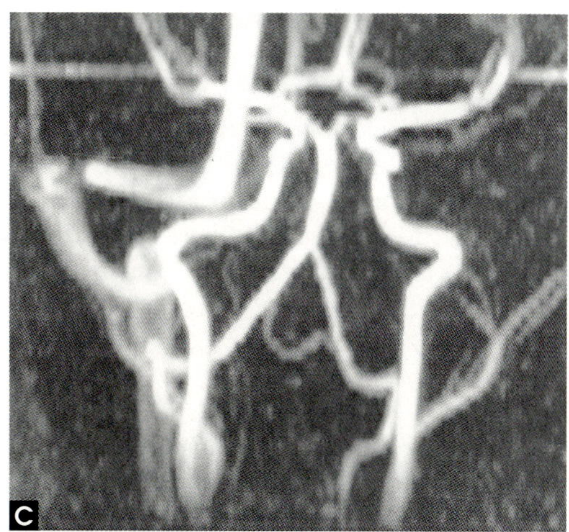

FIGURE 9.14

Phase-contrast magnetic resonance angiography in axial (**A**), oblique lateral (**B**), and frontal (**C**) projections shows overlapping of arterial and venous structures. Note that there is lateral sinus thrombosis in this child with left-sided mastoiditis. Note the expected position of the sinus in axial view (*arrows* in *A*). The irregular zone (*curved arrow* in *A*) in the opposite lateral sinus persisted on follow-up examinations, and presumably represents an arachnoid granulation.

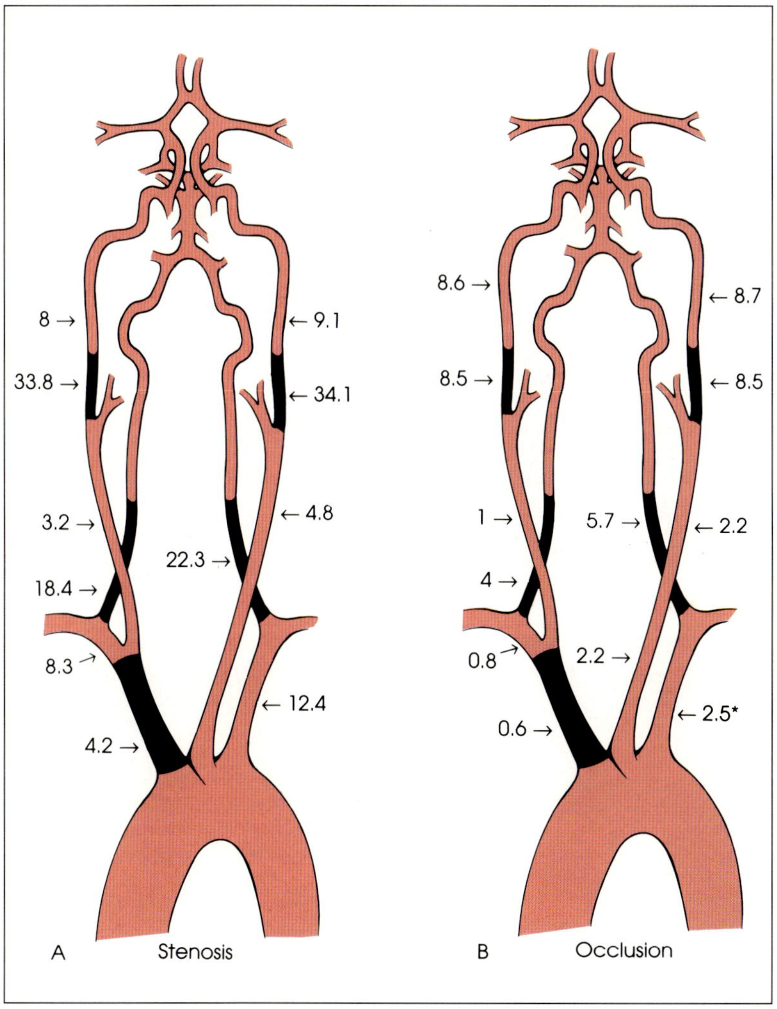

FIGURE 9.15

The most common sites of carotid artery stenosis (**A**) and occlusion (**B**). Values are percents. (*From* Imparato and Riles [42]; with permission.)

In two- or three-dimensional TOF MRA, a narrowed vessel will cause turbulence in blood flow and loss of the signal (Figures 9.16 and 9.17) [48–50]. The degree of stenosis of carotid lesions has corresponded similarly on MRA, CCA, and DSA [48–50], and recent studies have demonstrated 86% to 100% sensitivity and 90% to 92% specificity for lesions narrowed by 70% or more [44–48,50]. The data on MRA's detection of ulcerative plaques is limited and inconclusive [44,47,49,50]. Normal turbulence at the carotid siphon must be differentiated from pathologic narrowing, and the complex flow generated distal to the stenosis can lead to overestimation of atherosclerotic narrowing (Figures 9.4 and 9.5) [44,46,47, 49–51].

Angiographic atherosclerotic disease is recognized as a decrease in vessel diameter or, less commonly, a fusiform dilatation. Ulcerative plaques are confirmed by visualization of contrast material extending into the plaque. Indirect signs include a decrease in flow rate through affected vessels, retrograde filling of vessels distal to the occlusion, and formation of collateral circulation. An increased flow through the external carotid artery compared with the internal carotid can signify narrowing of the latter. Dissecting aneurysms and arteritis may mimic atherosclerotic narrowing [52,53].

The current feeling among radiologists is that patients with lesions narrowed by 60% or more on MRA should undergo CCA for preoperative evaluation. Those with low-grade stenosis on MRA may be followed up with yearly exams.

Intracranial Cerebrovascular Occlusive Disease

Thrombosis of atherosclerotic lesions accounts for most cases of intracranial ischemia; this estimate may vary by study and racial population. Preliminary studies demonstrate that three-dimensional TOF MRA can accurately detect occlusion of the larger intracranial vessels [54–57]. There was good correlation between physical findings, CCA, DSA, and MRA (Figure 9.18) [54–57]. Erroneous narrowing can be recorded at areas of complex flow, such as the carotid siphon or knee of the middle cerebral artery. The slow flow and the small volume of blood through distal intracranial vessels leads to saturation effects [10].

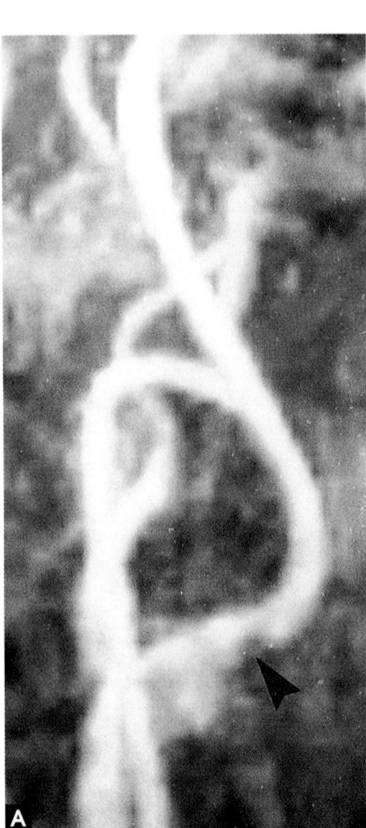

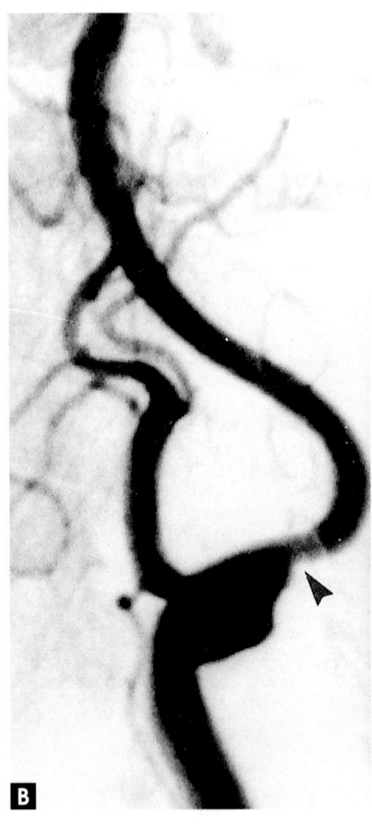

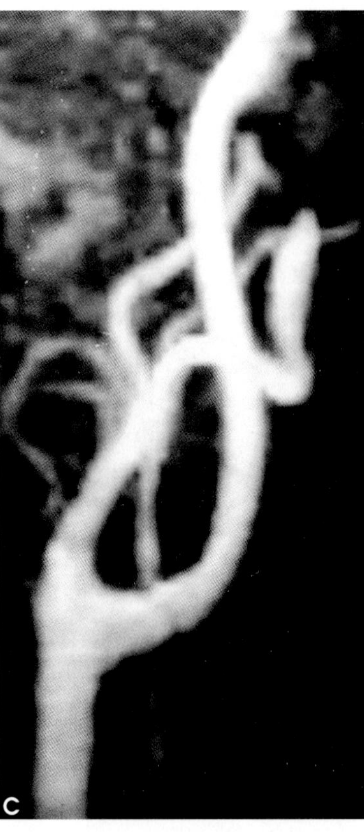

FIGURE 9.16

A, Lateral-view three-dimensional time-of-flight magnetic resonance angiogram demonstrates a moderate stenosis (*arrowhead*) at the internal carotid artery just distal to the bifurcation of the common carotid artery. **B,** Lateral-view digital subtraction angiogram shows the same lesion (*arrowhead*). **C,** Follow-up lateral-view three-dimensional time-of-flight magnetic resonance angiogram after carotid endarterectomy shows no evidence of stenosis or occlusion.

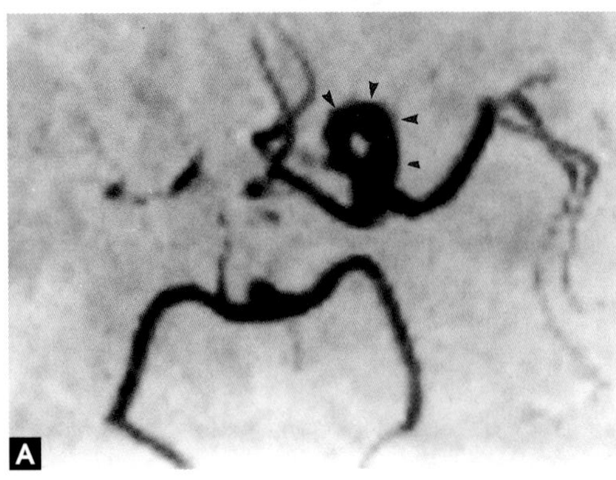

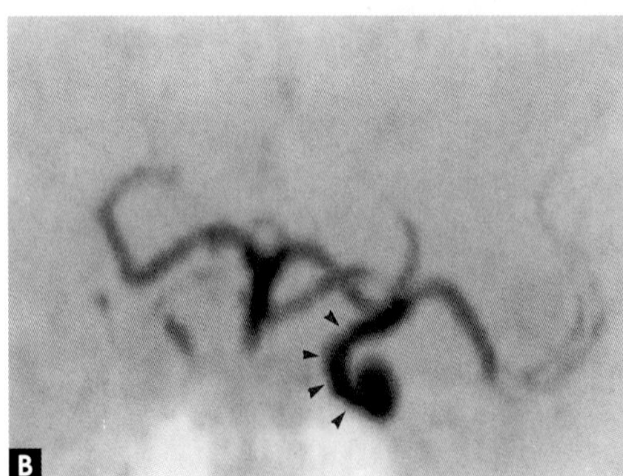

FIGURE 9.17

Base (**A**) and frontal (**B**) projections of a three-dimensional time-of-flight magnetic resonance angiogram (MRA) show decreased signal in the severely stenotic right internal carotid artery. There is partial filling by collateral flow from the ophthalmic artery (which is too small to be seen on the MRA). The normal left internal carotid is marked by *arrowheads* for orientation.

Inflammation of the cranial blood vessels (vasculitis) can also result in ischemia or stroke. The typical radiographic appearance of arteritis includes aneurysmal dilatation, narrowing or occlusion of arteries, beaded segments of arteries, and thrombosed vessels (Figure 9.19) [58]. Since vasculitis can involve vessels too small to be visualized by MRA (including leptomeningeal branches, those along the basal cistern, and distal cortical vessels), it is not used in evaluating this disorder [59].

Collateral Blood Flow

The degree of ischemia or the extent of infarct produced by intracranial and extracranial stenosis is dependent on collateral blood flow, which can involve all arteries of the head and neck. These arteries appear as a complex of fine, tortuous vessels on angiogram [60]. Three-dimensional PC MRA evaluation of collateral blood flow through the circle of Willis has correlated with angiographic and transcranial Doppler findings (Figure 9.20) [23,52,54–57, 61,62].

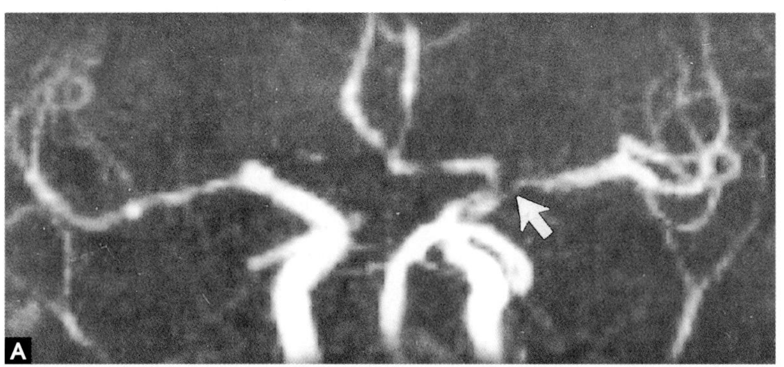

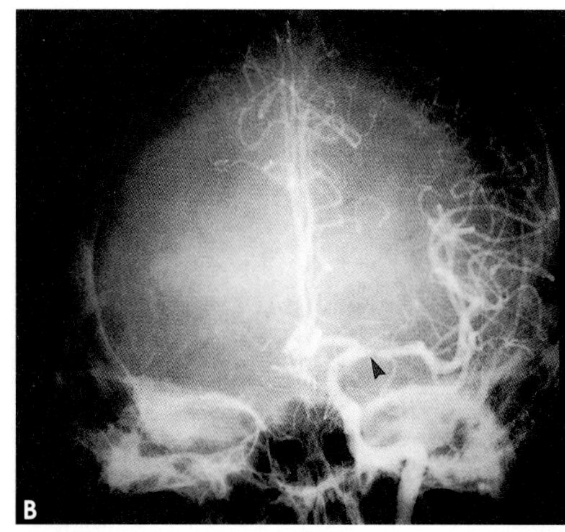

FIGURE 9.18

A, Frontal view of time-of-flight magnetic resonance angiography demonstrates left middle cerebral artery stenosis (*arrow*). Absence of the horizontal anterior cerebral artery was interpreted as focal stenosis in this vessel. **B,** Companion frontal view of left conventional cerebral angiography shows the left middle cerebral artery stenosis (*arrowhead*).

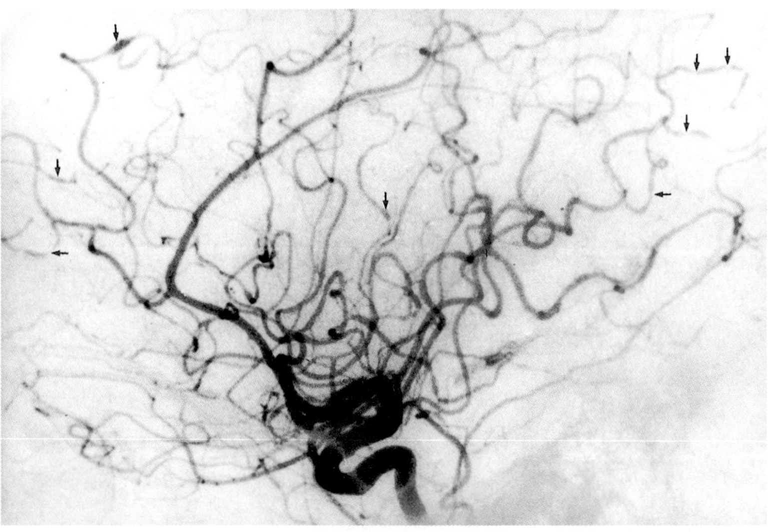

FIGURE 9.19

Lateral conventional cerebral angiographic view shows irregularity and beading of almost every tertiary cerebral artery (*arrows*) consistent with a diagnosis of arteritis. These vessels are too small to be discerned by current magnetic resonance angiography techniques.

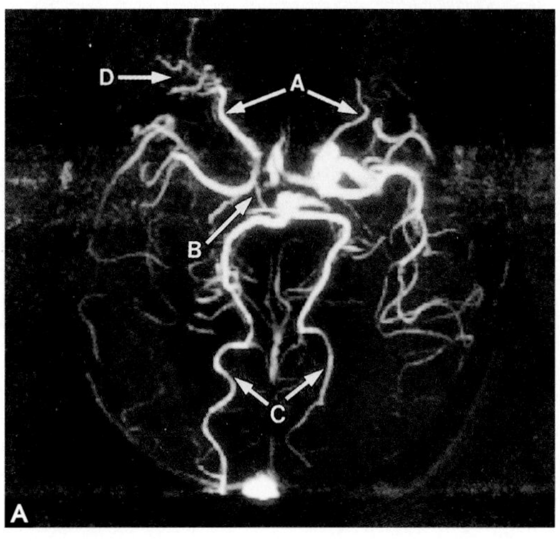

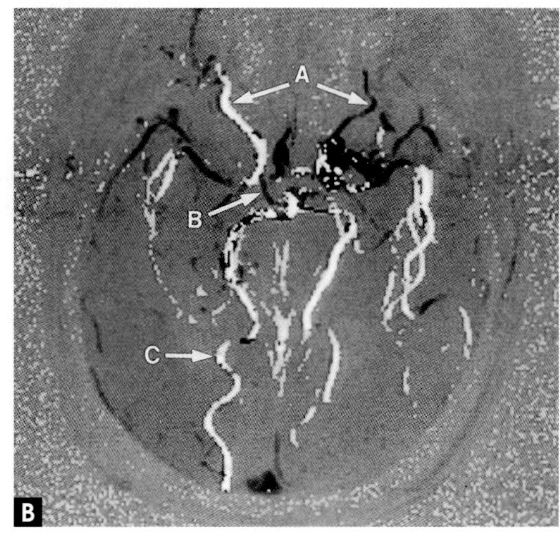

FIGURE 9.20

Three-dimensional phase-contrast magnetic resonance angiogram demonstrates collateral flow in a patient with an occluded right internal carotid artery. **A,** The right middle cerebral artery is being filled by an enlarged right posterior communicating artery and through the right ophthalmic artery via the right external carotid. **B,** The posterior-to-anterior flow of the right posterior communicating artery (*black*) and the anterior-to-posterior flow in the ophthalmic artery (*white*). A—ophthalmic artery; B—right posterior communicating artery; C—posterior cerebral artery; D—right external carotid artery. (*From* Pernicone and coworkers [23]; with permission.)

Vascular Malformations

Intracranial aneurysms and arteriovenous malformations (AVMs) rarely cause ischemic damage; however, their neurologic symptoms may mimic ischemic deficits. Early detection of these vascular anomalies through screening tests may have an impact on survival since a major bleed from an aneurysm carries a 50% mortality and AVMs have a 10% mortality [63,64].

Intracranial Aneurysms

Figure 9.21 summarizes the most frequent sites of saccular aneurysms [65]. Twenty percent of patients will have tandem lesions, most commonly in the same vessel or involving symmetric areas [66].

Three-dimensional TOF MRA and two- and three-dimensional PC MRA can detect aneurysms with diameters of 3 to 15 mm (Figures 9.22 and 9.23) [22,56–71]. The slow-flow saturation effects of aneurysms greater than 15 mm lead to unwanted signal loss (Figure 9.10), and subacute thrombus may falsely simulate flowing blood [9,67–69]. Although there is excellent anatomic correlation among MRA, CCA, and DSA, some discrepancies exist in the delineation of the dome, flow jet, and small adjacent vessels with MRA [67–69,71]. Until techniques improve, either CCA or DSA remains the gold standard for the preoperative evaluation of aneurysms.

Magnetic resonance angiography is currently used extensively after aneurysm obliteration. It has demonstrated the presence of residual flow and intraluminal thrombus after embolization and has confirmed the balloon's position after balloon occlusion of the aneurysm (Figures 9.23 and 9.24) [68]. No studies have shown vasospasm using MRA; therefore, tradi-

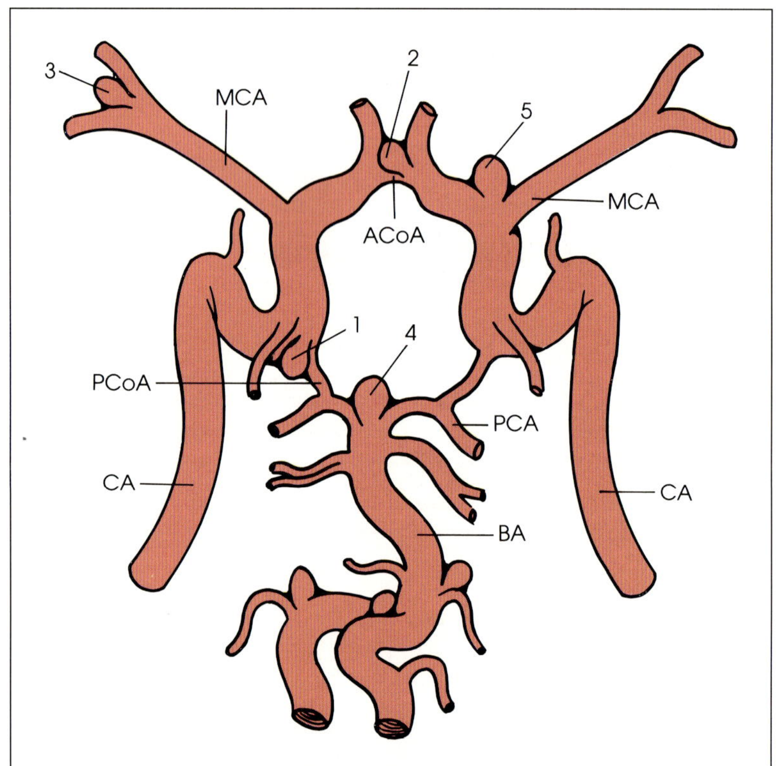

FIGURE 9.21

Ninety percent of all intracranial aneurysms occur around the circle of Willis near bifurcations. The most common locations include (**1**) the internal carotid artery (CA) at the posterior communicating artery (PCoA), (**2**) the anterior cerebral artery (ACA) at the anterior communicating artery (ACoA), (**3**) the bifurcation of the middle cerebral artery (MCA), (**4**) the posterior cerebral artery (PCA) and basilar artery (BA), and (**5**) the bifurcation of the MCA and ACA. Ten percent of aneurysms occur in the posterior circulation. (*Adapted from* Rhoton [65]; with permission.)

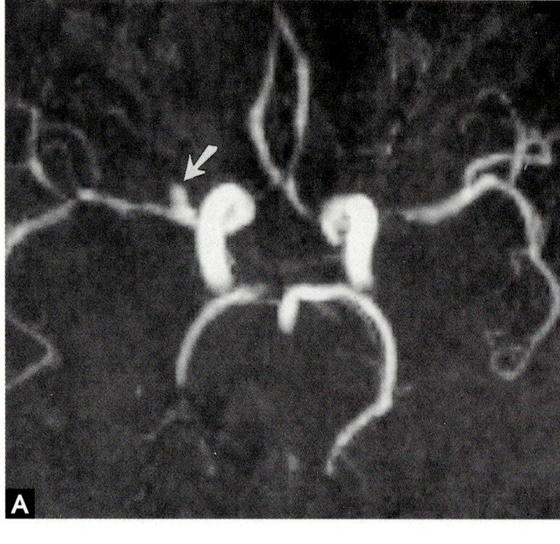

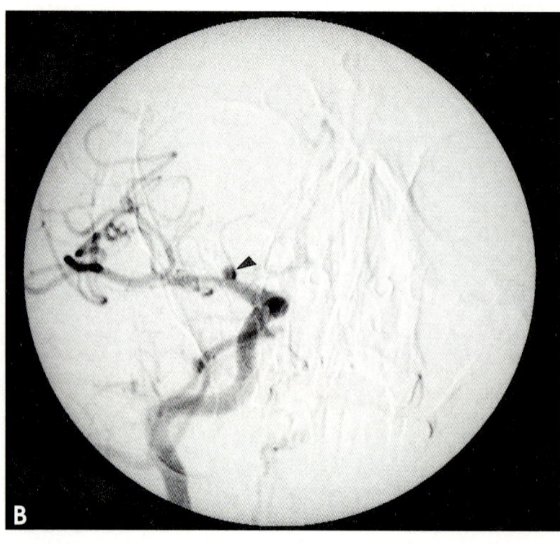

FIGURE 9.22

A, Time-of-flight magnetic resonance angiogram shows a small saccular aneurysm of the horizontal right middle cerebral artery (*arrow*). **B,** Companion digital subtraction angiography in a Waters frontal view confirms the presence of the aneurysm (*arrowhead*).

tional transcranial Doppler or CCA must be used to detect this complication.

Intracranial Arteriovenous Malformations

Cerebral AVMs are abnormal congenital connections between the intracranial arterial and venous systems that dilate over time. Ninety percent are located above the tentorium and 10% involve the posterior fossa. Fifty percent are 2.5 to 5 cm in diameter, 40% are smaller, and the remaining 10% exceed 5 cm in size [64].

Magnetic resonance angiography can effectively demonstrate important anatomic structures of AVMs. Two- and three-dimensional TOF MRA illustrate venous and nidus anatomy; three-dimensional PC MRA delineates arterial and nidus anatomy; and phase-encoding PC MRA can visualize all structures (Figures 9.5 and 9.25) [67,69,72,73].

Conventional cerebral angiographic findings in AVMs include dilated, tortuous feeding and draining vessels and tightly packed intrinsic vessels. The transit time through the malformation is rapid (Figure 9.26). CCA (with DSA) is superior to MRA because it furnishes distinct information concerning small malformations, details sequential blood flow, and better represents the supplying and draining vessels. It also offers quantitative

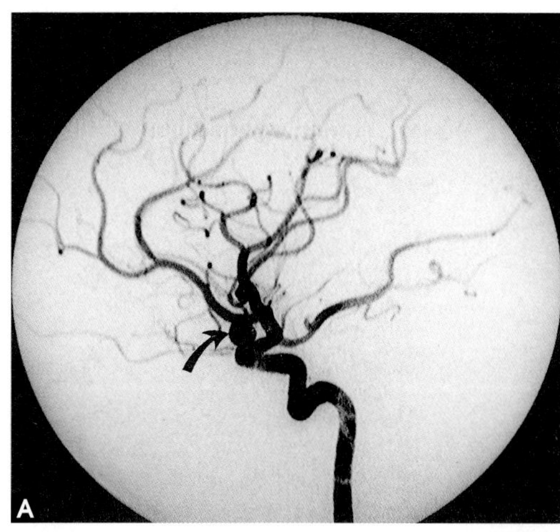

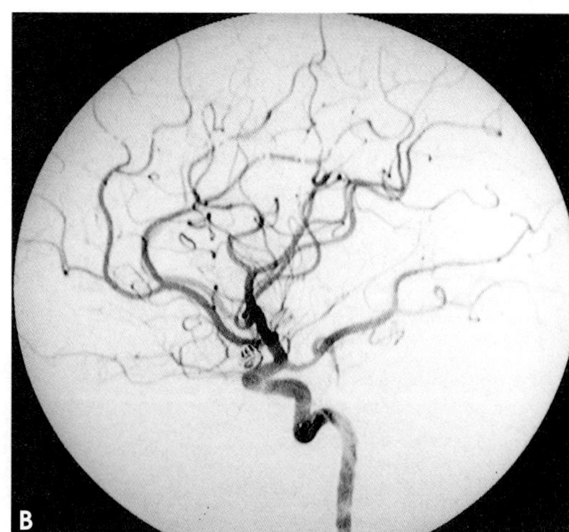

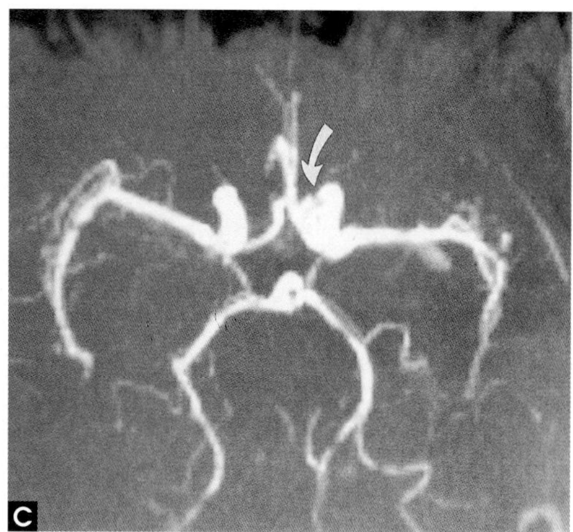

FIGURE 9.23

A 30-year-old woman with subarachnoid hemorrhage. **A,** Digital subtraction angiography (DSA) illustrated a 7-mm left paraophthalmic artery aneurysm (*arrow*). **B,** DSA after successful embolization of the aneurysm using a detachable coil. **C,** Follow-up three-dimensional time-of-flight magnetic resonance angiogram (MRA) demonstrates bright signal in the left paraophthalmic aneurysm (*arrow*), which could represent subacute clot or flow. A phase-contrast (PC) MRA or a T_1-weighted MR image is needed to distinguish flow (which would be hyperintense on PC MRA) from clot (which would not be seen on PC MRA, but would be hyperintense on T_1-weighted MR image).

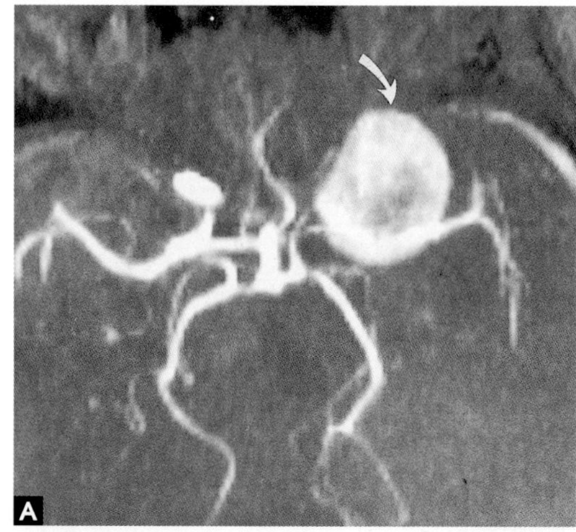

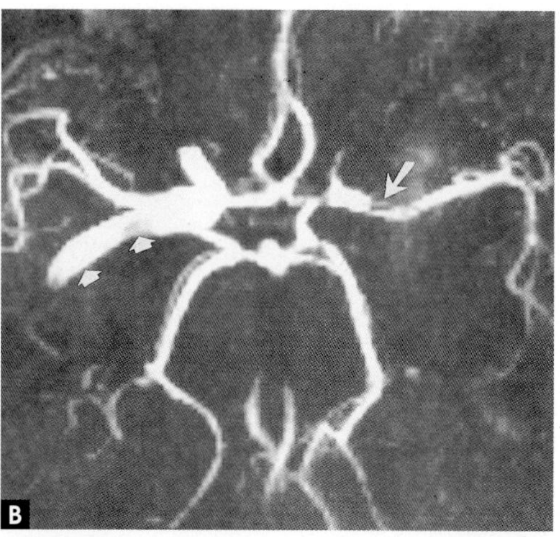

FIGURE 9.24

A, Base projection three-dimensional time-of-flight magnetic resonance angiogram (MRA) of a giant parasellar aneurysm (*arrow*) of the left internal carotid artery. **B**, Follow-up phase-contrast MRA after a left internal cerebral artery occlusion by detachable balloons and thrombogenic coils shows no flow through the aneurysm or the petrous and cavernous segment of the left internal carotid artery. Note the normal right petrous carotid artery on the opposite side (*short arrows*) for comparison. The horizontal segment of the middle cerebral artery is compressed by the clot within the aneurysm (*long arrow*).

data on arteriovenous circulation time and arterial stump pressure [1,2].

Arteriovenous malformations can be treated surgically, with angiographic embolization or balloon occlusion, and MRA would be an excellent noninvasive follow-up evaluation in these patients. No research studies have detailed this application, however.

CONCLUSIONS

Intra-arterial CCA remains the gold standard for the evaluation of most cerebrovascular pathology, but this technique is not without risk. MRA is evolving as a noninvasive imaging technique that may replace CCA and DSA, complement other diagnostic exams, and aid in posttherapeutic management of cerebrovascular disease. With advancement in gradient design, modification of acquisition programs, and improvement in image processing, the current technical limitations of MRA may be overcome.

ACKNOWLEDGMENTS

The authors wish to acknowledge the contribution of cases from The Methodist Hospital in Houston, Texas. We would also like to thank Jackie Bogan for her patience in typing and retyping this chapter.

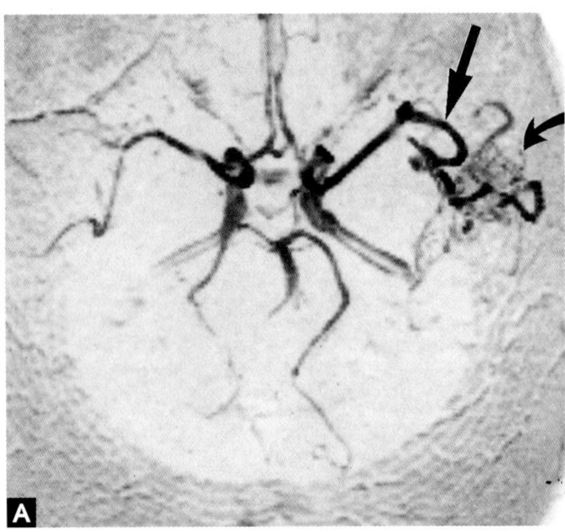

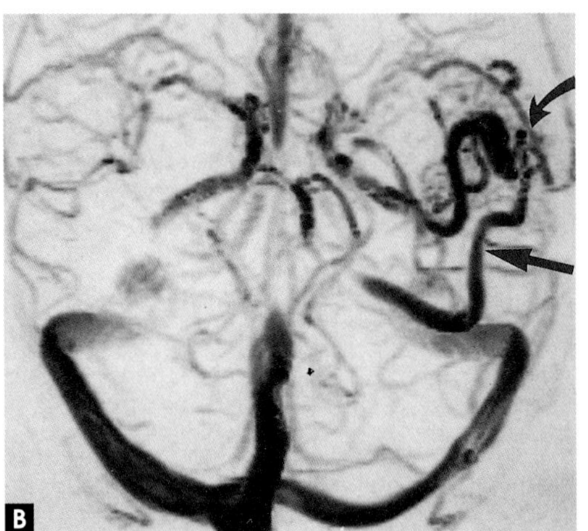

FIGURE 9.25

Left temporal arteriovenous malformation on axial magnetic resonance angiography. **A,** Three-dimensional time-of-flight (TOF) image depicts the feeding artery (*straight arrow*) and the nidus (*curved arrow*). **B,** Three-dimensional phase-contrast (PC) image with 20 cm/s encoding shows the nidus (*curved arrow*) and the venous drainage (*straight arrow*). The background noise is noted more intensely on the TOF image compared with the PC image. (*From* Huston and Ehman [9]; with permission.)

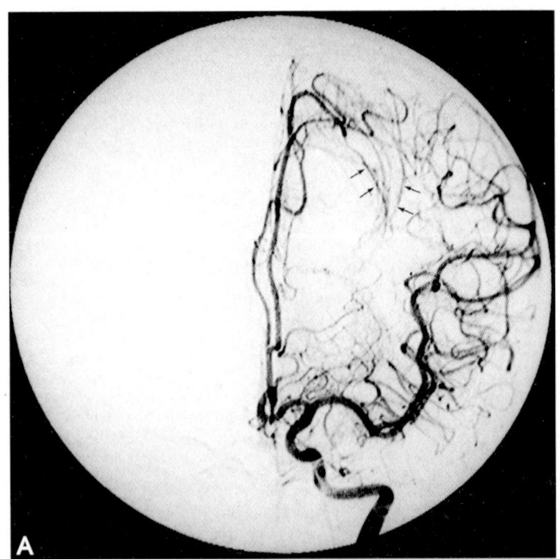

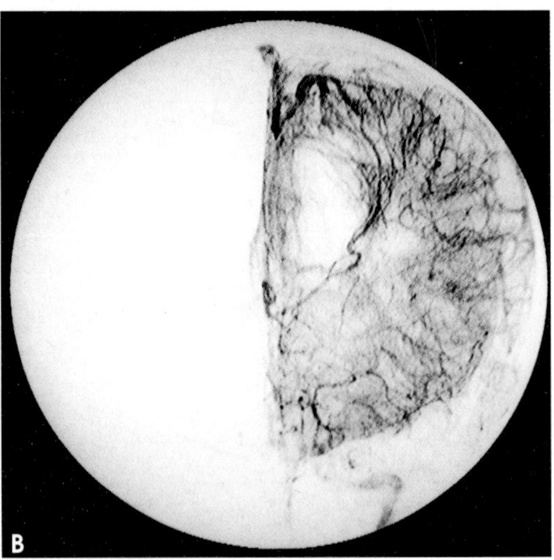

FIGURE 9.26

A, Digital subtraction angiography in a frontal projection demonstrates abnormal frontal arteries (*arrows*). **B,** Arteriovenous shunting and early venous drainage in an arteriovenous malformation. All of these vessels are too small to be visualized by current magnetic resonance angiographic (MRA) techniques. The mass effect on these anterior and middle cerebral vessels indicates the presence of hematoma. This precludes the use of time-of-flight MRA because the technique would interpret the clot as hyperintense signal, which could be mistaken as vascular flow. Phase-contrast MRA would only show the large vessels displaced by the hematoma.

REFERENCES

1. Huber P: Techniques of cerebral angiography. In *Cerebral Angiography.* New York: Thieme-Stratton, Inc.; 1982:5–14.
2. Osborn AG: Technical aspects of cerebral angiography. In *Introduction to Cerebral Angiography.* New York: Harper and Row; 1980:1–32.
3. Butler P: Digital Subtraction angiography: a neurosurgical perspective. *Br J Neurosurg* 1987, 1:323–333.
4. Kadir S: Digital subtraction angiography. In *Diagnostic Angiography.* Edited by Marke D. Philadelphia: WB Saunders; 1986:103–108.
5. Chien D, Edelman RR: Basic principles and clinical applications of magnetic resonance angiography. *Semin Roentgenol* 1992, 27:53–62.
6. Edelman RR: Basic principles of magnetic resonance angiography. *Cerebrovasc Intervent Radiol* 1992, 15:3–13.
7. Ruggieri PM, Masaryk TJ, Ross JS: Magnetic resonance angiography: cerebrovascular applications. *Stroke* 1992, 23:774–780.
8. Dumoulin CL: Phase-contrast magnetic resonance angiography. In *Neuroimaging Clinics of North America.* Edited by Drayer BP. Philadelphia: WB Saunders; 1992:657–675.
9. Huston J III, Ehman RL: Comparison of TOF and PC MR neuroangiographic techniques. *Radiographics* 1993, 13:5–19.
10. Ruggiere PM, Masaryk TJ, Ross JS, *et al.*: Intracranial magnetic resonance angiography. *Cerebrovasc Intervent Radiol* 1992, 15:71–81.
11. Pernicone JR, Siebert JE, Potchen EJ, *et al.*: Three-dimensional phase-contrast MR angiography in the head and neck: preliminary report. *AJNR* 1990, 11:457–466.
12. Hankey GJ, Warlow CP, Sellar RJ: Cerebral angiographic risk in mild cerebrovascular disease. *Stroke* 1990, 21:209–222.
13. Kadir S: Complications of angiography. In *Diagnostic Angiography.* Edited by Marke D. Philadelphia: WB Saunders; 1986:120–122.
14. Theodotou BC, Whaley R, Mahaley MS: Complications following transfemoral cerebral angiography for cerebral ischemia: report of 159 angiograms and correlation with surgical risk. *Surg Neurol* 1987, 28:90–92.
15. Quisling R: Cerebral Angiography. In *Neurological Surgery.* Edited by Youmans JR. Philadelphia: WB Saunders; 1990:239–252.
16. Grzyka U, Freitaf J, Zeumer H: Selective cerebral intra-arterial DSA: complication rate and control of risk factors. *Neuroradiology* 1990, 32:296–299.
17. Butler P: Digital substraction angiography: a neurosurgical perspective. *Br J Neurosurg* 1987, 1:323–333.
18. Polak JF: Noninvasive carotid evaluation: carpe diem. *Radiology* 1993, 186:329–331.
19. UK-TIA Study Group: Variation in the use of angiography and carotid endarterectomy by neurologists in the UK-TIA Aspirin Trial. *BMJ* 1983, 286:514–517.
20. Mas JL, Meder JF, Meary E, *et al.*: Magnetic resonance imaging in lateral sinus hypoplasia and thrombosis. *Stroke* 1990, 21:1350–1356.
21. Macchi PJ, Grossman RI, Gomori JM, *et al.*: High field MR imaging of cerebral venous thrombosis. *J Comput Assist Tomogr* 1986, 10:10–15.
22. Lin W, Haacke EM, Smith AS, *et al.*: Gadolinium-enhanced high resolution MRA with adaptive vessel tracking: preliminary results in the intracranial circulation. *Semin Magn Reson Imaging* 1992, 2:277–284.
23. Pernicone JR, Thorp KE, Ouimette MV, *et al.*: Magnetic resonance angiography in intracranial vascular disease. *Semin US CT MR* 1992, 13:256–273.
24. Tsuruda J, Saloner D, Norman D: Artifacts associated with MR neuroangiography. *AJNR* 1992, 13:1411–1422.
25. Turski P: *Vascular Magnetic Resonance Imaging.* Milwaukee, WI: GE Medical Systems; 1990.
26. Shellock FG, Kanal E: Policies, guidelines and recommendations for MR imaging safety and patient management. *J Magn Reson Image* 1991, 1:97–101.
27. Shellock FG: MR imaging of metallic implants and materials: a compilation of the literature. *AJR* 1988, 151:811–814.
28. Go KG, Kamman RL, Mooyaart EL: Interaction of metallic neurosurgical implants with MRI at 1.5 Tesla as a cause of image distortion and of hazardous movement of the implant. *Clin Neurol Neurosurg* 1989, 91:109–115.
29. Becker RL, Norfray JF, Teitelbaum GP, *et al.*: MR imaging in patients with intracranial aneurysm clips. *AJNR* 1988, 9:885–889.
30. Teitelbaum GP, Yee CA, Van Horn DD, *et al.*: Metallic ballistic fragments: MR imaging safety and artifacts. *Radiology* 1990, 175:855–859.
31. Ameri A, Bousser MG: Cerebral venous thrombosis. *Neurol Clin* 1992, 10:87–111.
32. Huber P: Thrombosis of the cerebral veins and venous sinuses. In *Cerebral Angiography.* New York: Thieme-Stratton Inc; 1982:492–496.
33. Yasargil MG, Damur M: Thrombosis of the cerebral veins and dural sinuses. In *Radiology of the Skull and Brain: Angiography.* Edited by Newton TH, Potts DG. St. Louis: CV Mosby; 1982:2375–2400.
34. Zouaoui A, Hidden G: Cerebral venous sinuses: anatomical variants or thrombosis? *Acta Anat* 1988, 133:318–324.
35. Johnson BA, Fram EK: Cerebral venous occlusive disease: pathophysiology, clinical manifestations and imaging. In *Neuroimaging Clinics of America.* Edited by Drayer BP. Philadelphia: WB Saunders; 1992:2:769–783.
36. Medlock MD, Olivero WC, Hanigan WC, *et al.*: Children with cerebral venous thrombosis diagnosed with magnetic resonance imaging and magnetic resonance angiography. *Neurosurgery* 1992, 31:870–876.
37. Padayachee TS, Bingham JB, Graves MJ, *et al.*: Dural sinus thrombosis: diagnosis and follow-up by magnetic resonance angiography and imaging. *Neuroradiology* 1991, 33:165–167.
38. Fram EK, Keller PJ, Drayer BP: MR angiography of cerebral venous occlusive disease. In *SMRI Book of Abstracts.* Edited by Gore J, Smith FW. Washington, D.C.: SMRI; 1990:98.
39. Ripe DJ, Boyko OB, Spritzer CE, *et al.*: Demonstration of dural sinus occlusion by the use of MR angiography. *AJNR* 1990, 11:199–201.
40. Wolf PA, Kannel WB, McGee DL: Epidemiology of strokes in North America. In *Stroke: Pathophysiology, Diagnosis and Management.* Edited by Barnett R, Mohr J, Stein B, *et al.*. New York: Churchill Livingstone; 1986:19–29.
41. *Stroke Update: US Dept. of Public Health, Health and Human Services.* Bethesda: National Institutes of Health; 1989:3–14.
42. Imparato AM, Riles TS: Peripheral arterial disease. In *Principles of Surgery.* Edited by Schwartz SI. New York: McGraw Hill; 1989:931–1010.
43. Masaryk TJ, Obuchowski NA: Noninvasive carotid imaging: caveat emptor. *Radiology* 1993, 2:325–328.
44. Mattle HP, Kent KC, Edelman RR, *et al.*: Evaluation of the extracranial carotid arteries: correlation of magnetic resonance angiography, duplex ultrasonography and conventional angiography. *J Vasc Surg* 1991, 13:838–845.
45. Zawadzki MB, Gillan G: Extracranial carotid magnetic resonance angiography. *Cerebrovasc Intervent Radiol* 1992, 15:82–90.
46. Anderson CM, Saloner D, Lee RE, *et al.*: Assessment of carotid artery stenosis by MR angiography: comparison of x-ray angiography and color-coded Doppler ultrasound. *AJNR* 1992, 13:989–1003.
47. Wilkerson DK, Keller I, Mezreich R: The comparative evaluation of three-dimensional magnetic resonance for carotid artery disease. *J Vasc Surg* 1991, 14:803–811.
48. Kido DK, Panzer RP, Szumowski J: Clinical evaluation of stenosis of the carotid bifurcation with magnetic resonance angiographic techniques. *Arch Neurol* 1991, 48:484–489.
49. Masaryk AM, Ross JS, DiCello MC, *et al.*: 3DFT MR angiography of the carotid bifurcation: potential and limitations as a screening examination. *Radiology* 1991, 179:797–804.

50. Heiserman JE, Drayer BP, Fram EK, *et al.*: Carotid artery stenosis: clinical efficacy of two-dimensional time of flight MR angiography. *Radiology* 1992, 182:761–768.

51. Warach S, Wei L, Ronthal M, *et al.*: Acute cerebral ischemia: evaluation with dynamic contrast-enhanced MR imaging and MR angiography. *Radiology* 1992, 182:41–47.

52. Osborne AG: External carotid artery. In *Introduction to Cerebral Angiography.* New York: Harper and Row; 1980:49–86.

53. Huber P: Angiographic findings and symptoms in vascular occlusion. In *Cerebral Angiography.* New York: Thieme-Stratton; 1982:257–260.

54. Heiserman JE, Drayer BP, Keller PJ, *et al.*: Intracranial vascular stenosis and occlusion: evaluation with three-dimensional time of flight MR angiography. *Radiology* 1992, 185:667–673.

55. Zimmerman RA, Bogdan AR, Gusnard DA: Pediatric magnetic resonance angiography: assessment of stroke. *Cerebrovasc Intervent Radiol* 1992, 15:60–64.

56. Wiznitzer M, Masaryk TJ: Cerebrovascular abnormalities in pediatric stroke: assessment using parenchymal angiographic magnetic resonance imaging. *Ann Neurol* 1991, 29:585–589.

57. Witznitzer M, Ruggieri PM, Masaryk TJ, *et al.*: Diagnosis of cerebrovascular disease in sickle cell anemia by magnetic resonance angiography. *J Pediatr* 1990, 117:551–555.

58. Ferris E: Arteritis. In *Radiology of the Skull and Brain: Angiography.* Edited by Newton TH, Potts DG. St. Louis: CV Mosby Company; 1974:2566–2597.

59. Katzmann R: Collagen vascular disease and systemic vasculitis. In *Textbook of Neurology*. Edited by Merritt HH. Philadelphia: Lea and Febiger; 1979:622–639.

60. Mishkin MM, Schreiber MN: Collateral circulation. In *Radiology of the Skull and Brain: Angiography.* Edited by Newton TH, Potts DG. St. Louis: CV Mosby Company; 1974:2344–2374.

61. Edelman RR, Mattle HP, O'Reilly GV, *et al.*: Magnetic resonance imaging of the flow dynamics in the circle of Willis. *Stroke* 1990, 21:56–65.

62. Pernicone JR, Siebert JE, Laird TA, *et al.*: Determination of blood flow direction using velocity phase image display with 3D phase contrast magnetic resonance angiography. *AJNR* 1992, in press.

63. Heros RC: Intracranial aneurysms: a review. *Minn Med* 1990, 73:27–32.

64. Luessenhop AJ: Cerebral arteriovenous malformations. Part 1. In *Contemporary Neurosurgery.* Edited by Tindall GT. Baltimore: Williams and Wilkins; 1989, 11:1–5.

65. Rhoton AL Jr: Microsurgical anatomy of saccular aneurysms. In *Neurosurgery.* Edited by Wilkins RH, Rengachary SS. New York: McGraw Hill; 1985, 9:1330.

66. Allcock JM: Aneurysms. In *Radiology of the Skull and Brain: Angiography.* Edited by Newton TH, Potts DG. St. Louis: CV Mosby Company; 1976:2435–2489.

67. Masaryk TJ, Modic MT, Ross MD, *et al.*: Intracranial circulation: preliminary results with three-dimensional MR angiography. *Radiology* 1989, 171:793–799.

68. Sevick RJ, Tsuruda JS, Schmalbrock P: Three-dimensional time-of-flight MR angiography in the evaluation of cerebral aneurysms. *J Comput Assist Tomogr* 1990, 14:874–881.

69. Huston J, Rufenacht DA, Ehman RL, *et al.*: Intracranial aneurysms and vascular malformations: comparison of time of flight and phase contrast MR angiography. *Radiology* 1991, 181:721–730.

70. Ross JS, Masaryk TJ, Modic MT, *et al.*: Intracranial aneurysm: evaluation by magnetic resonance angiography. *AJNR* 1990, 11:449–456.

71. Demaerel PH, Marchal G, Casteels I, *et al.*: Intracavernous aneurysm: superior demonstration by magnetic resonance angiography. *Neuroradiology* 1990, 32:322–324.

72. Mattle HP, Wentz KU: Selective magnetic resonance angiography of the head. *Cerebrovasc Intervent Radiol* 1992, 15:65–70.

73. Nussel F, Wegmuller H, Huber P: Comparison of magnetic resonance angiography, magnetic resonance imaging and conventional angiography in cerebral arteriovenous malformations. *Neuroradiology* 1991, 33:56–61.

Chapter 10

Imaging of Stroke with Single Photon Emission Computed Tomography

JOSEPH C. MASDEU

Single photon emission computed tomography (SPECT) was introduced in the early 1980s as an instrument for the evaluation of regional cerebral blood flow (rCBF) and receptor density studies [1,2]. For the performance of SPECT, a flow tracer or a receptor binding substance is tagged with a radionuclide and injected into the patient (Figure 10.1). Using a gamma camera and the techniques of computed tomography (CT), a three dimensional image of the distribution of a radionuclide in the brain is obtained (Figure 10.2). In the past, initial images, usually performed with Xe-133, have lacked enough anatomical resolution to be clinically useful. This situation has been corrected in the past few years with the advent of improved cameras and radiotracers. Perfusion studies are now being used for the study of cerebrovascular disease, the first application for which SPECT radiopharmaceuticals were approved by the Food and Drug Administration (FDA).

One of the major reasons for the growing interest in SPECT is that it represents a relatively inexpensive technique for performing functional neuroimaging. The older and more accurate modality for functional neuroimaging is positron emission tomography (PET). Unlike PET, SPECT cannot measure regional cerebral metabolism, but, in most clinical situations, it provides a qualitative estimate of regional cerebral perfusion, which in many neurologic disorders is tightly coupled with brain metabolism. Thus, SPECT, available in about 80% of the hospitals in the United States, provides functional information not available by CT or magnetic resonance (MR) imaging at a cost similar to that of CT.

Different radiopharmaceuticals have been used with SPECT for the study of cerebral perfusion. The radiotracer accumulates in different areas of the brain proportionally to the rate of delivery of nutrients to that volume of brain tissue and is described in units of mL/min/100 g. Work in animals and humans has demonstrated that under properly controlled conditions, SPECT data obtained with perfusion agents approximates perfusion closely enough to be meaningful in clinical and research studies [3]. Furthermore, most routine clinical applications of brain perfusion SPECT do not require quantitation of perfusion and rely exclusively on the generation of images that reflect tracer uptake and retention only.

Two brain perfusion radiopharmaceuticals have been approved by the FDA for clinical use. I-123 Isopropyl iodoamphetamine (IMP) distributes proportionally to rCBF over a wide range of flows but may be decreased with low plasma pH as in cerebral ischemia or acidosis [4]. Brain activity remains relatively constant

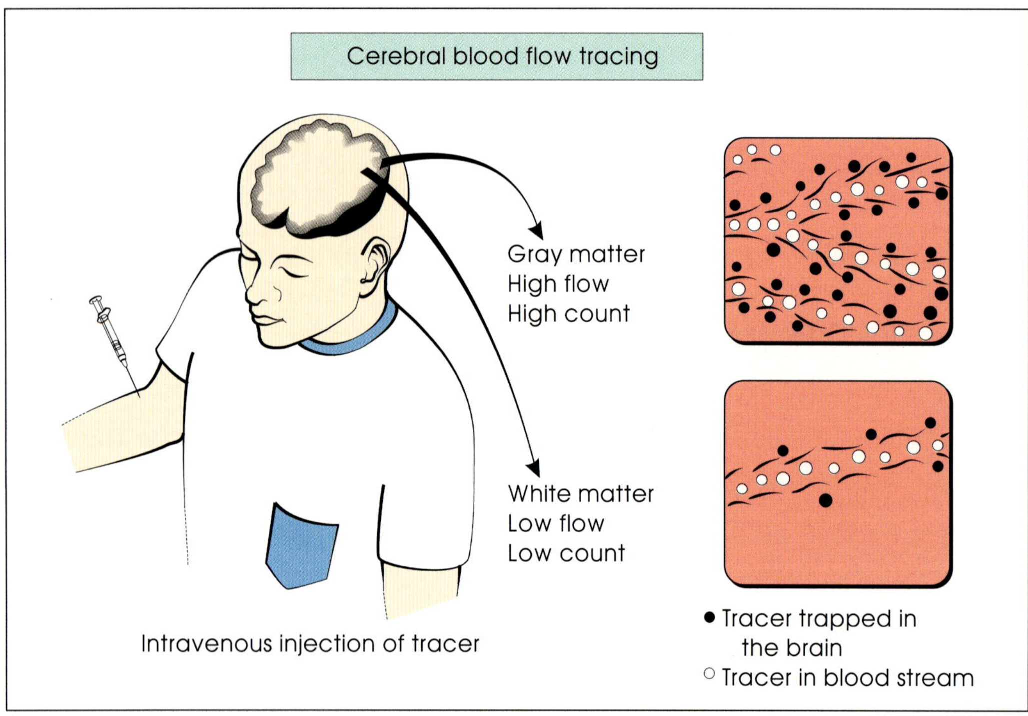

FIGURE 10.1

Injection of a single photon emission computed tomography (SPECT) perfusion agent. These agents, which are highly lipid soluble, tend to penetrate the blood-brain barrier and remain trapped in the perivascular space for many hours, enough to allow for imaging. Brain areas with high perfusion, such as the cerebral cortex, have higher counts than those with lower perfusion, such as the white matter.

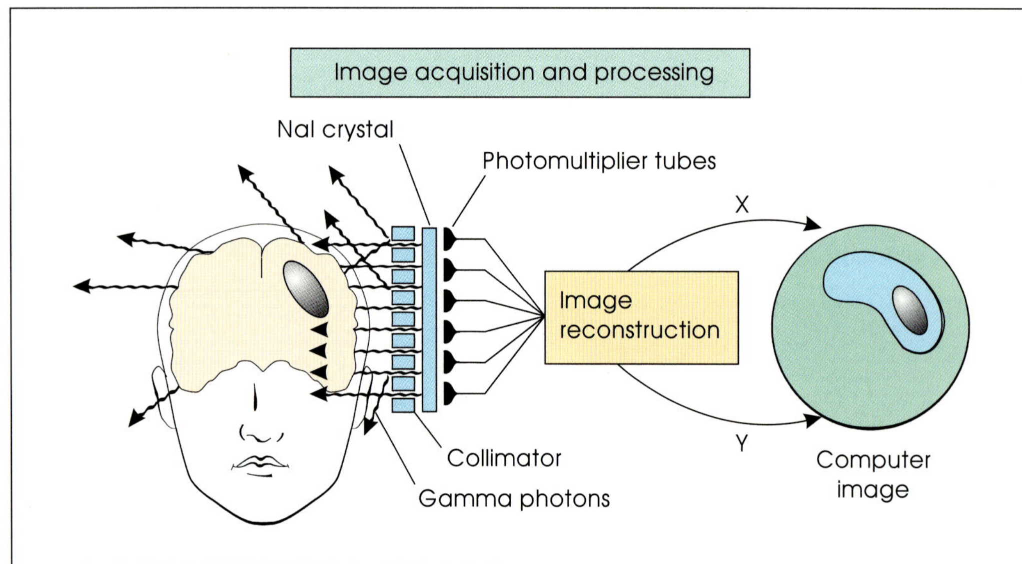

FIGURE 10.2

The distribution of a radionuclide in the brain is imaged by quantification of the photons that interact with sodium iodine (NaI) detectors. Careful collimation is essential for image quality. Mathematical algorithms similar to the ones used by other computed tomographic techniques, including Fourier transform, are used to reconstruct the distribution of the isotope in the brain.

from 20 minutes to at least 60 minutes after injection. Tc 99m Hexamethyl propylamine oxime (HMPAO), a lipid soluble macrocyclic amine, is available for routine clinical use [5]. Brain uptake is rapid and reaches its maximum within 10 minutes. Radiotracer distribution remains constant for many hours after injection. The radiopharmaceutical is chemically unstable *in vitro* by 30 minutes after preparation. A third radiopharmaceutical, Tc 99m ethyl dimer (ECD) is currently undergoing clinical evaluation and will probably be available in the coming year [6]. Its blood clearance is rapid, resulting in high brain to soft tissue activity ratios early after injection, which improve with time. Both Tc 99m HMPAO and Tc 99m ECD exhibit less brain extraction than I-123 IMP, but the more favorable dosimetry permits a substantially higher dose (20–30 MCi) and a higher photon flux. Radiolabeling with Tc 99m on-site followed by mandated quality control measures such as chromatography must be performed in an experienced nuclear medicine laboratory. These procedures are standard in all nuclear medicine services.

The inert gas xenon-133 has also been used to study rCBF. Xe-133 SPECT is performed after the inhalation to the gas and is based on clearance techniques that relate the change in radiotracer activity over time to blood flow [7]. The principal advantage over other tracers that remain in the brain is that rCBF can be measured quantitatively without arterial sampling. Xe-133 does have major limitations including poor spatial resolution and the need for specialized instrumentation. However, SPECT with Xe-133 is of particular interest for research in stroke, where effects related to abnormal perfusion coupled with decreased or increased tissue affinity for other radiotracers can yield SPECT patterns that are difficult to interpret.

SPECT IN STROKE

SPECT has a role in the evaluation of patients with stroke. It can help differentiate an ischemic event from postictal phenomena such as Todd's paresis. Initial data suggest that it may be useful in prognosticating the likelihood of an early stroke after a transient ischemic attack (TIA) and in separating small deep stroke from cortical stroke. After an acute stroke, early SPECT depicts the area of ischemia with greater accuracy than either CT or MR imaging. Reperfusion of an arterial territory after thrombolysis can be documented more easily and safely with SPECT than with angiography. SPECT before and after the injection of acetazolamide has been used to assess the vascular reserve in patients with severe stenosis of the proximal vessels of the cerebrovascular tree. Combined with transcranial Doppler studies, SPECT is useful to document ischemia after subarachnoid hemorrhage (SAH). It has also been used to assess the result of brain perfusion from arterial ligation intended to treat arteriovenous malformations (AVM) or aneurysms.

In many of these clinical situations, the information obtained with SPECT complements that obtained with CT (*eg*, when there is intracranial hemorrhage) and MR imaging/MR angiography, which provide information on structural damage to the brain and cerebral vasculature. Newer MR techniques, such as echo-planar imaging to study brain perfusion, can be used to detect ischemic areas very soon after stroke onset. Examples of the practical application of SPECT in cerebrovascular disease are reviewed below.

NONISCHEMIC NEUROLOGIC DEFICITS

Occasionally, the clinical situation arises of differentiating ischemia from epilepsy as the cause of a neurologic deficit, particularly in cases with a prolonged postictal state. Ischemia will cause an area of hypoperfusion on SPECT, whereas epileptic phenomena are often manifested by hyperperfusion (Figure 10.3). Differentiating ischemia from epilepsy is becoming paramount at a time when thrombolysis and other techniques to treat acute stroke are being evaluated. Increased perfusion of the hemisphere contralateral to the affected limbs has also been reported by SPECT imaging in some cases of infantile alternating hemiplegia [8].

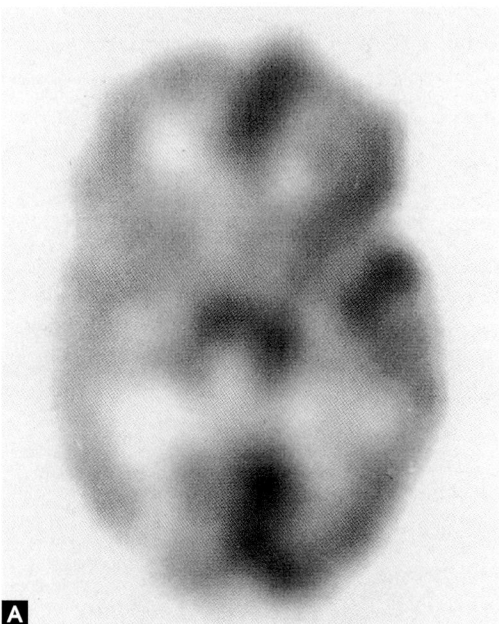

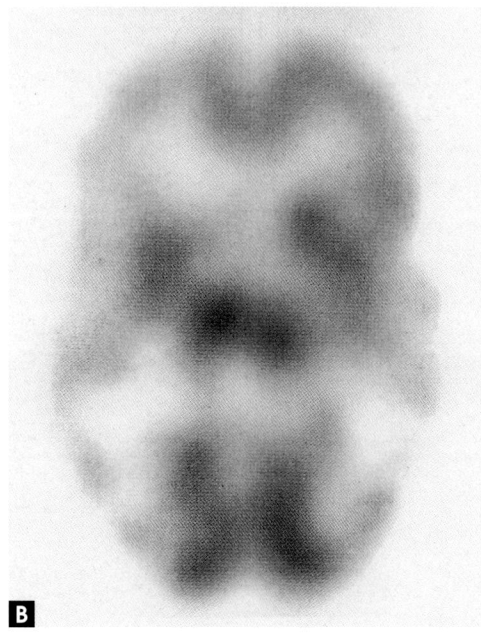

FIGURE 10.3

Peri-ictal hemiplegia. **A**, Axial single photon emission computed tomography (SPECT) showing increased perfusion of the left hemisphere obtained in a 58-year-old woman 26 hours after she was found in the street with a right-sided hemiplegia, global aphasia, and a gaze deviation to the left. Clinical findings persisted at the time of the above SPECT. Computed tomography was negative. Electroencephalogram obtained 12 hours before the SPECT had shown marked slowing over the left hemisphere but no epileptiform activity. Improvement ensued over a 1-week period, when the patient could give a history of having had a seizure disorder since her teens. **B**, Follow-up SPECT after the patient had improved showed symmetrical perfusion of the hemispheres.

TRANSIENT ISCHEMIC ATTACK

SPECT may be useful in identifying patients at especially high risk for stroke following a TIA. Bogousslavsky and coworkers [9] studied 12 patients within a week after a TIA using SPECT. Three of four who had a reduction in CBF of more than 30% suffered subsequent infarction in the first week following the TIA [9]. It is possible that patients with a negative SPECT had a lacunar event whereas those with a positive study were more likely to have experienced embolic ischemia with cortical involvement. Early recurrence is more frequent with embolic disease, often requiring anticoagulation, than with lacunar stroke.

The proportion of SPECT findings after a TIA is time dependent. As many as 60% of TIA patients will have abnormalities if examined on the day of admission, 40% by the second day [10], and the percentage continues to fall during the first week following the event [11]. The sensitivity of SPECT imaging in TIAs can be improved with the addition of reactivity testing with acetazolamide, which may also provide information on the mechanism of ischemia [12]. For instance, failure of perfusion increase in a vascular territory suggests stenosis or occlusion of the artery supplying that territory (Figure 10.4). The ability to identify patients with low flow states due to asymptomatic carotid disease may permit appropriate selection of cases for carotid endarterectomy.

Decreases in cerebrovascular reserve, measured as a diminished dilatory response to CO_2 or acetazolamide, is an indicator of perfusion failure [13]. The long half-life of most of the SPECT agents imposes technical obstacles to this procedure. This can be partially overcome by using multiple injections [12], reduced doses of radionuclides, and applying subtraction techniques [14]. By using two isotopes, a technetium agent for a baseline blood flow measurement, and an iodine agent for a postacetazolamide blood flow measurement, the separate distributions can be measured using two windows on some of the modern three-headed scanners. This greatly simplifies reactivity testing with SPECT and eliminates the need for multiple injections and subtraction techniques [15].

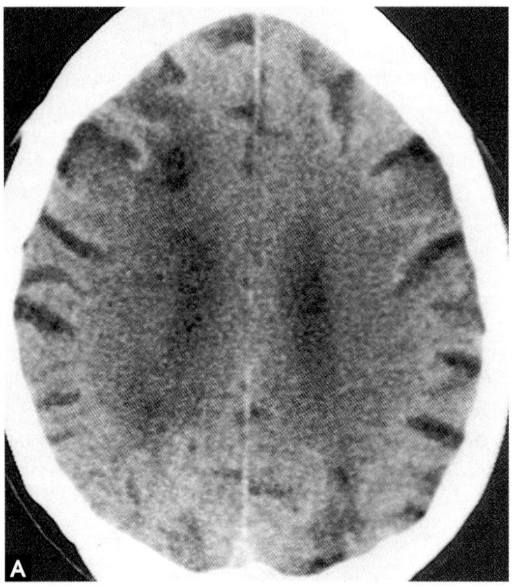

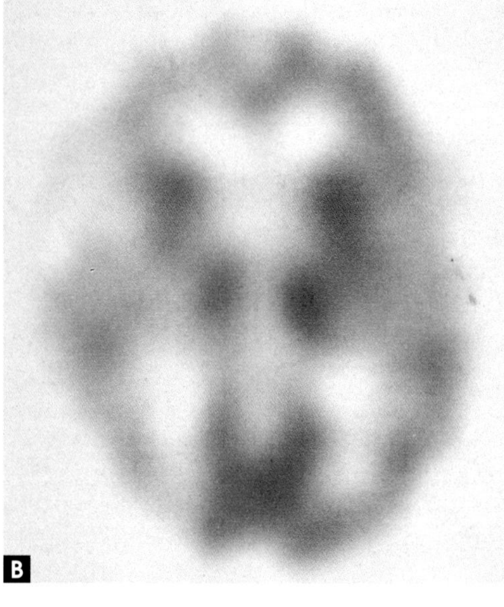

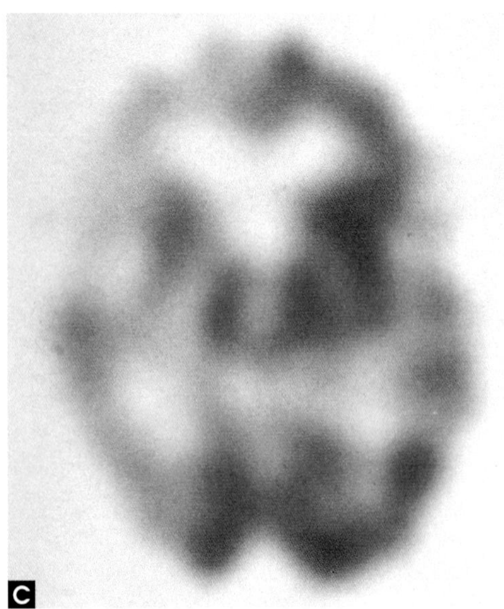

FIGURE 10.4

Use of acetazolamide challenge to assess vascular reserve and differentiate ischemia from diaschisis. **A**, A 51-year-old man had transient left arm weakness. A computed tomography scan showed hypodense areas in the watershed of the left hemispheric white matter. Duplex ultrasound revealed occlusion of the right internal carotid artery at the bifurcation. **B**, Hexamethylpropylamine oxime (HMPAO) single photon emission computed tomography (SPECT) before acetazolamide showed hypoperfusion of the right middle cerebral artery (MCA) territory and the thalamus (usually supplied by the posterior circulation). **C** and **D**, Two days later, SPECT was repeated after oral loading with acetazolamide. The difference between the hemispheres became more obvious. Perfusion of the previously hypoperfused right thalamus became normal (diaschisis), but not in the cortical distribution of the right MCA. Note the sharp difference between the ischemic territory of the MCA and the normal cortex supplied by the posterior cerebral artery from the posterior circulation.

The above-mentioned techniques are still investigational, but preliminary results suggest that reactivity testing may increase the sensitivity of detecting perfusion failure [16] and may have predictive value for early recurrent stroke or first stroke in asymptomatic patients [17,18]. The ability to determine stroke subtype accurately and hemodynamic status with physiologic imaging is likely to become central to the management of patients with cerebrovascular disease in the future [19,20].

ACUTE ISCHEMIC NEUROLOGIC DEFICIT

Precise information on which area of the brain is affected by ischemia cannot always be garnered from clinical features alone [21,22]. Information on localization and extent of the brain lesion can be important for management. For instance, acute anticoagulation is not indicated for lacunar stroke affecting deep structures but is indicated for cardiogenic emboli, which generally cause cortical infarction. Accurate definition of stroke subtype is important for treatment and prediction of recurrence, recovery, and mortality [23–25]. The need to rapidly and accurately differentiate stroke subtypes is becoming increasingly important as more specific stroke therapies evolve. Demonstration of hemodynamically significant carotid stenosis in the setting of an acute infarct may prompt the use of revascularization as opposed to anticoagulation or thrombolytic therapy.

Early after a stroke, CT is helpful to define brain hemorrhage. However, in ischemic stroke, CT is often negative. By 8 hours after an infarction, about 20% of the CT scans will be positive [26,27], whereas nearly 90% of SPECTs will be abnormal (Figure 10.5) [11,27–30]. Similar to PET, the defects seen on SPECT during the acute phase are usually equal to or larger, and better defined, than the lesion depicted by CT [31,32].

Magnetic resonance angiography is helpful to assess the status of major arteries supplying the brain, particularly in hemodynamic stroke due to atherothrombosis, but is less helpful when emboli have travelled distally to occlude the branches of major cerebral vessels [33]. Cortical areas of ischemia can be readily identified on SPECT (Figure 10.6). There are few human studies of MR imaging in acute and subacute stroke [34,35]. Several hours must pass before changes in the

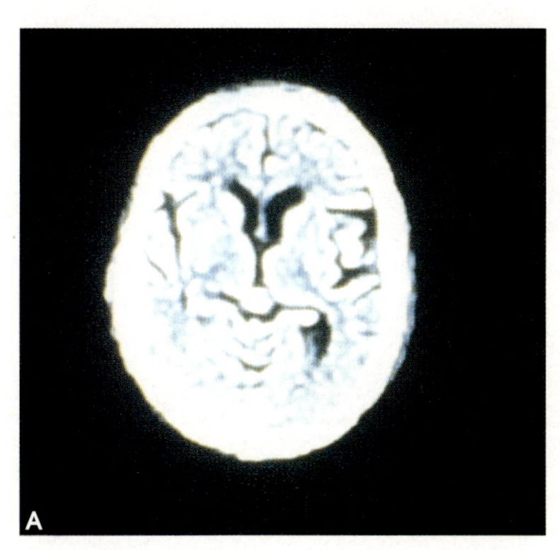

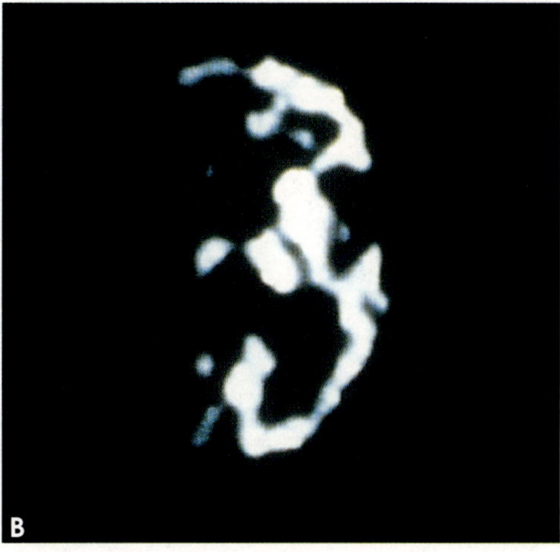

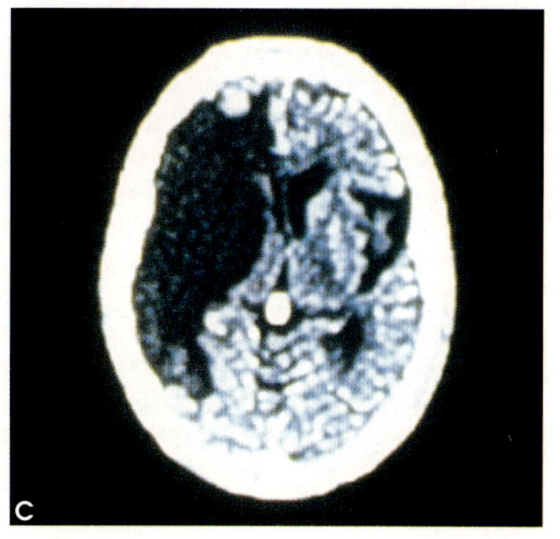

FIGURE 10.5

Acute stroke. Initial computed tomography (CT) (**A**) did not show the lesion, clearly depicted by single photon emission computed tomography (SPECT) (**B**). CT 3 days after stroke showing a large hemispheric infarction (**C**). (*Courtesy of* Dr. RS Tikofsky, Medical College of Wisconsin.)

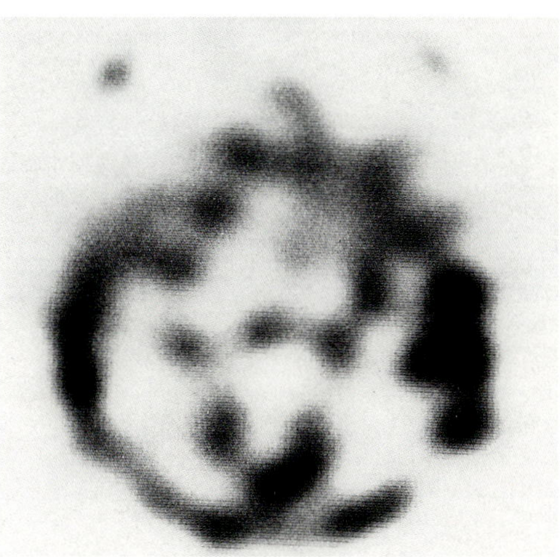

FIGURE 10.6

Cortical branch occlusion. Axial single photon emission computed tomography (SPECT) of a 74-year-old woman with a Wernicke's aphasia. Posterior to an area of hyperperfusion in the perisylvian region, there is an area of hypoperfusion in the posterior extent of the superior temporal and involving the angular gyrus. In this patient, the area of increased perfusion represented compensatory luxury perfusion in the neighboring cortex, rather than granulation tissue, as in Figure 10.8*E*.

water state and volume can be detected by MR imaging [36]. False-negative rates of 7% to 20% have been reported in MR imaging studies for acute stroke and depend on the size of the infarction and the strength of the magnet [35]. Contrast enhancement with Gd-DTPA and other techniques such as flow imaging (dynamic contrast enhancement), diffusion-perfusion studies, sodium imaging, and spectroscopy may improve the sensitivity and specificity of MR imaging during the minutes and hours following the onset of cerebral ischemia [20,37].

Beyond 72 hours the sensitivities of anatomic (CT and MR imaging) and functional imaging (SPECT) are nearly identical [6,38,39]. However, SPECT is more likely to miss lacunar and small deep infarcts, and CT or MR imaging is more likely to miss areas of selective neuronal loss without complete tissue destruction (Figure 10.7).

When interpreting the abnormalities seen on SPECT, it is important to consider the time since the onset of ischemia. Areas initially demonstrating hypoperfusion may be replaced by areas of hyperemia (Figure 10.8). Later, these same areas may again show decreased flow. It may be possible to have a relatively normal appearing scan during the transition between these periods. This is more likely to happen with HMPAO than with the I-123–labeled agents or with bicisate, which are poorly retained in areas of infarction even with inappropriately high flow relative to metabolic requirements.

Another application of SPECT in stroke is for monitoring the effect on cerebral perfusion of different therapeutic interventions (Figure 10.9). For example, in thrombolytic trials, it is important to determine if there is a clot in order to evaluate the effect of the medication. Currently, this requires angiography. If Tc 99m HMPAO is injected at the time of initiation of thrombolytic therapy, a follow-up scan, after the patient has received treatment and has stabilized, can demonstrate the *pretreatment* perfusion defect. Examination of this defect could then be correlated with efficacy of the medication. This application remains to be validated. When recanalization occurs, demonstration of reperfusion by SPECT may occur slowly over several days [40]. The pathophysiology underlying this observation and the implications for evaluating thrombolytic therapy need to be clarified.

Blood flow measurements may also be useful in monitoring currently used therapies. The effects of hemodilution can be quantitated [41]. Indications for the use of anticoagulation may be determined from SPECT studies. Larger infarcts are known to be at higher risk for bleeding complications. In the first days following infarction, SPECT scans accurately estimate the extent of the ischemic area and may help assess the bleeding risk in patients considered for anticoagulation. During anticoagulation, changes in the patency of an artery may also have important therapeutic consequences. Recanalization of large arteries may be associated with higher risk for hemorrhagic transformation. Flow into a previously ischemic area may suggest that lower levels of anticoagulation should be used.

FIGURE 10.7

Migraine-related infarction. Axial single photon emission computed tomography (SPECT) of a 25-year-old woman with classical migraines since age 18 who for 3 years had noted a permanent scotoma on the left visual field, which was detected on testing. Visual-evoked responses and magnetic resonance imaging were normal. SPECT shows an area of hypoperfusion in the vicinity of a hyperperfused area in the right calcarine cortex. Epileptogenic changes could give similar findings.

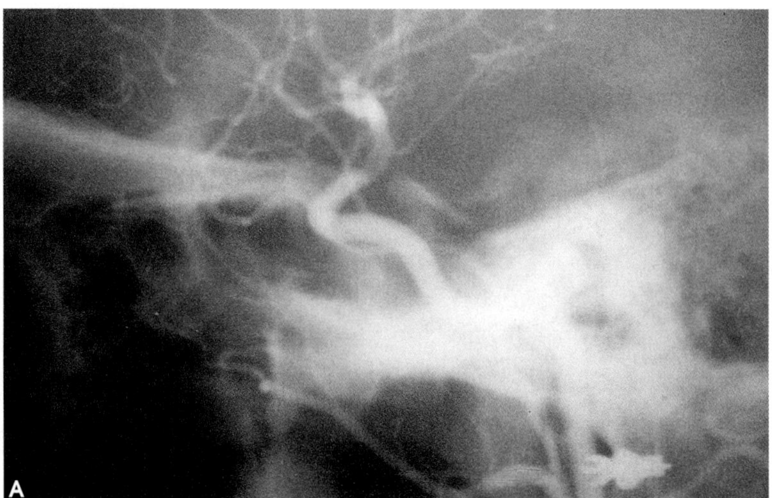

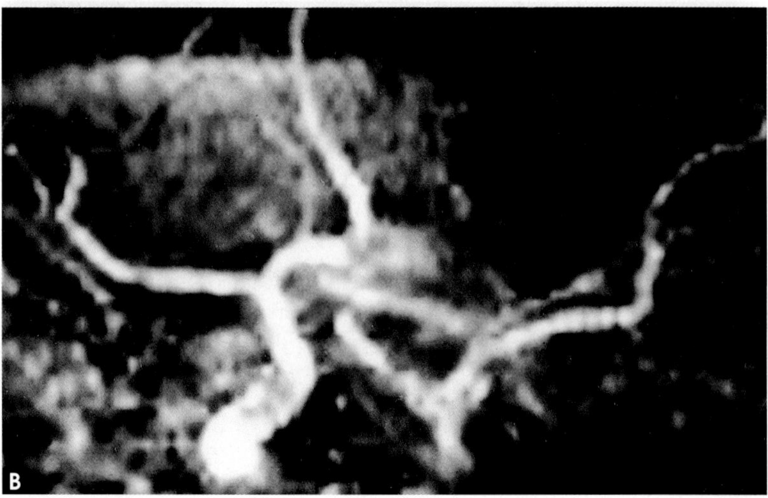

FIGURE 10.8

Acute stroke with late hyperemia. A 23-year-old woman had a left putaminal infarct due to dissection of the supraclinoid portion of the left internal carotid artery, appreciated on lateral angiography (**A**) and, subsequently, on magnetic resonance (MR) angiography (**B**). *(continued)*

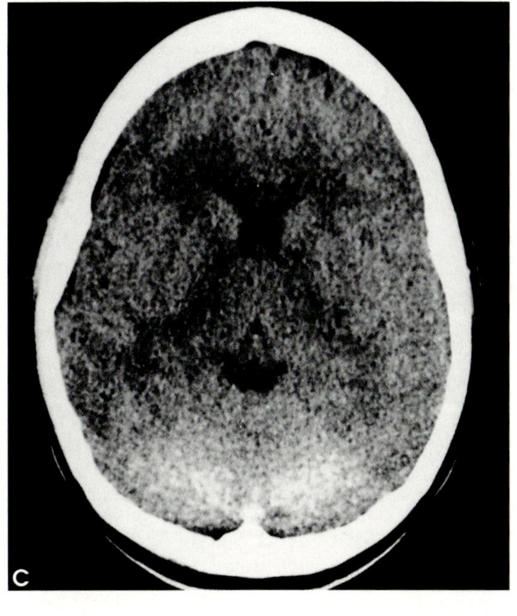

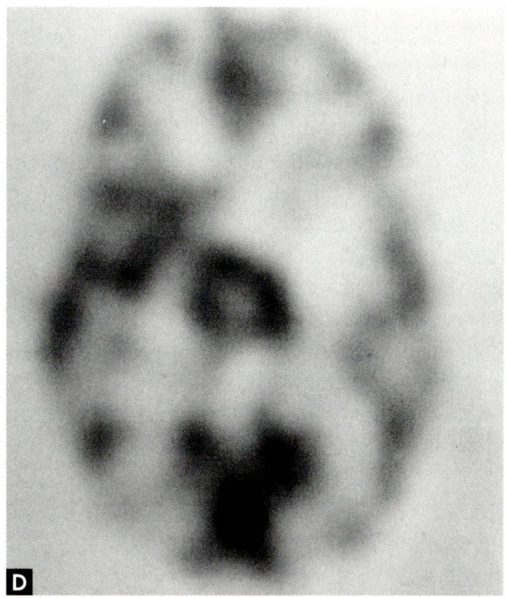

FIGURE 10.8

(*continued*) **C**, Early computed tomography (CT) was negative. **D**, Early single photon emission computed tomography (SPECT) at the same level as the CT showed hypoperfusion of the left basal ganglia and overlying frontal cortex. Repeat SPECT 3 weeks after the event showed an area of hyperperfusion corresponding to the organizing cerebral infarction (**E**), apparent on MR imaging (**F**).

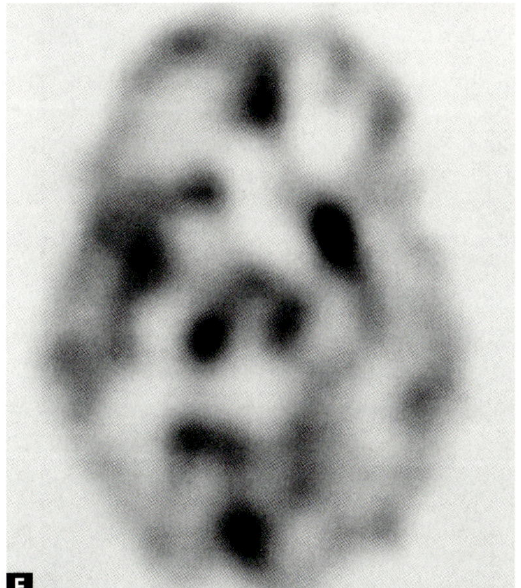

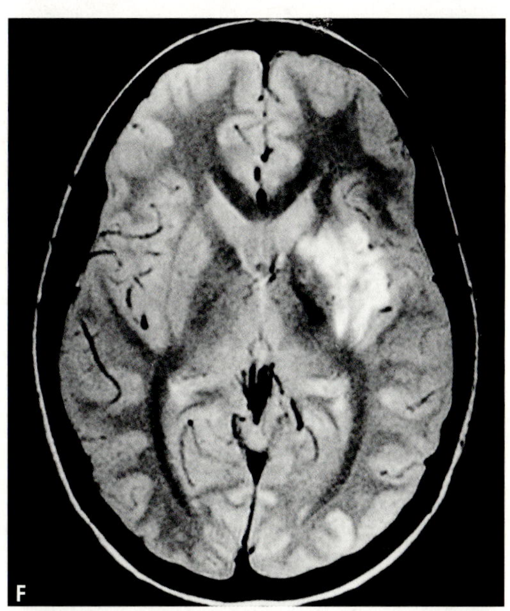

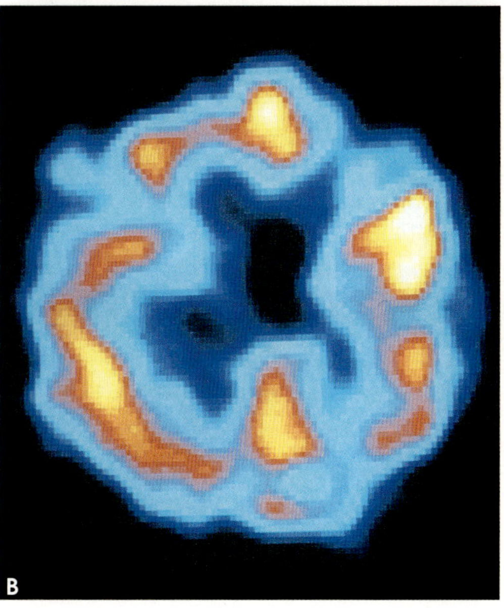

FIGURE 10.9

Thrombolysis after middle cerebral artery (MCA) occlusion. Single photon emission computed tomography (SPECT) obtained before (**A**) and after (**B**) thrombolysis in a 64-year-old woman with an acute left hemispheric infarct. Occlusion and reperfusion of the horizontal portion of the MCA was documented on angiography. (*Courtesy of* L. Brass, Yale University)

Subarachnoid Hemorrhage

Ischemia from vasospasm is a major cause of morbidity and mortality following subarachnoid hemorrhage [42]. In this setting, regional hypoperfusion on SPECT correlates with the presence and severity of delayed neurologic deficits [43]. SPECT facilitates the early diagnosis of cerebral hypoperfusion due to vasospasm and may help in differentiating hypoperfusion from other causes of deterioration after subarachnoid hemorrhage (Figure 10.10). Given that therapies exist for reducing the effects of vasospasm, the application of techniques for early and accurate diagnosis are of obvious importance. Given the ability of SPECT to detect surface ischemia, this technique, when combined with transcranial Doppler, may prove to be a sensitive screen for the early detection of vasospasm and delayed ischemic deficits in an entire hemisphere or an isolated cortical branch [43,44].

SPECT imaging has also been applied to the evaluation of arteriovenous malformations. This has been primarily in the evaluation of cerebrovascular steal both at rest and following acetazolamide administration [45]. The presence of severe steal has prompted staging of the surgical resection and encouraged embolization as a preliminary treatment [46].

ACKNOWLEDGMENT

Dr. Lawrence Brass, from Yale University, provided some of the material for this chapter, both in terms of text and images. Dr. Ronald S. Tikofsky, from the Section of Nuclear Medicine, Medical College of Wisconsin, provided Figures 10.5 and 10.10.

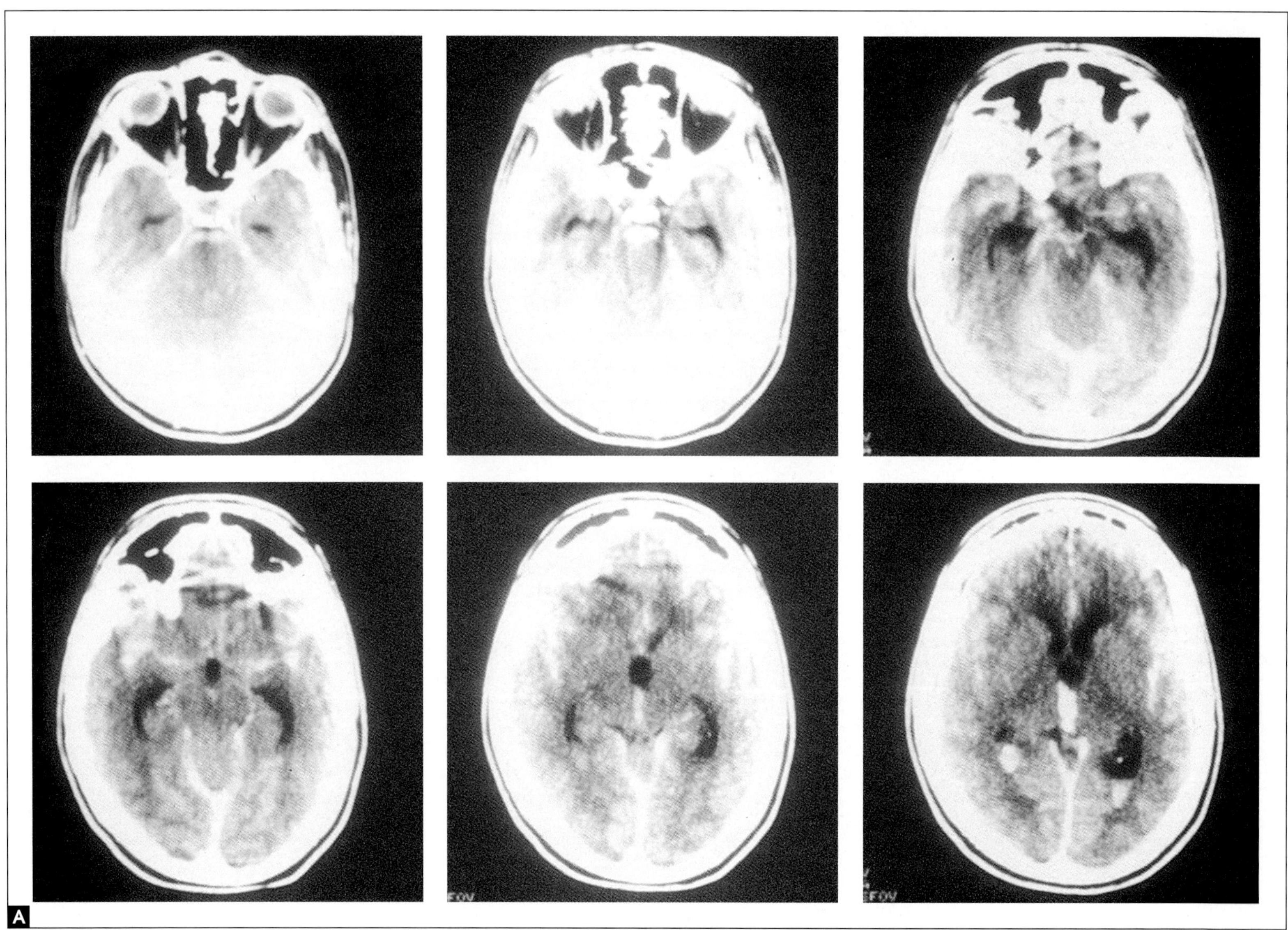

FIGURE 10.10

Vasospasm after subarachnoid hemorrhage. After massive subarachnoid hemorrhage on computed tomography (CT) (**A**), single photon emission computed tomography (SPECT) obtained on day 2 was normal (**B**) (*continued*)

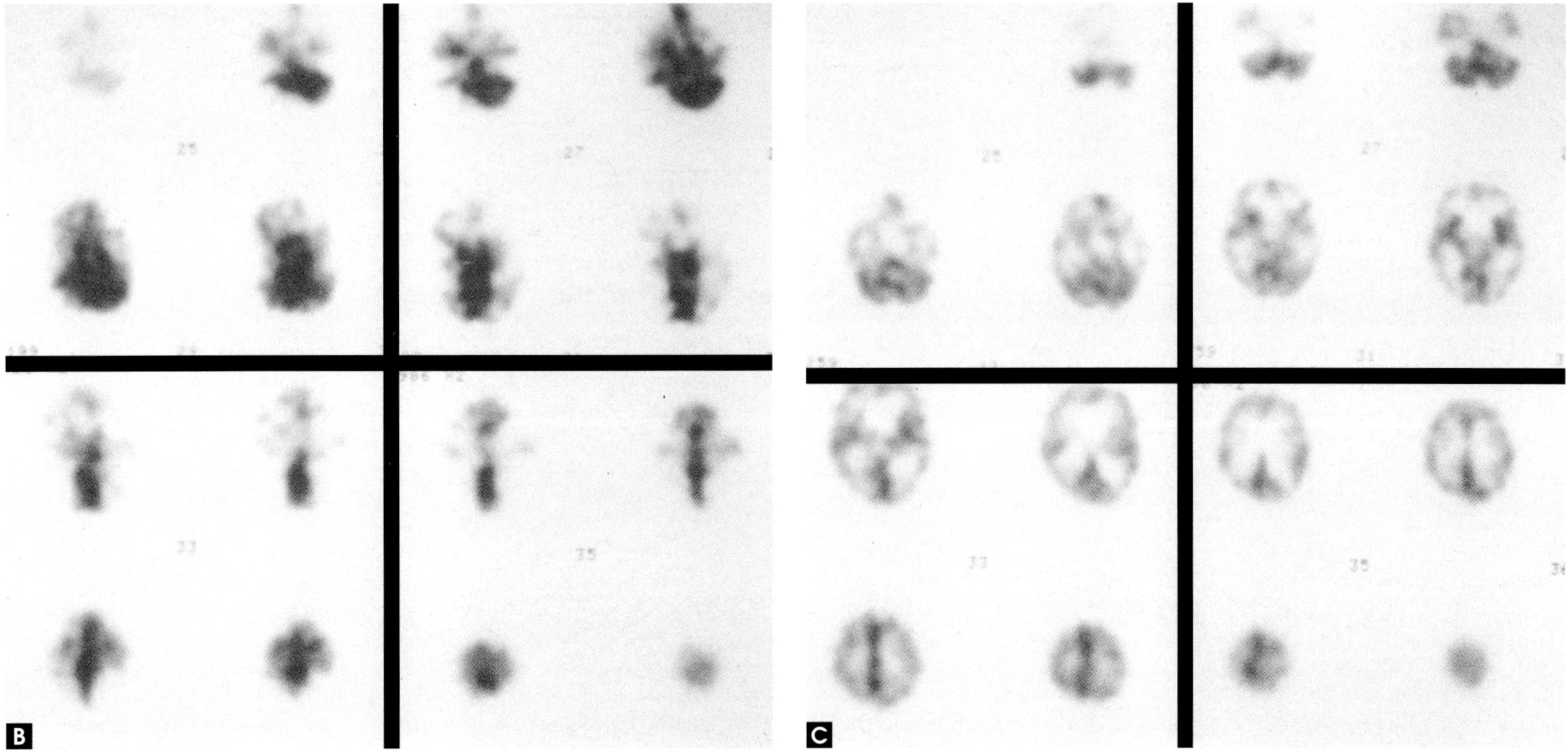

FIGURE 10.10

(*continued*), but SPECT on day 12 shows multiple perfusion defects in the hemispheres, particularly in the parietal watershed areas and in the right cerebellar hemisphere (**C**). (*Courtesy of* RS Tikofsky, Medical College of Wisconsin.)

REFERENCES

1. Piez CW, Holman BL: Single photon emission computed tomography. *Comp Radiology* 1985, 9:201–211.
2. English RJ, Brown SE, eds: *Single Photon Emission Computed Tomography: A Primer.* Second ed. New York: Society of Nuclear Medicine; 1990.
3. Kung HF: New technetium-99m-labeled brain perfusion imaging agents. *Semin Nucl Med* 1990, 20:150–158.
4. Kuhl DE, Barrco JR, Huang SC, *et al.*: Quantifying local cerebral blood flow *N*-isopropyl-p-I-123 iodoamphetamine (IMP) tomography. *J Nucl Med* 1982, 23:196–203.
5. Neirinckx RD, Canning LR, Piper IM, *et al.*: Technetium-99m d,1-HM-PAO: a new radiopharmaceutical for SPECT imaging of regional cerebral blood perfusion. *J Nucl Med* 1987, 28:191–202.
6. Holman BL, Hellman RS, Goldsmith SJ, *et al.*: Biodistribution, dosimetry, and clinical evaluation of technetium-99m ethyl cysteinate dimer in normal subjects and in patients with chronic cerebral infarction. *J Nucl Med* 1989, 30:1018–1024.
7. Devous MD, Stokey EM, Bonte FJ: Quantitative imaging of regional cerebral blood flow by dynamic single-photon tomography. In *Radionuclide Imaging of the Brain.* Edited by Holman BL. New York: Churchill Livingstone Inc.; 1985:135–162.
8. Aminian A, Strashun A, Rose A: Alternating hemiplegia of childhood: studies of regional cerebral blood flow using ^{99m}Tc-hexamethylpropylene amine oxime single-photon emission computed tomography. *Ann Neurol* 1993, 33:43–47.
9. Bogousslavsky J, Delaloye-Bischof A, Regli F, Delaloye B: Prolonged hypoperfusion and early stroke after transient ischemic attack. *Stroke* 1990, 21:40–46.
10. Hartmann A: Prolonged disturbances of regional cerebral blood flow in transient ischemic attacks. *Stroke* 1985, 16:932–939.
11. De Roo M, Mortelmans L, Devos P, *et al.*: Clinical experience with Tc-99m HM PAO high resolution SPECT of the brain in patients with cerebrovascular accidents. *Eur J Nucl Med* 1989, 15:9–15.
12. Chollet F, Celsis P, Clanet M, *et al.*: SPECT study of cerebral blood flow reactivity after acetazolamide in patients with transient ischemic attacks. *Stroke* 1989, 20:458–464.
13. Bonte FJ, Devous MDS, Reisch JS, *et al.*: The effect of acetazolamide on regional cerebral blood flow in patients with Alzheimer's disease or stroke as measured by single-photon emission computed tomography. *Invest Radiol* 1989, 24:99–103.
14. Momose T, Kosaka N, Nishikawa J, *et al.*: A new method for brain function study using Tc-99m HMPAO SPECT. *Radiation Med* 1989, 7:82–87.
15. Devous MD, Gassaway SK: Simultaneous SPECT imaging of Tc-99m- and I-123 labeled brain agents in patients using the PRISM scanner. *J Nucl Med* 1990, 31:877.
16. Burt RW, Witt RM, Cikrit DF, Reddy RV: Carotid artery disease: evaluation with acetazolamide-enhanced Tc-99m HMPAO SPECT. *Radiology* 1992, 182:461–466.
17. Cikrit DF, Burt RW, Dalsing MC, *et al.*: Acetazolamide enhanced single photon emission computed tomography (SPECT) evaluation of cerebral perfusion before and after carotid endarterectomy. *J Vasc Surg* 1992, 15:747–753.
18. Hasegawa Y, Yamaguchi T, Tsuchiya T, *et al.*: Sequential change of hemodynamic reserve in patients with major cerebral artery occlusion or severe stenosis. *Neuroradiology* 1992, 34:15–21.
19. Weiller C, Ringelstein EB, Reiche W, Buell U: Clinical and hemodynamic aspects of low-flow infarcts. *Stroke* 1991, 22:1117–1123.
20. Prichard JW, Brass LM: New anatomic and functional imaging methods. *Ann Neurol* 1992, 32:395–400.

21. Foulkes MA, Wolf PA, Price TR, *et al.*: The national stroke data bank: design, methods, and baseline characteristics. *Stroke* 1988, 19:547–554.
22. Mohr JP, Barnett HJM: Classification of ischemic stroke. In *Stroke.* Edited by Barnett HJM, Stein BM, Mohr JP, Yatsu FM. New York: Churchill Livingstone Inc; 1986:281–291.
23. Bogousslavsky J, Regli F: Borderzone infarctions distal to internal carotid artery occlusion: prognostic implications. *Ann Neurol* 1986, 20:346–350.
24. Schroder T: Hemodynamic significance of internal carotid artery disease. *Acta Neurol Scand* 1988, 77:353–372.
25. Sacco RL, Foulkes MA, Mohr JP, *et al.*: Determinants of early recurrence of cerebral infarction: Stroke Data Bank. *Stroke* 1989, 20:983–989.
26. Fieschi C, Argentino C, Lenzi GL, *et al.*: Clinical and instrumental evaluation of patients with ischemic stroke within the first six hours. *J Neurol Sci* 1989, 91:311–322.
27. Bose A, Pacia SV, Fayad P, *et al.*: Cerebral blood flow (CBF) imaging compared to CT during the initial 24 hours of cerebral infarction. *Neurology* 1990, 40(suppl 1):190.
28. Podreka I, Suess E, Goldenberg G, *et al.*: Initial experience with technetium-99m HM PAO brain SPECT. *J Nucl Med* 1987, 28:1657–1666.
29. Yeh SH, Liu RS, Hu HH, *et al.*: Brain SPECT imaging with Tc-99m hexamethylpropyleneamine oxime in the early detection of cerebral infarction: comparison with transmission computed tomography. *Nucl Med Commun* 1986, 7:873–878.
30. de Bruine JF, Limburg M, van Royen EA, *et al.*: SPECT brain imaging with 201 diethyldithiocarbamate in acute ischemic stroke. *Eur J Nucl Med* 1990, 17:248–251.
31. Berberich A, Buell U, Eclles A, *et al.*: Tc-99m hexamethylpropyleneamine oxide (HMPAO) SPECT in cerebrovascular disease (CVD). A comparison to transmission CT. *Radiology* 1986, 158:729–734.
32. Lee RG, Hill TC, Holman BL, Clouse ME: *N*-isopropyl-(I-123) p-iodoamphetamine brain scans with single-photon emission tomography: discordance with transmission computed tomography. *Radiology* 1982, 145:795–799.
33. Caplan L, Allam G, Teal P: The moving embolus. *J Neuroimag* 1993, 3:195–197.
34. Ramadan NM, Deveshwar R, Levine SR: Magnetic resonance and clinical cerebrovascular disease: an update. *Stroke* 1989, 20:1279–1283.
35. Alberts MJ, Faulstich ME, Gray L: Stroke with negative brain magnetic resonance imaging. *Stroke* 1992, 23:663–667.
36. Moseley ME, Cohen Y, Mintorovitch J, *et al.*: Early detection of regional cerebral ischemia in cats: comparison of diffusion- and T2-weighted MRI and spectroscopy. *Magnetic Reson Med* 1990, 14:330–346.
37. Fisher M, Sotak CH, Minematsu K, Li L: New magnetic resonance techniques for evaluating cerebrovascular disease. *Ann Neurol* 1992, 32:115–122.
38. Brott TG, Gelfand MJ, Williams CG, *et al.*: Frequency and patterns of abnormality detected by iodine-123 amine emission CT after cerebral infarction. *Radiology* 1986, 158:729–734.
39. Seiderer M, Krappel W, Moser E, *et al.*: Detection and quantification of chronic cerebrovascular disease: comparison of MR imaging, SPECT, and CT. *Radiology* 1989, 170:545–548.
40. Companioni JM, Lassen NA, Tfelt-Hansen P, Friberg L: Delayed reflow of an ischemic infarct after spontaneous thrombolysis studied by CBF tomography using SPECT and Tc-99m HMPAO. *Am J Physiol Imag* 1991, 6:167–171.
41. Vorstrup S, Andersen A, Juhler M, *et al.*: Hemodilution increases cerebral blood flow in acute ischemic stroke. *Stroke* 1989, 20:884–889.
42. Biller J, Godersky JC, Adams HC: Management of aneurysmal subarachnoid hemorrhage. *Stroke* 1988, 23:13–18.
43. Davis SM, Andrews JT, Lichtenstein M, *et al.*: Correlations between cerebral arterial velocities, blood flow, and delayed ischemia after subarachnoid hemorrhage. *Stroke* 1992, 23:492–497.
44. Caplan LR, Brass LM, DeWitt LD, *et al.*: Transcranial Doppler ultrasound: present status. *Neurology* 1990, 40:696–700.
45. Batjer HH, Devous MDS: The use of acetazolamide-enhanced regional cerebral blood flow measurement to predict the risk of arteriovenous malformation patients. *Neurosurgery* 1992, 31:213–217.
46. Batjer HH, Devous MD, Seibert GB, *et al.*: Intracranial arteriovenous malformation: relationships between clinical and radiological factors and ipsilateral steal severity. *Neurosurgery* 1989, 23:322–328.

Chapter 11

Echocardiography in the Assessment of Cerebrovascular Events

PHILIP R. LIEBSON
JEFFREY S. SOBLE
ALEXANDER L. NEUMANN

Because up to 20% of all strokes are associated with cardiac embolic sources [1–4], the role of echocardiography is paramount in evaluation of the heart after transient ischemic events or stroke. Transthoracic echocardiography (TTE) has been the most widely applied cardiac imaging procedure, but transesophageal echocardiography (TEE) allows higher resolution and better visualization of structures obscure to the transthoracic approach. This discussion will focus on the use of echocardiographic techniques to evaluate the presence of the most common causes of cardiac embolic events leading to stroke, including the detection of sources of arterial emboli from the ascending and transverse thoracic aorta (Figure 11.1).

The most likely cardiac precursors of embolic stroke include atrial fibrillation, mitral stenosis, acute myocardial infarction and ventricular aneurysm, and prosthetic cardiac valves (Tables 11.1 and 11.2) [5,6]. Other conditions in which cardiogenic embolic strokes can occur include paradoxic embolization through an atrial septal defect or patent foramen ovale, atrial septal aneurysm, aortic arch disease, left atrial myxoma, mitral valve prolapse, endocarditis, calcific aortic stenosis, and mitral annular calcification [7]. We will discuss the usefulness of TTE and TEE in identifying these abnormalities.

The frequency of cardiac embolic stroke varies with age, gender, and the presence of apparent clinical cardiac disease [2,8,9]. On the basis of the clinical characteristics of the cerebrovascular event, criteria have been recommended as evidence supporting a cardiogenic source of brain embolus [1,7,10]. These include evidence for potential cardiac sources listed above, minimal carotid atherosclerosis by ultrasound evaluation, nonla-

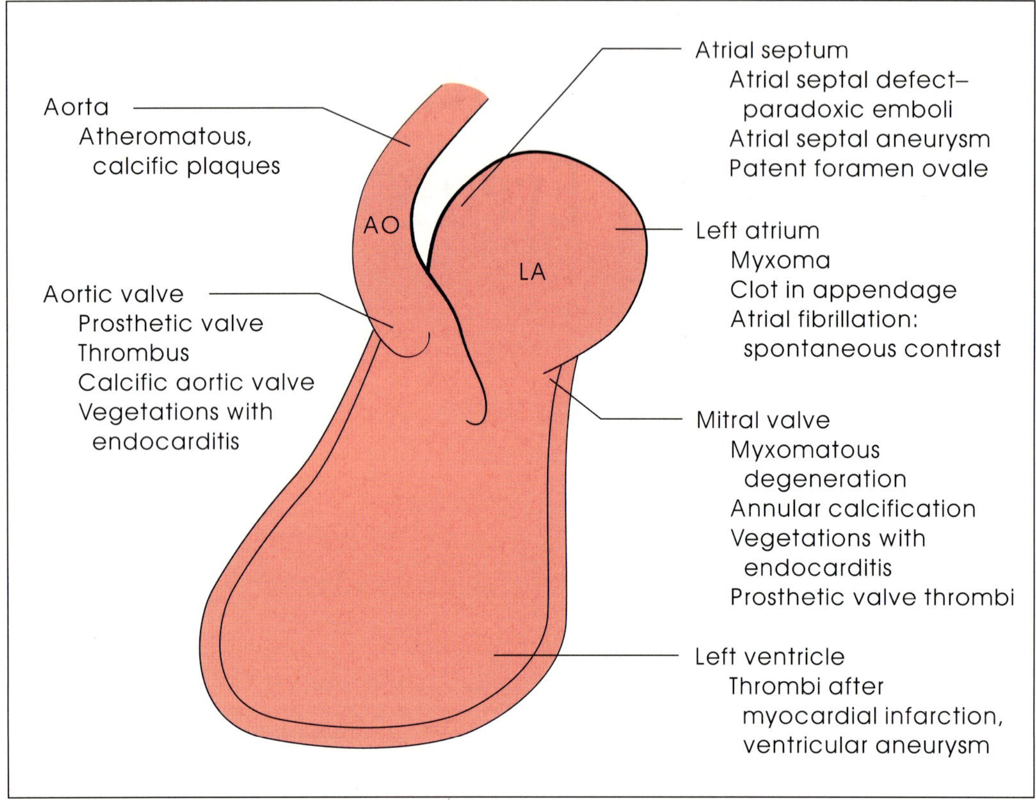

FIGURE 11.1

Location of the major abnormalities in the heart that may be associated with the cerebral embolization. Ao–aorta; LA–left atrium.

Table 11.1. Major and minor risk for cardiogenic embolism

Major
Prosthetic valve
Mitral stenosis
Atrial fibrillation
Recent myocardial infarction
Infective endocarditis
Left ventricular aneurysm
Dilated cardiomyopathy
Left ventricular thrombus
Minor
Mitral valve prolapse
Mitral annular calcification
Atrial septal aneurysm
Calcific aortic stenosis
Patent foramen ovale
Atrial septal defect

Table 11.2. Causes of cardiac sources of cerebral embolic events*

Cause	All events, %
Nonvalvular atrial fibrillation	45
Acute myocardial infarction	15
Ventricular arrhythmia	10
Prosthetic aortic, mitral valve	10
Rheumatic heart disease	10
Miscellaneous	10
Atrial myxoma, mitral valve prolapse, mitral annulus calcification, paradoxic embolism, endocarditis, aortic atheroma, clot, calcific aortic stenosis, dilated cardiomyopathy, ventricular aneurysm	

*From Cerebral Embolism Task Force [1]; with permission.

Table 11.3. Advantages of transthoracic (TTE) and transesophageal (TEE) echocardiography for cardiac sources of embolism*

Better defined by TEE	Usually seen by TTE
Prosthetic valve vegetations	Myxomatous mitral valve prolapse
Left atrial appendage clot	Large aortic and mitral valve vegetations
Spontaneous contrast in left atrium	Aortic and mitral stenosis
Small valvular vegetations	Mitral annular calcification
Aortic arch atheroma and thrombi	Left ventricular wall motion abnormalities
Patent foramen ovale, atrial septal defect	Left ventricular thickness
Atrial septal aneurysm	Dilated cardiomyopathy
Atrial myxoma	

*From Hart [7]; with permission.

cunar infarct, or possibly, lacunar infarct without evidence for diabetes or hypertension.

The establishment of a possible cardiac source of embolus does not rule out the presence of cerebrovascular disease itself as a cause. Approximately 25% of patients with cerebrovascular events and a possible cardiac source of embolus may have other potential sources of stroke [2,4]. For example, 10% to 20% of stroke patients with a presumed cardiac source of embolus have significant carotid stenosis [4]. Approximately one third of patients with an ischemic stroke have a potential cardiac source of embolus on the basis of echocardiography [5].

Methods other than echocardiography should be considered in the assessment of stroke patients with cardiac embolic sources. These include computed tomography (CT) and magnetic resonance (MR) imaging scanning of the heart. Echocardiography has the advantage of versatility, rapidity of assessment, and noninvasive approach, with little or no risk.

CLINICAL PERSPECTIVES IN THE EVALUATION OF CARDIAC SOURCE OF EMBOLISM

TTE may provide excellent visualization for diagnosis of left ventricular thrombus, mitral annular calcification, mitral and aortic valvular vegetation, and myxomatous mitral valve with prolapse. The disadvantages of TTE include inability to visualize adequately the left atrial appendage, incomplete evaluation of the interatrial septal defects, which are potential conduits for paradoxic embolism, and limited visibility of vegetations or valve disruption with prosthetic valves in the mitral or aortic position. These are situations in which TEE study appears to provide additional information [11]. Thus, these include the diagnosis of atrial appendage thrombus, evaluation of atrial septal defect, patent foramen ovale and atrial septal aneurysm, presence of small vegetations of the aortic and mitral valve as well as clot formation, and plaque formation in the ascending aorta and aortic arch. Because of its increased sensitivity compared with TTE, TEE is preferable as a cardiac imaging technique for evaluation of possible cardiac embolic sources for cerebrovascular events [3]. Discomfort to the patient and added cost of the procedure are disadvantages of TEE.

On the other hand, TEE, although a semi-invasive technique, provides higher frequency resolution and allows excellent visualization of the left atrium and atrial appendage, which may be visualized in 98% of subjects [3,12]. Biplane technique allows visualization of the ascending aorta for determining potential aortic sources for cerebrovascular events. A comparison of the advantages of transthoracic and transesophageal approaches is noted in Table 11.3.

Transesophageal echocardiography is accomplished by first anesthetizing the throat using a topical spray, and providing small doses of an intravenous amnestic agent. An endoscope is inserted into the mouth, swallowed, and positioned in the esophagus or stomach. A variety of views of the heart can be accomplished in a period of 10 to 15 minutes. Agitated saline injected into an antecubital vein by means of an intravenous indwelling catheter during the study will allow demonstration of even small atrial septal defects or patent foramen ovale by producing microbubbles that are echogenic and indicate blood flow patterns. During the study, a Valsalva maneuver is performed to increase the sensitivity of the test for right-to-left interatrial shunting. TEE can be accomplished in over 98% of patients by experienced operators [13]. There is evidence that TEE improves diagnostic yield over TTE by two to 10 times with regard to potential cardiac sources of embolism [13].

The yield of echocardiography, whether transthoracic or transesophageal, depends on the mode of selection of patients. In a series of unselected patients hospitalized for stroke, various yields have been obtained. In one group, none of the patients without clinical evidence of heart disease had a specific embolic source identified [14]. In another report of patients with cerebral ischemic events selected for either having had a cardiac embolic mechanism suspected or no probable mechanism for ischemia identified prior to echocardiography (*eg*, extracranial arterial disease, arteritis, or hematologic abnormalities), 6.5% had an intracardiac thrombus, 23% had potential cardiac embolic mechanism, and 70% had no cardiac abnormalities that could be construed as causing the cardiac embolism [15]. In a more select group referred for evaluation for cardiac embolism involving TTE, 40% had cardiac abnormalities that could possibly be a cause of cardiac embolism [16]. Use of TEE increased the yield to 58%.

Transesophageal echocardiography has markedly increased the yield for the detection of atrial thrombi [17]. A meta-analysis by Mugge and coworkers [12] of those patients with suspected cardiogenic embolism or atrial fibrillation demonstrated the presence of left atrial cavity thrombi in 7% and atrial appendage thrombi in 12% of patients subsequently proven by angiography, surgery, or autopsy [12]. TEE may also be an adjunct to patients with suspected mitral valve prolapse, a condition in which cardiac embolic cerebrovascular events may be increased, especially in the younger population. In one study, TEE showed cardiac pathologic findings in 45% of patients with normal transthoracic echocardiograms and showed evidence for mitral valve prolapse in some patients in which TTE was normal [18].

Transesophageal echocardiography identified the potential cardiac source of embolism in 57% of a study group presenting with unexplained stroke or transient ischemic attack (TIA) [13]. Only 15% of this group had a potential cardiac source using TTE. Three cardiac conditions in which TEE demonstrated abnormalities when transthoracic diagnosis was virtually absent were patent foramen ovale, left atrial thrombus, and left atrial spontaneous contrast. TEE identified one or more of these findings in 18 of 79 patients, TTE in only one. In patients with no clinical heart disease, diagnostic yield for potential cardiac sources of emboli in cerebral ischemia using TEE was almost 40%. Another study using TEE revealed potential cardiac sources of embolism in 41% of patients, of whom 27% had no clinical cardiovascular abnormalities. This compared with only 14% diagnostic yield by TTE [19].

Other situations in which TEE may provide insights into potential sources of cerebrovascular emboli include the diagnosis of ascending aortic dissection, aortic valve thickening, and mass lesions of mitral annulus or leaflets.

A review of TEE in the evaluation of stroke concluded that TEE was especially helpful in patients with stroke who were less than 45 years of age and in those without clinical evidence of heart disease [20]. Although TEE may be especially helpful in diagnosis of patent foramen ovale, spontaneous echocardiographic contrast in the left atrium, atrial septal aneurysm, and aortic atherosclerotic debris, these diagnoses are less likely to be associated with cerebrovascular events than intracardiac masses such as thrombi, myxomas, or vegetations. This concern is especially relevant to patients with cerebrovascular events who had no clinical cardiac disease. There are few guidelines for treatment in these cases, aside from the use of anticoagulants with intracardiac thrombi. Nonetheless, it is advisable to document the presence of these abnormalities until such time as prospective studies indicate beneficial effects of intervention in their presence.

SPECIFIC CARDIAC CONDITIONS

Atrial Fibrillation

The presence of atrial fibrillation is associated with increased stroke risk even in the absence of valvular deformity, as in rheumatic heart disease [10]. With atrial fibrillation, the incidence of TIAs or strokes, whether clinically apparent or silent, may be as high as 8% a year in patients over 60 years of age [2,21]. Nonrheumatic atrial fibrillation is most common in the elderly [22,23]. The value of echocardiography in apparent atrial fibrillation is the determination of either sluggish intra-atrial blood flow or atrial clot, both of which may be associated with increased risk for embolic strokes (Figures 11.2–11.4) [24–27]. Nonvalvular atrial fibrillation is associated with cerebral embolic events and accounts for almost half of cardiogenic embolic strokes [6]. Whether atrial fibrillation is associated with valvular disease or not, evidence for clot in the left atrium, including the left atrial appendage, appears to increase the risk for embolic events [26]. In examining Framingham data over 34 years of follow-up, Wolf and coworkers [23] assessed the independent predictability of nonrheumatic atrial fibrillation, hypertension, cardiac failure, and clinical coronary disease as risk predictors for stroke. The presence of atrial fibrillation increased the risk fivefold compared with the absence of this arrhythmia. This compares with only a twofold increase in coronary artery

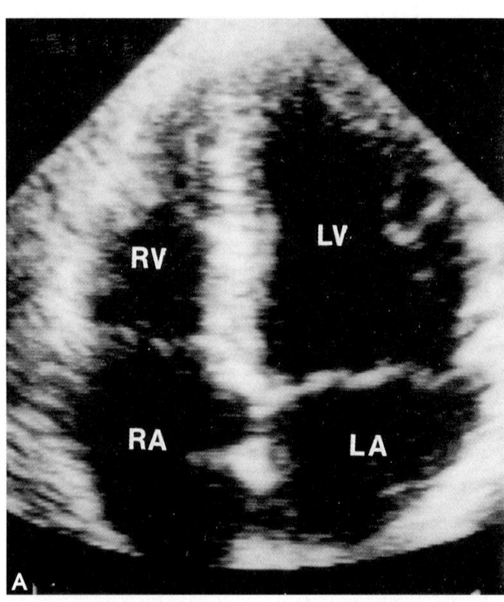

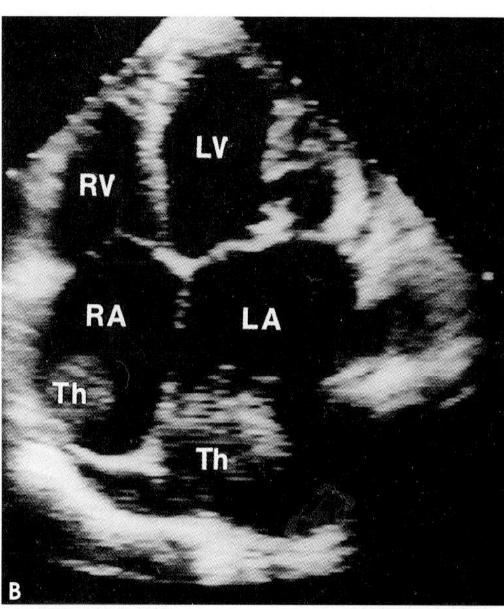

FIGURE 11.2

A, Transthoracic apical four-chamber (4C) view in ventricular systole. **B**, Similar 4C view showing right atrium (RA) and left atrium (LA) thrombi (Th). LV—left ventricle; RV—right ventricle.

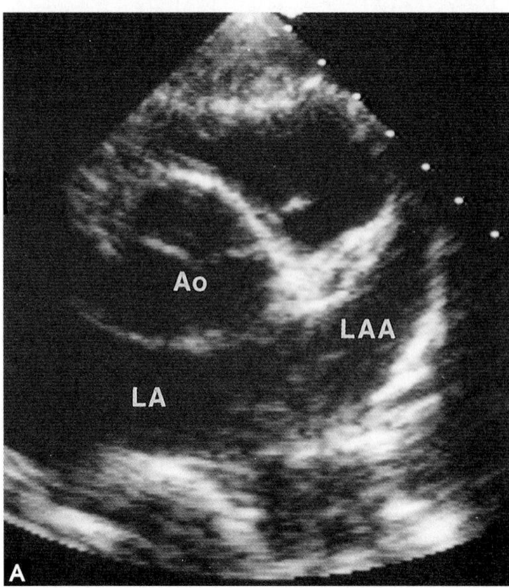

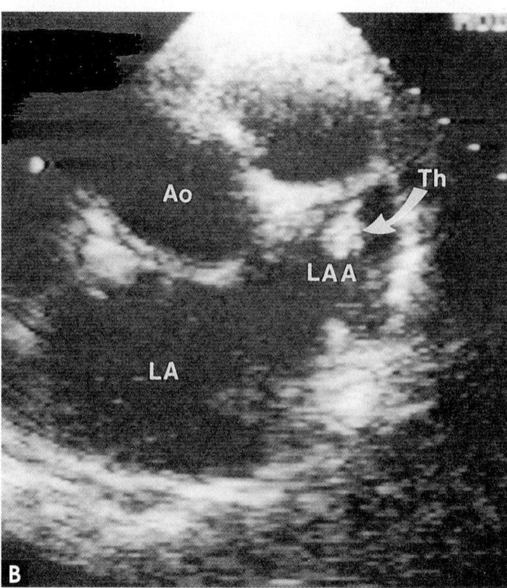

FIGURE 11.3

A, Transthoracic (TT) short axis view showing normal left atrium (LA) and left atrial appendage (LAA). **B**, Thrombus (Th) (*arrow*) in the LAA. The sensitivity for detection of LAA thrombi using TT views is very low, however. Ao—aorta.

disease, a threefold increase with hypertension, and a fourfold increase with cardiac failure compared with the respective absence of these conditions.

Meta-analysis of pooled studies indicates that TEE has increased the detection of left atrial thrombi especially those in the left atrial appendage [12]. The sensitivity of TTE is relatively low, 30% to 70%, for the detection of left atrial thrombi in suspected cardiogenic embolism (Figures 11.2 and 11.3) [17]. Thus, only approximately 3% of patients with suspected cardiogenic embolism were found to have left atrial appendage thrombi determined by TTE.

The sensitivity of TEE for the presence of left atrial thrombi is close to 100%, especially if biplane studies are used [3]. There are some pitfalls in that pectinate muscle scalloping within the appendage wall may be confused with thrombotic material [12].

Spontaneous echo contrast (SEC) is a smoke-like appearance of a chamber, usually associated with stasis and frequently found in the atria in atrial fibrillation (Figure 11.4). SEC has been associated with previous stroke or peripheral embolism in patients with atrial fibrillation, and may be seen also in mitral stenosis whether or not atrial fibrillation is present [24,25]. One study evaluating patients with mitral stenosis or atrial fibrillation demonstrated that the presence or absence of SEC in the left atrium was associated with a significantly higher 1-year incidence of stroke or peripheral embolism, the relative risk being as high as 10.6 with spontaneous contrast present [24].

Transesophageal echocardiography provides a better evaluation of SEC than TTE (Figure 11.4). Doppler evaluation of the flow in the atrial appendage may indicate risk for clot formation in the appendage [26]. It is possible that echocardiographic evidence for SEC may cause the physician to consider pharmacologic treatment using agents that have been reported to lower fibrinogen, such as ticlopidine, pentoxyfylline, propranolol, and nisoldipine [25].

Ischemic Heart Disease

Myocardial infarction and its consequences have constituted some of the more common associates with embolic stroke. It has been estimated that acute myocardial infarction and ventricular aneurysm, taken together, constitute up to 25% of all embolic stroke from cardiac sources [1]. Since acute myocardial infarction may be virtually asymptomatic in 10% to 20% of individuals, and ventricular aneurysm itself usually does not present with acute symptoms or signs, these diagnoses should be considered in the older age group even without clinical symptoms of ischemic heart disease. TTE is usually effective in demonstrating ventricular aneurysm and the presence of clot.

It is estimated that about 3% of patients with acute myocardial infarction experience ischemic stroke within 4 weeks, especially during the first 2 weeks following myocardial infarction [1,2]. These are predominantly in association with transmural anterior myocardial infarction and can be attributed to the presence of mural thrombi in the left ventricle in up to 35% of patients with transmural infarcts [28,29]. As many as 20% of patients with anterior myocardial infarction and mural thrombus may experience stroke within 4 weeks after infarct.

Left ventricular thrombi usually develop between 1 and 7 days following onset of myocardial infarction (Figure 11.5 and 11.6). Although 2-D echocardiography is highly specific for the detection of intracardiac thrombi, occasional technical difficulty can be found with TEE insofar as the left ventricular apex may not be clearly visualized because of position of the left ventricular in relation to the transducer. Ultrafast cardiac CT has been shown to be effective in providing additional information in these cases.

Since patients with ventricular aneurysms who experience cerebral ischemia may have other potential causes, such as arterial atheromatous disease, the relationship of the ventricular

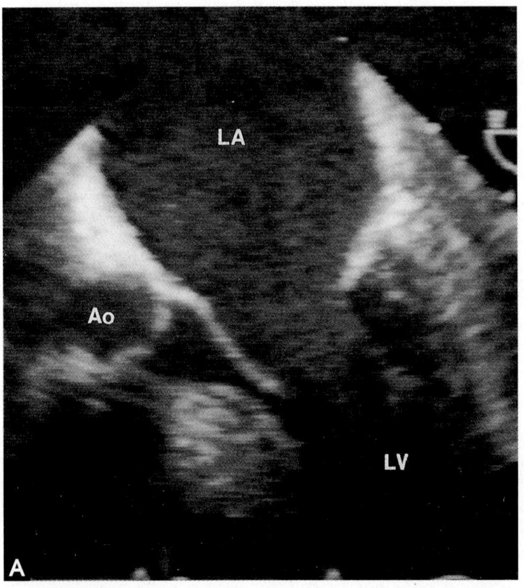

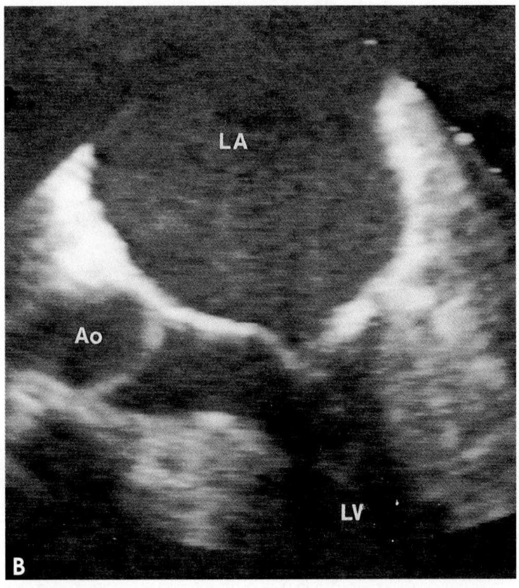

FIGURE 11.4

Transesophageal echo showing spontaneous echo contrast in the left atrium (LA). **A**, Ventricular diastole. Note mitral valve leaflets open. **B**, Ventricular systole. Note mitral valve leaflets closed. Ao—aorta; LV—left ventricle.

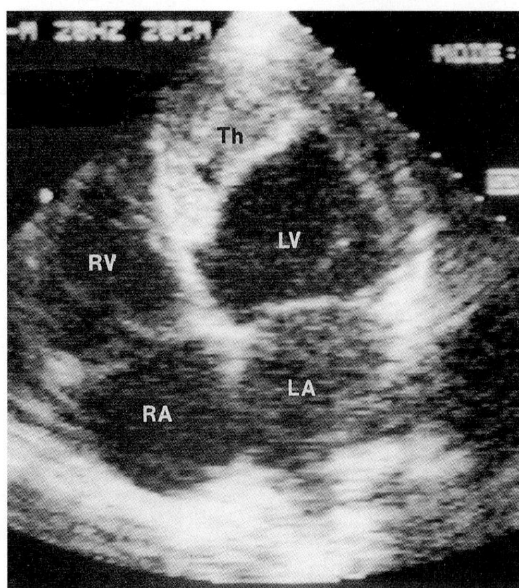

FIGURE 11.5

Transthoracic apical four-chamber view showing a large thrombus (Th) in the apex of the left ventricle (LV). LA—left atrium; RA—right atrium; RV—right ventricle.

aneurysm with stroke in any given patient may be coincidental. There may be an overlap in the diagnosis of ventricular aneurysm and dilated cardiomyopathy. The latter condition may be idiopathic or be associated with multiple myocardial infarcts. Embolism is more likely from thrombi that have mobility, central lucency, and protrude significantly [30].

Valvular Heart Disease

Several forms of valvular heart disease have been associated with cardioembolic stroke. Rarely, calcific emboli from a stenotic or sclerotic aortic valve have been reported to cause vision loss due to retinal embolization [31] (Figures 11.7 and 11.8). A bicuspid aortic valve may be a focus for calcification (Figure 11.9). Rheumatic mitral stenosis has long been recognized as a source of systemic arterial embolization, particularly in the setting of atrial fibrillation. Mitral stenosis is readily identified and characterized by TTE by the unique valve deformity and presence of an increased transvalvular gradient by Doppler study (Figure 11.10). TTE will detect about 50% of the left atrial thrombi, with more difficulty in identifying thrombus in the left atrial appendage [32–34] (Figure 11.11). TEE, on the other hand, will detect close to 100% of thrombi seen at the time of surgery, and provides excellent images of the left atrial appendage, as has been previously indicated (Figure 11.12) [35,36].

Mitral Annular Calcification

Mitral annular calcification (MAC) without stenosis has also been shown to carry a twofold increased risk of stroke independent of other risk factors [37] (Figure 11.12). MAC is commonly seen in elderly patients. It is identified by echocardiography as echo dense calcium deposits typically located along the posterior aspect of the mitral annulus and occasionally extending to involve the chordal structures of the posterior mitral leaflet. It must also be emphasized that mitral annular calcification is frequently associated with atrial fibrillation, which is an independent risk for a stroke. Mitral annular calcification is also associated with other cardiac conditions that may predispose to stroke, including atherosclerosis and congestive heart failure [38,39].

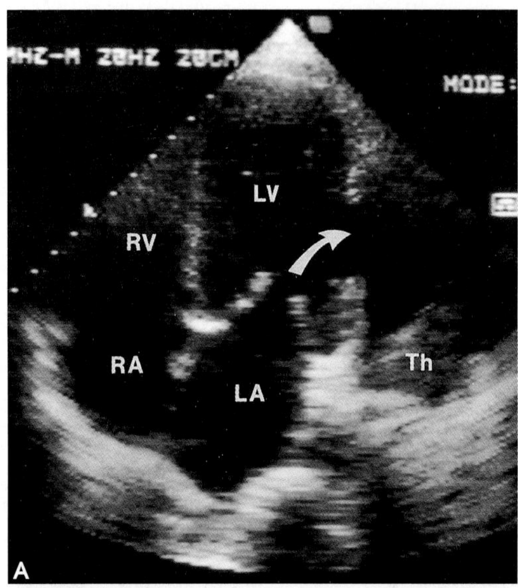

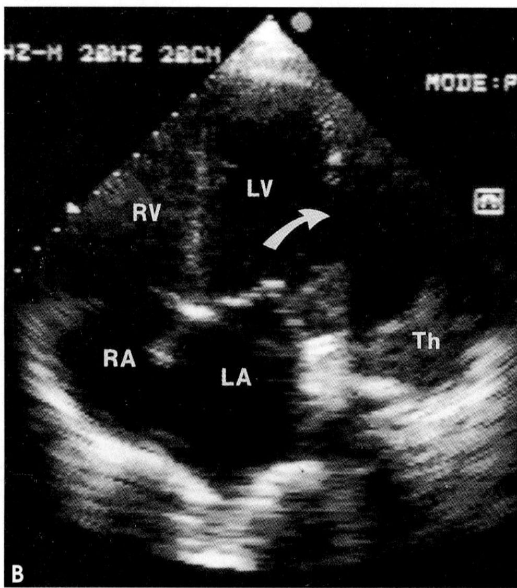

FIGURE 11.6

Left ventricular pseudoaneurysm with thrombus. **A** and **B**, Transthoracic four-chamber views showing a pseudoaneurysm with thrombus (Th). *Arrows* point to the ruptured lateral left ventricle (LV) wall leading to the pseudoaneurysm. **A**, Ventricular diastole. **B**, Ventricular systole. LA—left atrium; RA—right atrium; RV—right ventricle.

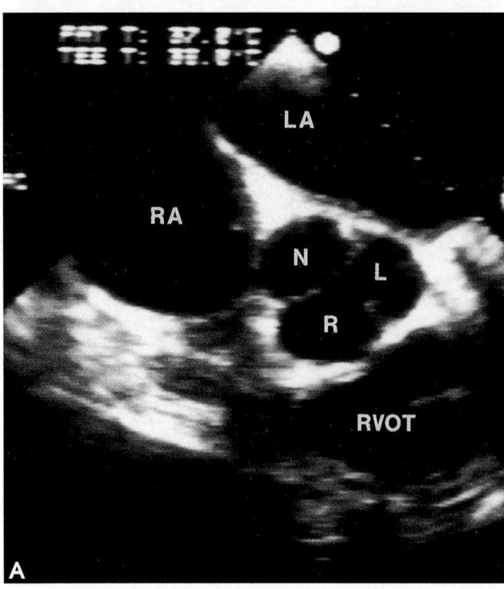

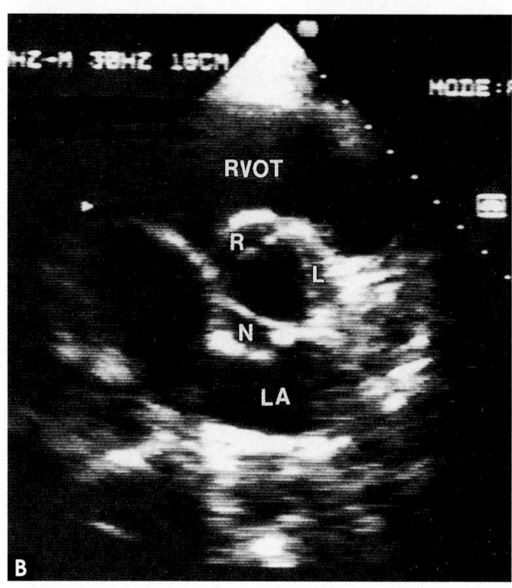

FIGURE 11.7

Normal aortic valve. **A**, Transesophageal echo of the normal aortic valve in diastole. **B**, Transthoracic short axis view of aortic valve open during ventricular systole. L—left coronary cusp; LA—left atrium; N—noncoronary cusp; R—right coronary cusp; RA—right atrium; RVOT—right ventricular outflow tract.

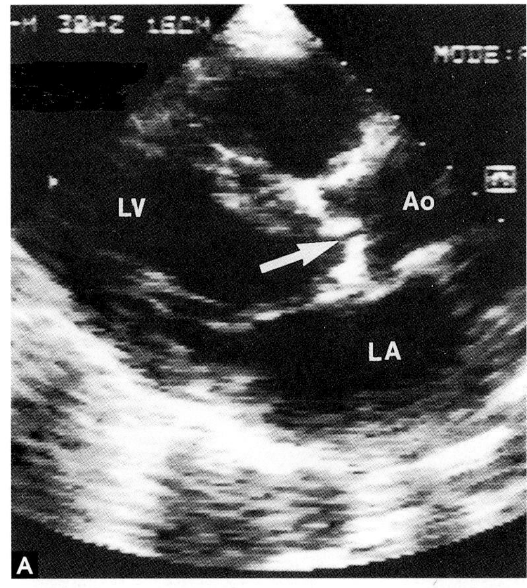

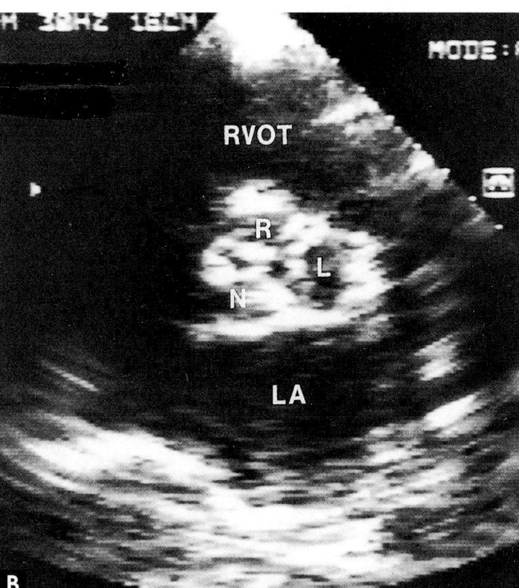

FIGURE 11.8

Aortic stenosis. **A**, Transthoracic long axis view with *arrow* pointed toward thick aortic valve with minimal opening in ventricular systole. **B**, Transthoracic short axis view showing the three very thick aortic valve cusps that hardly open. Ao—aorta; L—left coronary cusp; LA—left atrium; LV—left ventricle; N—noncoronary cusp; R—right coronary cusp; RVOT—right ventricular outflow tract.

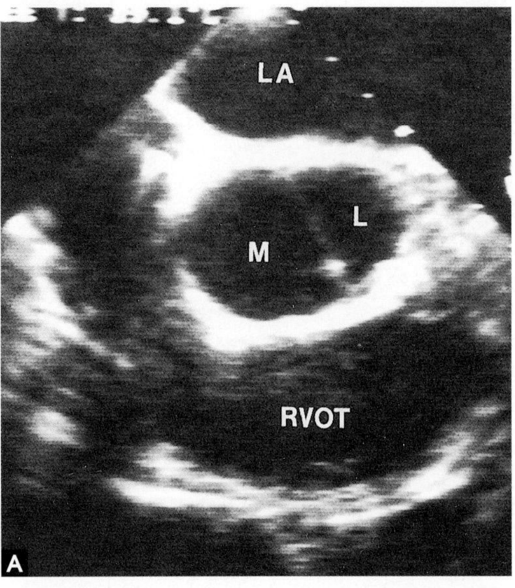

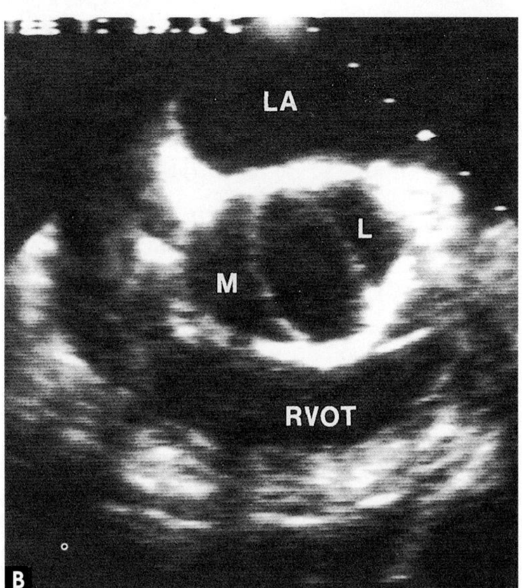

FIGURE 11.9

Bicuspid aortic valve transesophageal echo views. Bicuspid valves are associated with increased risk for vegetations and may be also associated with intracranial berry aneurysms. **A**, Diastole. **B**, Systole. Compare these with the normal aortic valve (Fig. 11.7). L—left coronary cusp; LA—left atrium; M—medial cusp; RVOT—right ventricular outflow track.

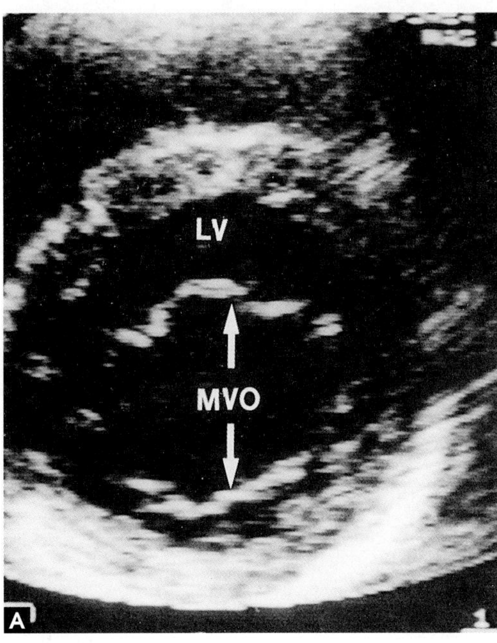

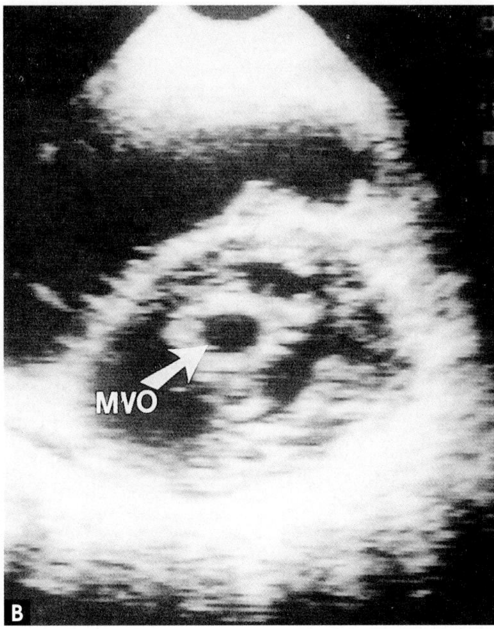

FIGURE 11.10

Mitral valve short axis views. **A**, Normal mitral valve opening (MVO) (*arrows*). **B**, MVO (*arrow*) in mitral stenosis. Normal mitral valve orifice area is >4 cm^2. Mitral valve orifice area in *B* is <1 cm^2. LV—left ventricle.

In conclusion, mitral annular calcification is probably a marker of other cardiac and cerebrovascular disease rather than a direct embolic source. It is possible, however, that mitral annular calcification could cause small emboli that may present as retinal or cerebral hemisphere ischemic events.

Mitral Valve Prolapse

Although the incidence of neurologic complications in mitral valve prolapse (MVP) is low [40,41], MVP has been found with increased frequency over the general population in younger patients with cryptogenic stroke [38,41–50]. For example, of 60 patients under 45 years of age with TIA or minor nonprogressing stroke, 40% had MVP compared with less than 7% of age-matched controls [42]. Incidence of stroke in patients with MVP in various series ranged from 0.1% to 14%, averaging less than 4%, with follow-ups of 2 to 6 years in these series [48]. The prevalence of MVP in various series ranged from 1.9% to 40% in unselected stroke patients, averaging 10.5% in six series totaling 736 patients [48]. For unexplained stroke, it varied from 2.9% to 21.5% in five series, averaging 8.4% [48]. MVP is diagnosed by echo when there is increased thickness of the mitral valve leaflets (>4 mm) with systolic bowing of one or more leaflets past the plane of the mitral annulus in the 2-D parasternal long axis view, or systolic posterior displacement by M-mode [51].

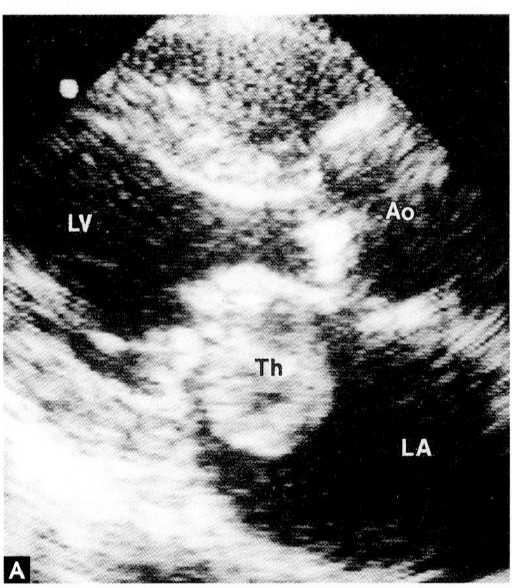

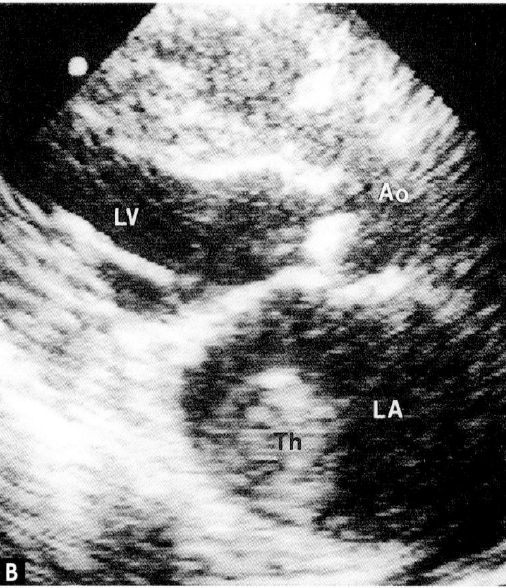

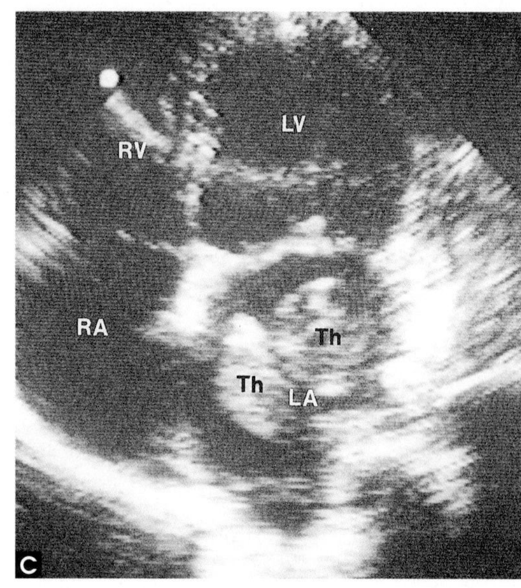

FIGURE 11.11

Mitral stenosis with left atrial ball thrombus. **A**, Transthoracic (TT) long axis (LAX) view showing thick anterior and posterior mitral leaflets and thrombus (Th) virtually occluding mitral orifice in ventricular diastole. **B**, TT LAX view in ventricular systole. Note that the thrombus is now deeper in the left atrium (LA). Note the very thick aortic valve in *A* and *B* (left of the aorta [Ao]). **C**, TT 4C view showing two thrombi in the LA with mitral stenosis. Thrombi may be formed when atrial fibrillation develops and when the LA dilates. LV—left ventricle; RA—right atrium; RV—right ventricle.

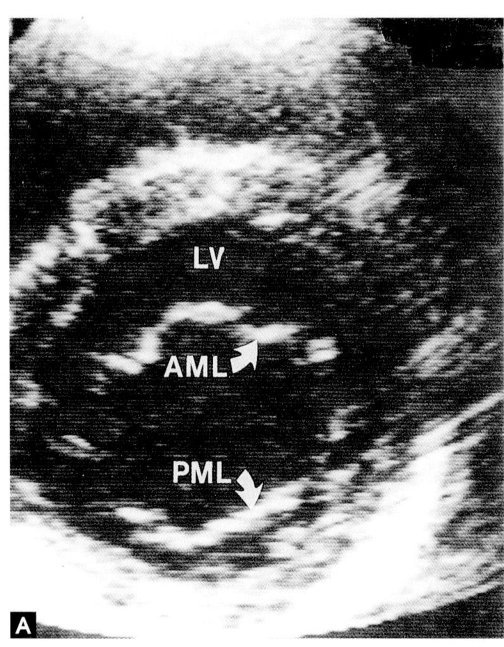

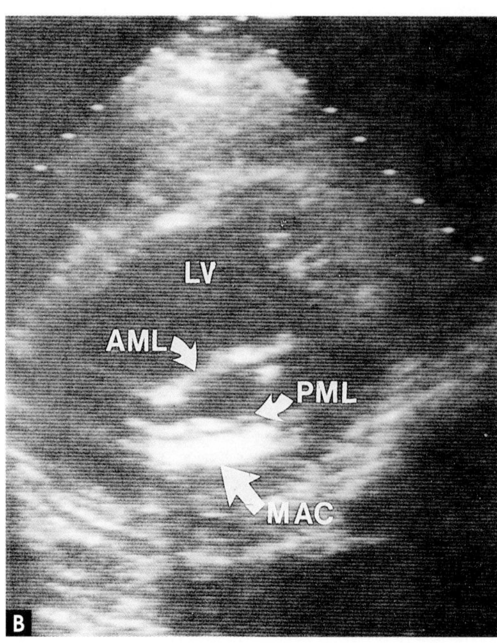

FIGURE 11.12

Transthoracic short axis views. **A**, Normal mitral valve in diastole. **B**, Heavy mitral annular calcification (MAC) below the posterior mitral leaflet (PML). Note that there is also restricted opening of the mitral valve in this case. *Arrows* point to anterior mitral leaflet (AML), PML, and MAC. LV—left ventricle.

This condition can be assessed by TTE using standard views (Figure 11.13). The incidence of mitral valve prolapse in stroke patients younger than 45 years of age is approximately 40% higher than in age-matched controls [42]. It is not only the presence of prolapse itself but the amount of valve thickening that may influence the possibility of embolic stroke [49]. Small fibrin deposits between the posterior leaflet and the atrial wall may lead to cerebral vascular events. It is unlikely, however, that even TEE resolution could depict these small lesions. Morphologic changes of the valve itself may be frequently seen using transesophageal approach in comparison with transthoracic echo. TEE can also assist in evaluation for atrial septal defect, which is associated with MVP.

Long-term studies have evaluated patients with idiopathic MVP diagnosed by clinical cineangiographic or echocardiographic criteria, or the combination. In one study of 300 patients with idiopathic MVP, 3.3% of patients followed over a period of 6 years developed a stroke [49]. None of these patients had coagulation disorders, paroxysmal atrial fibrillation, or used oral contraceptives. A more recent estimate by Hart and Easton of the incidence of stroke or TIA in young patients with mitral valve prolapse is less than 1%, and in older patients it accounts for only 1% of strokes [50].

Endocarditis: Vegetations, Abscesses, and Mycotic Aneurysms

Endocarditis of left-sided cardiac valves carries an established risk of embolization, and echocardiography plays a central role in the diagnosis and evaluation of valvular vegetations. Vegetations are visualized as echo densities adherent to the ventricular surface of the aortic valve or atrial surface of the mitral valve, are generally mobile, and demonstrate motion or vibration independent of the valve leaflets (Figures 11.14–11.18). In cases of suspected endocarditis, both transthoracic and trans-

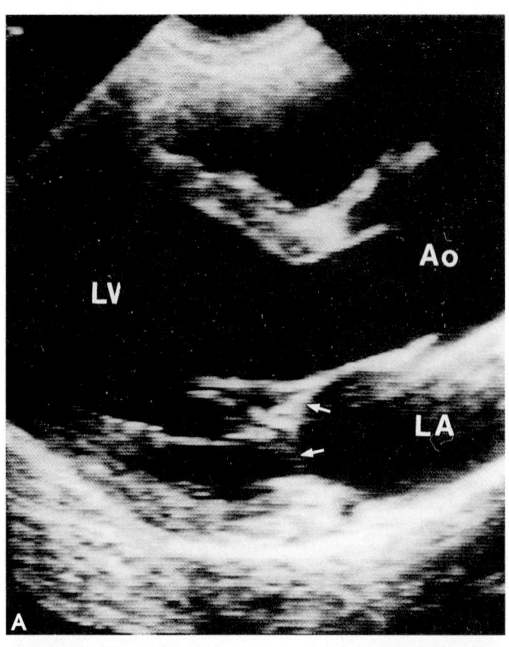

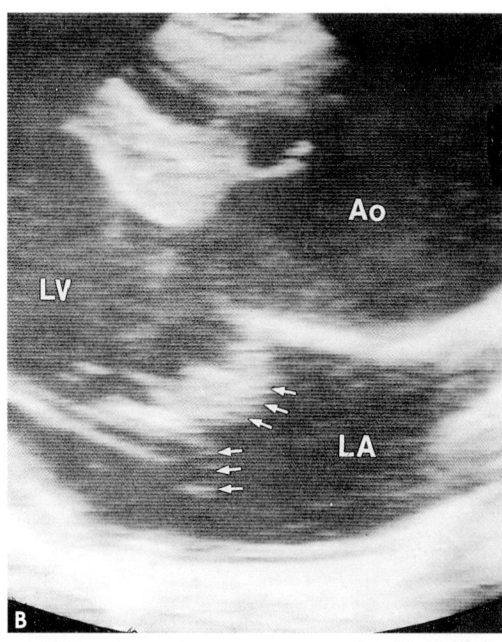

FIGURE 11.13

Transthoracic long axis views. **A**, Normal mitral valve closure (*arrows*) in ventricular systole. Note aortic valve above the left atrium (LA) is open. **B**, A patient with Marfan syndrome in ventricular systole. Note the dilated aorta (Ao), the myxomatous degeneration of mitral valve leaflets with considerable thickening and prolapse (*arrows*), and the thickened interventricular septum above the left ventricle (LV).

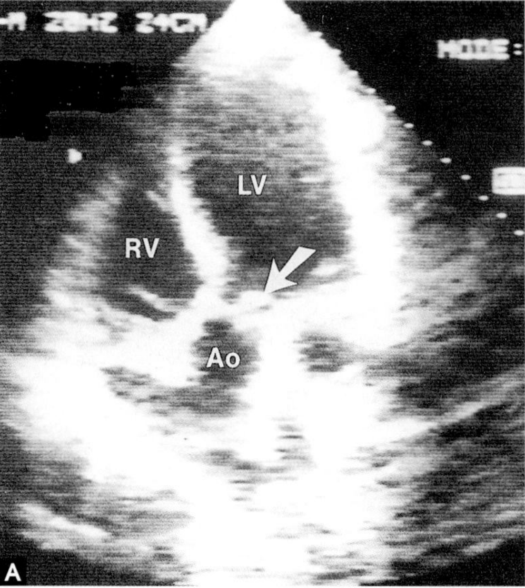

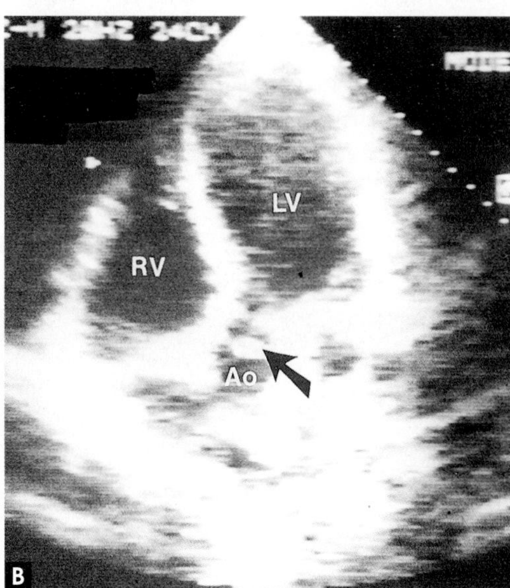

FIGURE 11.14

Transthoracic apical five-chamber view showing an aortic valve vegetation (*arrows*). **A**, Ventricle diastole. **B**, Ventricle systole. Ao—aorta; LV—left ventricle; RV—right ventricle.

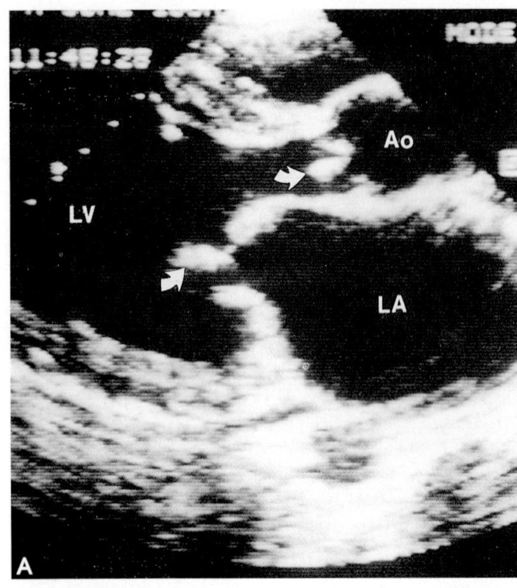

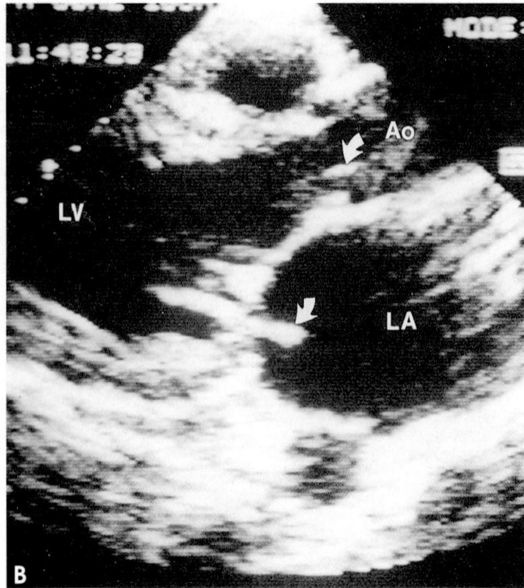

FIGURE 11.15

Transthoracic long axis views. Aortic and mitral valve vegetations (*arrows*). **A**, Ventricle diastole. **B**, Ventricle systole. Note how the vegetations change position during the cardiac cycle. Vegetations may be quite mobile, unlike mitral annular calcification and aortic valve stenosis. Ao—aorta; LA—left atrium; LV—left ventricle.

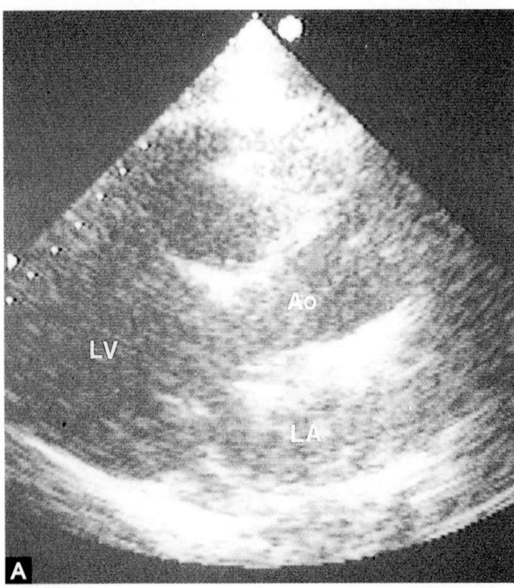

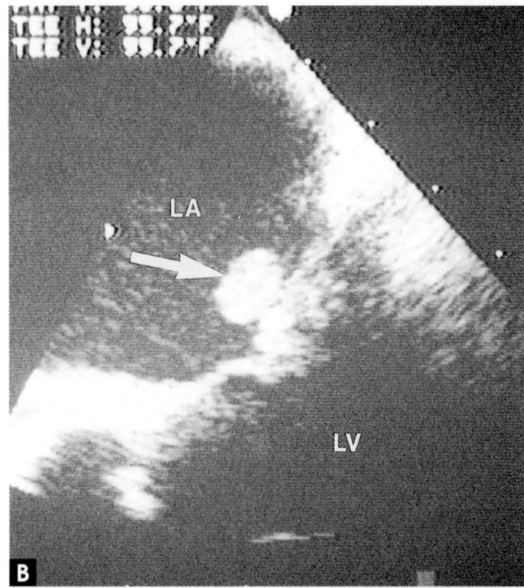

FIGURE 11.16

A, Transthoracic long axis view of poor quality in attempting to evaluate the presence of a vegetation. **B**, Transesophageal echocardiography clearly demonstrates a vegetation (*arrow*) on the left atrium (LA) side of the mitral valve. Ao—aorta; LV—left ventricle.

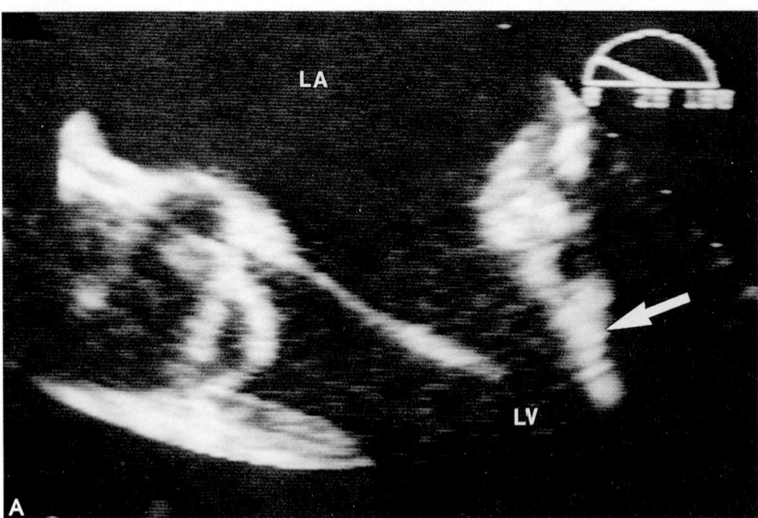

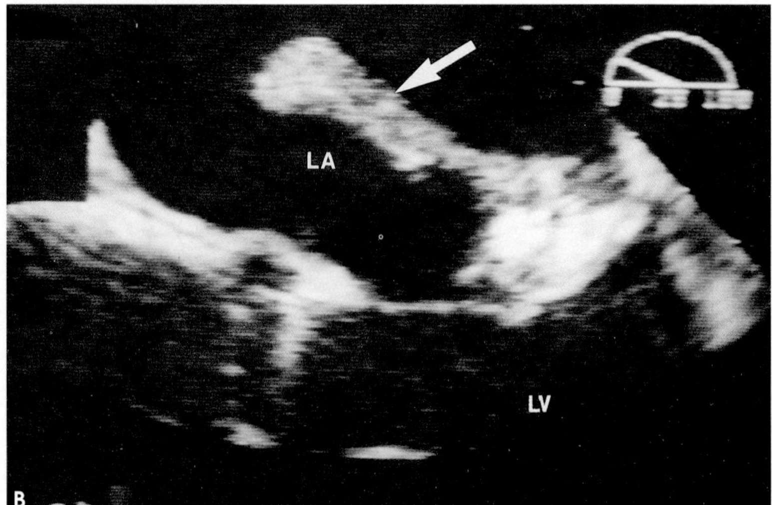

FIGURE 11.17

Transesophageal echocardiography showing mitral valve vegetation (*arrows*). **A**, Ventricular diastole. **B**, Ventricular systole. Note how the vegetation extends into the left ventricle (LV) during ventricular diastole and into the left atrium (LA) during ventricular systole, again demonstrating the considerable mobility of valvular vegetation.

esophageal echo have good specificity for vegetation, but transthoracic imaging carries a sensitivity in the range of 50% compared with over 90% for TEE [52–54]. Several studies have investigated the prognostic significance of the presence and morphology of valvular vegetations by echocardiography with regard to embolic phenomena. Larger, more mobile vegetations have been shown to carry an increased risk for embolization in some studies [54–56], although conflicting data exist [57–60]. In one study, vegetations which were 11 mm in size had a 50% cumulative risk of embolization, whereas 16-mm vegetations carried a 90% risk [55].

A 12-year study of neurologic complications of endocarditis suggested that neurologic complications occur with the same frequency in native and prosthetic valve endocarditis [61]. Streptococcal endocarditis appears to increase the risk of neurologic complications and mortality. In this series of 113 subjects with native valve endocarditis and 62 with prosthetic valve endocarditis, neurologic complications occurred in approximately the same percentage, 35% to 38%. Stroke was the most common neurologic complication. The majority of neurologic complications appear to occur before the onset of antibiotic treatment or shortly after the onset of antibiotic treatment, or usually within 8 days after the onset of antibiotic treatment. Recurrent ischemic episodes do not appear to be common after treatment has begun.

Ruptured cerebral mycotic aneurysms from infections account for about 5% of neurologic complications of infective endocarditis [62]. The risk of rupture of unsuspected mycotic aneurysm following a full course of antibiotics appears to be low. The mitral valve is commonly involved as a focus for mycotic aneurysm. In one series, it was involved in 52% of cases of mycotic aneurysm [62]. Echocardiography, especially TEE, is useful in the diagnosis of mycotic aneurysm in this location.

Endocarditis may not necessarily be infective. Marantic endocarditis may be seen on the aortic valve and produces bland emboli [63]. Mitral valve marantic endocarditis may be seen in systemic lupus erythematosus [7]. Marantic endocarditis should also be considered in patients with malignancies. Nonmalignant wasting diseases such as AIDS may also be associated with nonbacterial thrombotic endocarditis. Clinical diagnosis is made

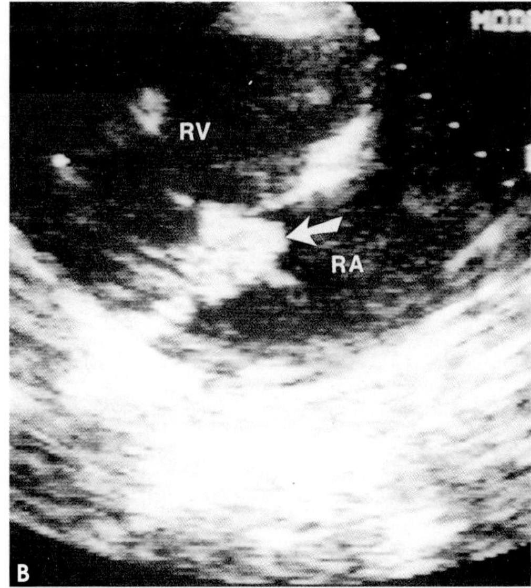

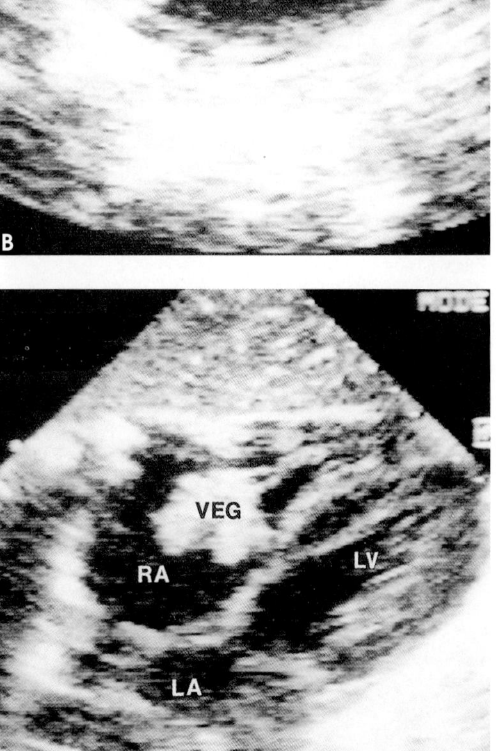

FIGURE 11.18

Transthoracic (TT) views of tricuspid valve vegetation (*arrows*). **A**, Parasternal right ventricle inflow tract view during ventricular diastole. **B**, Same view during ventricular systole with tricuspid valve closed. **C**, TT subcostal view during ventricular diastole. *Arrows* point to tricuspid valve vegetation. **D**, Same view during ventricular systole. Note the remarkably variable appearance of the vegetation (VEG) in different views during the cardiac cycle. These right-sided lesions could produce paradoxic emboli with patent foramen ovale or atrial septal defect. LA—left atrium; LV—left ventricle; RA—right atrium; RV—right ventricle.

by echocardiography since cardiac murmurs are not heard in many of these patients.

Prosthetic Valves

Prosthetic mitral and aortic valves can be sources of thromboembolism due to endocarditis or formation of thrombus on the valve (Figure 11.19). The risk of embolism is in the range of 2% to 4% in both patients with mechanical valves receiving warfarin and those with bioprosthetic valves who are not anticoagulated; ball-in-cage mechanical valves and valves in the mitral position are at increased risk [64–66]. TTE is limited in its ability to evaluate prosthetic valves by acoustic shadowing, particularly for mechanical valves in the mitral position [67,68]. In most situations where evaluation of prosthetic valve function is deemed clinically important, both transthoracic and transesophageal studies should be performed. TTE can be used to visualize the apex of the ball-in-cage valves better in the mitral position because the TTE beam is not obstructed by the base of the valve cage. Due to the proximity of the probe to the valves and favorable acoustic window, transesophageal imaging will reveal abnormalities not seen by TTE, including vegetations, thrombi, pieces of torn cloth, or areas of dehiscence, especially at the base of the valve prosthesis in the mitral position.

Abnormalities of the Interatrial Septum

Atrial Septal Defect, Patent Foramen Ovale

Several abnormalities of the interatrial septum have been associated with cerebral embolism. Atrial septal defect (ASD), particularly the secundum type (involving the fossa ovalis), is one of the most common congenital heart defects in adults. A patent foramen ovale (PFO) is an incomplete seal of the membrane or valve covering the fossa ovalis, leading to a small communication between the left and right atria (Figures 11.20 and 11.21). PFO is particularly common in the general population, since a probe can be passed through the margins of the fossa ovalis in approximately 25% of the adult population at autopsy [69]. A widely PFO is in essence an acquired form of ASD, and is due to either dilatation of the fossa ovalis secondary to right atrial distention or retraction of the valve due to left atrial dilatation.

Several studies have documented an increased incidence of PFO detected by echocardiography in patients with cryptogenic stroke, particularly in the younger population [70–73]. The incidence of PFO by echo in such patients is in the range of 40% to 60%. PFO may also be a risk factor for stroke in older age groups [74]. Normally, the gradient for blood flow across the interatrial septum is from left to right atrium throughout the cardiac cycle due to the higher filling pressure on the left side of the heart. Transient elevations of right atrial pressure can cause reversal of shunt flow during portions of the cardiac cycle or maneuvers such as cough or Valsalva [75]. Paradoxical embolism occurs due to passage of thrombi originating in the extremities across the interatrial septum to the systemic circulation.

This diagnosis is usually made with the injection of agitated saline as a contrast agent into a peripheral vein. TEE is much more sensitive than transthoracic assessment. Valsalva maneuver is routinely used to demonstrate the shunt. Contrast echocardiography appears to be more sensitive for the detection of PFO than oximetry or indicator dilution curves done during catheterization [76,77].

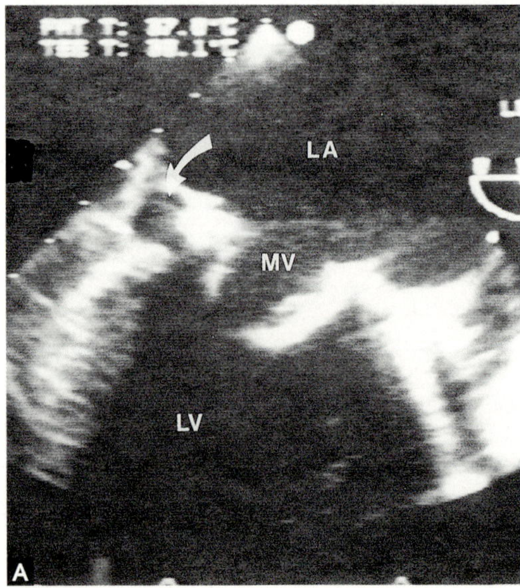

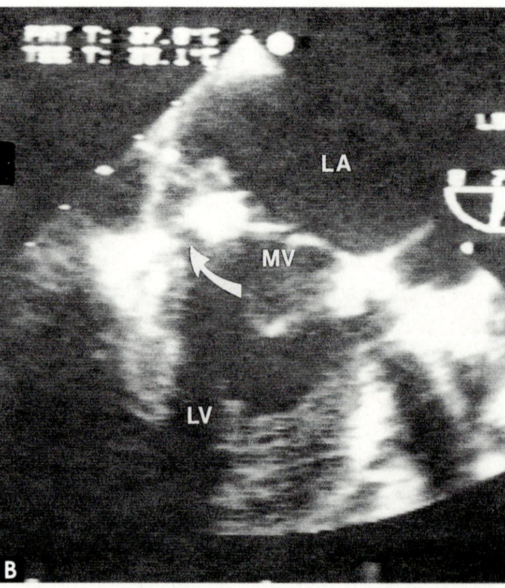

FIGURE 11.19

Transesophageal echocardiography (TEE) view showing dehiscence of a bioprosthetic mitral valve (*arrows*). **A**, Ventricular diastole. **B**, Ventricular systole. TEE is especially helpful in visualizing prosthetic disruptions in the mitral and aortic positions. LA—left atrium; LV—left ventricle; MV—mitral valve.

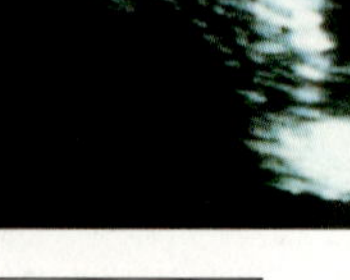

FIGURE 11.20

Transthoracic subcostal view showing a patent foramen ovale (PFO) (*arrow*). The *yellow color* indicates upward flow from the left atrium (LA) to the right atrium (RA) through the PFO in the interatrial septum. PFO may be associated with paradoxic emboli producing cerebral vascular events. RV—right ventricle.

In one study of 238 patients, 122 of whom had episodes of unexplained ischemic stroke or similar episodes explained by other cardiac abnormalities, PFO was diagnosed by contrast TEE in 21% compared with 19% by color Doppler TEE [72]. Contrast study using TTE demonstrated PFO in only 8% of subjects, compared with 22% determined by contrast TEE. Valsalva maneuver increases the yield of diagnosis of PFO. For example, in one series a PFO was found in 30% of patients presenting with nonhemorrhagic stroke or transient ischemic attacks under the age of 40 using contrast echocardiography. Use of Valsalva increased the diagnostic yield to 50%.

Atrial septal defects may be clinically silent and may be associated with cerebral embolization (Figure 11.22). In one series of stroke patients under the age of 50, eight of 11 had right to left shunts at the atrial level shown by contrast 2-D TTE [73]. In another series evaluated by TTE using 2-D contrast study, PFO was found in 40% of stroke patients and in 10% of an age-matched control group [70].

Contrast can be used to increase the sensitivity of echocardiography for the detection of ASD and, in particular, PFO. The injection of agitated saline into a peripheral vein creates echo contrast due to microbubbles within the right atrium and ventricle. These microbubbles are too large to pass through the pulmonary capillaries, but do not produce any significant obstruction to pulmonary vascular flow. Flow across the interatrial septum can be detected as negative contrast, or bubbles may pass into the left atrium with Valsalva maneuver. The presence of left-sided heart disease appears to decrease the rate of PFO detection by contrast echo, likely due to elevation of left atrial pressure [78].

Transesophageal echocardiography has a higher sensitivity for the diagnosis of ASD and PFO than does transthoracic echo, due to the high resolution images of the interatrial septum obtained from within the esophagus [13,77,79]. Color flow Doppler is generally diagnostic during TEE, but occasionally, with a small PFO, flow across the interatrial septum is only documented with contrast study.

Atrial Septal Aneurysm

Another abnormality associated with embolic stroke is atrial septal aneurysm (ASA) (Figure 11.23) [80,81]. In this condition, the valve

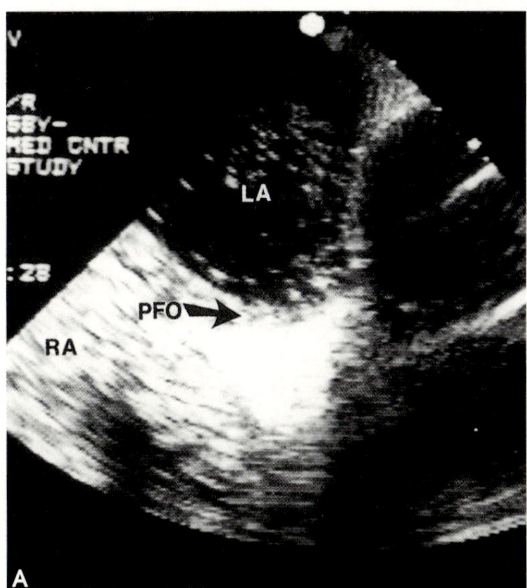

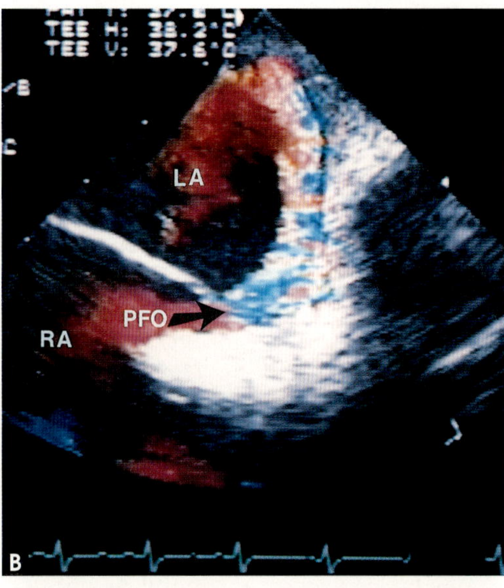

FIGURE 11.21

Patent foramen ovale (PFO) (*arrows*). Transesophageal echocardiography views. **A**, Echo contrast showing flow from the right atrium (RA) to the left atrium (LA) through the PFO. Note the remarkable echogenicity in the RA due to microbubbles from injected saline. Note the fewer but definitely evident microbubbles in the LA. Contrast material cannot get through the pulmonary capillary and thus would not appear in the left side of the heart unless there was a right to left intracardiac shunt. **B**, Use of color Doppler to show flow through the PFO. Note the speckled band indicating rather high velocity flow from RA to LA. RA pressure was considerably higher than LA pressure in this patient.

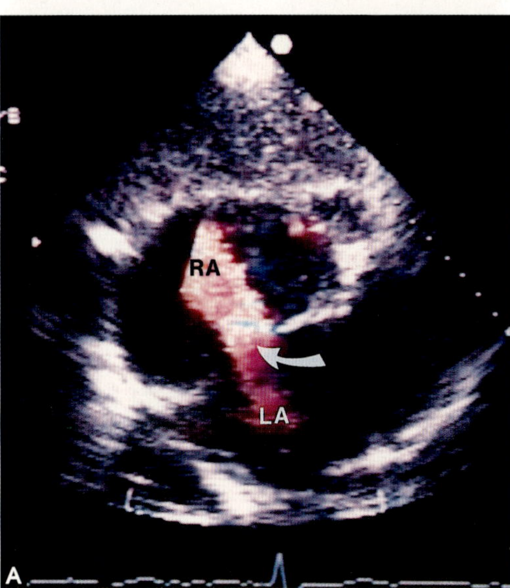

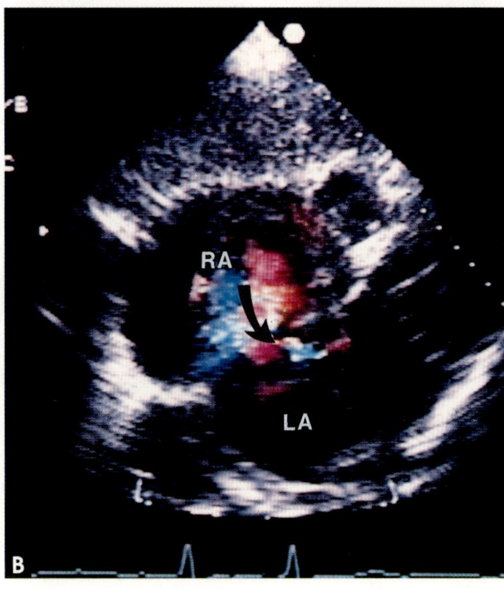

FIGURE 11.22

Transthoracic subcostal view. Secundum atrial septal defect with left to right shunt showing color Doppler flow. **A**, Left to right shunt. **B**, Right to left shunt in the same patient. *Arrows* point to the interatrial septum. Note the variation in flow patterns at different times in the cardiac cycle. LA—left atrium; RA—right atrium.

of the fossa ovalis is redundant and floppy; usually there is concomitant PFO, and not uncommonly MVP. Although there are no universally accepted dimensional criteria for the diagnosis of ASA, it has been suggested that the base and projection into the atrial chamber each should be at least 1.5 cm [82]. ASA is much more easily identified on TEE than with TTE [81,83]. The mechanism of thromboembolism is not well defined. Paradoxical embolism may certainly play a role in these patients with PFO, but the outpouching of the interatrial septum may also serve as a nidus for thrombus formation [83].

In several series, ASA has been associated with evidence for an embolic event in 20% to 28% of patients [84]. In those who have unexplained cerebral events who then undergo TEE, the prevalence of ASA is higher (15%) versus those patients with TEE performed for other reasons (3%–4%) [84]. TEE is superior to TTE in the evaluation of ASA. The prevalence of ASA is somewhat higher, in the 2% to 3% range, compared with TTE in the range of 0.15% to 0.3%.

In one series of 23 consecutive adult patients with ASAs determined by retrospective evaluation of echocardiograms, cerebrovascular events occurred in 43% [83]. In this series, thrombus was identified within the aneurysm in two patients. The mechanism of embolization may be either a primary thrombus formation within the aneurysm or paradoxic embolization through an interatrial communication. Contrast imaging was somewhat more sensitive, possibly because of atypical and rapidly changing jet direction within the bulging aneurysmal membrane during the cardiac cycle.

Other series have demonstrated a frequency of embolic phenomenon in 20% to 30% of patients with ASA [85]. The increased thickening of the aneurysmal membrane, demonstrated by transesophageal imaging, may be associated with myxomatous degeneration of the atrial septum, which may promote fibrin deposition, similar to the situation with mitral valve prolapse and finally causing microembolization. There is some evidence that ASA may be effectively treated by long-term anticoagulant therapy in those who have had an embolic event. Surgical resection of the aneurysm has also been considered, especially when repeated embolic events occur.

Cardiac Masses and Myxomas

Cardiac myxomas usually arise from the left atrium and are the most common primary tumor of the heart (Figure 11.24) [86]. Frequently, the mass is clinically silent until a cerebrovascular event occurs. Approximately 45% of left atrial myxomas are associated with peripheral emboli, of which one half cause cerebrovascular signs [86]. Thus, approximately 22% of patients with left atrial myxoma have clinical cerebrovascular emboli. On echo examination, an atrial myxoma is usually globular in appearance. It can be confused with thrombus or other tumors. Myxoma is usually attached by a stalk to the interatrial septum [87]. The usual site of attachment is in the area of the fossa ovalis. TEE is quite useful in determining the extent of the tumor and its attachments.

Lesions of Ascending Aorta and Aortic Arch

Echocardiography can be useful in evaluating lesions of the ascending aorta that may embolize. Since one third to one half of those patients with cerebral ischemia who have a possible cardiac source of embolus also have a localized carotid lesion [88], ultrasound of the carotids should be part of such an evaluation. Sources of potential cerebral embolization in the ascending aorta include aneurysm of the sinus of Valsalva near the aortic valve ascending aortic aneurysm, and protruding atheromas of the ascending and transverse aorta (Figures 11.25–11.28].

Assessment by TTE is limited, even though TTE may allow visualization of part of the ascending aorta and transverse arch. One study of 23 patients with thoracic aortic wall abnormalities considered responsible for a stroke or TIA on the basis of TEE did not demonstrate evidence for thoracic atheromatous lesions in over 30% of transthoracic studies [89].

There is ample evidence that atherosclerotic lesions may be a source of cerebral ischemia. In one series of 64 consecutive stroke patients referred for TEE who were thought by the neurology service to have embolus as a possible mechanism of stroke, and in which carotid ultrasound scanning was negative or inconclusive, 17% had complex intra-aortic debris that could have been a potential source embolus. This is compared with 4% of a

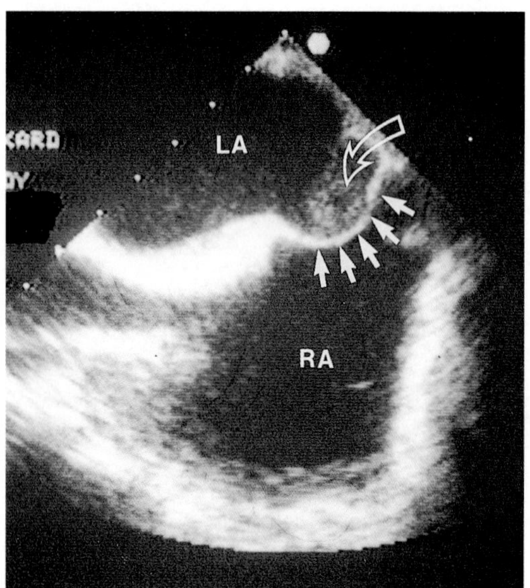

FIGURE 11.23

Transesophageal echocardiography view of an interatrial septal aneurysm. *Small arrows* point to the aneurysm protruding into the right atrium (RA). *Large arrow* indicates spontaneous echo contrast in the pouch of the aneurysm. Spontaneous echo contrast can lead to clot formation. These aneurysms are frequently associated with right to left shunting and thus can lead to cerebral vascular emboli. LA—left atrium.

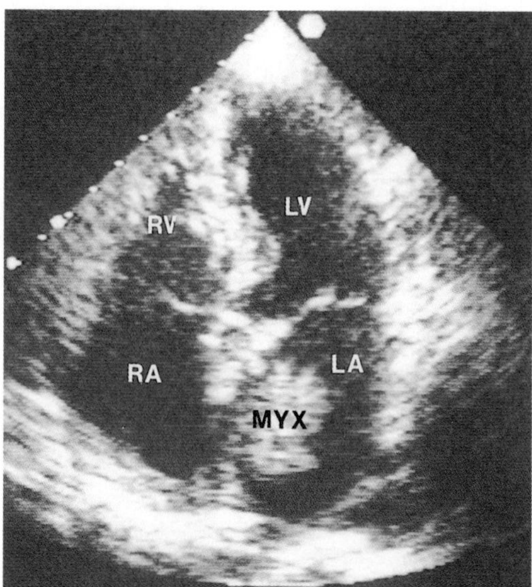

FIGURE 11.24

Transthoracic four chamber view showing myxoma (MYX) in the left atrium (LA). Atrial myxomas characteristically are attached to the interatrial septum as seen in this view. LV—left ventricle; RA—right atrium; RV—right ventricle.

consecutively evaluated control group who were referred for a TEE during the same time period for indications other than possible source of embolus or aortic dissection [91]. Complex lesions that may suggest a source of embolus include a protruding plaque extending greater than 0.75 to 1 cm into the aortic lumen, or an ulcerated plaque with ulcer cavity greater than 0.5 cm in depth, and plaque with adherent mobile thrombus [92,93].

Pedunculated and highly mobile intra-aortic atherosclerotic debris are more likely to produce embolic events than layered and immobile debris, 73% versus 12% in one study [92]. Treatment guidelines for patients with embolization associated with protruding aortic atherosclerosis have not been established, although anticoagulation would be suggested in situations in which a mobile thrombus is noted [92]. A recent prospective study of 94 patients (mean follow-up, 14 months) found that protruding aortic atheromas were associated with vascular events in 33% of patients. Those without protruding aortic atheromas had a 7% incidence of vascular events [94].

Protruding atheromas of the aortic arch may be common in patients over the age of 65 (Figure 11.27). One study in which intraoperative transesophageal evaluation was performed in 130

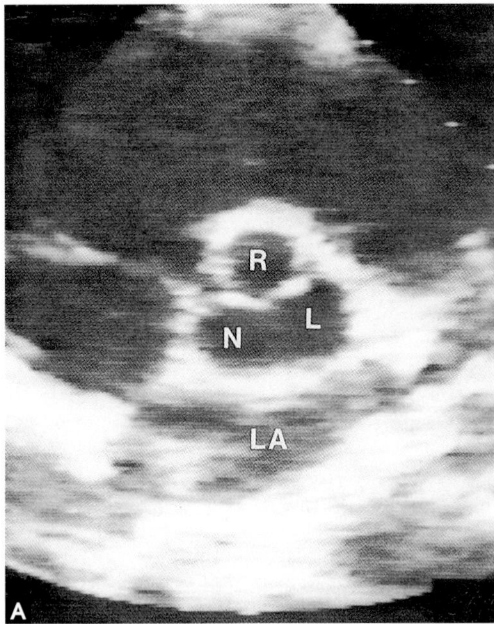

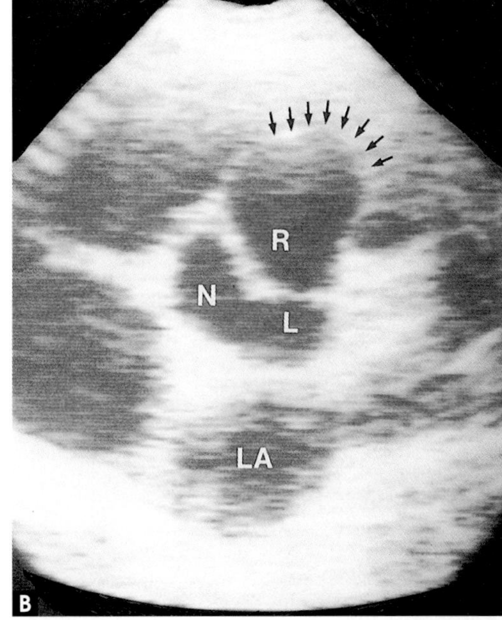

FIGURE 11.25

Transthoracic short axis views through the aortic valve. **A**, Normal aortic valve during ventricular diastole. **B**, Sinus of Valsalva aneurysm (*arrows*) involving the right coronary cusp. L—left coronary cusp; LA—left atrium; N—noncoronary cusp; R—right coronary cusp.

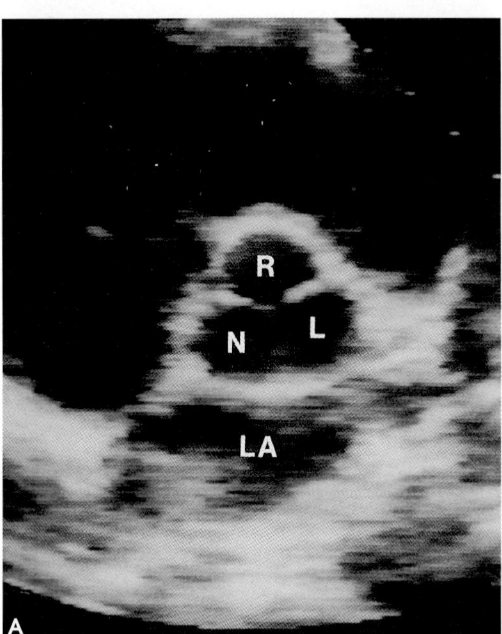

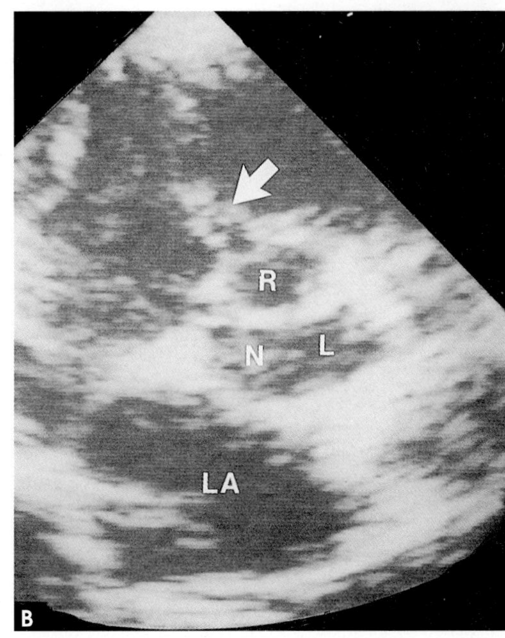

FIGURE 11.26

Transthoracic short axis views. **A**, Normal aortic valve in ventricular diastole. **B**, *Arrow* points to a ruptured sinus of Valsalva aneurysm. This could be associated with cerebral vascular emboli from thrombi forming in the base of the aneurysm. L—left coronary cusp; LA—left atrium; N—noncoronary cusp; R—right coronary cusp.

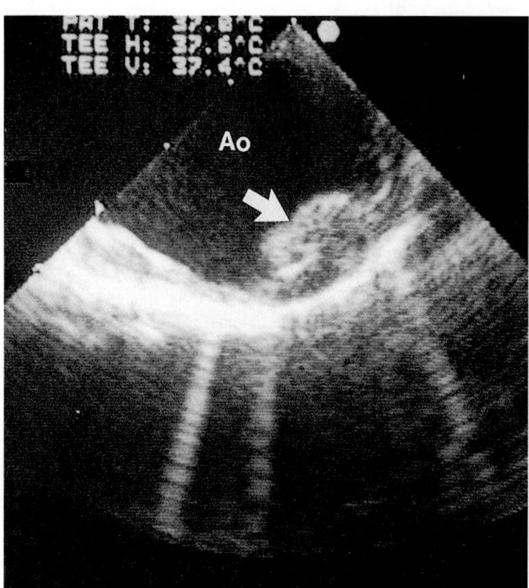

FIGURE 11.27

Transesophageal echocardiography view showing a protruding atheroma (*arrow*) in the aortic arch. Ao—aorta.

patients undergoing cardiopulmonary bypass surgery demonstrated that 18% had protruding atheromas in the aortic arch using intraoperative TEE. The incidence of stroke during cardiopulmonary bypass in this group was higher in patients with protruding atheromas than in those without protruding atheromas (15% vs 2%) [95]. TEE, especially using biplane technique, may be useful in evaluating the ascending and transverse aorta after initial screening by TTE.

The aortic arch can be adequately visualized in over 90% of patients using the transesophageal biplane approach [90]. Occasionally a large hiatal hernia or a distorted aortic arch may obstruct adequate thoracic imaging. A small area of the ascending aorta directly anterior to the left main stem bronchus may not be visualized by TEE. However, because of the diffuseness of thoracic aortic atheromata, it is unlikely that the presence of such disease would be missed. With regard to location, lesions in the aortic arch are more likely distal to the innominate artery, and thus would more likely affect the left side of the brain.

Unruptured aneurysm of the sinus of Valsalva has also been reported as a potential source of cerebrovascular embolism (Figure 11.25) [96]. This is a congenital aneurysm usually caused by the absence of the media in aortic wall near the sinus of Valsalva. Some of these aneurysms have intraluminal thrombus. The aneurysm can be readily visualized by transesophageal study.

Cerebrovascular events may be attributed to a thoracic aortic dissection (Figure 11.29). This is usually due to obstruction of carotid blood flow by the dissection, but embolic sources must also be considered. Transesophageal study can also be used for diagnosis of aortic dissection. Sensitivity for aortic descending dissection is close to 100%.

ACKNOWLEDGMENT

The authors acknowledge the excellent secretarial assistance of Shirley Johnson and Debra McDonald.

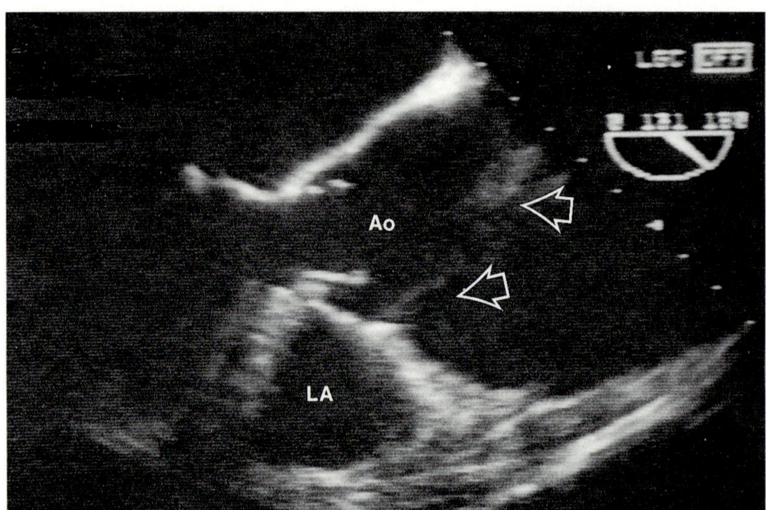

FIGURE 11.28

Transesophageal echocardiography long axis view showing ascending aortic aneurysm with spontaneous contrast (*arrows*). Ao—aorta; LA—left atrium.

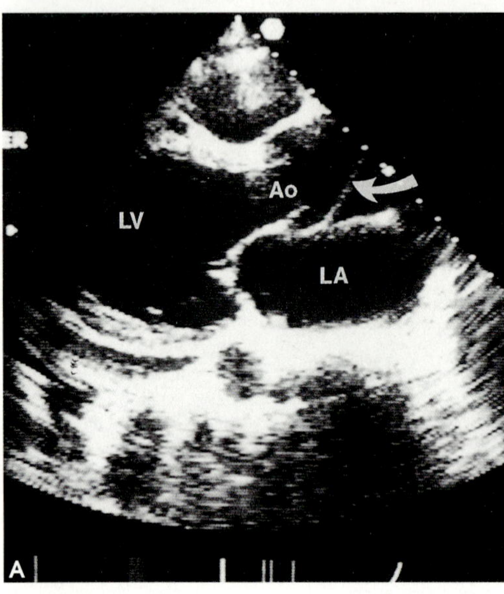

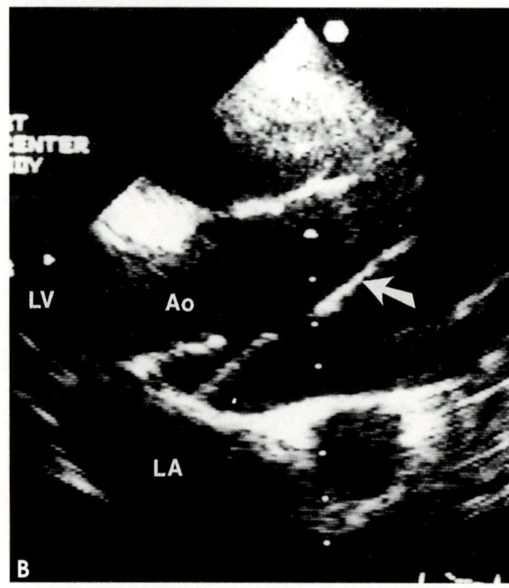

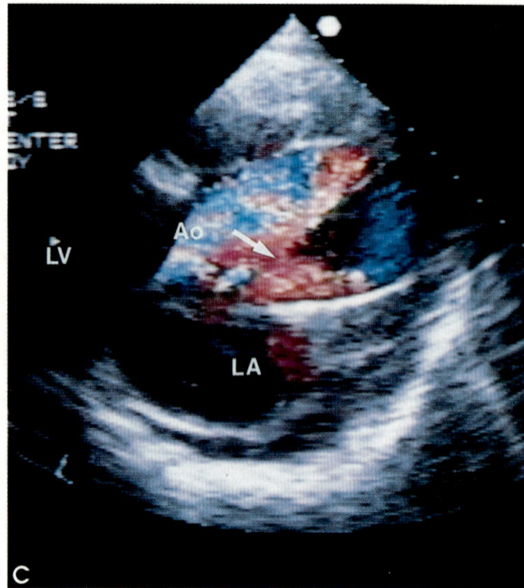

FIGURE 11.29

Ascending aortic dissection. **A**, Transthoracic long axis (TT LAX) view (*arrow* points to dissection) in proximal ascending aorta. **B**, Magnified view (*arrow* pointing to dissection). **C**, TT LAX color Doppler view showing flow from true lumen to false lumen (*arrow*). Such dissections can produce cerebral vascular events due to obstruction of the carotid arteries as the dissection extends into the aortic arch or from emboli resulting from clots in the dissection. Ao—aorta; LA—left atrium; LV—left ventricle.

REFERENCES

1. Cerebral Embolism Task Force: Cardiogenic brain embolism. *Arch Neurol* 1986, 43:71–84.
2. Cerebral Embolism Task Force: Cardiogenic brain embolism: the second report of the cerebral embolism task force. *Arch Neurol* 1989, 46:727–743.
3. Tegeler CH, Downes TR: Cardiac imaging in stroke. *Stroke* 1991, 22:1206–1211.
4. Bogousslavsky J, Cachin C, Regli F, *et al.*: Cardiac sources of embolism and cerebral infarction—clinical consequences and vascular concomitants: the Lausanne stroke registry. *Neurology* 1991, 41:855–859.
5. Asinger RW, Herzog CA, Dick CD: Echocardiography in the evaluation of cardiac sources of emboli: the role of transthoracic echocardiography. *Echocardiography* 1993, 10:373–396.
6. Mohr JP, Caplan LR, Melski JW, *et al.*: The Harvard Cooperative Stroke Registry: a prospective registry. *Neurology* 1978, 28:754–762.
7. Hart RG: Cardiogenic embolism to the brain. *Lancet* 1992, 339:589–593.
8. Boysen G, Nyboe J, Appleyard M, *et al.*: Stroke incidence and risk factors for stroke in Copenhagen, Denmark. *Stroke* 1988, 19:1345–1353.
9. Sacco R, Hauser WA, Mohr JP, Foulkes MA: One-year outcome after cerebral infarction in whites, blacks and hispanics. *Stroke* 1988, 22:305–311.
10. Gomez CR, Tulyapronchote R: Neurologists' perspective in the evaluation of ischemic stroke. *Echocardiography* 1993, 10:367–372.
11. Labovitz AJ: The increasing role of transesophageal echocardiography in unexplained cerebral ischemia. *Echocardiography* 1993, 10:363–365.
12. Mugge A, Kuhn H, Daniel WG: The role of transesophageal echocardiography in the detection of left atrial thrombi. *Echocardiography* 1993, 10:405–417.
13. Pearson AC, Labovitz AJ, Tatineni S, *et al.*: Superiority of transesophageal echocardiography in detecting cardiac source of embolism in patients with cerebral ischemia of uncertain etiology. *J Am Coll Cardiol* 1991, 17:66–72.
14. Greenland P, Knopman DS, Mikell FL, *et al.*: Echocardiography in diagnostic assessment of stroke. *Ann Intern Med* 1981, 95:51–53.
15. Lovett JL, Sandok BA, Giuliani ER, *et al.*: Two-dimensional echocardiography in patients with focal cerebral ischemia. *Ann Intern Med* 1981, 95:1–4.
16. Hofmann T, Kasper W, Meinertz T, *et al.*: Echocardiography evaluation of patients with clinically suspected arterial emboli. *Lancet* 1990, 336:1421–1424.
17. Pearson AC: Transthoracic echocardiography versus transesophageal echocardiography in detecting cardiac sources of embolism. *Echocardiography* 1993, 10:397–403.
18. Zenker G, Erbel R, Kramer G, *et al.*: Transesophageal two-dimensional echocardiography in young patients with cerebral ischemic events. *Stroke* 1988, 19:345–348.
19. Cujec B, Polasek P, Voll C, *et al.*: Transesophageal echocardiography in the detection of potential cardiac source of embolism in stroke patients. *Stroke* 1991, 22:727–733.
20. DeRook FA, Comess KA, Albers GW, *et al.*: Transesophageal echocardiography in the evaluation of stroke. *Ann Intern Med* 1992, 117:922–932.
21. The Stroke Prevention in Atrial Fibrillation Investigators: Predictors of thromboembolism in atrial fibrillation: II. Echocardiographic features of patients at risk. *Ann Intern Med* 1992, 116:6–12.
22. Moulton AW, Singer DE, Haas JS: Risk factors for stroke in patients with nonrheumatic atrial fibrillation: a case-control study. *Am J Med* 1991, 91:156–161.
23. Wolf PA, Abbott RD, Kannel WB: Atrial fibrillation as an independent risk factor for stroke: the Framingham study. *Stroke* 1991, 22:983–988.
24. Chimowitz MI, DeGeorgia MA, Poole M, *et al.*: Left atrial spontaneous echo contrast is highly associated with previous stroke in patients with atrial fibrillation or mitral stenosis. *Stroke* 1993, 24:1015–1019.
25. Black IW, Stewart WJ: The role of echocardiography in the evaluation of cardiac source of embolism. *Echocardiography* 1993, 10:429–439.
26. Vigna C, Russo A, DeRito V, *et al.*: Frequency of left atrial thrombi by transesophageal echocardiography in idiopathic and in ischemic dilated cardiomyopathy. *Am J Cardiol* 1992, 70:1500–1501.
27. Pop G, Sutherland GR, Koudstaal PJ, *et al.*: Transesophageal echocardiography in the detection of intracardiac embolic sources in patients with transient ischemic attacks. *Stroke* 1990, 1:560–565.
28. Nihoyannopoulos P, Smith GC, Maseri A, *et al.*: The natural history of left ventricular thrombus in myocardial infarction: a rationale in support of masterly inactivity. *J Am Coll Cardiol* 1989, 14:903–911.
29. Visser CA, Kan G, Meltzer RS, *et al.*: Embolic potential of left ventricular thrombus after myocardial infarction: a two-dimensional echocardiograpic study of 119 patients. *J Am Coll Cardiol* 1985, 5:1276–1280.
30. Haugland JM, Asinger RW, Mikell FL, *et al.*: Embolic potential of left ventricular thrombi detected by two-dimensional echocardiography. *Circulation* 1984, 70:588–598.
31. Holley KE, Bahn RC, McGoon DC, *et al.*: Spontaneous calcific embolization associated with calcific aortic stenosis. *Circulation* 1963, 27:197–202.
32. Bansal RC, Heywood JT, Applegate PM, *et al.*: Detection of left atrial thrombi by two-dimensional echocardiography and surgical correlation in 148 patients with mitral valve disease. *Am J Cardiol* 1989, 64:243–251.
33. Schweizer P, Bardos P, Erbel R, *et al.*: Detection of left atrial thrombi by echocardiography. *Br Heart J* 1981, 45:148–156.
34. Shrestha NK, Moreno FL, Narciso FV, *et al.*: Two-dimensional echocardiographic diagnosis of left atrial thrombus in rheumatic heart disease. *Circulation* 1983, 67:341–347.
35. Aschenberg W, Schlüter M, Kremer P, *et al.*: Transesophageal two-dimensional echocardiography for the detection of left atrial appendage thrombus. *J Am Coll Cardiol* 1986, 7:163–166.
36. Hwang JJ, Kuan P, Lin SC, *et al.*: Reappraisal by transesophageal echocardiography of the significance of left atrial thrombi in the prediction of systemic arterial embolization in rheumatic mitral valve disease. *Am J Cardiol* 1992, 70:769–773.
37. Benjamin EJ, Plehn JF, D'Agostino RB, *et al.*: Mitral annular calcification and the risk of stroke in an elderly cohort. *N Engl J Med* 1992, 327:374–379.
38. Aronow WS, Schoenfeld MR, Gutstein H: Frequency of thromboembolic stroke in persons ≥60 years of age with extracranial carotid arterial disease and/or mitral annular calcium. *Am J Cardiol* 1992, 70:123–124.
39. Furlan AJ, Cracium AR, Salcedo EE, *et al.*: Risk of stroke in patients with mitral annulus calcification. *Stroke* 1984, 15:801–803.
40. Nishimura RA, McGoon MD, Shub C, *et al.*: Echocardiographically documented mitral-valve prolapse. *N Engl J Med* 1985, 313:1305–1309.
41. Jones HR, Naggar CZ, Seljan MP, *et al.*: Mitral valve prolapse and cerebral ischemic events. *Stroke* 1982, 13:451–453.
42. Barnett HJ, Boughner DR, Taylor DW, *et al.*: Further evidence relating mitral-valve prolapse to cerebral ischemic events. *N Engl J Med* 1980, 302:139–144.
43. Bogousslavsky J, Regli F: Ischemic stroke in adults younger than 30 years of age. *Arch Neurol* 1987, 44:479–482.
44. DeBono DP, Warlow CP: Potential sources of emboli in patients with presumed transient cerebral or retinal ischemia. *Lancet* 1981, 14:343–345.
45. Kelley RE, Pina I, Lee SC: Cerebral ischemia and mitral valve prolapse: case control study of associated factors. *Stroke* 1988, 19:443–446.
46. Kouvaras G, Bacoulas G: Association of mitral valve leaflet prolapse with cerebral ischemic events in the young and early middle-aged patient. *Q J Med* 1985, 219:387–392.
47. Kostuk WJ, Boughner DR, Barnett HJM, *et al.*: Strokes: a complication of mitral-leaflet prolapse. *Lancet* 1977, 13:313–316.
48. Wolf PA, Sila CA: Cerebral ischemia with mitral valve prolapse. *Am Heart J* 1987, 113:1308–1315.
49. Duren DR, Becker AE, Dunning AJ: Long-term follow-up of idiopathic mitral valve prolapse in 300 patients: a prospective study. *J Am Coll Cardiol* 1988, 11:42–47.

50. Hart RG, Easton JD: Mitral valve prolapse and cerebral infarction. *Stroke* 1982, 13:429–430.
51. Devereux RB, Kramer-Fox R, Shear MK, *et al.*: Clinical and epidemiological issues in mitral valve prolapse. *Am Heart J* 1987, 113:1265–1280.
52. Shively BK, Gurule FT, Roldan CA, *et al.*: Diagnostic value of transesophageal compared with transthoracic echocardiography in infective endocarditis. *J Am Coll Cardiol* 1991, 18:391–397.
53. Sochowski RA, Chan KL: Implication of negative results on a monoplan transesophageal echocardiographic study in patients with suspected infective endocarditis. *J Am Coll Cardiol* 1993, 21:216–217.
54. Mügge A, Daniel WG, Frank G, *et al.*: Echocardiography in infective endocarditis: reassessment of prognostic implications of vegetation size determined by the transthoracic and the transesophageal approach. *J Am Coll Cardiol* 1989, 14:631–638.
55. Sanfilippo AJ, Picard MH, Newell JB, *et al.*: Echocardiographic assessment of patients with infectious endocarditis: prediction of risk for complications. *J Am Coll Cardiol* 1991, 18:1191–1199.
56. Davis RS, Strom JA, Frishman W, *et al.*: The demonstration of vegetations by echocardiography in bacterial endocarditis. *Am J Med* 1980, 69:57–63.
57. Steckelberg JM, Murphy JG, Ballard D, *et al.*: Emboli in infective endocarditis: the prognostic value of echocardiography. *Ann Intern Med* 1991, 114:635–640.
58. Buda AJ, Zotz RJ, LeMire MS, *et al.*: Prognostic significance of vegetations detected by two-dimensional echocardiography in infective endocarditis. *Am Heart J* 1986, 112:107–113.
59. Lutas EM, Roberts RB, Devereux RB, *et al.*: Relation between the presence of echocardiographic vegetations and the complication rate in infective endocarditis. *Am Heart J* 1986, 112:107–113.
60. Stewart JA, Silimperi D, Harris P, *et al.*: Echocardiographic documentation of vegetative lesions in infective endocarditis: clinical implications. *Circulation* 1980, 61:374–380.
61. Salgado AV, Furlan AJ, Keys TF, *et al.*: Neurologic complications of endocarditis: a 12-year experience. *Neurology* 1989, 39:173–178.
62. Salgado AV, Furlan AJ, Keys TF: Mycotic aneurysm, subarachnoid hemorrhage, and indications for cerebral angiography in infective endocarditis. *Stroke* 1987, 18:1057–1060.
63. Baron KD, Siquiera E, Hirano A: Cerebral embolism caused by nonbacterial thrombotic endocarditis. *Neurology* 1960, 10:391.
64. Saour JN, Sieck JO, Mamo LAR, *et al.*: Trial of different intensities of anticoagulation in patients with prosthetic heart valves. *N Engl J Med* 1990, 322:428–432.
65. Stein PD, Alpert JS, Copeland J, *et al.*: Antithrombotic therapy in patients with mechanical and biological prosthetic heart valves. *Chest* 1992, 102:445S–455S.
66. Bloomfield P, Wheatley DJ, Prescott RJ, *et al.*: Twelve-year comparison of a Bjork-Shiley mechanical heart valve with porcine bioprostheses. *N Engl J Med* 1991, 324:573–579.
67. Alton ME, Pasierski TJ, Orsinelli A, *et al.*: Comparison of transthoracic and transesophageal echocardiography in evaluation of 47 Starr-Edwards prosthetic valves. *J Am Coll Cardiol* 1992, 20:1503–1511.
68. Khandheria BK, Seward JB, Oh JK, *et al.*: Value and limitations of transesophageal echocardiography in assessment of mitral valve prosthesis. *Circulation* 1991, 83:1956–1968.
69. Perloff JK: Congenital heart disease in adults. In *Heart Disease*, 4th ed. Edited by Braunwald E. Philadelphia: WB Saunders; 1992:966–991.
70. Lechat P, Mas JL, Lascault G, *et al.*: Prevalence of patent foramen ovale in patients with stroke. *N Engl J Med* 1988, 318:1148–1152.
71. Webster WI, Smith HJ, Sharpe DN, *et al.*: Patent foramen ovale in young stroke patients. *Lancet* 1988, 2:11–12.
72. Hausmann D, Mugge A, Becht I, *et al.*: Diagnosis of patent foramen ovale by transesophageal echocardiography and association with cerebral and peripheral embolic events. *Am J Cardiol* 1992, 70:668–672.
73. Harvey JR, Teague SM, Anderson JL, *et al.*: Clinically silent atrial septal defects with evidence for cerebral embolization. *Ann Intern Med* 1986, 105:695–697.
74. DiTullio M, Sacco RL, Gopal A, *et al.*: Patent foramen ovale as a risk factor for cryptogenic stroke. *Ann Intern Med* 1992, 117:461–465.
75. Langholz D, Louie EK, Konstadt SN, *et al.*: Transesophageal echocardiographic demonstration of distinct mechanisms for right to left shunting across a patent foramen ovale in the absence of pulmonary hypertension. *J Am Coll Cardiol* 1991, 18:1172–1177.
76. Fraker TD Jr, Harris PJ, Behar VS, Kisslo JA: Detection and exclusion of interatrial shunts by two-dimensional echocardiography and peripheral venous injection. *Circulation* 1979, 59:379–384.
77. DiTullio M, Sacco RL, Venketasubramanian N, *et al.*: Comparison of diagnostic techniques for the detection of a patent foramen ovale in stroke patients. *Stroke* 1993, 24:1020–1024.
78. Siostrzonek P, Lang W, Zangeneh M, *et al.*: Significance of left-sided heart disease for the detection of patent foramen ovale by transesophageal contrast echocardiography. *J Am Coll Cardiol* 1992, 19:1192–1196.
79. Chen W, Kuan P, Lien W, *et al.*: Detection of patent foramen ovale by contrast transesophageal echocardiography. *Chest* 1992, 101:1515–1520.
80. Zabalgoitia-Reyes M, Herrera C, Gandhi DK, *et al.*: A possible mechanism for neurologic ischemic events in patient with atrial septal aneurysm. *Am J Cardiol* 1990, 66:761–764.
81. Pearson AC, Nagelhout D, Castello R, *et al.*: Atrial septal aneurysm and stroke: a transesophageal echocardiographic study. *J Am Coll Cardiol* 1991, 18:1223–1229.
82. Hanley PC, Tajik AJ, Hynes JK, *et al.*: Diagnosis and classification of atrial septal aneurysm by two-dimensional echocardiography: report of 80 consecutive cases. *J Am Coll Cardiol* 1985, 6:1370–1382.
83. Schneider B, Hanrath P, Vogel P, *et al.*: Improved morphologic characterization of atrial septal aneurysm by transesophageal echocardiography: relation to cerebrovascular events. *J Am Coll Cardiol* 1990, 16:1000–1009.
84. Kichura GM, Castello R: Abnormalities of the interatrial septum as a potential cardiac source of embolism. *Echocardiography* 1993, 10:441–449.
85. Belkin RN, Kisslo J: Atrial septal aneurysm: recognition and clinical relevance. *Am Heart J* 1990, 120:948–957.
86. Yufe R, Karpati G, Carpenter S: Cardiac myxoma: a diagnostic challenge for the neurologist. *Neurology* 1976, 26:1060–1065.
87. Mügge A, Daniel WG, Haverigh A, Lichtlen PR: Diagnosis of noninfective cardiac mass lesions by two-dimensional echocardiography: comparison of transthoracic transesophageal approaches. *Circulation* 1991, 83:70–78.
88. Bogousslavsky J, Hachinski VC, Boughner DR, *et al.*: Cardiac and arterial lesions in carotid transient ischemic attacks. *Arch Neurol* 1986, 43:223–228.
89. Rubin DC, Plotnick GD, Hawke MW: Intraaortic debris as a potential source of embolic stroke. *Am J Cardiol* 1992, 69:819–820.
90. Tunick PA, Perez JL, Kronzon I: Protruding atheromas in the thoracic aorta and systemic embolization. *Ann Intern Med* 1991, 115:423–427.
91. Rubin DC, Plotnick GD, Hawke MW: Intraaortic debris as a potential source of embolic stroke. *Am J Cardiol* 1992, 69:819–820.
92. Karalis DG, Chandrasekaran K, Victor MF, *et al.*: Recognition and embolic potential of intraaortic atherosclerotic debris. *J Am Coll Cardiol* 1991, 1:73–78.
93. Tunick PA, Perez JL, Kronzon I: Protruding atheromas in the thoracic aorta and systemic embolization. *Ann Intern Med* 1991, 115:423–427.
94. Tunick PA, Katz E, Freedberg R, *et al.*: High risk for vascular events in patients with protruding aortic atheromas: a prospective study [abstract]. *Circulation* 1993, 88:314.
95. Katz ES, Tunick PA, Rusinek H, *et al.*: Protruding aortic atheromas predict stroke in elderly patients undergoing cardiopulmonary bypass: a review of our experience with intraoperative transesophageal echocardiography. *J Am Coll Cardiol* 1992, 20:70–77.
96. Shahrabani RM, Jairaj PS: Unruptured aneurysm of the sinus of Valsalva: a potential source of cerebrovascular embolism. *Br Heart J* 1993, 69:266–267.

Chapter 12

Cardiac Diagnostics in Embolic Stroke and Preoperative Evaluation for Carotid Surgery

ROGER A. BILLHARDT
STUART W. ROSENBUSH

Emboli originating from the heart are believed to be the causative factor in 15% to 20% of strokes. It is important to search for an underlying cardiac disorder in stroke patients because it may be etiologically related to the presenting stroke, and because of the intrinsic value of identifying the heart problem itself. There may be therapeutic and prognostic implications for the neurologic and the cardiac diseases identified. Patients with cerebrovascular disease who are found to require surgical intervention will need a preoperative assessment of cardiac risk.

The two broad cardiac disease categories to consider in assessment of a patient with stroke are the anatomic-structural cardiac abnormalities and the arrhythmias (particularly atrial fibrillation), which could predispose to the development of thrombi within the heart. The cardiac abnormalities that have been associated with the presence of thromboemboli include many diseases that affect the heart walls and chambers or its valves (Figure 12.1) [1]. The relative frequency of these disorders in embolic stroke is shown in Figure 12.2 [2].

Atrial fibrillation has a unique position in the group of cardiac disorders that can produce cerebrovascular events. It is a very common arrhythmia and can occur in a very wide spectrum of conditions. The diagnostic characteristics of atrial fibrillation and the details of the relationship of atrial fibrillation to cerebrovascular events will be examined in detail.

ATRIAL FIBRILLATION

The detection of atrial fibrillation has importance on three different levels. First, the loss of atrial contraction and the usually very rapid ventricular rate often will have adverse hemodynamic consequences. Cardiac output will decrease, which may precipitate or aggravate myocardial ischemia or lead to congestive heart failure. Rarely, impairment of cerebral perfusion can occur, particularly in the presence of associated cerebrovascular disease. Second, the presence of atrial fibrillation implies the existence of an underlying causative medical disorder. Although a small percentage of people with atrial fibrillation are not found to have any identifiable etiology ("lone" atrial fibrillation), the majority do have an underlying cardiac or medical abnormality that is responsible for the arrhythmia. Third, and of greatest importance to neurologists, is the significant association between atrial fibrillation and the occurrence of cardioembolic strokes.

Conditions Associated with Atrial Fibrillation

Table 12.1 lists most of the more common conditions that can be associated with atrial fibrillation [3]. The risk of atrial fibrillation with each of these specific underlying conditions can vary widely, with a prevalence of less than 1% to as high as 75%. The highest prevalences are seen in mitral valve disease, congestive heart failure, coronary artery disease, and hypertension [4].

The contribution of the various heart disease categories to the overall atrial fibrillation population depends both on the prevalence of atrial fibrillation within the specific disease group as well as the actual prevalence of the disease itself. In the Framingham study [3], the cohort of those with any underlying heart problems had an average three to five times greater likelihood of developing atrial fibrillation. Those without overt heart problems but with the risk factors of hypertension, diabetes mellitus, left ventricular hypertrophy, and repolarization abnormalities on their electrocardiogram also had an increased risk of developing atrial fibrillation. In fact, because the group with risk factors alone was so much larger than the group with overt heart problems, the majority (70%) of the cases of atrial fibrillation were seen in the group consisting of those with risk factors alone [3].

Incidence in the General Population

The reported incidence of atrial fibrillation varies with the nature of the population studied. In the Framingham study [5], 5209 adult men and women were followed for 22 years for the development of chronic atrial fibrillation. An overall 2% chance of developing atrial fibrillation was observed over the two decades, with the incidence dramatically increasing with age (Table 12.2) [5].

Incidence in Patients with Stroke

Fifteen percent to 25% of patients diagnosed with stroke have atrial fibrillation. In the patients who developed stroke over the 30 years of follow-up in the Framingham study, the overall incidence of atrial fibrillation was 14.7%. This incidence was

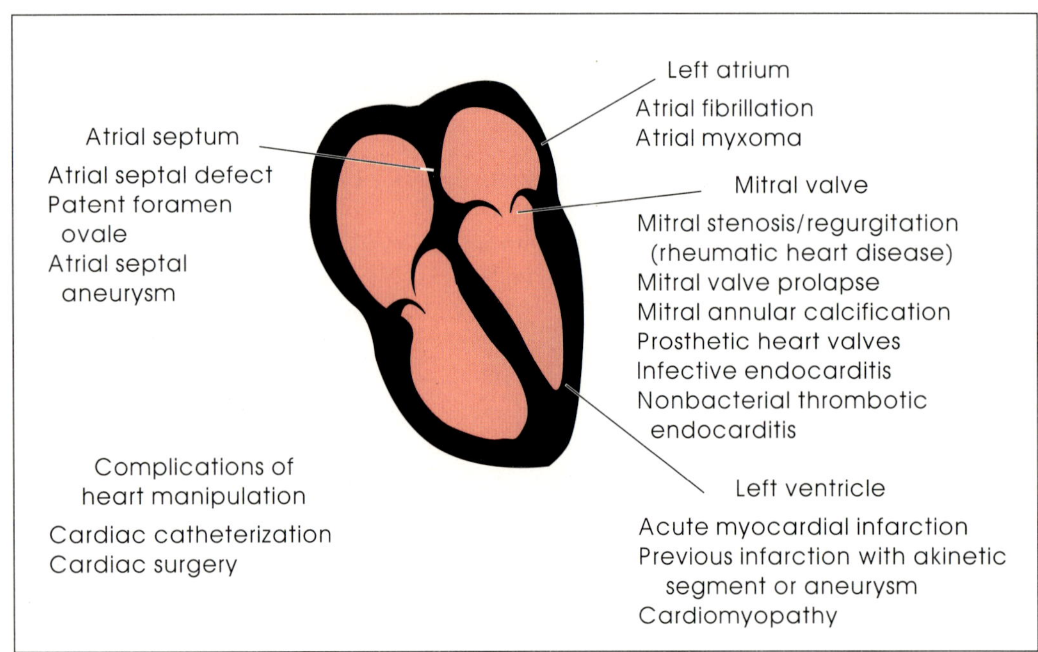

FIGURE 12.1
Cardiac sources of emboli.

observed to steadily increase with age (Table 12.3) [6]. Of the strokes seen in patients with atrial fibrillation, 66% to 75% are thought to be due to cardiogenic emboli [4,6].

Incidence of Stroke in Patients with Rheumatic or Nonvalvular Atrial Fibrillation

In patients with known atrial fibrillation, the incidence of stroke varies with the underlying heart disease. The incidence of stroke when the atrial fibrillation is associated with valvular rheumatic heart disease is 17 times greater than that of the control population. The incidence of stroke in patients with nonvalvular atrial fibrillation (NVAF) is approximately five to seven times greater than that found in the control population. Because of the higher prevalence of NVAF, it is the most common heart disease associated with cerebral emboli [7]. In addition to clinically recognized strokes, there is also a higher frequency of silent cerebral infarcts on CT scans in patients who have atrial fibrillation [8]. Patients with NVAF have historically been said to have an annual risk of thromboembolic events of about 3% to 6% per year [8]. A similar risk of 3% to 7% has been demonstrated in five recent randomized anticoagulation trials [9–13].

Risk Stratification of Nonvalvular Atrial Fibrillation Patients

Because NVAF is a commonly seen abnormality, and because of its significant association with strokes, attempts have been made to identify the higher risk patients with this arrhythmia. One of the larger recent studies, the Stroke Prevention in Atrial Fibrillation Trial (SPAF) [10], followed 1330 patients with NVAF for a mean of 1.3 years. Three independent risk factors for the development of thromboemboli were identified: recent (within 3 months) congestive heart failure, history of hypertension, and previous thromboembolism (Table 12.4) [14]. Nondiabetic patients without these risk factors had an even lower thromboembolism rate of 1.4% per year. Patients without any of the risk factors who were less than 60 years of age (*ie*, "lone" atrial fibrillation cases) had no thromboembolic events [14]. Another recent study, the Boston Area Anticoagulation Trial for Atrial Fibrillation [11], suggested that age and mitral annular calcification were clinical features associated with increased stroke risk [11].

Echocardiography has been used in the study of patients with NVAF to identify those patients who are at higher risk for stroke. Left atrial dimension, left ventricular function, and mitral valve characteristics have been evaluated but with inconsistent results.

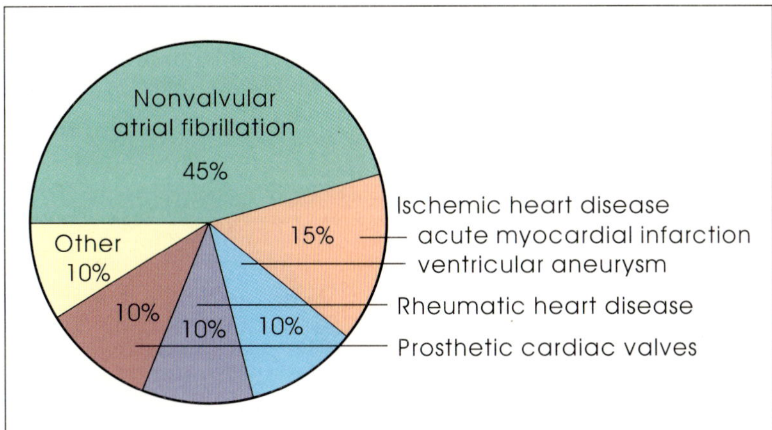

FIGURE 12.2

Relative frequency of cardiac disorders in embolic stroke.

Table 12.1. Conditions associated with atrial fibrillation

Cardiac	Extra-cardiac
Rheumatic mitral valve disease	Hyperthyroidism
Hypertension	Acute alcohol intake
Coronary artery disease	Cholinergic drug use
Acute myocardial infarction	Surgical/diagnostic procedures
Congestive heart failure	Pulmonary emboli
Mitral annular calcification	
Mitral valve prolapse	
Enlarged left atrium	
Cardiomyopathy	
Cardiovascular surgery	
Pericarditis	

Data from Kannel and Wolf [3].

Table 12.2. Cumulative 22-year incidence of atrial fibrillation*

Age group, *y*	Rate per 1000	
	Men	Women
25–34	2.6	2.2
35–44	19.7	6.4
45–54	26.1	31.8
55–64	37.9	29.9
Overall	21.5	17.1

**From* Kannel and coworkers [5]; with permission.

The Stroke Prevention in Atrial Fibrillation study findings suggested that left atrial size and left ventricular dysfunction are significant independent risk factors for stroke in NVAF [15].

Diagnosis of Atrial Fibrillation

Physical Examination

The presence of atrial fibrillation may be suspected on physical examination. The pulse is usually rapid and is totally irregular or "irregularly irregular." The pulse rate measured by palpation of the radial or other peripheral artery is less than the heart rate obtained by palpation or auscultation at the cardiac apex. This "pulse deficit" is caused by failure of some of the rapid beats to produce a pressure wave strong enough to be transmitted to the peripheral arteries. Other findings on examination include a variable first heart sound and a loss of the jugular venous pulse "A-wave."

Electrocardiography

The electrocardiogram is the primary method used to make a diagnosis of atrial fibrillation. In the presence of atrial fibrillation P-waves are absent, while small and irregular atrial oscillations called *F-waves* occurring at 350 to 600 per minute are present. These oscillations have a varying amplitude and morphology, and are usually best seen in leads II, III, and V1. The ventricular response is irregularly irregular; in patients who are not on medications and who have normal atrioventricular conduction, the rate is usually between 100 to 160 beats per minute (Figure 12.3) [16].

Holter Monitoring

If routine 12-lead electrocardiography does not demonstrate the presence of atrial fibrillation, longer periods of in-hospital monitoring or ambulatory electrocardiographic (Holter) monitoring should be performed where there is a suspicion of paroxysmal

Table 12.3. Percentage of strokes associated with atrial fibrillation according to age*

Age group, *y*	Strokes in atrial fibrillation, %
30–39	0.0
40–49	0.0
50–59	6.7
60–69	8.1
70–79	21.3
80–89	36.2
Total	14.7

**From* Wolf and coworkers [6]; with permission.

Table 12.4. Thromboembolic event rates by number of clinical risk factors*†

Clinical risk group	Thromboembolic rate per year, %
No risk factors	2.5
One risk factor	7.2
Two to three risk factors	17.6

**Data from* The Stroke Prevention in Atrial Fibrillation Investigators [14].
†Risk factors include history of hypertension, recent congestive heart failure, and previous thromboembolism.

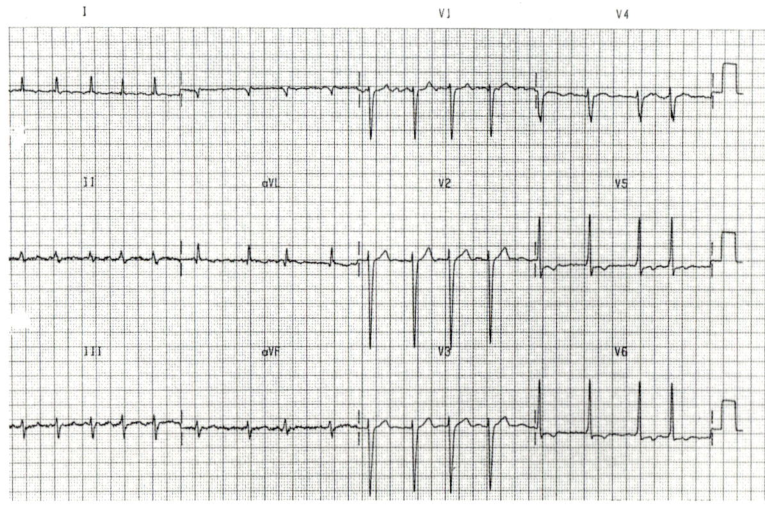

FIGURE 12.3

Twelve-lead electrocardiogram demonstrating atrial fibrillation. Note irregular rate and absence of P-waves.

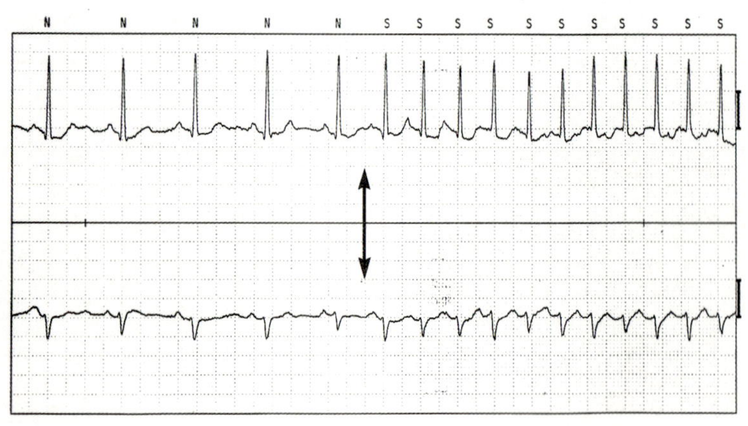

FIGURE 12.4

Two-channel ambulatory electrocardiographic (Holter) monitor capturing an episode of paroxysmal atrial fibrillation (*arrow*).

atrial fibrillation. This is particularly important in patients who do have an underlying cardiac lesion and certainly if cerebrovascular disease is not obviously present.

With the use of prolonged electrocardiographic monitoring, patients with paroxysmal atrial fibrillation may be identified (Figure 12.4). The few studies that have been performed in patients with ischemic strokes or transient ischemic attacks (TIAs) have reported a 0% to 4% incidence of detecting previously undiagnosed atrial fibrillation. In one study [17] evaluating patients with suspected systemic embolism, Holter monitoring was performed and found to be only marginally useful. All of the patients who were found to have atrial fibrillation on the Holter monitor either had a known history of atrial fibrillation in the past or had atrial fibrillation on their 12-lead electrocardiogram. The conclusion from this study was that Holter monitoring was not useful in detecting new patients with atrial fibrillation, but that it may be potentially useful in patients with a past history of atrial fibrillation, but who are in sinus rhythm at the time they are seen.

In a different study [18] evaluating a group of selected patients with carotid TIAs and without known atrial fibrillation, bursts of atrial fibrillation were detected in 2%. Additionally, another 11.1% of patients were found to have other significant arrhythmias [18]. In one other study [19] of patients with strokes or TIAs, previously undiagnosed significant arrhythmias were found in 6.5% of the patients who had Holter monitoring performed. In half of these patients the arrhythmia was atrial fibrillation and in the other half significant conduction defects were identified. Thus, in patients with cerebrovascular accidents, particularly if they are suspected of being cardioembolic in origin, electrocardiographic monitoring should be considered if the standard electrocardiogram does not demonstrate atrial fibrillation.

Anticoagulation in Nonvalvular Atrial Fibrillation

Five excellent randomized studies [9–13] have been performed in recent years to assess the efficacy of anticoagulation with warfarin in the prevention of thromboemboli in patients with NVAF. Although there were some differences in patient population, methods, and levels of anticoagulation, the results in terms of reduction in the risk of thromboemboli were consistent, and major bleeding complications were not excessive in any of the trials (Table 12.5).

Thus, with the exception of patients with lone atrial fibrillation who have been shown to have a low thromboembolism risk, the benefits of anticoagulation outweigh the risks. Therefore, according to the American College of Chest Physicians, "It is strongly recommended that long-term oral warfarin therapy (INR 2.0–3.0) be used in patients with atrial fibrillation who are eligible for anticoagulation, except in patients less than 60 years of age who have no associated cardiovascular disease ("lone AF")" [20]. Patients with lone atrial fibrillation less than 60 years of age in the Stroke Prevention in Atrial Fibrillation and Warfarin in the Prevention of Stroke Associated with Non-Rheumatologic Atrial Fibrillation studies had no thromboembolic events at all. In a Mayo Clinic population study these patients had an incidence of thromboembolic events of only 1.3% per year [21].

The role of aspirin is less clear at the time of this writing. The Placebo Controlled Randomized Trial of Warfarin and Aspirin for Prevention of Thromboembolic Complications in Chronic Atrial Fibrillation study did not show any clear-cut benefit of 75 mg of aspirin per day, but the Stroke Prevention in Atrial Fibrillation study did demonstrate an intermediate benefit of 325 mg of aspirin per day. However, aspirin was not effective in those over 75 years of age, and anticoagulation may be dangerous in this older group of patients. The role of aspirin may become better elucidated with further studies. The present American College of Chest Physicians recommendation continues: "Patients with atrial fibrillation who are poor candidates for anticoagulation therapy should be treated with aspirin at a dose of 325 mg per day" [20].

NONINVASIVE CARDIAC IMAGING

Magnetic Resonance Imaging

Magnetic resonance (MR) imaging is a technique well known to neurologists because of its powerful utility in the evaluation of neurologic disorders. Potential advantages of MR imaging in the study of the cardiovascular system include its excellent spatial resolution and its ability for tomographic imaging in any plane or in three dimensions [22].

Table 12.5. Studies assessing the efficacy of anticoagulation with warfarin in the prevention of thromboemboli in patients with nonvalvular atrial fibrillation*

	AFASAK (n=1007)	SPAF (n=1330)	BAATAF (n=420)	CAFA (n=378)†	SPINAF (n=525)
Reduction in relative risk of systemic thromboembolism‡	60% (P<0.05)	67% (P=0.01)	86% (P<0.05)	45% (P=0.30)	79% (P=0.001)
Annual incidence of major bleeding§	<1%	1.5%	<1%	2.5%	1.3%

**Data from* Peterson and coworkers [9], Stroke Prevention in Atrial Fibrillation (SPAF) [10], Boston Area Anticoagulation Trial for Atrial Fibrillation (BAATAF) [11], Connolly and coworkers [12], and Ezekowitz and coworkers [13].

†The Canadian Atrial Fibrillation Anticoagulation Study (CAFA) study was terminated early due to publication of two other positive studies of similar design and objective. (DuPont Pharmaceutical, Wilmington, DE; with permission.)

‡All study results are based on an intention to treat analysis. International Sensitivity Index varies from study to study. Data on file.

§Definition of major bleeding varies. In some cases blood transfusions were required in major and minor bleeding.

AFASAK—Copenhagen Atrial Fibrillation, Aspirin, and Anticoagulant Study; SPINAF—Stroke Prevention in Nonrheumatic Atrial Fibrillation.

Magnetic resonance imaging has been used in the evaluation of cardiovascular anatomy, function, and tissue characterization. Table 12.6 lists potential areas where cardiac MR imaging may be considered. However, because of its limited availability, expense, and the availability of other noninvasive techniques, cardiac MR imaging is not routinely used in clinical assessment.

Magnetic resonance imaging can be used to image cardiac masses and thrombi. Although echocardiography remains the primary diagnostic modality in evaluating suspected cardiac tumors or thrombi, MR imaging is occasionally useful as an adjunctive or confirmatory technique. MR imaging may be particularly useful in patients in whom adequate imaging is not possible with transthoracic or transesophageal echocardiography. MR imaging can also be used in the verification of intracardiac masses that are seen on echocardiography; it may help to exclude a mass in the presence of equivocal echocardiographic findings. In some patients with equivocal or unexplained echo findings, MR imaging has demonstrated alternative anatomic explanations for the echo findings. Tissue characterization of a mass with MR imaging may add some specificity to the diagnosis [26]. MR imaging may be useful in determining whether to operate on cardiac masses, and it may aid in the planning of the surgical procedure [27]. MR imaging sensitivity in diagnosing cardiac tumors has been reported to range from 80% to nearly 100% [28].

The sensitivity and specificity of MR imaging for cardiac thrombus is not known, but studies have demonstrated that intracardiac thrombus can be well visualized with MR imaging. It is often useful as an adjunctive technique to echocardiography [29]. At the same time, the underlying cardiac pathology can also be characterized [30] (Figure 12.5).

Table 12.6. Potential uses of cardiac magnetic resonance imaging*

Evaluation of cardiac anatomy
Ventricular size, wall thickness, mass
Ischemic heart disease, infarction, aneurysm, pseudoaneurysm
Pericardial diseases
Congenital heart disease
Intracardiac tumor
Intracardiac thrombus
Dissection of the aorta
Evaluation of coronary arteries
Native vessels
Coronary artery bypass grafts
Evaluation of cardiac function
Global ventricular function
Regional wall motion abnormalities
Valvular lesions
Shunts
Tissue characterization

**Data from* Mohiaddin and Longmore [22], White [23], Manning and coworkers [24], and Bateman and Whiting [25].

Magnetic resonance imaging is an extremely useful technique in the examination of the thoracic aorta because of its profound sensitivity to flow and its ability to produce direct transverse, coronal, sagittal, and oblique images. It is an extremely useful study for the diagnosis or exclusion of thoracic aortic dissection.

Three noninvasive imaging techniques are available for evaluation of aortic dissection: MR imaging, transesophageal echocardiography (TEE), and contrast-enhanced computed tomography (CT). In one comparative study all three of these techniques were shown to have excellent sensitivities (greater than 90%), and the specificity of MR imaging was significantly better than that of TEE or CT (97.8% vs 76.9% and 87.1%, respectively). The three techniques were equally effective in detecting thrombus in the aorta; MR imaging and TEE were effective in detecting an entry site and the presence of aortic regurgitation [31].

Because of its accuracy, safety, speed, and convenience, TEE should be considered first in cases of suspected dissection [32]. MR imaging may be less practical in seriously ill patients, but it is extremely accurate and its images are of very high quality. Therefore, one approach for evaluating patients with suspected dissection is to use TEE in patients who are considered to be too unstable to be moved and use MR imaging in more stable patients with acute or subacute lesions (Figure 12.6).

Cardiac X-Ray Computed Tomography

Cardiac CT, like MR imaging, can be used to define intracardiac clots or mobile masses (such as left atrial myxomas) with high success rates. CT has been largely relegated to a confirmatory test when questions are raised by echocardiography. Because of CT's ability to differentiate tissue densities, it can differentiate a clot from a tumor as in Figure 12.7.

Aortic dissection, an unusual cause of stroke, can also be evaluated by CT with intravenous contrast enhancement. Its specificity is higher than transesophageal echocardiography and similar to MR imaging for aortic dissection. However, it is not as effective as either of the other methods in defining the presence of aortic insufficiency due to the dissection, or in identifying the initial site of dissection [31].

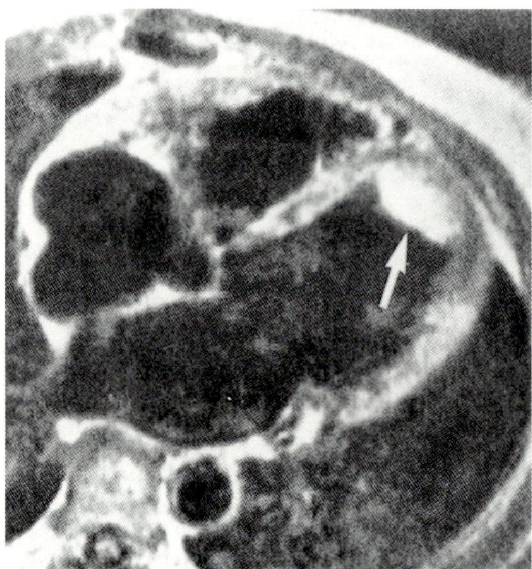

FIGURE 12.5

Magnetic resonance imaging demonstration of intracardiac thrombus. Left ventricular thrombus in a man with left ventricular failure and stroke. High-signal mass in apex of left ventricle consistent with thrombus (*arrow*). (Axial, T1-weighted scan.) (*From* Gomes and coworkers [30]; with permission.)

Radionuclide Angiocardiography

Radionuclide angiocardiography is a useful technique for assessing cardiac performance. It can be performed as a "first pass study" in which a radionuclide bolus is injected intravenously and followed (with a gamma camera) as it initially passes through the heart. More commonly, the radionuclide is used to label erythrocytes. (A common technique is to inject stannous pyrophosphate intravenously and subsequently follow this with an injection of a technetium pertechnetate radioactive label.) It is then allowed to reach a state of equilibrium with homogeneous distribution of the labeled erythrocytes within the circulation. The electrocardiogram is used to "gate" acquisition of the data. Cycles of data acquisition are triggered by the R-wave of the electrocardiogram and the cardiac cycle can be divided into time segments [33]. The data from hundreds of heartbeats are compiled for each cardiac cycle time segment. Following the acquisition of data, it is summed, processed, and displayed as a single representative cardiac cycle [34].

Images from the "gated" cardiac cycle time segments are viewed in a cinematic loop display. Usually multiple views are acquired and displayed. This technique is also called radionuclide ventriculography or multigated acquisition (MUGA) scanning. A subjective assessment of the size, position, and shape of the cardiac chambers and great vessels can be made by viewing the cinematic loop. Visual analysis of motion of the various ventricular segments is possible, allowing for qualitative evaluation of global and regional ventricular function. Quantitative analysis can also be performed.

Radionuclide angiocardiography is used to evaluate ventricular function in acute and chronic coronary artery disease, congestive heart failure, valvular heart disease, congenital heart disease, or unexplained symptoms. It provides a very accurate, relatively inexpensive, noninvasive method to measure ejection fraction. For patients in whom echocardiography gives inadequate visualization of ventricular wall motion or in whom a very accurate determination of ejection fraction is desired, radionuclide angiography should be performed.

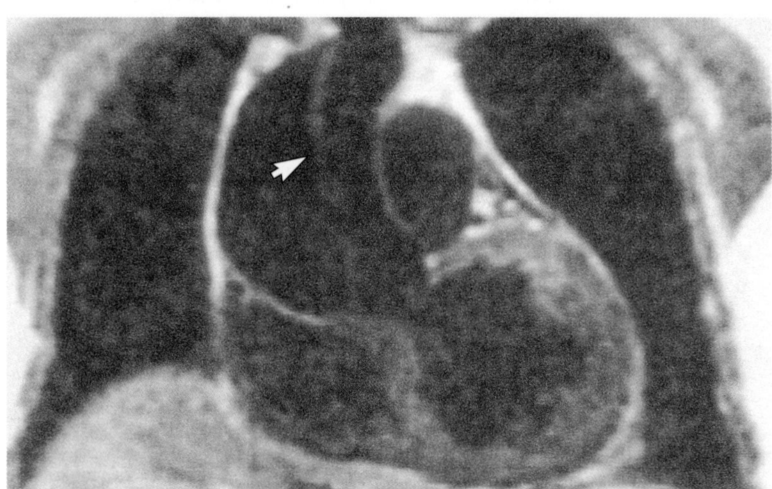

FIGURE 12.6

Magnetic resonance imaging study demonstrating proximal aortic dissection. Dilated ascending aorta with prominent line of dissection (*arrow*). (Electrocardiogram gated, T1-weighted, spin-echo, coronal section.)

Cardiac diseases that predispose to left ventricular thrombi, such as cardiomyopathy and myocardial infarction, can be evaluated with radionuclide angiography, particularly if echocardiography provides insufficient imaging. Intracardiac masses or thrombi are not generally visible with radionuclide angiography and this technique is not recommended for the detection of intracardiac masses or thrombi. Rarely, evidence for a mass or thrombus is suggested indirectly by the presence of a "filling defect" within the radioactively labeled blood pool of the ventricles (Figure 12.8).

CARDIAC EVALUATION FOR CAROTID ENDARTERECTOMY SURGERY

Carotid endarterectomy is an increasingly common treatment modality for asymptomatic severe carotid stenoses, and for 70% or greater symptomatic carotid artery stenosis causing mild stroke or transient ischemic episodes [35–38]. Clinical trials are continuing in an effort to define benefit for asymptomatic

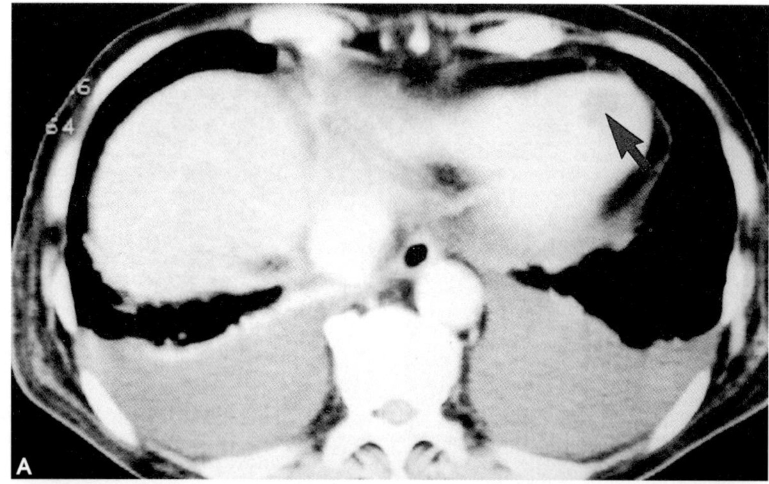

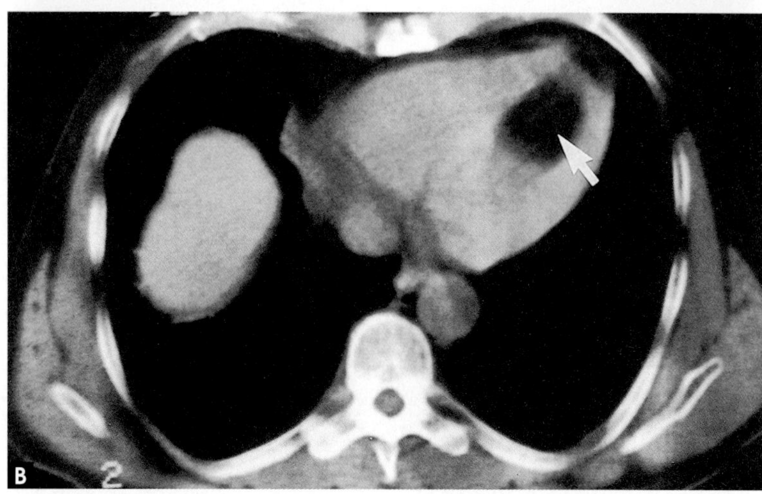

FIGURE 12.7

Gated cardiac radiograph computed tomography images of left ventricular thrombus (**A**) (*arrow*), and a left ventricular lipoma (**B**) (*arrow*). Note the ability to differentiate the fatty lipoma from thrombus due to their significantly different computed tomography densities. (*From* Kubicka and coworkers [36]; with permission from Mosby-Year Book, Inc.)

patients or those symptomatic patients with moderate stenosis. It is well known that peripheral vascular disease and carotid arterial disease are associated with an increased incidence of coronary artery disease [39]. This coronary artery disease may be clinically silent or associated with typical or atypical anginal symptoms. Ischemic cardiac events are a significant cause of morbidity following noncardiac surgery, resulting in an estimated 50,000 perioperative myocardial infarctions and more than 20,000 deaths per year [40]. The incidence of perioperative myocardial infarction in recent carotid endarterectomy trials ranged from 0.9% to 2%, even with preoperative cardiac screening and the exclusion of patients with myocardial infarction within 6 months, and those with unstable angina or congestive heart failure [35,36,38].

Ideally, the magnitude of cardiac risk for carotid surgery can be determined with noninvasive cardiac evaluation. In fact, history and physical risk factor stratification, electrocardiographic criteria, and stress testing are the primary modalities used clinically for preoperative evaluation. However, when clinical evidence for myocardial ischemia is present, invasive coronary angiography is often necessary.

History, Examination, and Electrocardiogram

Goldmann and coworkers [41] identified four historical or physical findings as independent risk factors for life-threatening and fatal cardiac complications in noncardiac surgical procedures: important valvular aortic stenosis, a preoperative third heart sound or jugular venous distention, myocardial infarction in the preceding 6 months, and poor general medical condition. Patients with angina at rest, angina pectoris with minimal exertion, or those with frequent episodes of typical angina throughout the day are at significant risk and require further evaluation before surgical therapy should be undertaken. Patients with a known history of angina who are asymptomatic after bypass surgery, angioplasty, or with medical management are at less of a risk for a myocardial event and may be cleared for surgery, but preoperative stress testing is often recommended.

Assessment of patients with atypical chest pain, or those asymptomatic patients with other risk factors (Table 12.7) but without recent infarction is more difficult. In the presence of an abnormal electrocardiogram, complex ventricular ectopy on the electrocardiogram (couplets, nonsustained ventricular tachycardia), significant murmurs of aortic stenosis or regurgitation,

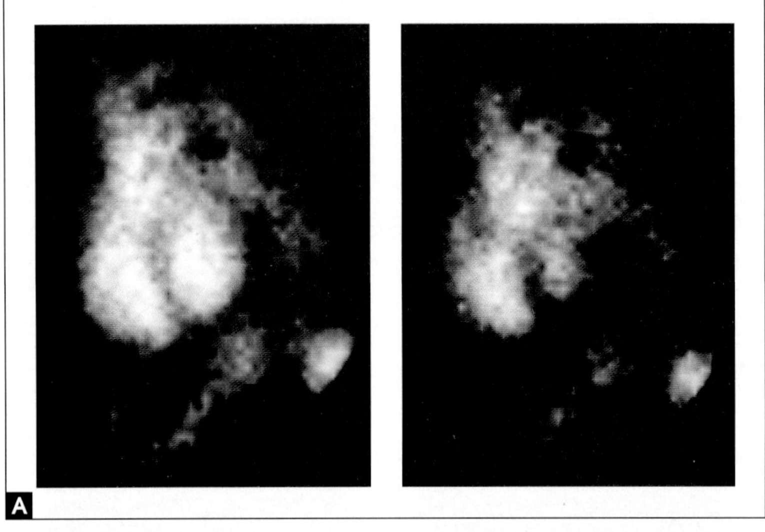

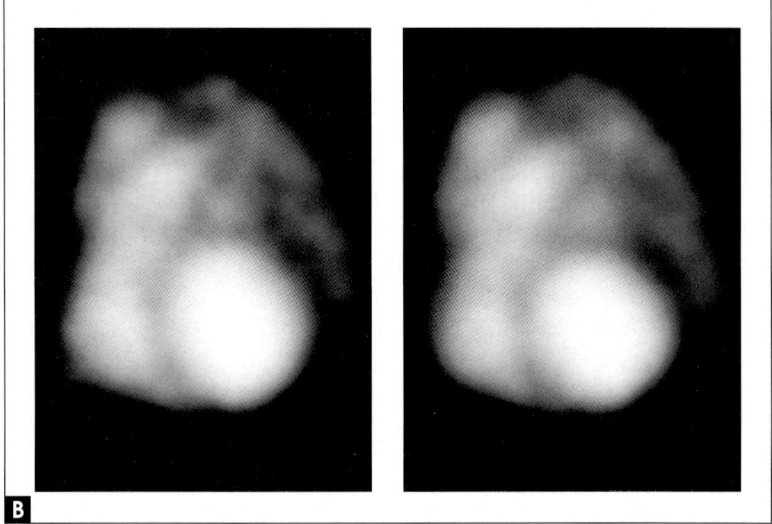

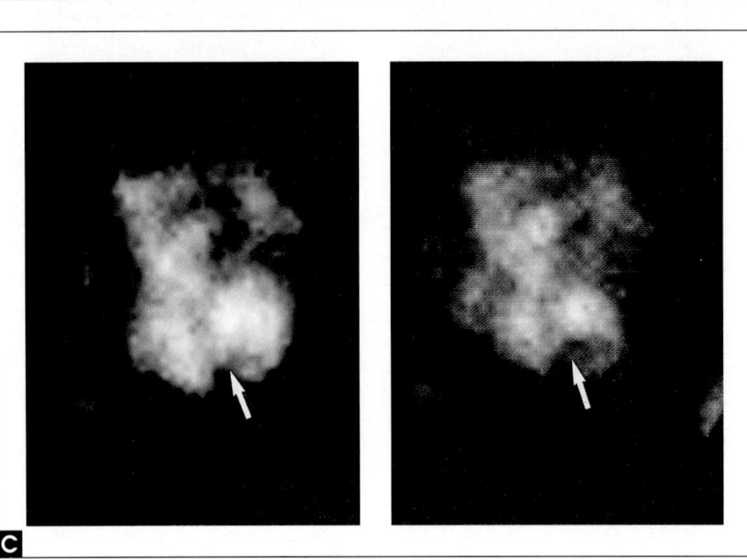

FIGURE 12.8

Radionuclide angiography. End-diastolic (*left*) and end-systolic (*right*) frames (in the left anterior oblique projection) of a normal subject (**A**), a patient with a dilated cardiomyopathy (**B**), and a patient with left ventricular thrombus (**C**) (*arrows*). (*Courtesy of* Amjad Ali, MD.)

significant mitral regurgitation, or signs of congestive heart failure, further noninvasive evaluation is necessary. Valvular heart disease severity can be assessed adequately in most instances with Doppler echocardiography, and this modality can also be useful in patients with congestive heart failure signs and symptoms.

Electrocardiographic findings of ST segment depressions of 1 mm or more at rest, diffuse T-wave inversions, left bundle branch block pattern, or pathologic Q-waves mandate further evaluation for ischemia and comparison with prior electrocardiograms. ST segment elevation in two contiguous leads indicates possible acute infarction, pericarditis, left ventricular aneurysm, left ventricular hypertrophy, or a normal variant known as early repolarization. Left ventricular hypertrophy on the electrocardiogram is a strong predictor of postoperative myocardial ischemia [42].

Patients without chest discomfort who have a normal electrocardiogram and who have no other risk factors may be cleared for surgery. Although silent ischemia is still a possibility in this group, the risk is small. See Figure 12.9 for a decision tree for cardiac evaluation prior to carotid surgery.

Table 12.7. Risk factors for postoperative ischemia

Risk factors
Diabetes mellitus
Renal failure, on dialysis
Hypertension with left ventricular hypertrophy
Angina pectoris
Recent myocardial infarction (within 6 months*)
Preoperative congestive heart failure
Significant aortic stenosis or regurgitation
Age >70
Poor preoperative medical condition

*Without post–myocardial infarction exercise testing or coronary angiography/intervention.

Stress Testing

Numerous options are available for myocardial stress testing. These include standard bicycle or treadmill stress studies with electrocardiographic monitoring, thallium-201 scintigraphic evaluation of myocardial perfusion with exercise, and exercise MUGA or echocardiographic studies. Pharmacologic stress testing can be used for patients who are not able to exercise.

Standard Exercise Testing

Electrocardiographic monitoring in standard exercise stress testing relies on the production of ST segment depression

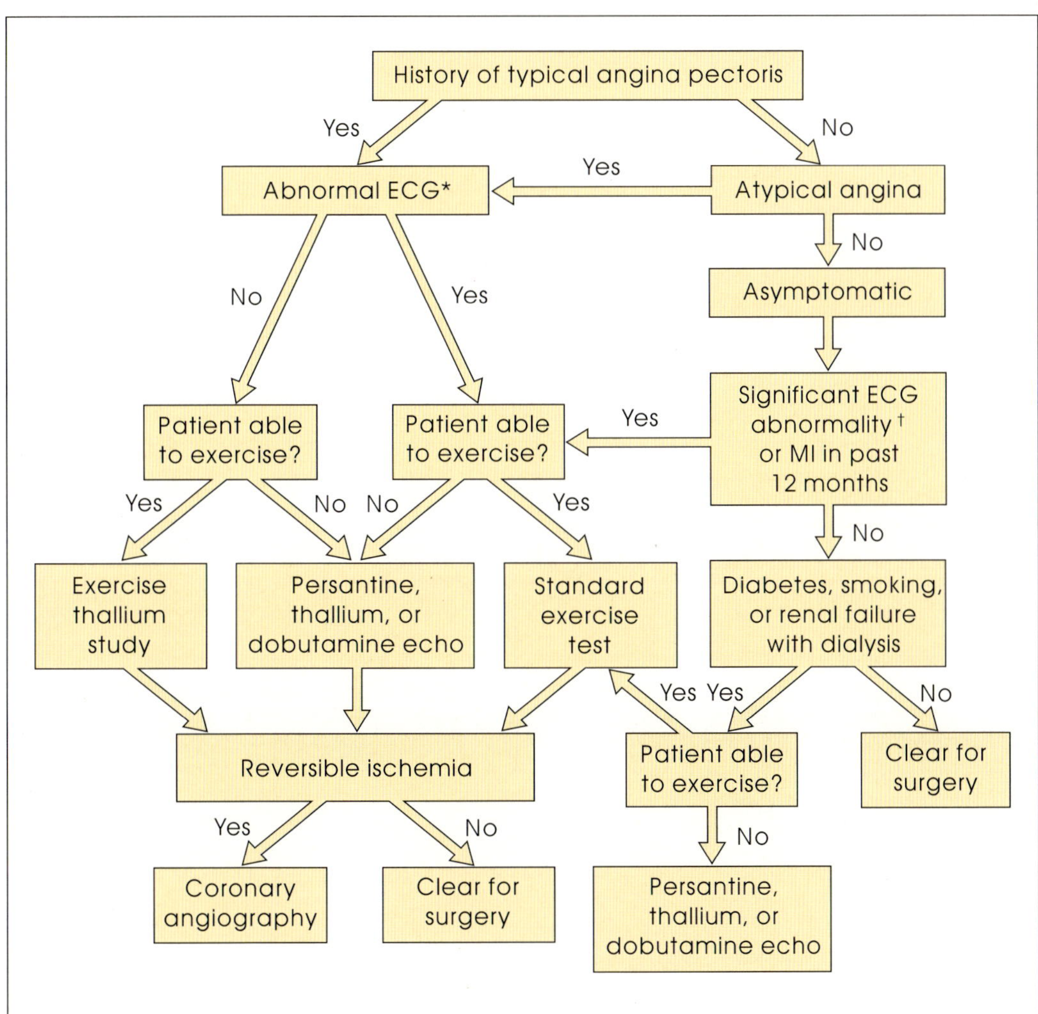

FIGURE 12.9

Decision tree for cardiac evaluation prior to carotid surgery. *Asterisk* indicates electrocardiogram (ECG) presence of left bundle branch block (LBBB), significant base ST segment abnormalities, and left ventricular hypertrophy with strain. *Dagger* indicates LBBB, anterior infarction or aneurysm pattern, and ischemic ST-T changes. MI—myocardial infarction.

caused by subendocardial ischemia. The increased myocardial oxygen demand of exercise produces QRS repolarization changes from isoelectric ST segments at rest to 1 mm or greater horizontal or downsloping ST segment depression with exercise in the presence of coronary artery stenoses (Figure 12.10). The electrocardiographic diagnosis of coronary artery disease is less reliable in the presence of repolarization (ST segment) abnormalities at rest with digitalis use or in the presence of left ventricular hypertrophy with strain. Similarly the resting repolarization changes present with left bundle branch block conduction make regular stress testing nondiagnostic.

With a normal resting electrocardiogram, the sensitivity and specificity for electrocardiographic stress testing is 66% and 77%, respectively [43]. A normal, adequate-intensity stress study indicates a low risk of an adverse cardiovascular event in the perioperative period. However, an equivocal study or one in which less than 85% of the maximal predicted heart rate for age has been reached warrants further investigation, usually by exercise or pharmacologic stress scintigraphy. Positive studies may be further evaluated by exercise scintigraphy or by coronary angiography.

Exercise Scintigraphic Perfusion Stress Testing

Thallium-201 is a potassium analogue that is avidly absorbed by normal myocardium. Technetium-99m labeled isonitriles (Cardiolite [DuPont Pharma Radiopharmaceuticals] is the most widely used) have been recently introduced because of purportedly better imaging qualities. They too are taken up by normal myocardium as potassium is absorbed. The gamma rays emitted by these compounds allow imaging of the myocardium with gamma camera technology that is widely available. Both thallium-201 and Cardiolite myocardial uptake is flow dependent; therefore, areas of myocardium perfused by stenotic coronary arteries will show relatively less pharmaceutical uptake and fewer scintigraphic counts than the myocardium receiving increased flow and exercise-induced hyperemia from a normal, non flow-limiting coronary artery. Since thallium imaging can take advantage of redistribution of the isotope into ischemic, but still viable myocardium, and thereby differentiate between ischemic and infarcted muscle, thallium remains the most widely used radiopharmaceutical for cardiac stress testing. Cardiolite requires a reinjection 24 hours after stress to determine "reversibility" (from ischemic to nonischemic) and thereby differentiate ischemia from infarction. However, alternate injection protocols can allow same-day evaluation [44].

Scintigraphic stress testing is performed in concert with electrocardiographic ST segment monitoring during exercise, with injection of the radiopharmaceutical at peak exercise. The combination of positive ischemic response on electrocardiogram and a reversible thallium defect is a good indication that coronary artery disease is present and surgical risk is increased [45,46]. The use of single photon emission computed tomography (SPECT) processed images in concert with planar thallium or Cardiolite images enhances the sensitivity of exercise scintigraphy [47], but may reduce its specificity. Large reversible perfusion defects (Figure 12.11), increased lung uptake of the radiopharmaceutical, and multiple areas showing redistribution or reversibility are scintigraphic variables indicating high-risk coronary anatomy [48].

Patients with significant reversible thallium or Cardiolite perfusion defects should undergo coronary angiography. Patients with small or equivocal defects, or those patients with fixed defects and no reversible ischemic areas on scanning, may be cleared for surgery.

Pharmacologic Stress Perfusion Scintigraphy

A maximal or near maximal exercise effort is required to allow the full diagnostic capability of stress scintigraphy to be realized. Patients who are unable to raise their heart rates to 85% of their age-predicted maximal rates are more likely to have nondiagnostic or false-negative cardiac perfusion scans [49]. The major reasons for the inability to reach the target heart rate are listed in Table 12.8.

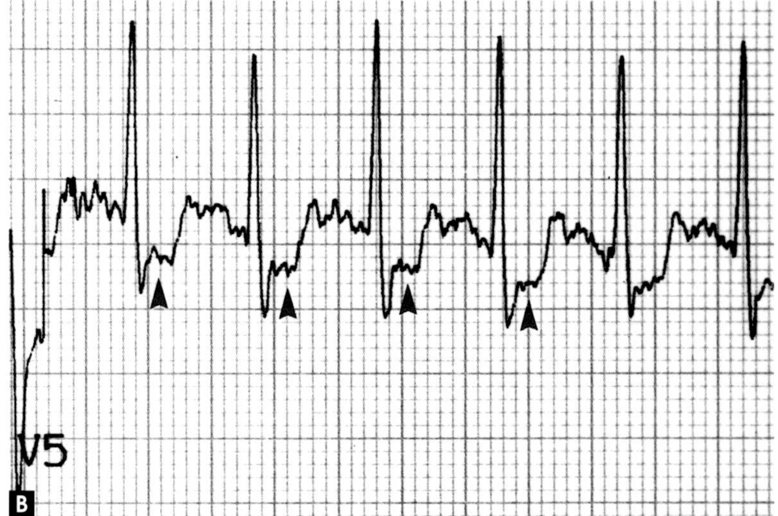

FIGURE 12.10

A, Resting lead V5 electrocardiogram showing normal, isoelectric baseline ST segments (*arrows*). **B**, Lead V5 tracing at peak treadmill exercise showing 3-mm horizontal ST segment depression (*arrows*). This change demonstrates significant exercise-induced subendocardial ischemia and is the hallmark of a positive electrocardiogram exercise stress test.

Pharmacologic stress makes reaching a target heart rate unnecessary. The most commonly used pharmacologic agents for cardiac perfusion testing are dipyridamole and adenosine. They are delivered intravenously, and because these agents may not result in diagnostic ST segment abnormalities on electrocardiographic monitoring, scintigraphic perfusion defects are the primary endpoints for diagnosing coronary artery disease. Both dipyridamole and adenosine cause three- to fivefold increases in coronary blood flow to regions perfused by normal coronary arteries in the doses used for stress testing. No such increase in flow occurs in the myocardium served by a stenotic vessel. Therefore, the marked increase in radionuclide counts in myocardium perfused by arteries with normal vasodilating capacity contrast with the fewer counts reaching the myocardium served by a diseased artery. When the pharmacologically induced myocardial hyperemia subsides, counts visible in the viable but less well perfused myocardium will equilibrate with regions that have normal coronary flow, and the stress-induced defects will appear to "reperfuse" [50,51].

Dipyridamole thallium-201 stress imaging is equivalent to exercise stress imaging in detecting coronary artery disease [52–54]. Significant prognostic information is provided by dipyridamole scintigraphy as well [55–57], and perioperative risk for a myocardial event can be assessed by such imaging [58–60]. Thus, a reversible thallium defect with dipyridamole stress would indicate the need for coronary angiography prior to carotid endarterectomy. While the use of adenosine as a stress agent would be expected to give similar results as dipyridamole-induced myocardial hyperemia, it has not been as widely studied. In addition, adenosine has not yet been approved for myocardial perfusion imaging stress by the Food and Drug Administration. One difficulty in assessing the presence of coronary artery disease is the artifactual septal defects that frequently appear with exercise scintigraphy in patients with left bundle branch block conduction. A recent study by O'Keefe and coworkers [61] showed that the use of adenosine thallium scanning reduced septal artifacts and improved the specificity in diagnosing coronary disease in patients with left bundle branch block.

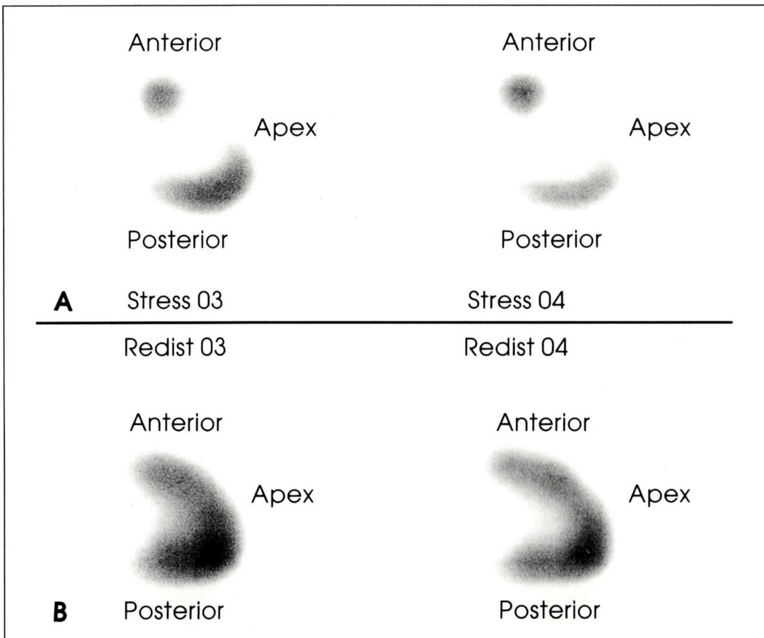

FIGURE 12.11

A, Exercise thallium study with a significant anterolateral perfusion defect indicating ischemia or infarction in the distribution of the left anterior descending coronary artery. **B**, Resting thallium scan 3 hours after exercise showing redistribution of radionuclide into the anterolateral left ventricular segment, thereby confirming that the exercise perfusion defect was due to reversible ischemia, not infarction. (*Scan courtesy* of Amjad Ali, MD.)

Stress Echocardiography

Exercise or pharmacologic stress echocardiography is another modality for diagnosing coronary artery disease. Wall motion abnormalities not present at rest, but occurring with exercise, as indicated by a decrease in systolic thickening of one or more left ventricular segments with stress, are associated with the presence of coronary artery disease (Figure 12.12) [62,63]. Comparison of exercise echocardiography and thallium-201 scintigraphy have shown comparable diagnostic accuracy [64]. Exercise or pharmacologic stress echocardiography has also been shown to be similar to scintigraphic scanning in women, whereas exercise MUGA scans are more diagnostic in men than in women [65]. The usual pharmacologic agents used with echocardiography are dipyridamole and dobutamine. Some patients may not have adequate echocardiographic interrib "windows" to allow a diagnostic study.

Stress Radionuclide Angiography (or Multigated Acquisition) Studies

The physiologic basis for exercise radionuclide angiography (RNA) scanning is similar to that of stress echocardiography. Segmental wall motion abnormalities with exercise are used to infer the presence of coronary artery disease. Since RNA scanning can also provide precise left ventricular ejection fractions, the failure of the ejection fraction to increase by more than 5% has also been used as a diagnostic clue for coronary artery disease [66].

Both RNA and electrocardiographic stress techniques can define regions of previous myocardial infarction by the presence of resting wall motion or wall thickening abnormalities, respectively. However, these techniques are not used as widely clinically for defining preoperative cardiac risk as are radionuclide flow scanning techniques (Table 12.9).

Table 12.8. Reasons for submaximal stress test heart rates
Drugs which cause resting bradycardia and blunt the rise in heart rate (beta blockers, diltiazem, verapamil, amiodarone)
Severe orthopedic problems making exercise painful
Peripheral vascular disease causing intermittent claudication
Neurologic abnormalities (prior stroke, peripheral neuropathy, Parkinson's disease)
Deconditioning
Poor motivation or inability to follow directions
Fear of the testing procedure

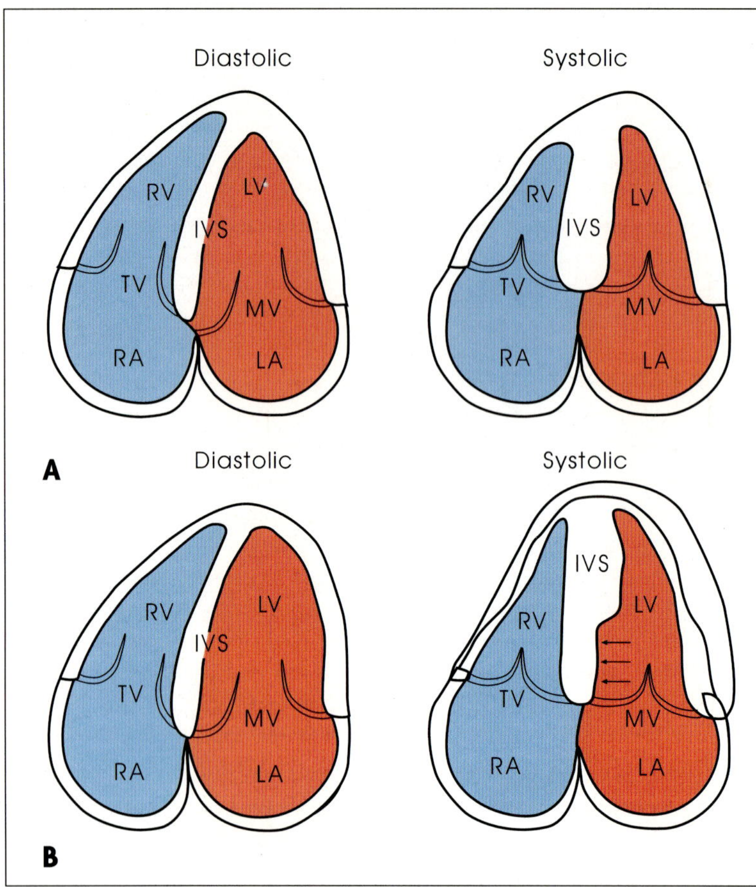

FIGURE 12.12

Schematic representation of systolic and diastolic apical four chamber stress echocardiographic views. **A**, At rest with normal segmental left ventricular wall thickening. **B**, Immediately postexercise with lack of systolic thickening, indicating ischemia in the inferoseptal region of the left ventricle (*arrows*). IVS—interventricular septum; LA—left atrium, LV—left ventricle; MV—mitral valve; RA—right atrium; RV—right ventricle; TV—tricuspid valve.

Table 12.9. Comparison of stress testing modalities

Testing modality	Advantages	Disadvantages
Electrocardiogram exercise stress	Inexpensive, well defined endpoints, widely available, no radiation exposure	Relatively low predictive accuracy particularly in women, requires near-normal resting electrocardiogram, patient must be able to exercise, does not provide anatomic detail
Exercise perfusion scintigraphy	Gives information on perfusion, anatomic detail available, differentiates viable and infarcted tissue, widely validated for preoperative risk stratification	Expensive, false-positive results in left bundle branch block*, radiation exposure, repeat imaging required, patient must be able to exercise
Pharmacologic stress perfusion scintigraphy	Same as for exercise perfusion scintigraphy, fewer false-positive results with left bundle branch block†, useful when patient cannot exercise	Expensive, radiation exposure, repeat imaging required, potential pharmacologic side effects, dipyridamole or adenosine cannot be used in patients taking dipyridamole, theophylline, or methyl xanthines
Exercise or pharmacologic stress echocardiography	No repeat imaging required, gives anatomic detail, less expensive than radionuclide testing, differentiates viable and infarcted tissue	Not widely validated for preoperative risk stratification, patient may not have an adequate echocardiographic "window," potentially high false-positive rates in nonischemic cardiac disease, does not give perfusion information
Exercise or pharmacologic radionuclide angiocardiography	No repeat imaging required, gives anatomic detail, less expensive than perfusion testing, differentiates viable and infarcted tissue	Not widely validated for preoperative risk stratification, more diagnostic for men than women‡, does not give perfusion information, radiation exposure

**Data from* Gomes and coworkers [30].
†Data from O'Keefe and coworkers [61].
‡Data from Wenger and coworkers [65].

Holter Monitoring

Ischemic ST segment changes recorded by continuous Holter monitoring preoperatively and postoperatively can identify those noncardiac surgery patients who will develop myocardial ischemic events [40,42]. This form of monitoring is currently being used experimentally to define preoperative risk factors. It has not been widely validated. Holter monitoring to evaluate ventricular arrhythmias in high-risk preoperative patients demonstrated a high incidence of nonsustained ventricular tachycardia and frequent ventricular ectopics, but this did not correlate with a worse postsurgical outcome [67].

Ultrafast X-Ray Computed Tomography

Ultrafast CT can display the calcifications often present in coronary artery segments with significant or insignificant coronary atherosclerosis. The presence of coronary calcification is predictive of the presence of histopathologic coronary artery disease. However, there is no direct correlation between the amount of calcification present by CT and the severity of coronary atherosclerosis [68]. This technique remains experimental.

REFERENCES

1. Sandok BA: Evaluation of patients with suspected cardioembolic brain infarction. In *The Heart and Stroke. Exploring Mutual Cerebrovascular and Cardiovascular Issues.* Edited by Furlan AJ. London, New York: Springer-Verlag; 1987:37–45.
2. Cerebral Embolism Task Force: Cardiogenic brain embolism. *Arch Neurol* 1986, 43:71–84.
3. Kannel WB, Wolf PA: Epidemiology of atrial fibrillation. In *Atrial Fibrillation. Mechanisms and Management.* Edited by Falk RH. New York: Raven Press; 1992:81–92.
4. Wipf JE, Lipsky BA: Atrial fibrillation: thromboembolic risk and indications for anticoagulation. *Arch Intern Med* 1990, 150:1598–1603.
5. Kannel WB, Abbott RD, Savage DD, *et al.*: Epidemiologic features of chronic atrial fibrillation: the Framingham study. *N Engl J Med* 1982, 306:1018–1022.
6. Wolf PA, Abbott RD, Kannel WB: Atrial fibrillation: a major contributor to stroke in the elderly: the Framingham study. *Arch Intern Med* 1987, 147:1561–1564.
7. Wolf PA, Dawber TR, Thomas HE Jr, *et al.*: Epidemiologic assessment of chronic atrial fibrillation and risk of stroke: the Framingham study. *Neurology* 1978, 28:973–977.
8. Peterson P: Progress reviews: thromboembolic complications in atrial fibrillation. *Stroke* 1990, 21:4–13.
9. Peterson P, Godtfredsen J, Boysen G, *et al.*: Placebo-controlled, randomized trial of warfarin and aspirin for prevention of thromboembolic complications in chronic atrial fibrillation: the Copenhagen AFASAK study. *Lancet* 1989, 1:175–178.
10. Stroke Prevention In Atrial Fibrillation Investigators: Stroke prevention in atrial fibrillation study: final results. *Circulation* 1991, 84:527–539.
11. The Boston Area Anticoagulation Trial For Atrial Fibrillation Investigators: The effect of low-dose warfarin on the risk of stroke in patients with nonrheumatic atrial fibrillation. *N Engl J Med* 1990, 323:1505–1511.
12. Connolly SJ, Laupacis A, Gent M, *et al.*: Canadian atrial fibrillation anticoagulation (CAFA) study. *J Am Coll Cardiol* 1991, 18:349–355.
13. Ezekowitz MD, Bridgers SL, James KE, *et al.*: Warfarin in the prevention of stroke associated with nonrheumatic atrial fibrillation. *N Engl J Med* 1992, 327:1406–1412.
14. The Stroke Prevention In Atrial Fibrillation Investigators: Predictors of thromboembolism in atrial fibrillation: I. clinical features of patients at risk. *Ann Intern Med* 1992, 116:1–5.
15. The Stroke Prevention In Atrial Fibrillation Investigators: Predictors of thromboembolism in atrial fibrillation: II. echocardiographic features of patients at risk. *Ann Intern Med* 1992, 116:6–12.
16. Zipes DP: Specific arrhythmias: diagnosis and treatment. In *Heart Disease. A Textbook of Cardiovascular Medicine.* Edited by Braunwald E. Philadelphia: W.B. Saunders; 1992:682–683.
17. Come PC, Riley MF, Bivas NK: Roles of echocardiography and arrhythmia monitoring in the evaluation of patients with suspected systemic embolism. *Ann Neurol* 1983, 13:527–531.
18. Bogousslavsky J, Hachinski VC, Boughner DR, *et al.*: Cardiac and arterial lesions in carotid transient ischemic attacks. *Arch Neurol* 1986, 43:223–228.
19. Rem JA, Hachinski VC, Boughner DR, *et al.*: Value of cardiac monitoring and echocardiography in TIA and stroke patients. *Stroke* 1985, 16:950–956.
20. Laupacis A, Albers G, Dunn M, *et al.*: Antithrombotic therapy in atrial fibrillation. *Chest* 1992, 102(suppl):426s–433s.
21. Kopecky SL, Gersh BJ, McGoon MD, *et al.*: The natural history of lone atrial fibrillation: a population-based study over three decades. *N Engl J Med* 1987, 317:669–674.
22. Mohiaddin RH, Longmore DB: Functional aspects of cardiovascular nuclear magnetic resonance imaging: techniques and application. *Circulation* 1993, 88:264–281.
23. White RD: Functional cine MRI of cardiovascular disease. *Cardio* 1990:45–62.
24. Manning WJ, Li W, Edelman RR: A preliminary report comparing magnetic resonance coronary angiography with conventional angiography. *N Engl J Med* 1993, 328:828–832.
25. Bateman TM, Whiting JS: Imaging techniques for the evaluation of coronary artery bypass grafts. In *Comparative Cardiac Imaging.* Edited by Brundage BH. Rockville: Aspen Publications; 1990:269–279.
26. Winkler M, Higgins CB: Suspected intracardiac masses: evaluation with MR imaging. *Radiology* 1987, 165:117–122.
27. Lund JT, Ehman RL, Julsrud PR, *et al.*: Cardiac masses: assessment by MR imaging. *Am J Roentgenol* 1989, 152:469–473.
28. Siegel MJ, Weber CK: Cardiac and paracardiac masses. In *Cardiovascular Magnetic Resonance Imaging.* Edited by Gutierrez FR, Brown JJ, Mirowitz SA. St. Louis: Mosby Yearbook; 1992:112–123.
29. Dooms GC, Higgins CB: MR imaging of cardiac thrombi. *J Comput Assist Tomogr* 1986, 10:415–420.
30. Gomes AS, Lois JF, Child JS, *et al.*: Cardiac tumors and thrombus: evaluation with MR imaging. *Am J Roentgenol* 1987, 149:895–899.
31. Nienaber CA, Von Kodolitsch Y, Nicolas V, *et al.*: The diagnosis of thoracic aortic dissection by noninvasive imaging procedures. *N Engl J Med* 1993, 328:1–9.
32. Cigarroa JE, Isselbacher EM, De Sanctis RW, *et al.*: Diagnostic imaging in the evaluation of suspected aortic dissection: old standards and new directions. *N Engl J Med* 1993, 328:35–43.
33. Zaret BL, Wackers FT, Soufer R: Nuclear cardiology. In *Heart Disease: A Textbook of Cerebrovascular Medicine.* Edited by Braunwald E. Philadelphia: W.B. Saunders; 1992:276–311.
34. Burnett KR, Lyons KP: Gated blood scintigraphy of the LV. In *Cardiovascular Nuclear Medicine.* Edited by Lyons KP. Norwalk, CT: Appleton & Lang; 1988:53–94.
35. North American Symptomatic Carotid Endarterectomy Trial Collaborators: Beneficial effect of carotid endarterectomy in symptomatic patients with high-grade carotid stenosis. *N Engl J Med* 1991, 325:445–453.

36. Kubicka R, Smith C, Piccione W, *et al.*: Cardiac tumors. *Postgrad Radiol* 1993, 13(4): 237–249.
37. European Carotid Surgery Trialists' Collaborative Group: MRC European carotid surgery trial: interim results for symptomatic patients with severe (70–99%) or with mild (10–29%) carotid stenosis. *Lancet* 1991, 337:1235–1243.
38. Mayberg MR, Wilson SE, Yatsu F, *et al.*: Carotid endarterectomy and prevention of cerebral ischemia in symptomatic carotid stenosis. *JAMA* 1991, 266:3289–3294.
39. Chambers BR, Norris JW: Outcome in patients with asymptomatic neck bruits. *N Engl J Med* 1986, 315:860–865.
40. Mangano DT, Browner WS, Hollenberg M, *et al.*: Association of perioperative myocardial ischemia with cardiac morbidity and mortality in men undergoing noncardiac surgery. *N Engl J Med* 1990, 232:1781–1788.
41. Goldman L, Caldera DL, Nussbaum SR, *et al.*: Multifactorial index of cardiac risk in noncardiac surgical procedures. *N Engl J Med* 1977, 297:845–850.
42. Hollenberg M, Mangano DT, Browner WS, *et al.*: Predictors of postoperative ischemia in patients undergoing noncardiac surgery. *N Engl J Med* 1992, 268:205–209.
43. Gianrossi R, Detrano R, Mulvihill D, *et al.*: Exercise-induced ST depression in the diagnosis of coronary artery disease: a meta-analysis. *Circulation* 1989, 80:87–98.
44. Taillefer R, Gagnon A, La Flamme L, *et al.*: Same-day injections of Tc-99m methoxy isobutyl isonitrile (hexamibi) for myocardial tomographic imaging: comparison between rest-stress and stress-rest injection. *Eur J Nucl Med* 1989, 15:113–117.
45. Ladenheim MC, Pollock BH, Rozanski A, *et al.*: Extent and severity of myocardial hypoperfusion in patients with suspected coronary artery disease. *J Am Coll Cardiol* 1986, 7:464–471.
46. Koss JH, Kobren SM, Greenwald AM, *et al.*: Role of exercise thallium-201 myocardial perfusion scintigraphy in predicting prognosis in suspected coronary artery disease. *Am J Cardiol* 1987, 59:531–534.
47. Maddahi J, Van Train K, Prigent F, *et al.*: Quantitative single photon emission computed thallium-201 tomography for detection and localization of coronary artery disease: optimization and prospective validation of a new technique. *J Am Coll Cardiol* 1989, 14:1689–1699.
48. Kaul S: A look at 15 years of planar thallium-201 imaging. *Am Heart J* 1989, 118:581–601.
49. Iskandrian AS, Heo J, Kong B, *et al.*: Effect of exercise level on the ability of thallium-201 tomographic imaging in detecting coronary artery disease: analysis of 461 patients. *J Am Coll Cardiol* 1989, 14:1477–1486.
50. Beller GA, Holzgrefe HH, Watson DD: Effects of dipyridamole-induced vasodilatation on myocardial uptake and clearance kinetics of thallium-201. *Circulation* 1983, 68:1328–1338.
51. Beller GA: Pharmacologic stress imaging. *JAMA* 1991, 265:633–638.
52. Varma SK, Watson DD, Beller GA: Quantitative comparison of thallium-201 scintigraphy after exercise and dipyridamole in coronary artery disease. *Am J Cardiol* 1989, 64:871–877.
53. Josephson MA, Brown BG, Hecht HS, *et al.*: Noninvasive detection and localization of coronary stenoses in patients: comparison of resting dipyridamole and exercise thallium-201 myocardial perfusion imaging. *Am Heart J* 1982, 103:1008–1018.
54. Albro PC, Gould KL, Westcott RJ, *et al.*: Noninvasive assessment of coronary stenoses by myocardial imaging during pharmacologic coronary vasodilatation. III. Clinical trial. *Am J Cardiol* 1978, 42:751–760.
55. Hendel RC, Layden JJ, Lippo JA: Prognostic value of dipyridamole thallium scintigraphy for evaluation of ischemic heart disease. *J Am Coll Cardiol* 1990, 15:109–116.
56. Younis LT, Byers S, Shaw L, *et al.*: Prognostic importance of silent myocardial ischemia detected by intravenous dipyridamole thallium myocardial imaging in asymptomatic patients with coronary artery disease. *J Am Coll Cardiol* 1989, 14:1635–1641.
57. Levinson JR, Boucher CA, Coley CM, *et al.*: Usefulness of semiquantitative analysis of dipyridamole-thallium 201 redistribution for improving risk stratification before vascular surgery. *Am J Cardiol* 1990, 66:406–410.
58. Wong T, Detsky AS: Preoperative cardiac risk assessment for patients having peripheral vascular surgery. *Ann Intern Med* 1992, 116:743–753.
59. Eagle KA, Coley CM, Newell JB, *et al.*: Combining clinical and thallium data optimizes preoperative assessment of cardiac risk before major vascular surgery. *Ann Intern Med* 1989, 110:859–866.
60. Boucher CA, Brewster DC, Darling RC, *et al.*: Determinations of cardiac risk by dipyridamole-thallium imaging before peripheral vascular surgery. *N Engl J Med* 1985, 312:389–394.
61. O'Keefe JH, Bateman TM, Barnhart CS: Adenosine thallium-201 is superior to exercise thallium-201 for detecting coronary artery disease in patients with left bundle branch block. *J Am Coll Cardiol* 1993, 21:1332–1338.
62. Morganroth J, Chen CC, David D, *et al.*: Exercise cross-sectional echocardiographic diagnosis of coronary artery disease. *Am J Cardiol* 1981, 47:20–26.
63. Wann LS, Childress RH, Dillon JC, *et al.*: Exercise cross-sectional echocardiography in ischemic heart disease. *Circulation* 1979, 60:1300–1308.
64. Quinones MA, Verani MS, Haichin RM, *et al.*: Exercise echocardiography versus thallium-201 single photon emission computed tomography in evaluation of coronary artery disease: analysis of 292 patients. *Circulation* 1992, 85:1026–1031.
65. Wenger NK, Speroff L, Packard B: Cardiovascular health and disease in women. *N Engl J Med* 1993, 329:247–256.
66. Iskandrian AS, Hakki A-H, De Pace NL, *et al.*: Evaluation of left ventricular function by radionuclide angiography during exercise in normal subjects and in patients with chronic coronary heart disease. *J Am Coll Cardiol* 1983, 1:1518–1529.
67. O'Kelly MB, Browner WS, Massie B, *et al.*: Ventricular arrhythmias in patients undergoing noncardiac surgery. *JAMA* 1992, 268:217–221.
68. Simons BD, Schwartz RS, Edwards WD, *et al.*: Noninvasive definition of anatomic coronary artery disease by ultrafast computed tomographic scanning: a qualitative pathologic comparison study. *J Am Coll Cardiol* 1993, 20:1118–1126.

Chapter 13

Hematologic Evaluation of the Stroke Patient

MAURA BRAGONI
EDWARD FELDMANN

Stroke treatment is determined by the underlying pathophysiologic process, whether the stroke is ischemic or hemorrhagic. Hematologic abnormalities may be a primary or secondary mechanism of stroke, and therefore deserve appropriate evaluation in every patient. In some patients, very specific therapies are administered because the stroke is associated with a particular hematologic disorder.

Information regarding hematologic abnormalities associated with stroke is increasing dramatically. In the past, only a few hematologic disorders were discussed as possible risk factors for stroke, such as elevated fibrinogen or hematocrit, platelet hyperaggregability, hypercoagulable states such as polycythemia vera or disseminated intravascular coagulation (DIC), hyperlipidemia, diabetes mellitus, and hyperuricemia.

Modern techniques have begun to explore the regulation of the coagulation system, such as the function of antithrombin III (AT III). Proteins that interfere with the coagulation system, such as antiphospholipid antibodies, have been identified. Genetic disorders, whose pathogenetic mechanisms are still unclear, such as the syndrome characterized by mitochondrial myopathy, encephalopathy, lactic acidosis, and stroke-like episodes (MELAS), can also be detected.

Most stroke patients can be adequately managed with routine hematologic testing. Exhaustive hematologic evaluations are pursued only in selected patients where particular clinical features of stroke presentation or laboratory tests suggest that more thorough evaluation is warranted. All treatable stroke patients deserve appropriate, aggressive evaluation.

EPIDEMIOLOGY

There are numerous roadblocks to clarifying the role played by the hematologic disorders in stroke. The precise cause of stroke in an individual patient may be difficult to establish. A hematologic abnormality detected after a stroke does not imply that it caused the stroke. Causality may be more reasonably presumed if the hematologic alteration predates the stroke, persists after the acute phase, or is detectable in relatives of the patient [1].

The prevalence of hematologic disorders in stroke and nonstroke populations is not well studied. In the stroke literature, the data typically reflect patient selection, when hematologic data exist at all. Prevalence data are more thorough in young stroke patients, or in older patients in whom the cause of the stroke was initially unclear. The paucity of data on the prevalence of hematologic abnormalities in the general population and of epidemiologic study in stroke patients makes it difficult to clarify the role played by hematologic findings.

The role of hematologic disorders in stroke is further obscured by the concomitant presence of other stroke risk factors. Young patients often have no other risk factors, making it easier to study the contribution of the hematologic abnormalities. How important are the hematologic alterations when other

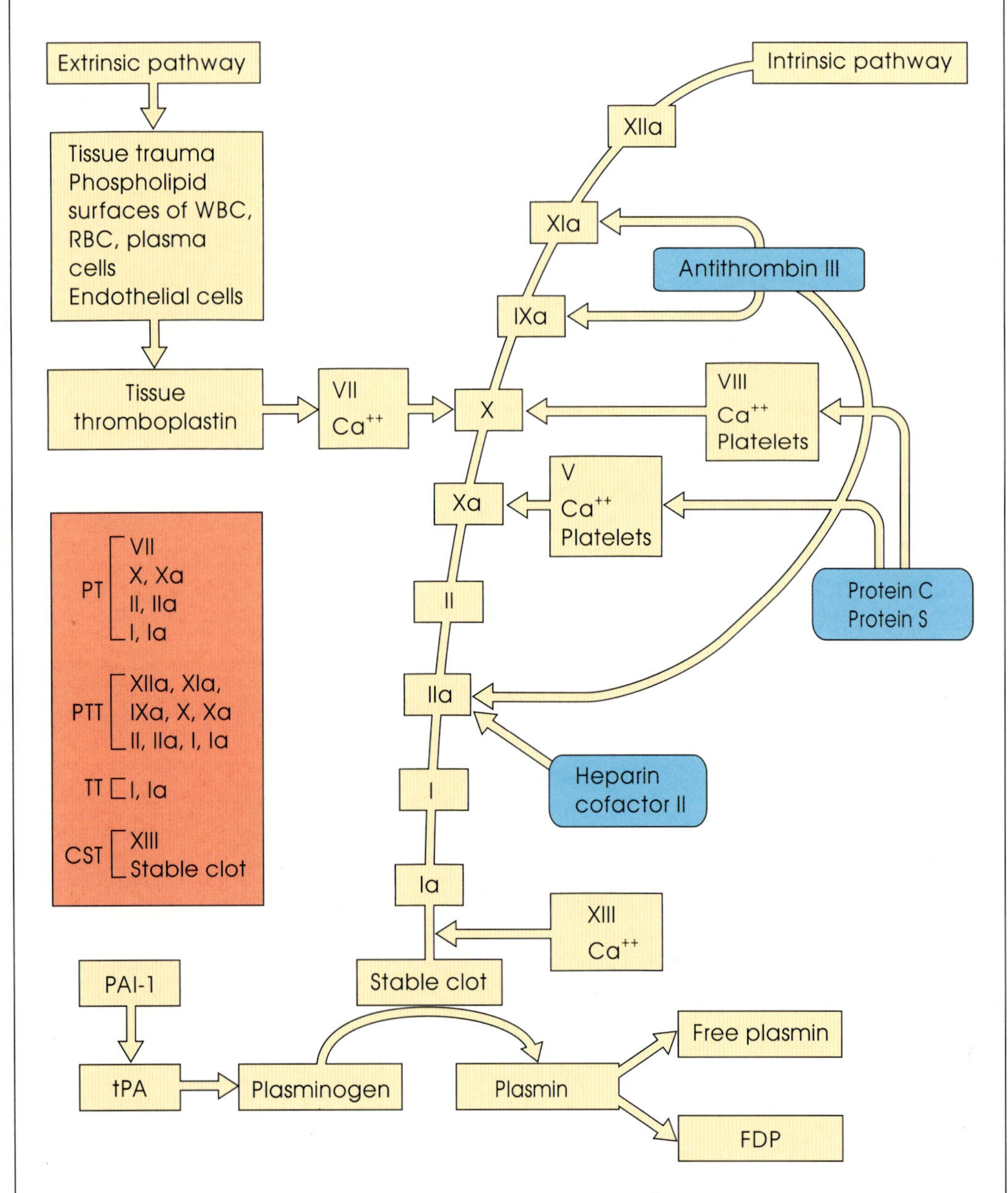

FIGURE 13.1

The human coagulation system and the laboratory tests that assess its function. The blood tests are indicated in *red* along with the coagulation factors they assess. The coagulation inhibitors are indicated in *blue*, along with the specific coagulation factors they inhibit. CST—clot stability test; FDP—fibrinogen degradation product; PAI-1—plasminogen activator inhibitor; PT—prothrombin time; PTT—partial thromboplastin time; RBC—red blood cells; tPA—tissue plasminogen activator; TT—thromboplastin time; WBC—white blood cells.

risk factors are present? There are few data directed at this issue, in young or in older patients. Moreover, the prevalence of the hematologic abnormalities may vary by stroke mechanism, further complicating the issue. For example, thrombotic stroke may more often be associated with hematologic disorders than embolic stroke.

MAJOR COAGULATION MECHANISMS

The major features of the human coagulation system, as well as the specific laboratory tests designed to access them, are outlined in Figure 13.1. The two coagulation pathways with inhibitory factors such as AT III, protein C, protein S, and heparin cofactor II are illustrated. The fibrinolytic system is also included in the figure. The specific hematologic tests that may be performed in order to identify abnormalities of the system are also illustrated. The tests are matched with the specific factors they assess. These tests do not measure the serum level of the coagulation factors, which can be performed separately.

HEMATOLOGIC DISORDERS ASSOCIATED WITH STROKE

Tables 13.1 through 13.8 list the key factors in the human coagulation system. For each factor, the related hematologic disorders associated with stroke are listed.

Table 13.1. Platelet disorders in stroke

Functional alterations	Diseases
Hyperaggregability	Sticky platelet syndrome
Hypoaggregability	Glanzmann's thrombasthenia, antiplatelet drugs, uremia, paraproteinemia
Adhesion deficit	Bernard-Soulier syndrome
Increased platelets	Essential thrombocythemia, thrombocytosis
Decreased platelets	TTP, thrombocytopenia, ITP, alloimmune thrombocytopenic purpura, HITP types I and II, hemolytic uremic syndrome, Wiskott-Aldrich syndrome, thrombocytopenia with absent radius syndrome

HITP—heparin-induced thrombocytopenia; ITP—idiopathic (immune) thrombocytopenic purpura; TTP—thrombotic thrombocytopenic purpura.

Table 13.2. Erythrocyte disorders in stroke

Functional alterations
- Paroxysmal nocturnal hemoglobinuria
- Enhanced aggregability

Increased erythrocytes
- Polycythemia vera
- Secondary polycythemia

Decreased erythrocytes
- Anemia

Stroke Features

To provide a basis for selective hematologic testing of individual patients based on their presentation, the clinical and laboratory features associated with stroke and the individual hematologic disorders are discussed in the sections that follow. The systemic clues alerting the clinician to the presence of a particular hematologic disorder are listed in Tables 13.9 through 13.16, while the text discusses the neurologic features.

The presence of a hematologic disorder in a stroke patient is suspected from the clinical presentation of either the hematologic disorder or the stroke. In some situations, such as stroke associated with acute nonlymphoblastic leukemia (ANLL), the hematologic disorder will already have been symptomatic. However, the hematologic disorder, aside from its association with stroke, may be otherwise asymptomatic. Clues such as age provide an initial direction for evaluation in these patients. For example, children with stroke should be tested for organic acidemias or MELAS. Alternatively, peculiar features of the stroke, such as a predilection for venous thromboses, will provide clues to the diagnosis.

Note that widely differing hematologic diseases, congenital or acquired, may be associated with the same type of stroke. For example, Leigh's disease and the antiphospholipid antibody syndrome may both be associated with ischemic stroke. On the other hand, the same disease may be found either in ischemic or hemorrhagic stroke. For example, Fabry's disease, essential thrombocythemia, or leukemia may be seen either in ischemic or hemorrhagic stroke.

PLATELET DISORDERS AND STROKE

Table 13.9 lists the systemic features of platelet disorders associated with stroke.

Table 13.3. Leukocyte disorders in stroke

Increased leukocytes
- Leukemia: ANLL, ALL
- Lymphoma: Hodgkins, non-Hodgkins

Decreased leukocytes
- Chronic familial cerebral vasculopathy

ALL—acute lymphoblastic leukemia; ANLL—acute nonlymphocytic leukemia (acute promyelocytic leukemia, acute myelomonocytic leukemia, acute myeloblastic leukemia, acute monocytic leukemia).

Table 13.4. Plasma cell disorders in stroke

Increased plasma cells and protein
- Waldenstrom's macroglobulinemia
- Myeloma

Increased protein
- Cryoglobulinemia

Functional Alterations of Platelets

The sticky platelet syndrome is present in migraine patients. It is associated with ischemic stroke [2]. Glanzmann's thrombasthenia and the Bernard-Soulier syndrome are congenital disorders of platelet function associated with hemorrhagic stroke in young patients [3]. Abnormal platelet aggregation, secondary to absent or defective receptors for fibrinogen and von Willebrand's factor on the platelet membrane, leads to bleeding in Glanzmann's thromboasthenia. Defective platelet adhesion due to absent or defective receptors for von Willebrand's factor on platelet membrane leads to bleeding in the Bernard-Soulier syndrome. Acquired conditions, such as uremia, paraproteinemia, or the use of antiplatelet drugs such as aspirin may be associated with hemorrhagic stroke [3]. While the occurrence of intracerebral hemorrhage during aspirin use has been described, an epidemiologic association of aspirin with intracerebral hemorrhage has not been conclusively demonstrated [4].

Table 13.5. Hemoglobin disorders in stroke

HbSC	HbSA
Hemoglobin SC disease	Sickle cell trait
HbSS	Thalassemia β
Sickle cell anemia	Cooley's anemia
	β variants

Hb—hemoglobin.

Table 13.6. Coagulation factor disorders in stroke

Coagulation factor inhibitor deficiency
- AT III
- Protein C
- Protein S
- Heparin cofactor II

Coagulation factor deficiency
- Factor VII
- Factor VIII (hemophilia A)
- von Willebrand's factor (von Willebrand's disease)
- Factor IX (Christmas disease)
- Factor XI
- Factor XII
- Factor XIII
- Fibrinogen (afibrinogenemia, DIC)

Coagulation factor excess
- Factor VIII
- Fibrinogen

Deficiency of regulatory clotting factors
- Vitamin K

Serum disorders of uncertain mechanism
- Decrease A/G ratio
- Plasma hyperviscosity

A/G ratio—serum albumin/globulin ratio; AT III—antithrombin III; DIC—disseminated intravascular coagulation.

Increased Platelet Count

Essential thrombocythemia is a myeloproliferative disorder associated with either ischemic or hemorrhagic stroke in men aged 40 to 50 years. Transient ischemic attacks (TIAs) and transient monocular blindness are also reported. The ischemic events may be associated with cortical vein or sinus thrombosis [5] or arterial occlusions [6]. Thrombocytosis may occur in association with TIAs and ischemic stroke [7]. The platelet count associated with ischemic stroke in both essential thrombocythemia and thrombocytosis ranges between 600×10^9 and 1345×10^9 L [5–7].

Decreased Platelet Count

Thrombotic thrombocytopenic purpura (TTP) is an acquired disease with abrupt onset characterized by variable neurologic manifestations including headache, mental changes, seizures, visual symptoms, cranial nerve palsies, numbness, vertigo, and coma. TIA and both ischemic and hemorrhagic stroke may occur. Occlusive platelet thrombi found in the cerebral microcirculation are believed to cause ischemic stroke in these patients [8].

Thrombocytopenia occurs in several acquired conditions such as disseminated intravascular coagulation (DIC), myeloproliferative diseases, and aplastic anemia. Bleeding is related to the number of platelets, ranging from 20 to 25×10^9/L for spontaneous hemorrhages [9], to less than 100×10^9/L as reported in postoperative neurosurgery patients [10]. Any hemorrhagic cerebral event may occur, including intracerebral hemorrhage, subarachnoid hemorrhage, or subdural hematoma.

Table 13.7. Fibrinolytic disorders in stroke

Decreased fibrinolysis
- Plasminogen deficiency
- Vascular plasminogen activator deficiency
- L(pa) increase
- Antifibrinolytic drugs: tranexamic acid, aminocaproic acid

Increased fibrinolysis
- Fibrinolytic drugs: streptokinase, urokinase, t-PA

L(pa)—cholesterol-rich lipoprotein; t-PA—tissue-type plasminogen activator.

Table 13.8. Uncertain pathogenic mechanisms in stroke

Congenital diseases
- Fabry's disease
- Leigh's disease
- MELAS
- Homocystinuria/homocysteinemia
- Familial hypo-α-lipoproteinemia
- Organic acidemias: methylmalonic acidemias, propionic acidemias, isovaleric acidemias

Immunologic disorders
- Antiphospholipid antibody syndrome: aCL, LAC

aCL—anticardiolipin antibody; LAC—lupus anticoagulant; MELAS—mitochondrial myopathy, encephalopathy, lactic acidosis, stroke-like episodes.

Alloimmune thrombocytopenia and immune thrombocytopenic purpura (ITP) are immunologic disorders in which thrombocytopenia causes hemorrhagic events, such as intracerebral hemorrhage, subarachnoid hemorrhage, or subdural hematoma [11]. In alloimmune thrombocytopenia, hemorrhages in utero are also reported [12,13].

Heparin-induced thrombocytopenia type I is rarely implicated in systemic or cerebral thromboembolic events. Type II is more frequently associated with ischemic stroke. Thrombosis secondary to platelet-aggregating antibodies is believed to be responsible for ischemic stroke in this disorder. Severe thrombocytopenia, to values even less than 10×10^9/L, has been reported in association with thromboembolic events [14]. The ischemic event may occur in the anterior or posterior circulation, and arteries or veins may be affected. Superior sagittal sinus thrombosis is frequently described [15]. TIA may also occur. Hemorrhagic stroke during treatment with heparin is also noted, but the mechanism seems to be related to the direct effect of the drug on the coagulation system.

Thrombocytopenia associated with the hemolytic uremic syndrome is an acquired condition in which variable neurologic signs are described. Behavioral changes, seizures (tonic-clonic), cortical blindness, dizziness, diplopia, cranial nerve palsy, cerebellar ataxia, and coma are the most relevant neurologic features. Both ischemic and hemorrhagic events are described. Platelet aggregates and thrombi in the cerebral microcirculation, presumably secondary to endothelial cell injury, have been described in patients with ischemic stroke in this disorder [16].

Thrombocytopenia with absent radius syndrome and Wiskott-Aldrich syndrome are genetic diseases in which hemorrhagic strokes may affect children or young adults [17].

Table 13.9. Systemic features of platelet disorders associated with stroke

Disease	Clinical features	Associated laboratory features
Sticky platelet syndrome	Young, family history of coronary artery disease	PLT hyperaggregability
Glanzmann's thrombasthenia	Autosomal recessive, epistaxis, bruising, gastrointestinal bleeding, menorrhagia	PLT hypoaggregability
Uremia	Renal failure	PLT hypoaggregability
Antiplatelet drugs	History of aspirin use	PLT hypoaggregability
Paraproteinemia	Mild splenomegaly, hepatomegaly, peripheral lymphoadenopathy, weakness, renal impairment, bleeding, signs of organ infiltration, infections	PLT hypoaggregability, anemia, monoclonal or polyclonal Ig (serum electrophoresis)
Bernard-Soulier syndrome	Autosomal recessive, epistaxis, bleeding from mucous membranes, bruises, rarely bleeding in joints	Giant platelets, mild thrombocytopenia
Essential thrombocythemia	5th–6th decade, higher prevalence in men, easy bruising and bleeding, DVT, PE, emboli to the digits, splenomegaly	PLT > 1,000,000/mm^3, increased megakaryocyte count
Thrombocytosis	Iron-deficiency anemia and myeloproliferative disorders, thrombotic tendency	Laboratory signs of primary disease
TTP	Adult, higher prevalence in women, abrupt, fever, weakness, arthralgia, jaundice, renal abnormalities, abdominal distress, tachycardia, purpura, bleeding, eventually clinical signs of DIC	LDH and bilirubin increase, microangiopathic hemolytic anemia, erythrocyte fragmentation in peripheral smear, reticulocytosis, proteinuria, laboratory signs of DIC
Thrombocytopenia	Aplastic anemia, acute leukemia, DIC	PLT < 20–25,000/mm^3
ITP	"Adult" type: chronic, idiopathic, or secondary to lymphoproliferative diseases, autoimmune diseases, HIV infection; "childhood" type: acute, self-limited, follows a minor virus infection, adult and child may be affected by either type	Anti-PLT autoantibody, thrombocytopenia
Alloimmune thrombocytopenic purpura	Newborn antigen PLT^{A1}–positive, from antigen PLT^{A1}–negative mother	Thrombocytopenia
HITP Type I	Onset 1–5 days after starting heparin, rare thromboembolic events	PLT > 50,000/mm^3
HITP Type II	Onset 2 weeks after starting heparin, sooner if secondary exposure, skin necrosis precedes the HITP, thromboembolic events and hemorrhages, high-dose and type related: bovine-lung-heparin	Anti-PLT–antibody, PLT < 10–50,000/mm^3, PLT count may be normal
Thrombocytopenia during hemolytic uremic syndrome	Acquired, childhood, renal impairment, hypertension, vitreous hemorrhage, retinal infarction	Microangiopathic hemolytic anemia, thrombocytopenia
Wiskott-Aldrich syndrome	X-linked recessive, young, eczema, infections, myeloproliferative disorders	Thrombocytopenia, altered lymphocytes function
Thrombocytopenia with absent radius syndrome	Autosomal recessive, young, skeletal, renal cardiac malformations, aplasia/hypoplasia of radius	Megakaryocyte deficit, thrombocytopenia

DIC—disseminated intravascular coagulation; DVT—deep vein thrombosis, HITP—heparin-induced thrombocytopenia; ITP—idiopathic thrombocytopenic purpura; LDH—lactic dehydrogenase; PE—pulmonary emboli; PLT—platelet; TTP—thrombotic thrombocytopenic purpura.

ERYTHROCYTE DISORDERS AND STROKE

Table 13.10 lists the systemic features of the erythrocyte disorders associated with stroke.

Functional Alterations of Erythrocytes

Paroxysmal nocturnal hemoglobinuria is associated with TIA and ischemic and hemorrhagic stroke, especially in young adults. A mechanism responsible for ischemic stroke has not been identified in this disorder. Cerebral vein involvement is typical [18]. Conclusive data on arterial thrombosis are lacking [1]. Cerebrovascular complications and portal vein thrombosis are the usual causes of death in these patients. Recently, enhanced erythrocyte aggregability has been linked to cerebral ischemia, either in the acute phase or in the chronic phase of an ischemic stroke [19].

Increased Erythrocyte Count

Polycythemia vera is a myeloproliferative condition affecting elderly patients. Both ischemic and hemorrhagic stroke may occur. Arterial or venous vessels may be affected by the thromboembolic event. Among the hemorrhagic complications, intracerebral hemorrhage, subarachnoid hemorrhage, subdural, and extradural hematoma are described. The occurrence of ischemic stroke is dependent on age. Men aged 51 to 60 years and women older than 70 years show an increased risk of thrombotic events compared with younger patients [20]. The risk of stroke seems to correlate positively with an increased hematocrit value. Stroke risk increases as hematocrit rises from 44% to 59%, and the risk is even higher with a hematocrit value over 60% [20]. Other workers could not demonstrate a clear correlation between hematocrit and higher risk of stroke [21]. Serum hyperviscosity has also been linked to stroke in polycythemia [22]. Secondary polycythemia is implicated in causing ischemic stroke, but less frequently than polycythemia vera [1].

Decreased Erythrocyte Count

The occurrence of ischemic stroke is reported during severe anemia associated with iron deficiency. Impaired oxygen-

Table 13.10. Systemic features of erythrocyte disorders associated with stroke

Disease	Clinical features	Associated laboratory features
Paroxysmal nocturnal hemoglobinuria	Acquired, age 25–40 years, thrombosis of portal vein	Chronic hemolytic anemia, thrombocytopenia, granulocytopenia, hemoglobinuria of early morning
Enhanced aggregability	No particular general features	Erythrocyte hyperaggregability, increased serum globulin level, increased fibrinogen
Polycythemia vera	Old age, plethora, severe pruritis, coronary artery disease, conjunctival and retinal blood vessel congestion, DVT, PE, peptic ulcers with gastrointestinal bleeding, splenomegaly	Hematocrit increase, increased leukocyte , PLT, marrow cellularity, and megakaryocyte counts
Secondary polycythemia	Middle age, male sex, smoker, hypertension, obesity, thromboembolic events caused by stress, chronic pulmonary disease, cardiovascular disease, hemoglobinopathy, inappropriate erythropoietin production	Hematocrit increase
Anemia	Pallor, weakness, increased heart rate	Hemoglobin 7–7.5 mg/dL, may be associated with thrombocytosis

DVT—deep vein thrombosis; PE—pulmonary emboli; PLT—platelets.

Table 13.11. Systemic features of leukocyte disorders associated with stroke

Disease	Clinical features	Associated laboratory features
ANLL	Weakness, pallor, bruising hemorrhage, infections, splenomegaly, hepatomegaly; APL: DIC and bleeding; AMOL/AMML: skin infiltrates, gum hypertrophy	Anemia, thrombocytopenia, leukopenia, increased blasts
ALL	Pallor, weakness, bleeding, infections, splenomegaly, hepatomegaly, lymphoadenopathy, thymus enlargement	Anemia, thrombocytopenia, leukopenia, increased blasts
Lymphoma	Lymphadenopathy, organ infiltration	Anemia, leukopenia, thrombocytopenia, LDH, AST, ALT, and CK increase
Chronic familial cerebral vasculopathy	Young adulthood, familial incidence	Decreased number and abnormal peripheral B-lymphocytes

ALL—acute lymphoblastic leukemia; ALT—alanine aminotransferase; AMML—acute myelomonocytic leukemia; AMOL—acute monocytic leukemia; ANLL—acute nonlymphocytic leukemia; APL—acute promyelocytic leukemia; AST—aspartate aminotransferase; CK—creatine kinase; DIC—disseminated intravascular coagulation; LDH—lactic dehydrogenase.

carrying capacity of blood and a marked thrombocytosis can lead to ischemic cerebral vascular symptoms [23]. A hemoglobin level of 7.5 g/dL, associated with severe atherosclerosis of the carotid arteries, has also been associated with stroke [3]. Ischemic cerebral thrombosis may occur in the arteries or in the veins.

LEUKOCYTE DISORDERS AND STROKE

Table 13.11 lists the systemic features of leukocyte disorders associated with stroke.

Increased Leukocyte Count

Acute nonlymphoblastic leukemia (or myelogenous leukemia), including promyelocytic leukemia, myelomonocytic leukemia, myeloblastic leukemia, and monocytic leukemia, is associated with intracranial hemorrhage and ischemic stroke, the latter being less frequent. Among the hemorrhages, the most frequent type seems to be cerebral hemorrhage, usually involving the white matter [24]. The mechanism of the neurologic events may be related to the occurrence of DIC, septic infarction, or the hyperviscosity syndrome. DIC is often a very early complication of promyelocytic leukemia, causing intracerebral hemorrhage followed by death in up to 60% of these patients [24]. The hyperviscosity syndrome is marked by auditory and visual disturbances, headache, ataxia, somnolence, and coma. Generally, it occurs when the leukocyte count is over 200,000/mm^3. Myelogenous leukemia is the common culprit [3].

Acute lymphoblastic leukemia is associated with hemorrhagic and ischemic stroke, the incidence of both complications being approximately the same. Severe leukocytosis plays an important role in causing intracerebral hemorrhage in acute lymphoblastic leukemia as the leukemic nodules disrupt blood vessel walls [24]. Thrombocytopenia is also involved in the pathogenesis of hemorrhagic stroke [25]. Disseminated intravascular coagulation and septic infarctions are the basis for ischemic complications [24]. Lymphoma may be associated with thrombosis of cortical veins and sinuses. Superior sagittal sinus thrombosis is the most common cerebrovascular complication of this disorder [25]. Direct infiltration or compression of the sinus by tumor causes sinus thrombosis [24]. Ischemic stroke secondary to disseminated intravascular coagulation and septic infarction has also been described in patients with lymphoma [24].

Decreased Leukocyte Count

Chronic familial cerebral vasculopathy is an uncommon disease classified among the amyloidoses, characterized by familial incidence, recurrent stroke, and dementia, and is associated with a low count of abnormal B-lymphocytes in the peripheral blood [17]. Amyloid deposition in cerebral vessels leads to progressive disruption of the vessel walls, obliteration of the lumen, and recurrent stroke.

PLASMA CELL DISORDERS AND STROKE

Table 13.12 lists the systemic features of plasma cell disorders associated with stroke.

Increased Plasma Cell Count

Waldenstrom's macroglobulinemia and myeloma are associated with ischemic stroke, intracerebral hemorrhage, and subarachnoid hemorrhage [3]. Headache, confusion, lethargy, and coma may also occur. The pathogenesis of these symptoms is believed to be the hyperviscosity seen with both diseases. A progressive, symmetrical peripheral neuropathy is also described.

Cryoglobulinemia, in particular mixed cryoglobulinemia, is associated with ischemic stroke, caused presumably by cerebral vasculitis [26,27].

HEMOGLOBIN DISORDERS AND STROKE

Table 13.13 describes the systemic features of hemoglobin disorders associated with stroke.

Sickle Cell Disorders

Hemoglobin sickle C (SC) disease, double heterozygous sickling hemoglobinopathy, may be associated with ischemic stroke, mental retardation, chorea, radiculopathy, vertigo, seizures, stupor, and coma [28].

Different patterns of neurologic complications may be observed in SC anemia because of the different phenotypic expressions of the disease. Either ischemic or hemorrhagic stroke may occur. Ischemic complications may be related either to an occlusive vasculopathy involving the distal intracranial segment of the

Table 13.12. Systemic features of plasma cell disorders associated with stroke

Disease	Clinical features	Associated laboratory features
Waldenstrom's macroglobulinemia	Older men, insidious, pallor, splenomegaly, hepatomegaly, peripheral lymphoadenopathy, retinal hemorrhage, venous congestion with vascular segmentation, bruising, purpura, epistaxis, gastrointestinal hemorrhages	Anemia, increased mast-cells, ESR increase, IgM monoclonal protein, hyperviscosity
Myeloma	Ages 60–70 years, history of bone pain, weakness, renal impairment, bleeding, signs of organ infiltration, infections	Anemia, Ig electrophoresis peak, ESR increase, hypercalcemia, hyperviscosity
Cryoglobulinemia	Raynaud's phenomenon, digital pain, skin ulcerations with cold, purpura, infections, vasculitis, glomerulonephritis, lymphoproliferative disorders may be associated	Monclonal (IgG, IgA, IgM) or polyclonal cryoglobulins

ESR—erythrocyte sedimentation rate.

internal carotid arteries, the proximal middle and anterior cerebral arteries, or to thromboembolic events. The occlusive vasculopathy is characterized by fibrous proliferation of the intima, which may cause the formation of thrombi. Among children, hemorrhagic complications secondary to fragmentation of the elastic lamina of the vessels have also been described [3]. The ischemic stroke is more frequent among children, and the hemorrhagic stroke more frequent among adults. Subarachnoid hemorrhage in young adults is usually related to ruptured aneurysms. Both large [29] and small arteries may be involved by the thromboembolic events. Thromboembolic events are secondary to sickling. Hypoxia, infection, acidosis, and dehydration may precipitate a sickling crisis [3]. Cranial neuropathies, spinal infarction, hypopituitarism, optic atrophy, and seizures are also described.

Ischemic stroke has also been described in sickle cell trait. It has been linked to low oxygen concentrations or acidosis, such as during anesthesia [30], but other reports describe ischemic stroke in the absence of these conditions [31].

Thalassemia

Ischemic arterial strokes may occur during the course of Cooley's anemia [32,33], thalassemia intermedia, and thalassemia minima. The latter is considered a very uncommon cause of ischemic events. Both children and young adults with Cooley's anemia may be affected. In thalassemia intermedia, the ischemic event often occurs after transfusions or splenectomy. Prolonged thrombocytosis, observed after splenectomy, is involved in the pathogenesis of thromboembolic events seen in these patients. The precise mechanisms that lead to stroke are not clear [34].

COAGULATION FACTOR DISORDERS AND STROKE

Table 13.14 lists the systemic features of coagulation factor disorders associated with stroke.

Coagulation Factor Deficiency

Deficiency of AT III, protein C, or protein S may be congenital or acquired. In either situation, TIA, amaurosis fugax, and ischemic stroke are described [35]. Both arteries and veins may be involved. The ischemic event may occur in the young, even in newborns [36], as well as in the elderly.

Ischemic arterial stroke, TIA, and venous thrombosis are associated with congenital heparin cofactor II deficiency. AT III levels are normal. Defective thrombin inhibition secondary to heparin cofactor II deficiency has been suggested as the cause of the thrombotic complications [37].

Factor VII deficiency may be acquired or congenital [38,39]. Superficial bleeding due to defective activation of the extrinsic coagulation pathway is the typical presentation of this disease. A high rate of intracranial hemorrhages has also been described in these patients. Presumably, the natural absence of collagen in the brain also results in defective function of the intrinsic coagulation pathway in these patients [38]. Recurrent ischemic stroke has also been described in association with factor VII deficit but the pathogenic mechanism is unclear [39].

Hemophilia A, von Willebrand's disease, and Christmas disease may cause hemorrhagic stroke. The pathogenesis of bleeding in these types of hemophilia is the deficit of coagulation factors required to activate the coagulation pathway, as shown in Figure 13.1. Delayed bleeding after trauma, often

Table 13.13. Systemic features of the hemoglobin disorders associated with stroke

Disease	Clinical features	Associated laboratory features
Hemoglobin sickle C disease	Double heterozygous, proliferative retinotherapy, infarction of orbital bone: lid edema, proptosis, headache, hip and shoulder necrosis	HbSC electrophoresis, critical sickling begins at 30% of venous PO_2
Sickle C anemia	Homozygous, gallstones, painful episodes in one or more areas, priapism, leg ulcers, metacarpal and metatarsal bone periostitis in childhood, nephrotic syndrome, infections, progressive nonfunctional splenomegaly, proliferative retinopathy in < 5%, exacerbated by hypnoxia, dehydration, acidosis, and infections	HbSS β^6 glutamine-valine, hemolytic anemia, hyperbilirubinemia, mild sicklings at 100% of venous PO_2, severe sickling at 50%–65% of venous PO_2
Sickle cell trait	Heterozygous, generally asymptomatic, hematuria, thromboembolic events during severe anoxemia	HbSA for β^s gene, hematuria
Cooley's anemia	Homozygous, severe symptomatology, "mongloid" facies, extramedullary hematopoiesis, spleno-hepatomegaly, endocrinopathies (delayed puberty, diabetes mellitus), gallstones, infections, obligatory transfusions	β-Hemoglobinopathy, severe chronic hemolytic anemia
Thalassemia minima	Heterozygous, no clinical signs	Mild hemolytic anemia
Thalassemia intermedia	Mild symptomatology, pulmonary thrombosis, thrombocytosis and platelet function altered after transfusions/splenectomy	β Variants: mixed heterozygosity for different types of Hb; anemia

Hb—hemoglobin.

Table 13.14. Systemic features of coagulation factor disorders associated with stroke

Disease	Clinical features	Associated laboratory features
AT III deficit	Autosomal dominant: family history of thrombotic complications; acquired condition: DIC, surgery, preeclampsia, renal disease, liver diseases, inflammatory bowel disease, hemodialysis, plasmapheresis, drugs, malignancies, APL, malnutrition, or gastrointestinal loss; prothrombotic state, venous thrombosis, atypical sites of atrial thrombosis, PE	AT III deficiency
Protein C deficit	Autosomal dominant, homozygous: newborns die from pupura fulminans; heterozygous: family history of thrombotic complications; acquired condition: see list for AT III; prothrombotic state, venous thrombosis, atypical sites of arterial thrombosis, PE	Protein C deficiency type I: decreased concentration/abnormal function; type II: abnormal function
Protein S deficit	Autosomal dominant: family history of thrombotic complications; acquired conditions: see list for AT III; prothrombotic state, venous thrombosis, atypical sites of arterial thrombosis, PE	Protein S deficiency
Heparin cofactor II deficit	Autosomal dominant: family history of thrombotic complications; prothrombotic state, venous thrombosis, atypical sites of arterial thrombosis, PE	Heparin cofactor II deficiency
Factor VII deficit	Autosomal recessive: homozygous, heterozygous; DVT, PE, epistaxis, gingival bleeding, bruising, menorrhagia	PT, serum level deficiency
Hemophilia A	X-linked/recessive, more prevalent in the young, severity of bleeding related to factor level: (< 1%): spontaneous; (> 5%): minor trauma; (> 10%): trauma and surgery; hematuria, hemarthrosis, hematomas, bruising, postoperative bleeding	PTT, serum level deficiency
von Willebrand's disease	Autosomal dominant (chromosome 12), autosomal recessive, more prevalent in the young, epistaxis, bleeding from mucous membranes (rarely in joints), bruises, menorrhagia, angiodysplasia of intestinal vessels, mitral valve prolapse	Bleeding time, PTT, serum level deficiency
Christmas disease (hemophilia B)	X-linked recessive, more prevalent in young than adults, female carriers may be affected, hematuria, hemarthrosis, hematoma, bruising, severe postoperative bleeding	PTT, serum level deficiency
Factor XI deficit	Autosomal recessive, more prevalent in young than adults, severe postsurgical bleeding	PTT
Factor XII deficit	Autosomal recessive, more prevalent in young than adults, thrombotic tendency	PTT, serum level deficiency
Factor XIII deficit	Autosomal recessive, more prevalent in the young than adults, umbilical bleeding at birth, spontaneous abortion, posttrauma hemorrhages, poor wound healing	CST
Afibrinogenemia	Autosomal recessive: homozygous, heterozygous; more prevalent in the young than adults, variable symptomatology, umbilical bleeding at birth, mucous membrane bleeding, posttrauma and postsurgical hemorrhages, PE	TT, mild thrombocytopenia, fibrinogen level decreased
Fibrogen deficit during DIC	Caused by the following: tissue damage: trauma, surgery, heat stroke, burns, dissecting aneurysm, neuroleptic malignant syndrome, infections; immunologic disturbances: allograft rejection, immune complex disorders, incompatible blood transfusion; obstetrical complications: abruptio placentae, amniotic fluid embolism, eclampsia, retained fetal product; metabolic disorders: diabetic ketoacidosis; neoplasms: leukemia, mucin secreting adenocarcinoma; miscellaneous: cyanotic congenital heart disease, shock, snake venom, fat embolism; signs of primary disease, thrombosis of different organs, oozing, purpura, massive hemorrhages	PT, PTT, FDP, fibrinogen level decreased
Vitamin K deficiency	Acquired/congenital, easy bruising, oozing after venipuncture, hematomas, hematuria, gingival, gastrointestinal bleeding, hepatomegaly	Anemia, PT, PTT, deficiency of factor II, VII, IX, X
Factor VIII increase	Recurrent PE, venous thrombophlebitis	Increased serum level
Fibrinogen increase	Atherosclerotic complications, recurrent myocardial infarctions	Fibrinogen excess
Increased plasma viscosity	Atherosclerotic complications, recurrent myocardial infarctions	Plasmatic hyperviscosity
Decreased ratio A/G	Atherosclerotic complications, recurrent myocardial infarctions	Serum globulin increase, serum albumin decrease

A/G—serum ratio between albumin and globulin; APL—acute promyelocytic leukemia; AT III—antithrombin III; CST—clot stability test; DIC—disseminated intravascular coagulation; DVT—deep vein thrombosis; FDP—fibrinogen degradation products; PE—pulmonary emboli; PT—prothrombin time; PTT—partial thromboplastin time; TT—thromboplastin time.

described in hemophilic patients, is due to the unstable network of fibrin formed in these disorders. Intracerebral hemorrhage, subarachnoid hemorrhage, subdural, and extradural hematomas are described [40]. Bleeding may be spontaneous or after trauma in hemophilia A and Christmas disease. In von Willebrand's disease, bleeding is usually, but not always, linked to trauma. Patients of any age may be affected by these conditions. An association with hypertension and cerebral hemorrhage in the elderly is described in hemophilia A [3], as well as seizures and mental retardation. Peripheral nerve lesions affecting ulnar, radial, median, and femoral nerves are also described secondary to intramuscular bleeding. Spinal bleeding is also reported [40].

Factor XI deficiency is considered a very uncommon cause of hemorrhagic stroke. Defective activation of the intrinsic coagulation pathway causes hemorrhagic stroke [17]. Factor XII deficiency is associated with ischemic stroke [41], but the pathogenic mechanism is unknown. Factor XIII deficiency is usually associated with hemorrhagic stroke probably secondary to the formation of a defective stable clot typical of this disease. Trauma may precede the stroke [17].

Afibrinogenemia [17] is a genetic quantitative fibrinogen deficiency, which may be associated with hemorrhagic stroke [42]. Disturbed platelet adhesion and aggregation associated with fibrinogen deficiency are involved in the pathogenesis of cerebral hemorrhage. Cerebral hemorrhage may occur either in young or old patients. During DIC, an acquired deficit of fibrinogen occurs. Ischemic and hemorrhagic stroke, in particular intracerebral, intraventricular, and subarachnoid hemorrhages, are described. Superior sagittal sinus thrombosis is also common [25].

Vitamin K deficiency may cause hemorrhagic stroke by decreasing the amount of vitamin K–dependent coagulation factors (Table 13.14). Subarachnoid and subdural hemorrhages associated with lethargy, coma, and seizures have been described in newborns and infants [43]. Causes include severe dietary deficiency, antibiotic therapy depleting the intestinal flora, parenteral nutrition, biliary tract obstruction, severe liver diseases, and congenital deficiency [44].

The pathogenic mechanism of stroke for most of the disorders listed below is not completely clarified.

Coagulation Factor Increase

An increased level of factor VIII, in particular over five times the normal level, has been associated with ischemic stroke, but the pathogenic mechanism is unclear [45]. Recently, apparently unrelated abnormalities such as an increased fibrinogen, a decreased albumin/globulin ratio, and plasma hyperviscosity have been found in recurrent stroke in cerebrovascular patients. These findings have been described together or alone in several studies [46–49].

FIBRINOLYTIC DISORDERS AND STROKE

Table 13.15 lists the systemic features of fibrinolytic disorders associated with stroke.

Fibrinolytic Factor Deficiency

A deficit of plasminogen or plasminogen activator, the latter being less common, may be associated with ischemic stroke. Cortical venous infarcts are described [17]. An increase of lipoprotein (a) [Lp(a)], a cholesterol rich lipoprotein that increases the level of plasminogen activator inhibitor (PAI-1), has recently been associated with hemorrhagic and ischemic stroke [50,51].

Antifibrinolytic therapy with epsilon-aminocaproic acid or tranexamic acid may be complicated by ischemic stroke [52,53]. Other neurologic complications include a higher incidence of hydrocephalus after subarachnoid hemorrhage [54].

Fibrinolytic Factor Excess

Fibrinolytic therapy with streptokinase, urokinase, or tissue-type plasminogen activator may be associated with hemorrhagic stroke [55,56].

HEMATOLOGIC DISORDERS OF UNCERTAIN MECHANISM AND STROKE

Table 13.16 describes the systemic features of some hematologic disorders of uncertain mechanism associated with stroke.

Congenital Diseases

Fabry's disease may be associated with ischemic or hemorrhagic stroke of unknown pathogenesis. Both young and adult patients may be affected. Small or large vessels, occasionally multifocal, may be involved. Hemorrhagic stroke may be associated with hypertension or, rarely, with cerebral aneurysms

Table 13.15. Systemic features of fibrinolytic disorders associated with stroke

Disease	Clinical features	Associated laboratory features
Deficit of plasminogen	Autosomal dominant: heterozygous; venous thrombosis	Plasminogen deficiency
Deficit of vascular plasminogen activator	Autosomal dominant, venous thrombosis, PE	Plasminogen activator deficiency
Lp(a)	Coronary artery disease	Lp(a) excess
Tranexamic acid	Diarrhea	
Aminocaproic acid	Fulminant myopathy; rhabdomiolysis	Myoglobinuria
Streptokinase urokinase t-PA	Used for myocardial infarction, venous and arterial thrombosis of the limbs, PE	

Lp(a)—cholesterol-rich lipoprotein; PE—pulmonary embolism; t-PA—tissue-type plasminogen activator.

[17]. Paresthesias, pain of the limbs, mental retardation, personality changes, and seizures are the most common neurologic features. Heterozygous females may also be affected by these complications.

Leigh's disease may be complicated by ischemic stroke. The histopathologic findings are characterized by necrotizing destruction of parenchyma, proliferation of capillaries, and secondary gliosis. A clear explanation for the pathogenesis of ischemic stroke is still lacking. Either young or adult patients may be affected. A sporadic form of Leigh's disease has been described [57]. Bilateral optic atrophy, peripheral neuropathy, seizures, ataxia, and progressive deterioration of brainstem function are the most common symptoms in affected children with the inherited disease, as well as in the sporadic adult form.

MELAS syndrome is associated with ischemic stroke but the pathogenesis is unknown [58]. The abrupt onset of cortical blindness, deafness, hemiparesis, or hemianopsia in a child or young adult who had previously normal development should lead to suspicion of this disease. Seizures, myoclonic epilepsy [59], ophthalmoplegia [60], and intellectual impairment [58] are common features.

Either congenital homocystinuria or acquired homocysteinemia may be associated with ischemic stroke and TIA [61]. Atherosclerotic stenoses and occlusions of large vessels are common, particularly involving the carotid arteries and other large intracranial arteries [62]. Homozygous patients may also present with mental retardation [63].

Familial hypo-α-lipoproteinemia is associated with stroke in childhood and young patients. The pathogenic mechanism of the stroke in this disease is unknown. Organic acidemias, in particular methylmalonic, propionic, and isovaleric acidemias, are associated with stroke in children and young adults. Both ischemic and hemorrhagic stroke have been described. A few reports describe the occurrence of cerebellar hemorrhage [64,65]. The pathogenesis of stroke in these acidemias is unknown.

The antiphospholipid antibody syndrome is associated with ischemic stroke [66,67] in young adults. Both large and medium arteries and the veins of the brain are involved. Either recurrent venous thrombosis, arterial thrombosis, or embolism may occur [68]. TIA, monocular, or bilateral visual disturbances are also associated with this syndrome [69]. More than one mechanism appears to be involved in the pathogenesis of stroke in the antiphospholipid antibody syndrome. Microvascular occlusion due to platelet fibrin clots, suggesting possible in situ thrombosis, has been observed in these patients. Also, the cardiac valve abnormalities commonly seen in this syndrome may cause ischemic brain damage via embolism [35]. Potential mechanisms of coagulopathy include antibody interference with β-glycoprotein I (a natural inhibitor of coagulation); antibody damage to endothelium; disordered function of protein C, protein S, or, antithrombin III; and defective prostacyclin release. Paradoxically, thrombotic events are strongly associated with thrombocytopenia.

Table 13.16. Systemic features of hematologic disorders of uncertain mechanism associated with stroke

Disease	Clinical features	Associated laboratory features
Fabry's disease	X-linked, males and heterozygous females, angiokeratomas in mucous membranes and skin, corneal opacities, renal impairment in middle age, coronary artery disease	Leukocyte α-galactoside activity deficiency
Leigh's disease	Autosomal recessive/X-linked recessive, childhood, episodes of lactic acidosis in infancy, sporadic disease: young adults	Pyruvic and lactic acidemia, plasma amino acid levels, serum electrolyte
MELAS	Genetics variable, short-stature, initial development normal, muscle weakness, mitochondrial myopathy	Pyruvic and lactic acidemia, urinary amino acid determination, serum electrolyte determination
Homocystinuria/homocystinemia	Autosomal recessive; homozygous: children/young; clinical features: marfanoid habitus, ectopia lentis, myopia, malar flush, livedo reticularis, premature athersclerosis, peripheral venous/arterial thrombosis, osteporosis; heterozygous: young/adult; clinical features: renovascular hypertension, occlusive arterial disease, "claudicatio intermittens," venous thrombosis; caused by vitamin B12/folate deficit: adult; clinical features: coronary artery disease, atherosclerotic disease	CBS deficiency, plasma homocystine and methionine level increase, vitamin B12 and folate deficit
Familial hypo-α lipoproteinemia	Coronary artery disease in childhood or young adult	Lipoprotein determination
Organic acidemia	Autosomal recessive, neonatal period or childhood vomiting, metabolic acidosis, lethargy	PLT and leukocyte decrease, urinary and plasma increase of the specific amino acid, hyperammonemia
Antiphospholipid antibody syndrome	Young adult, migraine with or without aura, livedo reticularis, miscarriages, DVT, atypical sites of arterial thrombosis, PE, mitral valave abnormalities, Libman-Sacks endocarditis	LAC, aCL, ESR increase, VDRL false-posivity, thrombocytopenia, increased PTT

aCL—anticardiolipin antibody; CBS—cystathionine β-synthetase; DVT— deep vein thrombosis; ESR—erythrocyte sedimentation rate; LAC—lupus anticoagulant; MELAS—mitochondrial myopathy, encephalopathy, lactic acidosis, stroke-like episodes; PLT—platelet; PTT—partial thromboplastin time; VDRL—Venereal Disease Research Laboratory.

WHEN AND HOW TO PURSUE A HEMATOLOGIC EVALUATION

Routine Evaluation

A routine hematologic evaluation should be performed in every patient presenting with hemorrhagic or ischemic stroke. The routine tests are listed in Table 13.17. These tests may suggest the presence of an underlying hematologic disorder.

Extensive Evaluation

Extensive testing (Table 13.18) should be performed when routine tests are abnormal, or when routine tests are normal but the clinical presentation raises suspicion of an underlying hematologic disorder. Routine tests will usually be abnormal in patients with severe DIC or myeloproliferative disorders causing stroke. On the other hand, young patients with a disorder such as heterozygous afibrinogenemia might present with normal routine tests, requiring the performance of a thromboplastin time to establish the diagnosis. Young stroke patients typically require extensive testing. In older patients, extensive testing should also be performed despite a normal routine screening battery with unexplained recurrent stroke when the clinical presentation is unusual, such as venous infarction, when no conventional risk factors for stroke are present, or when there is a family history of cerebrovascular disease or pertinent hematologic disorder. Table 13.18 lists the extensive hematologic tests performed in the evaluation of such stroke patients.

Clinical Approach

This final section illustrates an algorithmic clinical approach to evaluating stroke patients for hematologic disorders. The algorithms correlate the systemic clinical features of stroke patients with the tests required to diagnose possible underlying hematologic disorders. The algorithms list only extensive testing, while routine testing should be performed in every patient and is illustrated in Table 13.17. In each algorithm, the systemic features are

Table 13.17. Blood tests performed in the routine evaluation of the stroke patient

Test	Disorders diagnosed
Platelet count	Essential thrombocythemia, TTP, ITP, thrombocytopenia, thrombocytosis, Bernard-Soulier syndrome
Erythrocyte count	Polycythemia, anemia
Hematocrit	Polycythemia, anemia
Leukocyte count	ANLL, ALL chronic familial cerebral vasculopathy
Serum protein electrophoresis	Myeloma, Waldenstrom's macroglobulinemia, decreased A/G ratio
Hemoglobin %	Polycythemia, anemia
Bleeding time	von Willebrand's disease, aspirin use
PT	Factor VII deficiency, afibrinogenemia, DIC, vitamin K deficit
PTT	Hemophilia A, von Willebrand's disease, Christmas disease, factor XII deficit, afibrinogenemia, DIC, vitamin K deficit, antiphospholipid antibody syndrome

A/G—serum ratio between albumin and globulin; ALL—acute lymphoblastic leukemia; ANLL—acute nonlymphoblastic leukemia; DIC—disseminated intravascular coagula tion; ITP—idiopathic thrombocytopenic purpura; PT—prothrombin time; PTT—partial thromboplastin time; TTP—thrombotic thrombocytopenic purpura.

Table 13.18. Tests performed in the extensive hematologic evaluation of stroke patients and the disorders diagnosed

Test	Disorders diagnosed
Platelet aggregation test	HITP, sticky platelet syndrome, Glanzmann's thromboasthenia
Ham's test	Paroxysmal nocturnal hemoglobinuria
Erythrocyte mass study with ^{51}CR	Polycythemia vera
Immunoglobulin electrophoresis	Myeloma, Waldenstrom's macroglobulinemia, cryoglobulinemia
Cold precipitable Ig test	Cryoglobulinemia
Hemoglobin electrophoresis	SSA, sickle cell trait, β-thalassemia, hemoglobin SC disease
Functional assay for AT III	AT III deficiency
Functional assay for protein C	Protein C deficiency
Electro-immunoassay of protein-free S antigen	Protein S deficiency
Heparin cofactor II activity	Heparin cofactor II deficiency
Factor VII level	Factor VII deficiency or excess
Factor VIII level	Hemophila A, factor VIII excess
Factor XII level	Factor XII deficiency
Clot stability test	Factor XIII deficiency
Fibrinogen level	DIC, fibrinogen abnormalities
FDP	DIC
Thromboplastin time	Afibrinogenemia
Plasma viscosity	Plasma hyperviscosity
Plasminogen level	Plasminogen deficit
Functional assay for lipoprotein Lp(a)	Lp(a) excess
Leukocyte α-galactosidase determination	Fabry's disease
Pyruvate and lactate serum level	Leigh's disease, MELAS
Plasma amino acid levels (also after methionine load)	Leigh's disease, organic acidemias, homocystinuria/homocystinemia
Fibroblast cystationine-β synthase activity	Homocystinuria/homocystinemia
Serum electrolytes	Leigh's disease, MELAS
Vitamin B12 and folate level	Acquired homocystinemia
Ammonemia	Propionic and methylmalonic acidemias
Urinary organic acid quantitation	Leigh's disease, MELAS, homocystinuria, acidemias
Electroimmunoassay for lipoproteins	Familial hypo-α-lipoproteinemia
LAC/aCL	Antiphospholipid antibody syndrome

aCL—anticardiolipin antibody; AT III—antithrombin III; DIC—disseminated intravascular coagulation; FDP—fibrinogen degradation products; Ham's test—erythrocyte lysis during complement activation by acidification; HITP—heparin-induced thrombocytopenia; LAC—lupus anticoagulant; Lp(a)—cholesterol-rich lipoprotein; MELAS—mitochondrial myopathy, encephalopathy, lactic acidosis, stroke-like episodes; SSA—sickle cell anemia.

grouped according to the nature of the underlying hematologic disease. In the algorithm for ischemic stroke (Figure 13.2), systemic features are grouped in relation to congenital, immunologic, and coagulation disorders. In the algorithm for hemorrhagic stroke (Figure 13.3), the systemic features are grouped in relation to congenital, coagulation, and acquired disorders.

This approach is a simplified guide for the evaluation of possible hematologic disorders associated with stroke. It cannot substitute for a more individualized approach, as every patient may have a different clinical presentation. For example, an older patient may present with Leigh's disease because this disorder may have a sporadic presentation. This occurrence is not illustrated in the algorithms, but must be considered in an adult patient with a progressive, deteriorating presentation associated with ocular involvement. Moreover, when a high clinical index of suspicion exists, the physician may perform the entire extensive testing battery, despite the lack of clues to narrow down the diagnostic possibilities.

Young patients must undergo extensive testing in most situations. In older patients, extensive testing should be performed when no other risk factors are detectable, with venous or atypical sites of arterial thromboses, when recurrent stroke occurs, when easy bruising or hemorrhages occur, or when a positive family history for severe and recurrent vascular disorders is present. We must also keep in mind that any stroke subtype may be the result of any one of a number of disorders, and that

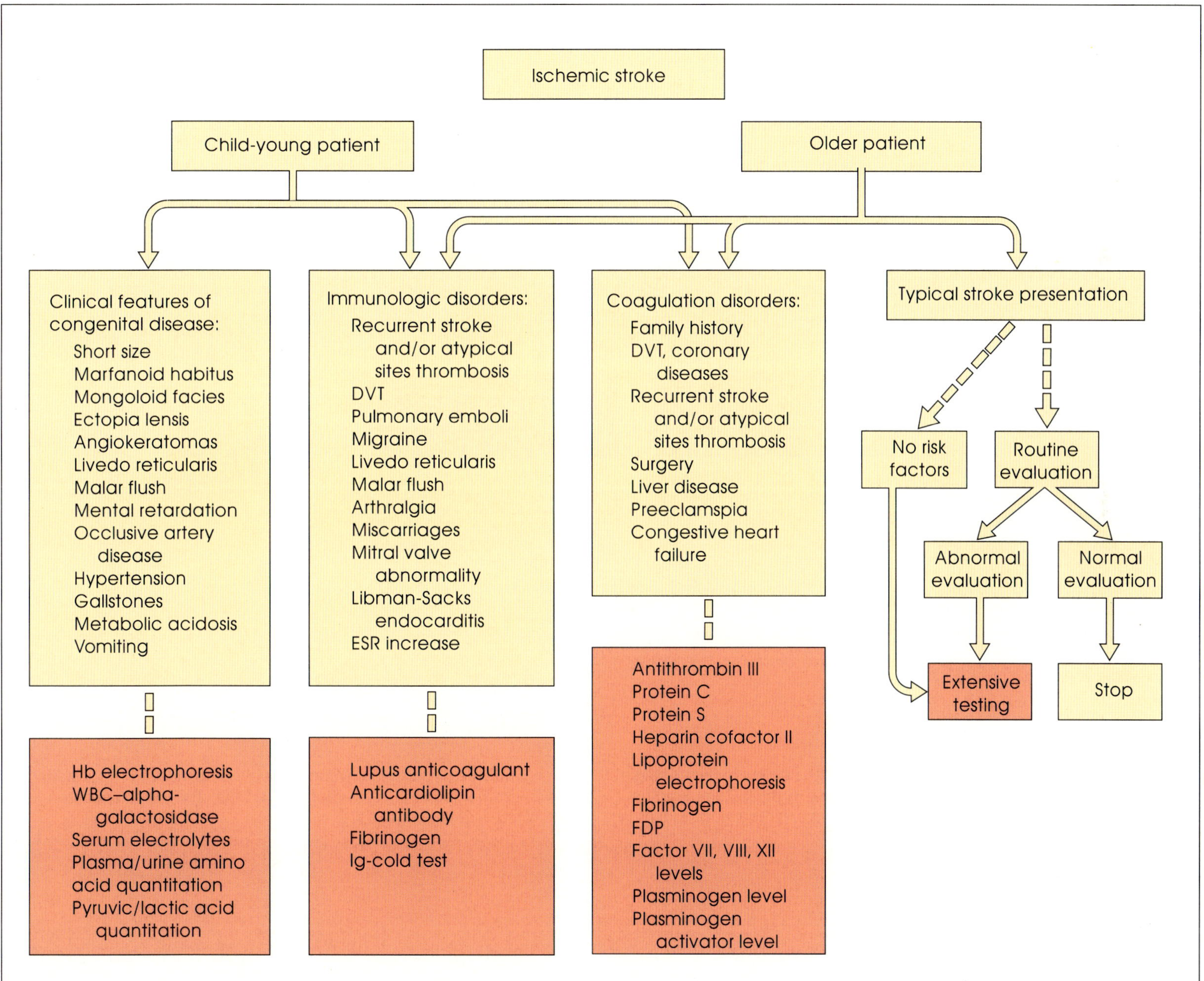

FIGURE 13.2

Clinical and laboratory approach for hematologic evaluation in ischemic stroke. Note that only extensive testing is illustrated in the picture. Routine testing should be performed in every patient. Shown in *red* are the extensive tests that may be performed in young and old patients. DVT—deep vein thrombosis; ESR—erythrocyte sedimentation rate; FDP—fibrinogen degradation product; Hb—hemoglobin; WBC—white blood cell.

a search for the cause of stroke might be difficult in particular patients.

Figure 13.2 illustrates the clinical features and subsequent tests to be performed in the evaluation of children, young adults, and elderly persons with ischemic stroke. As illustrated, all young patients are submitted to extensive testing in this schema. Older patients are extensively tested only under certain conditions. Figure 13.3 illustrates the clinical features and subsequent testing to be performed in children, young adults, and elderly persons with hemorrhagic stroke.

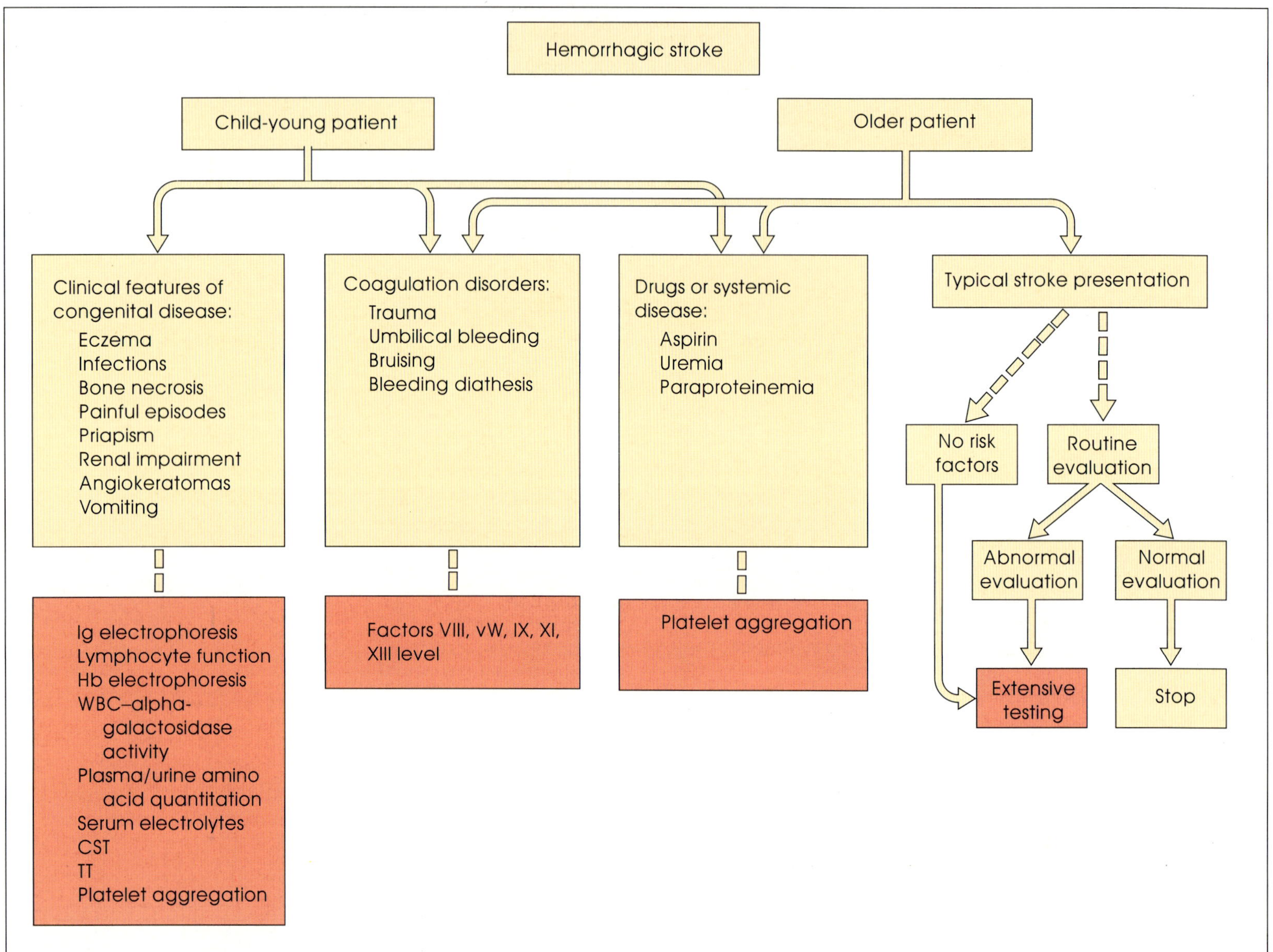

FIGURE 13.3

Clinical and laboratory approach for hematologic evaluation in hemorrhagic stroke. Note that only extensive testing is illustrated in the picture. Routine testing should be performed in every patient. Shown in *red* are the extensive tests that may be performed in young and old patients. CST—clot stability test; Hb—hemoglobin; TT—thromboplastin time; vW—von Willebrand factor; WBC—white blood cell.

REFERENCES

1. Hart RG, Kanter MC: Hematological disorders and ischemic stroke: a selective review. *Stroke* 1990, 21:1111–1121.
2. Check W: Possible platelet syndrome suggested in early stroke. *JAMA* 1984, 252:597–598.
3. Davies-Jones GAB: Neurological manifestations of hematological disorders. In *Neurology and General Medicine*, 1st ed. Edited by Aminoff MJ. New York: Churchill Livingstone Inc; 1989:187–210.
4. Steering Committee of the Physicians' Health Study Research Group: Final report on the aspirin component of the ongoing Physicians' Health Study. *N Engl J Med* 1989, 321:129–135.
5. McDonald TD, Tatemichi TK, Kranzler SJ, *et al.*: Thrombosis of the superior sagittal sinus associated with essential thrombocytosis followed by MRI during anticoagulant therapy. *Neurology* 1989, 39:1554–1555.
6. Benassi G, Ricci P, Calbucci F, *et al.*: Slowly progressive ischemic stroke as first manifestation of essential thrombocythemia. *Stroke* 1989, 20:1271–1272.
7. Preston FE, Martin JF, Stewart R, *et al.*: Thrombocytosis, circulating platelet aggregates, and neurological dysfunction. *BMJ* 1979, 2:1561–1563.
8. Ridolfi RL, Bell WR: Thrombotic thrombocytopenc purpura: report of 25 cases and review of the literature. *Medicine* 1985, 60:413–428.
9. Shafer AI: Thrombocytopenia and disorders of platelet function. In *Internal Medicine*, 3rd ed. Edited by Stein JH. Boston: Little, Brown and Company; 1990:1041–1048.
10. Chan KH, Mann KS, Chan TK: The significance of thrombocytopenia in the development of postoperative intracranial hematoma. *J Neurosurg* 1989, 71:38–41.
11. Crowell RM, Ojemann RG, Ogilvy CS: Spontaneous brain hemorrhage: surgical considerations. In *Stroke*. 2nd ed. Edited by Barnet HJM, Mohr JP, Stein B, Yatsu FM. New York: Churchill Livingstone Inc.; 1992:1169–1187.
12. Giovangrandi Y, Daffos F, Kaplan C, *et al.*: Very early intracranial hemorrhage in alloimmune fetal thrombocytopenia. *Lancet* 1990, 336:310.
13. Bussel JB, Tanli S, de C Peterson H: Favorable neurological outcome in 7 cases of perinatal intracranial hemorrhage due to immune thrombocytopenia. *Am J Pediatr Hemat-Oncology* 1991, 13:156–159.
14. Becker PS, Miller VT: Heparin-induced thrombocytopenia. *Stroke* 1989, 20:1449–1459.
15. Kyritsis AP, Williams EC, Schutta HS: Cerebral venous thrombosis due to heparin-induced thrombocytopenia. *Stroke* 1990, 21:1503–1505.
16. Sheth KJ, Swick HM, Haworth N: Neurological involvement in hemolytic-uremic syndrome. *Ann Neurol* 1986, 19:90–93.
17. Natawicz M, Kelley R: Mendelian etiologies of stroke. *Ann Neurol* 1987, 22:175–192.
18. Stern BJ, Kitter S, Sloan M, *et al.*: Stroke in the young (part I). *Maryland Med J* 1991, 40:453–462.
19. Tanahashi N, Gotoh Furio, Tomita M, *et al.*: Enhanced erythrocytes aggregability in occlusive cerebrovascular disease. *Stroke* 1989, 20:1202–1207.
20. Pearson TC, Wetherley-Mein G: Vascular occlusive episodes and venous haematocrit in primary proliferative polycythemia. *Lancet* 1978, 9:1219–1222.
21. Berk PD, Goldberg JD, Donovan PB, *et al.*: Therapeutic recommendations in polycythemia vera based on polycythemia vera study group protocols. *Semin Hematol* 1986, 23:132–143.
22. Schafer AI: The hypercoagulable state. *Ann Intern Med* 1985, 102:814–828.
23. Alexander MB: Iron deficiency anemia, thrombocytosis and cerebrovascular accident. *South Med J* 1983, 76:662–663.
24. Graus R, Rogers L, Posner JB: Cerebrovascular complications in patients with cancer. *Medicine* 1985, 64:16–35.
25. Stern BJ, Kitter S, Sloan M, *et al.*: Stroke in the young (part II). *Maryland Med J* 1991, 40:565–571.
26. Gorevic PD, Kassab HJ, Levo Y, *et al.*: Mixed cryoglobulinemia: clinical aspects and long-term follow-up of 40 patients. *Am J Med* 1980, 69:287–308.
27. Abramsky O, Slavin S: Neurologic manifestations in patients with mixed cryoglobulinemia. *Neurology* 1974, 24:245–249.
28. Roderic HF, Bruce HP: Neurological complications of hemoglobin SC disease. *Arch Neurol* 1984, 41:289–292.
29. Stockman JA, Nigro MA, Miskin MM, *et al.*: Occlusion of large cerebral vessels in sickle-cell anemia. *N Engl J Med* 1972, 287:846–849.
30. Dalal FY, Schmidt GB, Bennett EJ, *et al.*: Sickle-cell trait. *Br J Anaesth* 1974, 46:387–388.
31. Reyes MG: Subcortical cerebral infarctions in sickle-cell trait. *J Neurol Neurosurg Psych* 1989, 52:516–518.
32. Logothesis J, Constantoulakis M, Economidou J, *et al.*: Thalassemia major (homozygous β-thalassemia). *Neurology* 1972, 22:294–304.
33. Sinniah D, Vignaendra V, Ahmad K: Neurological complications of β-thalassemia major. *Arch Dis Child* 1977, 52:977–979.
34. Wong V, Yu YL, Liang RHS, *et al.*: Cerebral thrombosis in β-thalassemia/hemoglobin E disease. *Stroke* 1990, 21:812–816.
35. Coull BC, Goodnight SH: Antiphospholipid antibodies and coagulation disorders in ischemic stroke. In *Stroke*. 2nd ed. Edited by Barnet HJM, Mohr JP, Stein B, Yatsu FM. New York: Churchill Livingstone Inc.; 1992:859–873.
36. Seligsohn RI, Berger A, Abend M, *et al.*: Homozygous protein C deficiency manifested by massive venous thrombosis in the newborn. *N Engl J Med* 1984, 310:559–562.
37. Tran TH, Marbet GA, Duckert F, *et al.*: Association of hereditary heparin cofactor II deficiency with thrombosis. *Lancet* 1985, 24:413–414.
38. Matthey KK, Koerper MA, Ablin AR: Intracranial hemorrhage in congenital factor VII deficiency. *J Pediatr* 1979, 94:413–415.
39. Lefrere JJ, Chaunu MP, Conard J, *et al.*: Congenital factor VII deficiency and cerebrovascular stroke. *Lancet* 1985, 2:1006–1007.
40. Eister ME, Gill FM, Blatt PM, *et al.*: Central nervous system bleeding in hemophiliacs. *Blood* 1978, 51:1179–1188.
41. Goodnough LT, Saito H, Ratnoff OD: Thrombosis or myocardial infarction in congenital clotting factor abnormalities and chronic thrombocytopenias: a report of 21 patients and a review of 50 previously reported cases. *Medicine* 1983, 62:248–255.
42. Montgomery R, Natelson SE: Afibrinogenemia with intracerebral hematoma. *Am J Dis Child* 1977, 131:555–556.
43. Bhanchet P, Tuchinda S, Hathirat P, *et al.*: A bleeding syndrome in infants due to acquired prothrombin complex deficiency: a survey of 93 affected infants. *Clin Pediatr* 1977, 16:992–998.
44. White GC: Disorders of blood coagulation. In *Internal Medicine*, 3rd ed. Edited by Stein JH. Boston, Toronto, London: Little, Brown and Company; 1990:1048–1063.
45. Kosik KS, Furie B: Thrombotic stroke associated with elevated plasma factor VIII. *Ann Neurol* 1980, 8:435–437.
46. Beamer N, Coull BM, Sexton G, *et al.*: Fibrinogen and the albumin-globulin ratio in recurrent stroke. *Stroke* 1993, 24:1133–1139.
47. Resch KL, Ernst E, Matrai A, *et al.*: Fibrinogen and viscosity as risk factors for subsequent cardiovascular events in stroke survivors. *Ann Intern Med* 1992, 117:371–375.
48. Coull BM, Beamer N, de Garmo P, *et al.*: Chronic blood hyperviscosity in subjects with acute stroke, transient ischemic attack, and risk factors for stroke. *Stroke* 1991, 22:162–168.
49. Wilhelmsen L, Svardsudd K, Korsan-Bengsten K, *et al.*: Fibrinogen as a risk factor for stroke and myocardial infarction. *N Engl J Med* 1984, 311:501–505.

50. Woo J, Lau E, Lam CWK, *et al.*: Hypertension, lipoprotein(a), and apolipoprotein A-I as risk factors for stroke in the Chinese. *Stroke* 1991, 22:203–208.
51. Zenker G, Költringer P, Bone G, *et al.*: Lipoprotein(a) as a strong indicator for cerebrovascular disease. *Stroke* 1986, 17:942–945.
52. Kassel NF, Torner JC, Adams HP: Antifibrinolytic therapy in the acute period following aneurysmal subarachnoid hemorrhage: preliminary observations from the Cooperative Aneurysm Study. *J Neurosurg* 1984, 61:225–230.
53. Vermeulen M, Lindsay KW, Murray GD, *et al.*: Antifibrinolytic treatment in subarachnoid hemorrhage. *N Engl J Med* 1984, 311:432–437.
54. Graff-Radford NR, Torner J, Adams HP, *et al.*: Factors associated with hydrocephalus after subarachnoid hemorrhage: a report of the Cooperative Aneurysm Study. *Arch Neurol* 1989, 46:744–752.
55. Kase CS, Mohr JP, Caplan LR: Intracerebral hemorrhage. In *Stroke.* 2nd ed. Edited by Barnet HJM, Mohr JP, Stein B, Yatsu FM. New York: Churchill Livingstone Inc.; 1992:561–616.
56. The TIMI Study Group: Comparison of invasive and conservative strategies after treatment with intravenous tissue plasminogen activator in acute myocardial infarction: results of the Thrombolysis in Myocardial Infarction (TIMI) Phase II Trial. *N Engl J Med* 1989, 320:618–627.
57. Kalimo H, Lundberg PO, Olsson Y: Familial subacute necrotizing encephalomyelopathy of the adult form (adult Leigh syndrome). *Ann Neurol* 1979, 6:200–206.
58. Kuriyama M, Umezaki H, Fukuda Y, *et al.*: Mitochondrial encephalomyopathy with lactate-pyruvate elevation and brain infarctions. *Neurology (Cleveland)* 1984, 34:72–77.
59. Fitzimons RB, Clifton-Bligh P, Wolfenden WH: Mitochondrial myopathy and lactic acidemia with myoclonic epilepsy, ataxia and hypothalamic infertility: a variant of Ramsay-Hunt syndrome? *J Neurol Neurosurg Psych* 1981, 4479–4492.
60. Lou HC, Reske-Nielsen E: Progressive external ophthalmoplegia: evidence for a disorder in pyruvate-lactate metabolism. *Arch Neurol* 1976, 33:455–456.
61. Coull BM, Malinow MR, Beamer N, *et al.*: Elevated plasma homocysteine concentration as a possible independent risk factor for stroke. *Stroke* 1990, 21:572–576.
62. Boers GHJ, Smals AGH, Trijbels FJM, *et al.*: Heterozygosity for homocystinuria in premature peripheral and cerebral occlusive arterial disease. *N Engl J Med* 1985, 313:709–715.
63. Thoene JG: Disorders of amino acid metabolism. In *Internal Medicine.* 3rd ed. Edited by Stein JH. Boston: Little, Brown and Company; 1990:2301–2310.
64. Dave P, Curless RG, Steinman RG: Cerebellar hemorrhage complicating methylmalonic and propionic acidemia. *Arch Neurol* 1984, 41:1293–1296.
65. Fischer AQ, Challa VR, Burton BK, *et al.*: Cerebellar hemorrhage complicating isovaleric acidemia: a case report. *Neurology* 1981, 31:746–748.
66. Hess DC: Stroke associated with antiphospholipid antibodies. *Stroke* 1992, 23(suppl I):23–28.
67. Brey RL, Hart RG, Sherman DG, *et al.*: Antiphospholipid antibodies and cerebral ischemia in young people. *Neurology* 1990, 40:1190–1196.
68. Levine SR, Brey RL, Joseph CLM, *et al.*: Risk of recurrent thromboembolic events in patients with focal cerebral ischemia and antiphospholipid antibodies. *Stroke* 1992, 23(suppl I):29–32.
69. Levine SR, Deegan MJ, Futrel N, *et al.*: Cerebrovascular and neurologic disease associated with antiphospholipid antibodies: 48 cases. *Neurology* 1990, 40:1181–1189.

Chapter 14

Management of Medical Complications in Cerebrovascular Disease

JAMES T. PATRICK
JOSÉ BILLER

Approximately 500,000 people suffer a new or recurrent stroke each year. Of the 350,000 survivors, approximately 31% require assistance with care and 71% have impaired vocational capacity; thus, the mortality and morbidity from stroke is substantial. Current therapies for acute stroke are being developed, and their effectiveness may be enhanced by rapid application. Assuming the patient survives the ictal event—hemorrhagic or ischemic stroke—then death results from complications including herniation, pneumonia, or myocardial infarction. Intervening morbid complications include seizures and behavioral changes. Minimizing or preventing these medical complications will increase the opportunity for the patient to be restored to his or her former functional and environmental status.

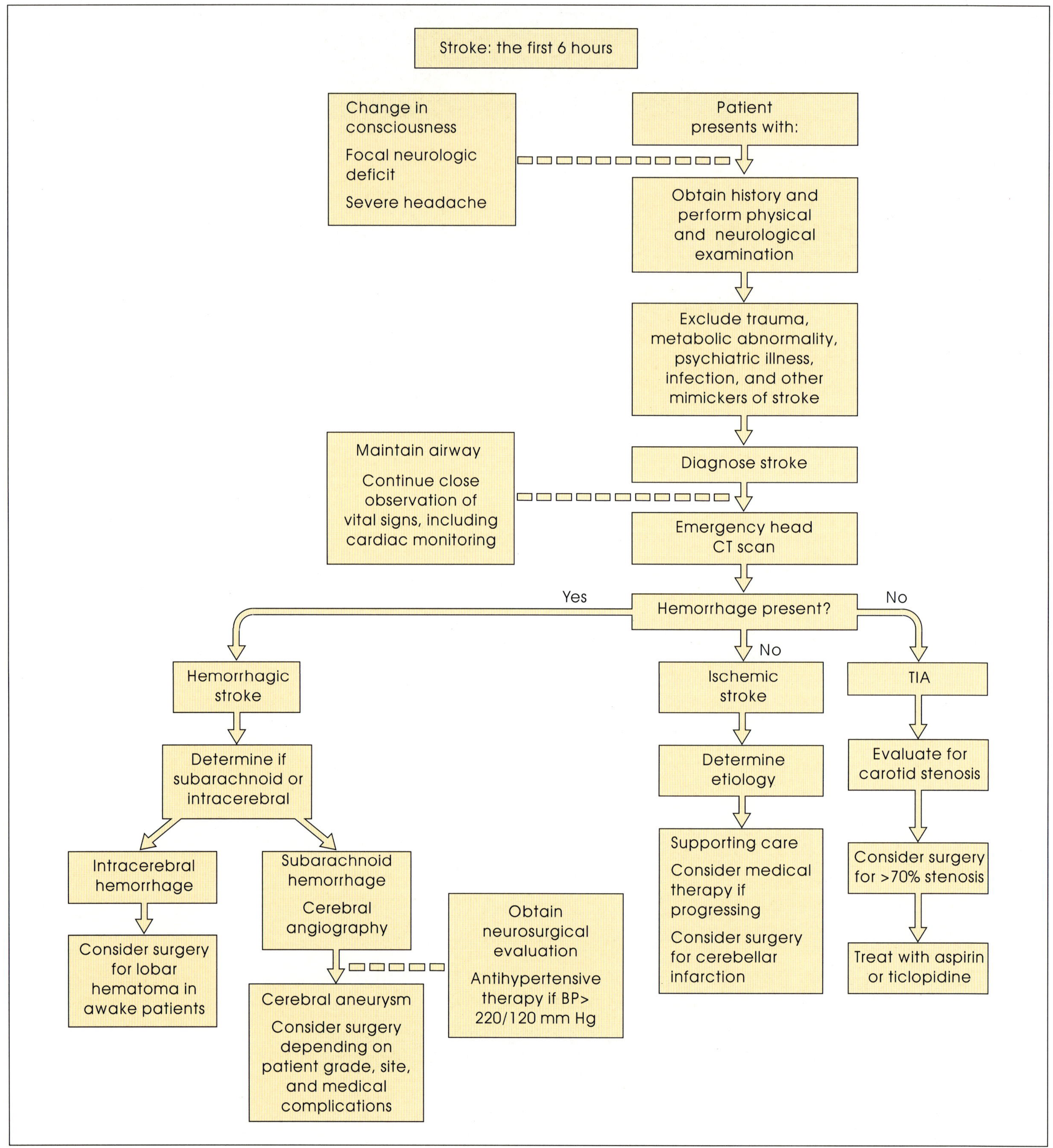

FIGURE 14.1

Flow diagram for the evaluation and initial management of suspected stroke. BP—blood pressure; CT—computed tomography; TIA—transient ischemic attack. (*From* National Stroke Association Consensus Statement [2]; with permission.)

Stroke is a major cause of death and disability [1]. Because general medical complications are common following stroke, the primary care physician must be well versed in their recognition and treatment. In this chapter, we review poststroke complications and their treatment.

EVALUATION AND INITIAL MANAGEMENT

Rapid diagnosis and initiation of treatment of the stroke patient are requisite to maximize recovery. Differentiation of ischemic versus hemorrhagic stroke is necessary because the treatment differs significantly for each condition. Cranial computed tomography (CT) without contrast is employed to differentiate ischemic from hemorrhagic stroke and to identify disorders that mimic stroke such as tumor, abscess, and hematoma (subdural or epidural). The National Stroke Association protocol for the evaluation and initial management of suspected stroke is presented in Figure 14.1 [2].

Initially, respiratory and cardiovascular stabilization are achieved in conjunction with examination of the neurologic, cardiac, and vascular systems. Screening studies include the following: serum sodium, potassium, chloride, carbon dioxide, blood urea nitrogen, creatinine, glucose, calcium, magnesium, phosphorus, cholesterol, triglycerides, Veneral Disease Research Laboratory (VDRL) reactivity, and erythrocyte sedimentation rate; complete blood cell count with differential, platelet count, prothrombin time, and partial thromboplastin time; urine analysis; plain chest radiograph; 12-lead electrocardiogram; and CT.

Following the diagnosis of acute stroke, the patient is admitted to a specialized intensive care or stroke unit for additional evaluation, initiation of specific treatments, and prevention of complications. The most frequent mechanisms of ischemic stroke include atherothrombosis of the extra- and intracranial carotid and vertebrobasilar systems by arteriogenic emboli or hemodynamic insufficiency, small artery occlusive disease, cardio- and aortogenic emboli, prothrombotic states, and arterial dissection. Based on the suspected mechanism of stroke, additional evaluation may include carotid-vertebral ultrasound duplex imaging, transcranial Doppler ultrasound, transthoracic echocardiography, transesophageal echocardiography, CT, magnetic resonance imaging, magnetic resonance angiography, and conventional cerebral angiography. Based on stroke etiology, specific treatment is initiated. Various diagnostic studies and treatments are discussed in subsequent chapters.

Medical complications may arise immediately following acute stroke; some of these complications are life-threatening and include brain herniation, cardiac dysfunction, and pneumonia (Table 14.1) [3]. The following discussion addresses the diagnosis, treatment, and prevention of medical complications attending acute stroke.

MEDICAL COMPLICATIONS

Respiratory

Pneumonia

Mortality from pneumonia occurs in 15% to 25% of acute stroke patients; it is the most common cause of nonneurologic death with a peak incidence at 2 to 4 weeks [3–5]. The etiology of pneumonia is multifactorial. Conditions predisposing to pneumonia include recumbent position, atelectasis and poor mobilization of secretions, and decreased respiratory drive and chest movements ipsilateral to hemiparesis [6,7]. Many cases of pneumonia are due to aspiration of oropharyngeal contents. Video fluoroscopy reveals that approximately 50% of patients with ischemic stroke experience aspiration [8]. Thus, pending the demonstration of intact oropharyngeal function, oral feedings are withheld. If dysfunction is present, then a temporary enteral feeding tube is placed.

The signs and symptoms of pneumonia include fever, dyspnea, an increase in volume or change in texture of the sputum, and pulmonary consolidation. Evaluation includes complete blood count (CBC) with differential, chest radiograph, sputum gram stain with culture and sensitivity, and blood culture. Empiric antibiotic treatment is initiated pending identification of the infectious agent. The more common agents include species of *Pseudomonas*, *Staphylococcus*, and *Klebsiella*; less common agents include *Escherichia coli* and species of *Serratia* and *Proteus* [9].

Sinusitis

A not infrequent complication of nasotracheal tubes (NTT) and nasogastric tubes (NGT) is sinusitis that may lead to sepsis [10–12]. Placement of large bore NTT for airway maintenance and ventilation, and NGT for secretion control frequently occurs in the emergent treatment of stroke patients. Patients receiving corticosteroids or those with diabetes mellitus are at increased risk for infection. The diagnosis is based on CT of the sinuses and tracheal and sinus microbial cultures. The more common nosocomial organisms include *Staphylococcus aureus*, enterococci, and gram-negative bacilli (*eg*, *Pseudomonas aeruginosa*). Treatment consists of discontinuing the NTT or NGT, decongestants, antibiotics, and drainage if indicated [10].

Inadvertent Nasotracheal Intubation

Placement of small bore nasoenteric feeding tubes (NET) for nutrition occurs frequently in stroke patients. Complications in

Table 14.1. Comparison between mechanisms of death during the first week and the second to fourth week in 180 patients with supratentorial lesions*

	Infarction		Hemorrhage	
Cause of death	First week	2–4th week	First week	2–4th week
Transtentorial herniation	36	6	42	2
Pneumonia	0	28	1	2
Cardiac dysfunction	7	17	0	2
Pulmonary embolism	0	4	0	0
Sudden death	2	8	0	0
Septicemia	1	4	0	0
Unknown	0	12	1	3
Brain stem extension (of hematoma)	—	—	1	1
Total	46	79	45	10

**From* Silver and coworkers [3]; with permission.

placing the flexible silastic tube with a stiff guidewire include esophagogastric perforation and tracheobronchial intubation [13,14]. If the NET is positioned centrally within the tracheobronchial tree, then no untoward effect occurs if the tube is removed prior to initiation of alimentation; however, if the NET is positioned peripherally within the tracheobronchial tree, puncturing of the pleura may occur with attendant pneumothorax. Inadvertent misplacement of the NET may occur due to the patient's decreased level of consciousness or gag reflex. Cuffed endotracheal and tracheostomy tubes do not protect against NET misplacement. Evaluation of NET position is best achieved with abdominal plain films. Bedside aspiration of fluid, which can be difficult through a small bore tube, must be pH tested; clear fluid is an insufficient indicator of gastric aspirate, as evidenced by a report of a misplaced NET yielding clear cerebrospinal fluid [15]. Injection of air into a misplaced NET is not recommended because auscultatory sounds can be misleading, due to the adjacency of the left lung and stomach, and dangerous, resulting in pneumothorax.

Neurogenic Pulmonary Edema

Neurogenic pulmonary edema (NPE) occurs when there is a severe central nervous system (CNS) insult and attendant increased pulmonary capillary permeability resulting in a protein-rich transudate that occupies the alveolar spaces [16–18]. The insult can be subarachnoid hemorrhage, head injury, seizure, or ischemic stroke. Several mechanisms can cause an increase in pulmonary capillary hydrostatic pressure and thus, pulmonary edema. These mechanisms include left atrial hypertension, systemic hypertension, and pulmonary venoconstriction. However, in NPE, in addition to increased capillary hydrostatic pressure, there is an opening of endothelial tight junctions resulting in extravasation of protein into the interstitial space and then, when the lymphatic drainage capacity is exceeded, into the alveolar space. The alteration in tight junctions is ascribed to sympathetic overactivity due to the CNS insult [19,20]. Treatment includes optimization of hemodynamic and oxygenation status using positive end-expiratory pressure (PEEP) and α-adrenergic blockers.

Cardiac

Cardiac dysfunction is frequently associated with stroke; it may be the cause of, coexistent with, or a consequence of stroke. Cardiac dysfunction can manifest as electrocardiography (ECG) changes, arrhythmias, or ischemia. ECG changes include tall P waves, prolonged QT interval, ST wave depression or inversion, and peaked or inverted T waves and U waves. Arrhythmias include sinus bradycardia, wandering atrial pacemaker, paroxysmal atrial pacemaker, nodal bradycardia, ectopic atrial and ventricular activity, AV block, AV dissociation, and atrial fibrillation [21]. Ischemia may manifest as elevations in CK-MB isoenzymes.

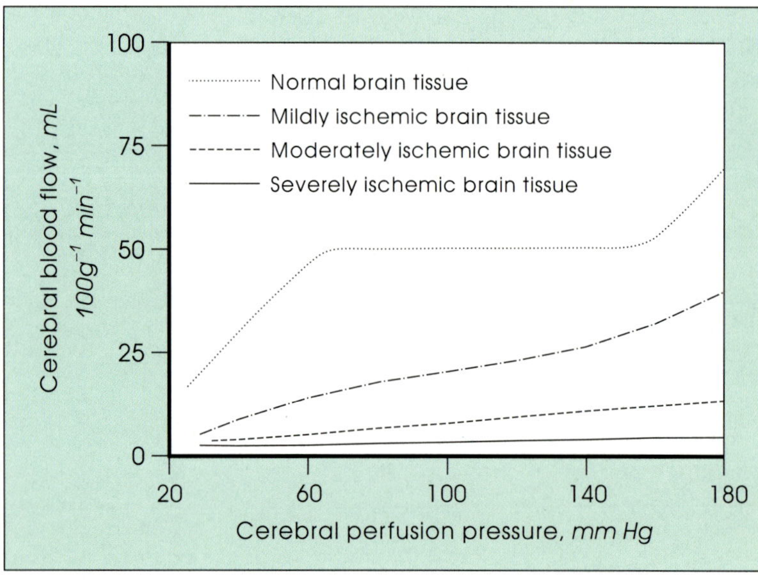

FIGURE 14.2

Effect of focal brain ischemia on autoregulation (from data obtained in spontaneously hypertensive rats [25]). The normal curve is based on data obtained in humans [26]. (*From* Powers [24]; with permission.)

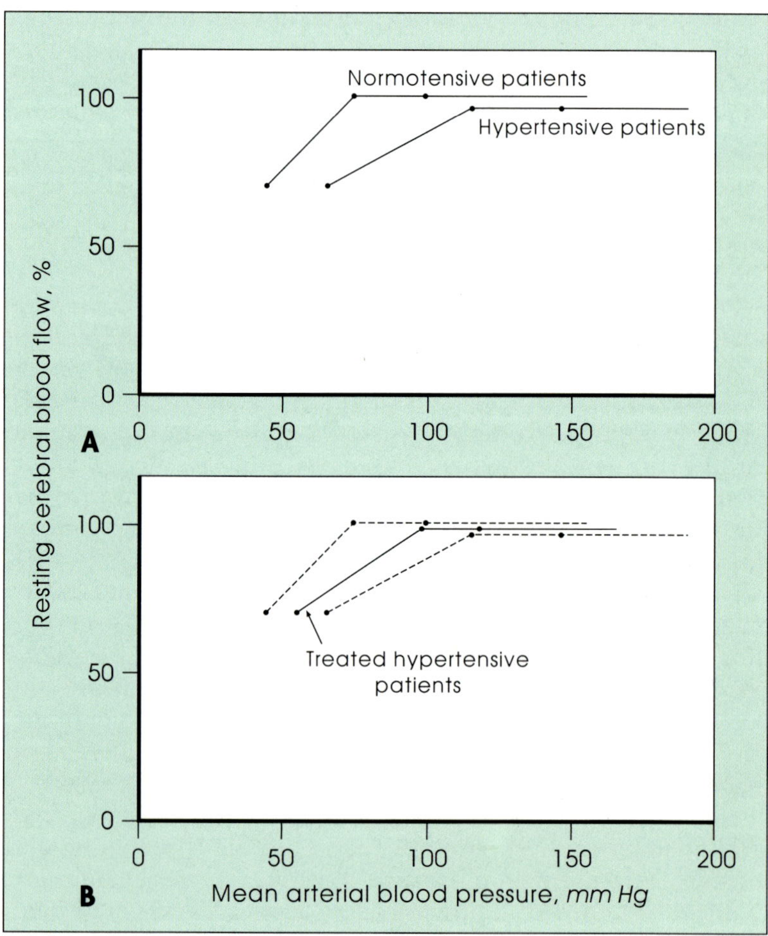

FIGURE 14.3

A, Mean curves of autoregulation of cerebral blood flow (CBF) in normotensive and severely hypertensive human subjects. Each curve is defined by the mean values of resting blood pressure, the lower limit of CBF autoregulation, and the lowest tolerated blood pressure. The curve from the hypertensive patients is shifted to the right on the blood pressure axis. **B**, Mean curve of CBF autoregulation in patients with a formerly severe hypertension that at the time of the study was effectively controlled by antihypertensive treatment. The curve falls between the two curves above, which are shown by dotted lines. (*From* Strandgaard [27]; with permission.)

Cardiac dysfunction occurs with ischemic stroke, hemorrhagic stroke, and subarachnoid hemorrhage. Patient prognosis is worse for stroke-associated ischemic heart or cardiac arrhythmias than preexistent ischemic changes or arrhythmias. Norris and coworkers [22] reported that 11% of stroke patients had elevated CK-MB isoenzymes that correlated with ECG changes and arrhythmias. Temporally related cardiac effects were the result and not the cause of stroke. A suggested mechanism for the cardiac effects is as follows: the stroke induces an excessive CNS noradrenergic sympathetic activation that elicits a positive inotropic and chronotropic effect, necessitating increased myocardial oxygen demand and resulting in cardiac dysfunction [23].

Due to the high frequency of stroke-associated cardiac dysfunction, cardiac monitoring for 24 to 48 hours following hospital admission is indicated. If ECG changes occur, then serial CK and LDH isoenzymes are obtained. Ischemic changes are usually treated with beta blockers, calcium channel blockers, or nitrates.

Vascular

Systemic Hypertension

Arterial hypertension immediately following stroke is a common occurrence. However, blood pressure usually returns spontaneously to the prestroke level within a few days. Patients with poststroke hypertension have increased early mortality; however, a causal relationship has not been established. Management of the usually transient hypertension is controversial. The objective is to maintain adequate cerebral blood flow (CBF) in the presence of impaired autoregulation. Assuming that cerebrovascular resistance is minimal, then CBF is directly proportional to cerebral perfusion pressure (CPP), which is the difference between the mean arterial pressure (MAP) and intracranial pressure (ICP). Thus, in the stroke patient, decreasing the MAP can significantly reduce CBF. The usual goal is to maintain a CPP of at least 50 to 60 mm Hg. However, in mildly, moderately, or severely ischemic brain tissue (Figure 14.2), a significantly greater CPP may be required to maintain neuronal integrity (CBF > 10–12 mL/100 g/min) and electrical activity (CBF > 20 mL/100 g min) [24]. Chronically hypertensive patients are at increased risk for exacerbation of ischemic stroke because their autoregulatory curve is shifted to the right, *ie*, dysautoregulation occurs at a higher MAP in the hypertensive versus normotensive patient (Figure 14.3) (Table 14.2) [27,28]. If end organ damage is present, *eg*, cardiac or renal, then acute reduction of blood pressure is indicated. If neurologic symptoms worsen, however, then restoration of blood pressure is warranted.

If urgent blood pressure reduction is indicated, then α- or β-adrenergic blockers can be employed, *eg*, labetalol 10 mg intravenously over 1 to 2 minutes. The dose may be repeated or doubled every 10 to 20 minutes until a satisfactory blood pressure reduction is achieved or until a cumulative dose of 300 mg has been administered [29]. Recent studies indicate that sodium nitroprusside, calcium channel blockers, and hydralazine cause cerebrovasodilation and may increase ICP [30].

Venous Thrombosis and Pulmonary Embolism

Lower extremity venous thrombosis is a common occurrence in stroke patients. In the absence of prophylaxis, deep venous thrombosis (DVT) develops in 60% to 75% of the patients and lethal pulmonary embolism (PE) occurs in 5%. Risk factors for DVT include immobility, paralysis, obesity, congestive heart failure, lower extremity venous disease, pregnancy, and estrogen use. Symptoms and signs of DVT are unreliable for making a diagnosis; thus, a low threshold for the employment of ancillary tests is warranted. Symptoms of PE include dyspnea, chest pain, and apprehension. Signs of PE include tachypnea (> 20/min), tachycardia (> 100/min), and fever (> 38.5°C). Evaluation for PE includes arterial blood gases that indicate an increased PO_2(A-a) gradient, arterial hypoxemia (PO_2 < 80 mm Hg), and hypocapnia. ECG reveals sinus tachycardia and right heart strain. Chest radiograph is usually unremarkable except perhaps for subsegmental atelectasis. Ventilation-perfusion (V-Q) scan is obtained on stable patients. Lower extremity venous duplex ultrasonography is performed to support a diagnosis of PE when the V-Q scan is nondiagnostic. Pulmonary angiography is performed when the noninvasive studies are indeterminate and there is a high index of suspicion for PE. Treatment to prevent continued embolization is intravenous heparin (activated partial thromboplastin time [aPTT] 1.5–2.5 times control)

Table 14.2. Autoregulation of cerebral blood flow in normotensive and hypertensive patients*†

Group	MAP, *mm Hg* Control	MAP, *mm Hg* Lower limit of autoregulation	MAP, *mm Hg* Lowest tolerated	Percent of resting MAP, *mm Hg* Lower limit of autoregulation	Percent of resting MAP, *mm Hg* Lowest tolerated
Normotensive (*n*=10)	98±10	73±9	43±8	74±12	45±12
Hypertensive (*n*=13)	145±17	113±17‡§	65±10‡	79±10	45±6
Controlled hypertensive (*n*=9)	116±18	96±17	53±17	72±29	46±16

*From Gifford [28]; with permission.
†Values given as mean ± SD.
‡*P*<0.01 for difference between normotensive and hypertensive patients.
§*P*<0.01 for difference between controlled and uncontrolled hypertensive patients.
MAP—mean arterial pressure.

followed by oral warfarin (international normalized ratio [INR] 2.0–3.0), which is continued for approximately 3 months. Indications for inferior vena cava interruption include a contraindication to anticoagulation or recurrent emboli despite adequate anticoagulation.

Four randomized trials [31–34] of low-dose subcutaneous heparin (LDH) or low molecular weight (LMW) heparin and heparinoids for DVT prophylaxis in patients with ischemic stroke have been reported. Both were effective with relative risk reductions of 45% and 79% for LDH and LMW heparin, respectively. Thus, DVT prophylaxis with LDH or LMW heparin is recommended; if anticoagulant treatment is contraindicated, then intermittent pneumatic compression boots are recommended.

Central Nervous System

Cerebral Edema

Cerebral edema with attendant herniation is the leading cause of death within the first week following ischemic or hemorrhagic stroke (Figure 14.4) [3]. Silver and coworkers [3] reported mortality based on the type and location of the stroke: ischemic supratentorial 15% and infratentorial 18%; and hemorrhagic supratentorial 58% and infratentorial 31% (Table 14.3) [3]. Initially, intracellular cytotoxic edema develops; subsequently, interstitial vasogenic edema is superimposed. Edema peaks at 2 to 5 days following the insult. Cerebral edema, via increasing ICP, is deleterious based on two mechanisms: increased ICP results in decreased CPP and CBF, thus exacerbating existing ischemia, and increased ICP results in parenchymal shifts (herniations). These

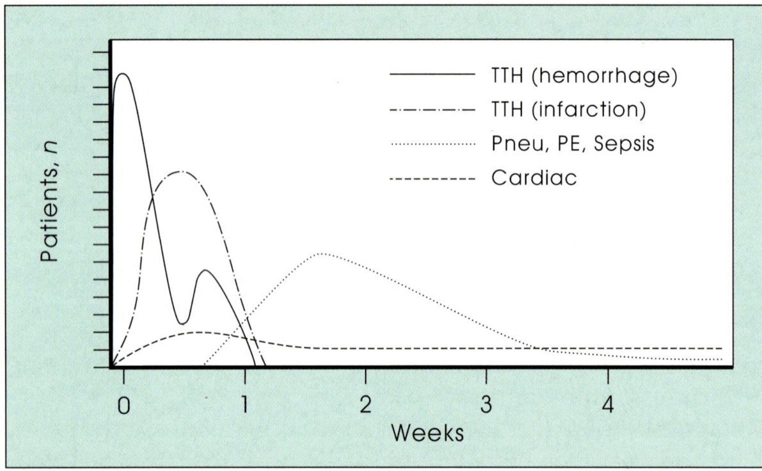

FIGURE 14.4

Diagrammatic representation of the causes of death following supratentorial infarction and hemorrhage. PE—pulmonary thromboembolism; Pneu—pneumonia; TTH—transtentorial herniation. (*From* Silver and coworkers [3]; with permission.)

Table 14.3. Mortality at 30 days by stroke type in 1073 consecutive patients admitted with completed strokes*

Stroke type	Deaths, *n*	Total, *n*	Mortality, %
Supratentorial			
Infarction	125	814	15
Hemorrhage	55	93	58
Infratentorial			
Infarction	28	153	18
Hemorrhage	4	13	31
Total	212	1073	20

**From* Silver and coworkers [3]; with permission.

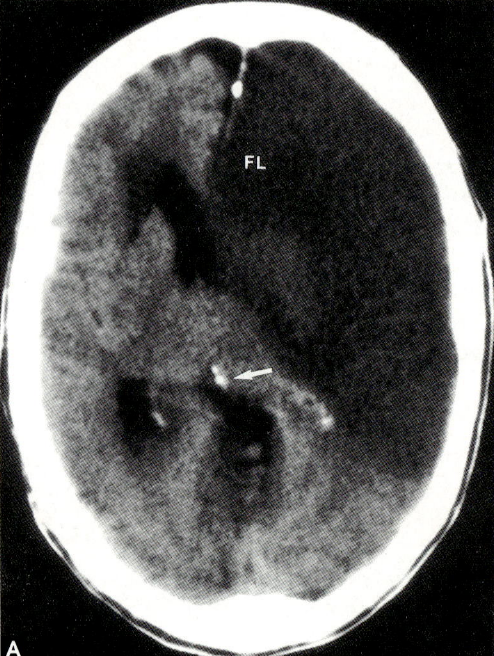

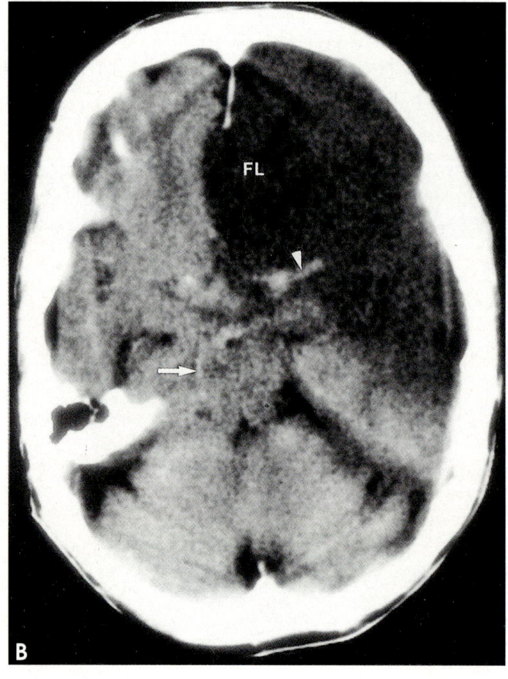

FIGURE 14.5

Cranial computed tomograms, without intravenous contrast, at the level of the lateral ventricles (**A**) and midbrain (**B**) from an 81-year-old woman who suffered a left internal carotid artery occlusion with infarction in the middle and anterior cerebral artery territories. *Scan A* shows significant edema (*low density*) with displacement across the midline of the left frontal lobe (FL) and pineal gland (*arrow*); also, effacement of the left anterior horn and compression of the left atrium. *Scan B* shows "high density sign," indicative of thrombosis, in the left middle (*arrowhead*) and right posterior (*arrow*) cerebral arteries; also, significant edema (*low density*) with displacement of the left FL across the midline. (Scans with right hemisphere on left side.)

herniations, which cause compression, stretching, and tearing of arteries and veins, result in additional ischemic and hemorrhagic infarctions to critical structures such as the brainstem cardiorespiratory center (Figures 14.5 and 14.6). Clinical manifestations of intracranial hypertension from cerebral edema include the following: drowsiness, headache, nausea and vomiting, papilledema, pupillary abnormalities, abducens nerve palsy, periodic respiratory pattern, ipsilateral extensor planter response, and spontaneous posturing.

Traditional treatment includes the following: positioning the head in the midline (to facilitate jugular venous return); elevating the head of the bed to 30 degrees (to decrease intracranial venous volume); hyperventilation to a PCO_2 of 25 to 30 mm Hg (to vasoconstrict intracranial arterioles); and inducing an osmotic diuresis with mannitol (1 g/kg intravenously over 30 minutes followed by 0.25–0.5 g/kg every 4 hours to obtain a serum osmolality of 310–320 mOsm/kg) without or with the loop diuretic furosemide (to decrease intracranial extracellular fluid volume). Steroids have not proven useful and may increase morbidity (stress ulcers, infection, hyperglycemia) [35]. Barbiturates appear to be ineffective. For cerebellar strokes with edema and herniation, ventriculostomy or posterior fossa decompression may be life saving.

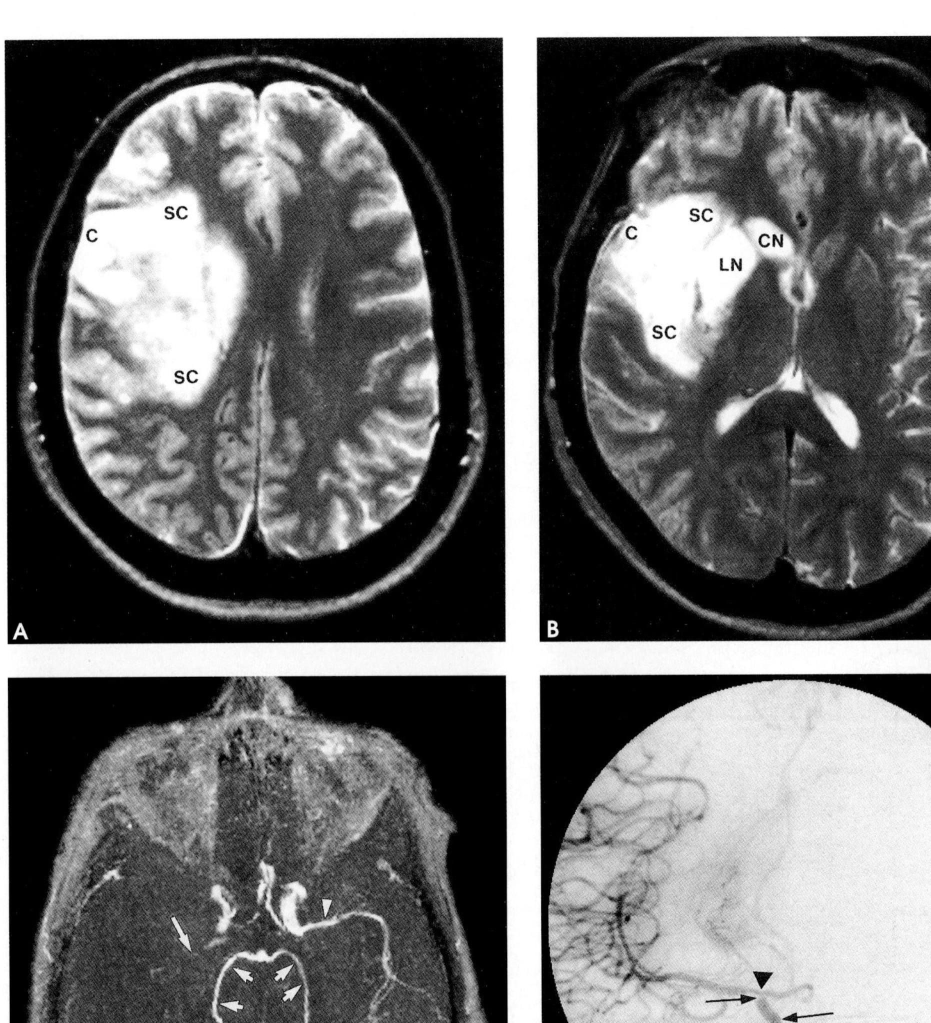

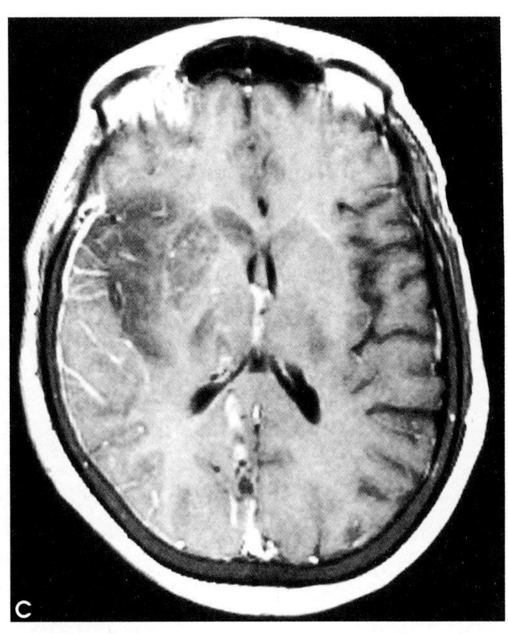

FIGURE 14.6

Magnetic resonance images (MRI) without contrast (T2-weighted) and with contrast (T1-weighted), magnetic resonance angiogram (MRA) (phase contrast), and digital subtraction angiogram from a 56-year-old woman who suffered a right internal carotid artery occlusion. **A**, MRI at the level of the lateral ventricles shows significant edema (*high intensity*) in the right cortical (C) and subcortical (SC) areas with a midline shift from right to left. **B**, MRI at the level of the basal ganglia shows edema (*high intensity*) in the right caudate nucleus (CN), lenticular nucleus (LN), SC, and C areas with a midline shift, from right to left, of the third ventricle. **C**, MRI at the same level as *B*, shows contrast enhancement (*high intensity*) of the vasculature in the edematous areas. **D**, MRA at the level of the midbrain shows no signal from the right (*arrow*) versus signal from the left (*arrowhead*) middle cerebral artery; signals (*high intensity*) are present from the posterior cerebral arteries (*double arrows*). **E**, Angiogram anterior-posterior view, shows severe stenosis of the terminal (*arrow*) right internal carotid artery (*double arrows*) at the origin (*arrowhead*) of the right middle cerebral artery. (MRI, MRA, and angiogram with right hemisphere on left side.)

Seizures

Poststroke seizures occur in 5% to 20% of patients [36]. Gupta and coworkers [37] reported that 33% of the patients experienced the first seizure within the first 2 weeks poststroke and of those seizures 90% occurred within the first 24 hours. Seventy-five percent of the patients experienced the first seizure within the first year and only 2% of the patients developed seizures after 2 years. Kilpatrick and coworkers [38] reported the following association of type of cerebrovascular event and seizure frequency: lobar hemorrhage, 15%; subarachnoid hemorrhage, 9%; transient ischemic attack, 4%; cortical infarction, 1%; and lacunar or deep hemorrhage, 0%.

Holmes [39] reported the following frequency of EEG activity in poststroke seizures: focal spikes, 78%; focal slow waves, 20%; diffuse slow waves, 10%; and normal, 5%. Early onset seizures are usually focal with secondary generalization whereas late onset seizures are usually generalized (tonic-clonic). Monotherapy with conventional anticonvulsant agents is usually successful.

Behavioral Changes

Behavioral changes commonly occur in stroke patients based on self-perception of deficits and location of brain damage. Reactive depression is due to the recognition of deficits in language, sensorimotor function, and activities of daily living [40]. Brain damage alters the noradrenergic and serotonergic transmitter systems that may underlie depression. Depression occurs in 26% to 60% of stroke patients. Fifty percent of patients with thromboembolic or hemorrhagic stroke develop depression within 2 weeks of the ictus [41]. Without treatment, depression will persist for many months and impede rehabilitative efforts [42,43]. Depression is more frequent with frontal lobe strokes (left greater than right) and it is more severe when the stroke is closer to the frontal pole [41,43]. The severity of depression is not directly related to the degree of Broca's aphasia. Depression may be masked by psychosomatic complaints of nonspecific head, face, extremity, or joint pain. Treatment includes a coordinated effort from the medical team and family support group. Pharmacotherapy with nortriptyline is useful [44]; treatment is initiated with a low dose at bedtime that is slowly increased over 2 to 3 weeks. Onset of the antidepressant effect is within 2 to 3 weeks. Based on the quinidine-like effects of nortriptyline, a pretreatment ECG is obtained. The anticholinergic side effects may exacerbate urinary outlet obstruction and narrow angle glaucoma.

Other behavioral changes that complicate recovery include frustration, anger, and labile affect (inappropriate crying and laughing). Poststroke aphasia and neglect may be improved by dopamine agonists such as bromocriptine.

Peripheral Nervous System

Compression neuropathy occurs in affected extremities. Due to hypesthesia or paresis, detection of the superimposed neuropathy may be difficult pending return of sensory-motor function to the extremity. The peroneal nerve may be compressed against the head of the fibula resulting in foot drop. Ulnar nerve compression at the elbow may occur, especially in wheelchair-bound patients. Traction brachial plexopathy may occur from a paretic subluxed shoulder; support for the extremity should be provided to avoid this complication.

Fluids, Electrolytes, and Glucose

Stroke patients are at risk for fluid, electrolyte, and glucose abnormalities throughout their hospitalization. At admission, intravenous access is obtained and maintenance fluids of 0.45 or 0.9 normal saline, depending on cardiovascular status, are initiated. In the absence of significant cerebral edema or elevated intracranial pressure, serum osmolality is maintained within normal limits (280–295 mOsm/kg).

Hyponatremia can have many causes including vomiting, diarrhea, gastric suctioning, fever, and diaphoresis. The syndrome of inappropriate antidiuretic hormone secretion occurs in stroke patients. It is characterized by excessive release of antidiuretic hormone resulting in hypervolemia, hypotonia, hyponatremia, and natriuresis. Treatment includes fluid restriction; the condition is usually self-limited. Excessively rapid correction of hyponatremia may result in osmotic myelinolysis (*eg,* central pontine myelinolysis) . Hyponatremia can occur also as the result of a central salt wasting syndrome. Stroke patients at increased risk include those with subarachnoid hemorrhage. Patients with central salt wasting syndrome have hyponatremia but decreased blood volumes. Infusions of isotonic saline, colloids, and packed red cells may be required to restore circulatory blood volume and normalize serum sodium.

Some animal and human studies indicate that ictal hyperglycemia exacerbates ischemic stroke by increasing anaerobic metabolism (with attendant lactic acid production), and altering phosphorus metabolism [45,46]. In addition, because glucose readily traverses the blood-brain barrier, elevated plasma concentrations can worsen cerebral edema. Based on these adverse effects, it is recommended that serum glucose be maintained at or below 125 to 150 mg/dL.

Gastrointestinal

Dysphagia occurs in approximately 30% of patients with stroke (hemispheric or brainstem). Video fluoroscopy is useful in identifying the swallowing phases that are abnormal (Figure 14.7). Therapy should address head position, selection of foods, and avoidance of aspiration. Bowel incontinence may occur due to loss of sensation and sphincter control. Increasing fiber in the diet and use of diapers to minimize skin maceration is recommended. Constipation may initially occur due to adynamic ileus. A bowel regimen, including softeners, laxatives, suppositories, and enemas is recommended to avoid constipation and impaction.

Gastrointestinal stress ulcers occur in stroke patients. In the absence of enteral feeding, prophylaxis with a histamine type 2 (H2) blocker or antacid is recommended. Alternatively, sucralfate, a complex of sucrose octasulfate and aluminum hydroxide, may be an effective prophylaxis for stress ulcers and decrease the risk of nosocomial pneumonia by maintaining the natural gastric acid barrier against bacterial overgrowth [47].

Urinary

Urinary retention and incontinence occur in stroke patients due to loss of volitional control or sphincter dyssynergy. Unless it is necessary for monitoring fluid and electrolyte status, indwelling catheters should be avoided. In the presence of an absolutely closed catheter system, significant bacteriuria occurs at a rate of 3% to 5% per day; thus, after 10 days, 50% of all catheterized patients will have significant bacteriuria [48]. Breaks in the catheter system, one or more per day, may double the infection rate [49]. Antibiotic prophylaxis, systemic, local, or topical, is ineffective and results in antibiotic-resistant organisms [49,50]. In the presence of an indwelling catheter, treatment of asymptomatic bacteriuria is usually not indicated; however, for significant clinical infection with pyuria and fever, treatment is recommended. If retention or incontinence occurs in the absence of an indwelling catheter, then the following treatment may be employed: in addition to intermittent catheterization, male patients may use a condom catheter and female patients may receive diapers to decrease wetness and reduce skin maceration.

Dermatologic

According to the National Survey of Stroke, approximately 15% of stroke patients develop pressure sores [51]. Pressure sores develop on weight-bearing immobile or hypesthetic body surfaces as follows: the occiput, scapulae, sacrum, and heels in supine patients; the ear, shoulder, greater trochanter, and malleoli in side-lying patients; and ischii for wheelchair-bound patients [52]. Additional contributing factors include obesity, moisture (from perspiration, urine, and feces), spasticity, infection, and nutritional deficiency [53]. Pressure sores, due to compressive ischemia of the skin and subcutaneous tissues, are avoided by frequent (every 2 hours or more) repositioning of the head, trunk, and extreminities [53]. Patients at greater risk, *eg*, severe hemiplegic, stuporous, or comatose patients, should be placed on an air- or fluid-filled mattress.

REHABILITATION

Rehabilitation has been defined as "the continuing and comprehensive team effort to restore an individual to his or her former functional and environmental status, or alternatively, to maintain or maximize remaining function" [54]. As previously noted, 31% of stroke survivors require assistance with care, 20% need help walking, and 71% have some impaired vocational capacity 7 years after the stroke [1]. Rehabilitative evaluation and treatment are initiated as soon as the patient is medically and neurologically stable [55,56]; details of rehabilitation are discussed in subsequent chapters.

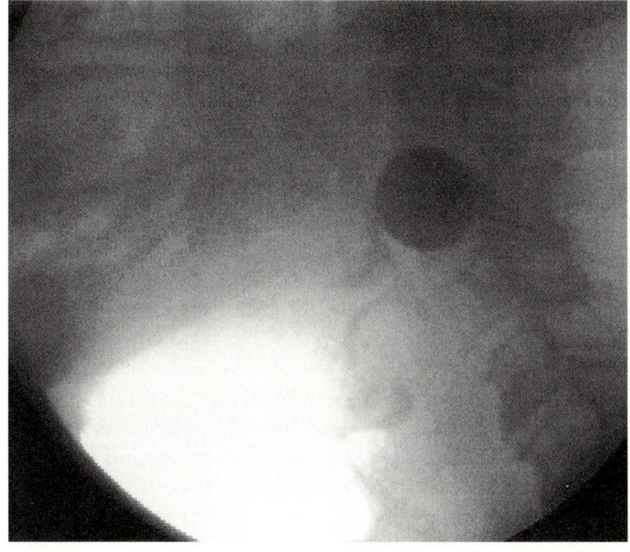

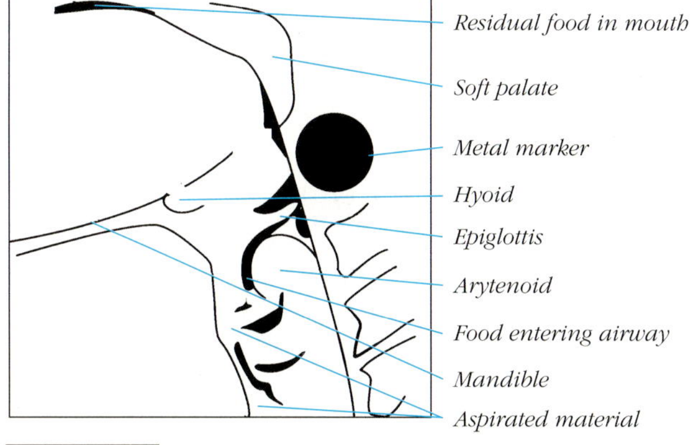

FIGURE 14.7

Videoprint and labelled tracing of a lateral radiographic view of the oropharynx during swallowing in a patient who is aspirating a significant amount of thick liquid because of reduced airway closure. (*Courtesy of* Jerilyn Logemann, PhD.)

REFERENCES

1. American Heart Association: *1992 Heart and Stroke Facts*. Dallas: American Heart Association; 1992.
2. National Stroke Association Consensus Statement: Stroke: the first six hours. Emergency evaluation. *Stroke Clin Upd* 1993, 6(1).
3. Silver FL, Norris JW, Lewis AJ, *et al.*: Early mortality following stroke: a prospective review. *Stroke* 1984, 15:492–496.
4. Bounds JV, Wiebers DO, Whisnant JP, *et al.*: Mechanisms and timing of deaths from cerebral infarction. *Stroke* 1981, 12:474–477.
5. Brown M, Glassenberg M: Mortality factors in patients with acute stroke. *JAMA* 1973, 224:1493–1495.
6. Fluck DC: Chest movements in hemiplegia. *Clin Sci* 1966, 31:383–388.
7. Przedborski S, Brunko E, Hubert M, *et al.*: The effect of acute hemiplegia on intercostal muscle activity. *Neurology* 1988, 38:1882–1884.
8. Horner J, Massey EW, Riski JE, *et al.*: Aspiration following stroke: clinical correlates and outcome. *Neurology* 1988, 38:1359–1362.
9. Horan TC, White JW, Jarvis WL, *et al.*: Nosocomial infection surveillance, 1984. *MMWR* 1986, 35:17SS–29SS.
10. Kronberg FG, Goodwin WJ: Sinusitis in intensive care unit patients. *Laryngoscope* 1985, 95:936–938.
11. Deutschman CS, Wilton PB, Sinow J, *et al.*: Paranasal sinusitis: a common complication of nasotracheal intubation in neurosurgical patients. *Neurosurgery* 1985, 17:296–299.
12. Perlman D, Caplan ES: Nosocomial sinusitis: a new and complex threat. *J Crit Ill* 1987, 2:19–25.
13. McWey RE, Curry NS, Schabel SI, *et al.*: Complications of nasoenteric feeding tubes. *Am J Surg* 1988, 155:253–257.

14. Carey T, Holcombe B: Endotracheal intubation as a risk factor for complications of nasoenteric tube insertion. *Crit Care Med* 1991, 19:427–429.
15. Bouzarth WF: Intracranial nasogastric tube insertion. *J Trauma* 1978, 18:818–819.
16. Malik AB: Mechanisms of neurogenic pulmonary edema. *Circ Res* 1985, 57:1–18.
17. Theodore J, Robin ED: Pathogenesis of neurogenic pulmonary edema. *Lancet* 1975, 2:749–751.
18. Simon RP: Neurogenic pulmonary edema. *Neurol Clin* 1993, 11:309–323.
19. Rosell S: Neuronal control of microvessels. *Ann Rev Physiol* 1980, 42:359–371.
20. Simon RP, Bayne LL: Pulmonary lymphatic flow alterations during intracranial hypertension in sheep. *Ann Neurol* 1984, 15:188–194.
21. Oppenheimmer SM, Hachinski VC: The cardiac consequences of stroke. *Neurol Clin* 1992, 10:167–176.
22. Norris JW, Hachinski VC, Myers MG, *et al.*: Serum cardiac enzymes in stroke. *Stroke* 1979, 10:548–553.
23. Rona G: Catecholamine cardiotoxicity. *J Mol Cell Cardiol* 1985, 17:291–306.
24. Powers WJ: Hemodynamics and metabolism in ischemic cerebrovascular disease. *Neurol Clin* 1992, 10:31–48.
25. Dirnagl U, Pulsinelli W: Autoregulation of cerebral blood flow in experimental focal brain ischemia. *J Cereb Blood Flow Metab* 1990, 10:327–336.
26. Strandgaard S, Oleson J, Skinhoj E, *et al.*: Autoregulation of brain circulation in severe arterial hypertension. *BMJ* 1973, 1:507–510.
27. Strandgaard S: Autoregulation of cerebral blood flow in hypertensive patients: the modifying influence of prolonged antihypertensive treatment on the tolerance to acute drug-induced hypotension. *Circulation* 1976, 53:720–727.
28. Gifford RW: Management of hypertensive crises. *JAMA* 1991, 266:829–835.
29. Brott T: Prevention and management of medical complications of the hospitalized elderly stroke patient. *Clin Geriatr Med* 1991, 7:475–482.
30. Hayashi M, Kobayashi H, Kawano H, *et al.*: Treatment of systemic hypertension and intracranial hypertension in cases of brain hemorrhage. *Stroke* 1988, 19:314–321.
31. McCarthy ST, Turner JJ, Robertson D, *et al.*: Low dose heparin as a prophylaxis against deep vein thrombosis after acute stroke. *Lancet* 1977, 2:800–801.
32. Turpie AGG, Levine MN, Hirsh J, *et al.*: A double-blind randomized trial of ORG 10172 low molecular weight heparinoid in the prevention of deep vein thrombosis in thrombotic stroke. *Lancet* 1987, 1:523–526.
33. Prins MH, den Ottolander GJH, Gelsema R, *et al.*: Deep vein thrombosis prophylaxis with a low molecular weight heparin (Kabi 2165) in stroke patients. *Thromb Haemost* 1987, 58(suppl):117.
34. Turpie AGG, Levine MN, Powers PJ, *et al.*: A double-blind randomized trial of ORG 10172 low molecular weight heparinoid versus unfractionated heparin in the prevention of deep vein thrombosis in patients with thrombotic stroke. *Thromb Haemost* 1991, 65:753.
35. Norris JW: Steroid therapy in acute cerebral infarction. *Arch Neurol* 1976, 33:69–71.
36. Olsen TS, Hogenhaven H, Thage O: Epilepsy after stroke. *Neurology* 1987, 37:1209–1211.
37. Gupta SR, Naheedey MH, Elias D, *et al.*: Postinfarction seizures: a clinical study. *Stroke* 1988, 19:1477–1481.
38. Kilpatrick CJ, Davis SM, Tress BM, *et al.*: Epileptic seizures in acute stroke. *Arch Neurol* 1990, 47:157–160.
39. Holmes GL: The electroencephalogram as a predictor of seizures following cerebral infarction. *Clin Electroencephalogr* 1980, 11:83–86.
40. Binder LM: Emotional problems after stroke. *Stroke* 1984, 15:174–177.
41. Robinson RG, Starr LB, Kubos KL, *et al.*: A two-year longitudinal study of post-stroke mood disorders: findings during the initial evaluation. *Stroke* 1983, 14:736–741.
42. Robinson RG, Starr LB, Price TR: A two-year longitudinal study of mood disorders following stroke: prevention and duration at six months follow-up. *Br J Psych* 1984, 144:256–262.
43. Robinson RG, Price TR: Post-stroke depressive disorders: a follow-up of 103 outpatients. *Stroke* 1982, 13:635–641.
44. Lipsey JR, Robinson RG, Pearlson GD, *et al.*: Nortriptyline treatment of poststroke depression: a double-blind treatment trial. *Lancet* 1984, 1:297–300.
45. Pulsinelli W, Levy DE, Sigsbee B, *et al.*: Increased damage after ischemic stroke in patients with hyperglycemia with or without established diabetes mellitus. *Am J Med* 1983, 74:540–543.
46. Chew W, Kucharczyk J, Moseley M, *et al.*: Hyperglycemia augments ischemic brain injury: in vivo MR imaging/spectroscopic study with nicardipine in cats with occluded middle cerebral arteries. *Am J Neuroradiol* 1991, 12:611–620.
47. Driks MR, Craven DE, Celli BR, *et al.*: Nosocomial pneumonia in intubated patients given sucralfate as compared with antacids or histamine type 2 blockers. *N Engl J Med* 1987, 317:1376–1382.
48. Garibaldi RA, Burke JP, Dickman ML: Factors predisposing to bacteriuria during indwelling urinary catheterization. *N Engl J Med* 1974, 291:215–219.
49. Warren JW, Platt R, Thomas RJ, *et al.*: Antibiotic irrigation and catheter-associated urinary tract infections. *N Engl J Med* 1978, 299:570–573.
50. Burke JP, Garibaldi RA, Britt MR, *et al.*: Prevention of catheter-associated urinary tract infections: efficacy of daily meatal care regimens. *Am J Med* 1981, 70:655–658.
51. Walker AE, Robins M, Weinfeld FD: Clinical findings. In Weinfeld FD, ed. *The National Survey of Stroke. Stroke* 1981, 12(suppl 1):I-13–I-37.
52. Roth EJ: Medical complications encountered in stroke rehabilitation. *Phys Med Rehab Clin North Am* 1991, 2:563–578.
53. Reuler J, Cooney T: The pressure sore: pathophysiology and principles of management. *Ann Intern Med* 1981, 94:661–666.
54. Hirschberg GG, Lewis L, Vaughn P: Levels and places of rehabilitation. In *Rehabilitation: A Manual for the Care of the Disabled and Elderly*. Edited by Hirschberg GG, Lewis L, Vaughn P. Rehabilitation. Philadelphia: J.B. Lippincott; 1976:143.
55. Roth EJ: The elderly stroke patient: principles and practices of rehabilitation management. *Top Geriatr Rehabil* 1988, 3:27–61.
56. Reding MJ, McDowell FH: Stroke rehabilitation. *Neurol Clin* 1987, 5:601–630.

Chapter 15

The Use of Antiplatelet Drugs to Prevent Stroke

L. JAAP KAPPELLE
HAROLD P. ADAMS, JR

Patients with symptoms of vascular disease are at risk for recurrent vascular events (Figure 15.1). In 1953, Craven [1] proposed that administration of aspirin might prevent ischemic cardiovascular events because it inhibits platelet aggregation (Figures 15.2 and 15.3). Since then, the drug has achieved great popularity. Because of its antipyretic and analgesic effects, relatively good tolerance, accessibility, and low cost, aspirin is the most commonly used drug today. In the United States alone, between 20 and 30 billion tablets are ingested each year [2]. In addition, there are several other antiplatelet agents (Tables 15.1 and 15.2). The Antiplatelet Trialists' Collaboration has defined antiplatelet agents as those drugs whose primary mode of action on the vascular system is the inhibition of platelet aggrega-

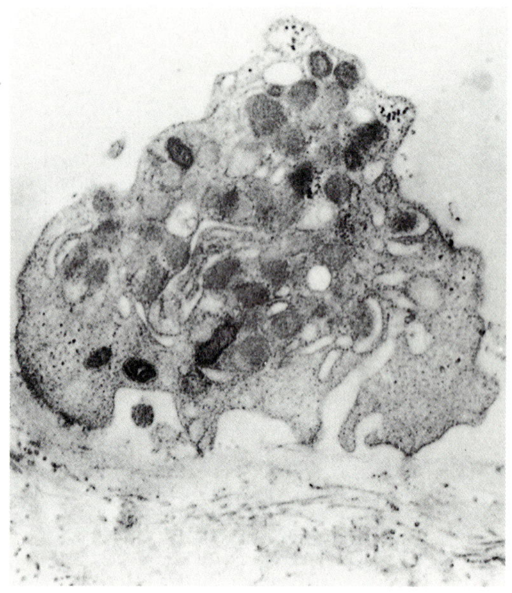

FIGURE 15.1

Platelet interaction with subendothelium of a human umbilical artery. Following damage of the vessel wall blood platelets adhere to the exposed subendothelium. (*Courtesy of* H.K. Nieuwenhuis, MD.)

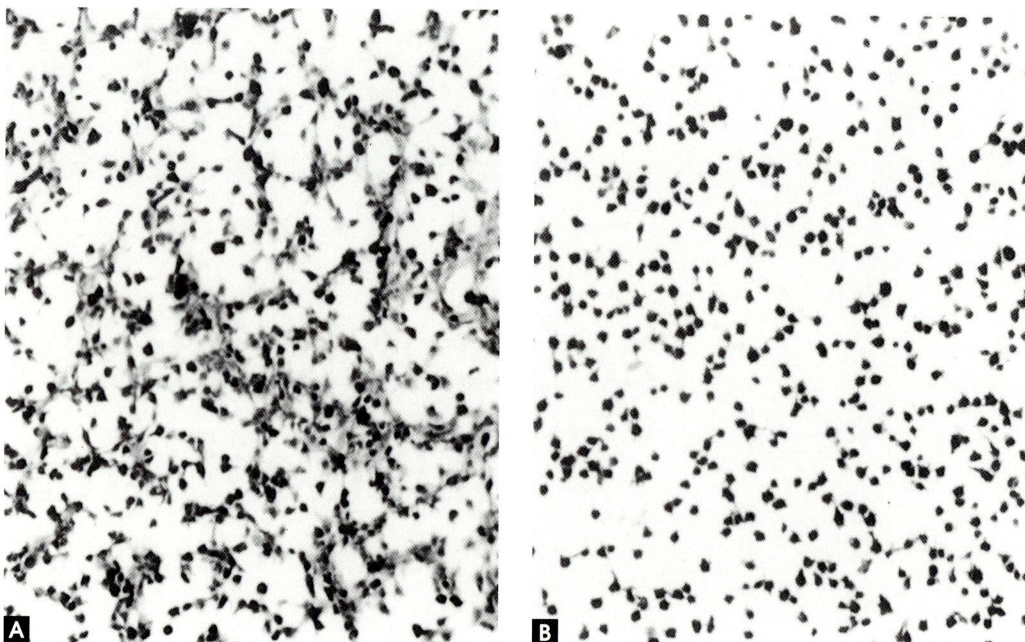

FIGURE 15.2

Platelet interaction with endothelial cell matrix. **A**, Spreading of platelets. **B**, Inhibition of platelet spreading by a platelet-function inhibitor. (*Courtesy of* H.K. Nieuwenhuis, MD.)

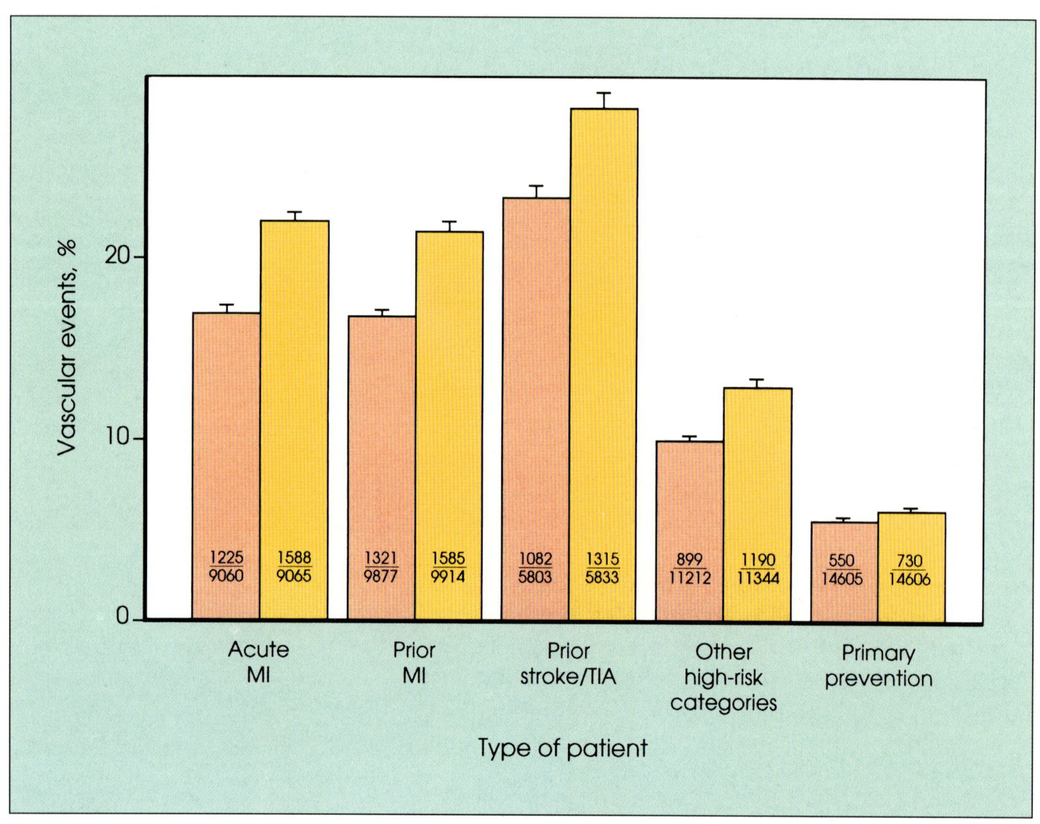

FIGURE 15.3

Absolute rates of vascular death, nonfatal myocardial infarction (MI), or nonfatal stroke, represented by underlined numbers on bars, in randomized trials of prolonged antiplatelet therapy (*orange bars*) versus control (*yellow bars*) in high risk categories and in primary prevention. TIA—transient ischemic attack. (*From* Fuster and coworkers [2] and Antiplatelet Trialists' Collaboration [3]; with permission.)

Table 15.1. Antiplatelet aggregating drugs*

Drugs of proven usefullness
Aspirin
Ticlopidine
Drugs of unproven efficacy
Dipyridamole
Sulfinpyrazone
Drugs to be tested
Clopidogrel

*Suloctidil is no longer available because of its toxicity.

tion and adherence [3]. Meta-analysis has demonstrated that they are of proven efficacy for reducing the risk of major vascular events (Figures 15.4 and 15.5) [3,4]. The calculated reduction in stroke risk is 24% among patients enrolled in high risk trials [3]. Antiplatelet-aggregating drugs are considered the yardstick with which other interventions to prevent stroke are compared.

Table 15.2. Mechanism of action of antiplatelet drugs that are used in clinical practice

Drug	Mechanism of action
Aspirin	Inhibits cyclooxygenase
Ticlopidine	Inhibits ADP
Clopidogrel	Inhibits ADP
Sulfinpyrazone	Suppresses cyclooxygenase (reversible)
Dipyridamole	Inhibits phosphodiesterase

While aspirin is the most widely studied drug, ticlopidine is also effective in stroke prevention [5,6].

Several controversies about antiplatelet therapy in stroke prevention persist. In the past there was controversy about the usefulness of aspirin in women, but present evidence suggests that it is effective in both sexes [7–9]. Currently, the chief controversy is about the best dose of aspirin for stroke prevention. Some experts recommend a low dose (30 to 325 mg/d) [10–12], while others recommend high doses (975 to 1300 mg/d) [13,14]. Unfortunately, there are no clinical trials in which the usefulness of low-dose aspirin and high-dose aspirin have been adequately compared [15–19].

Both ticlopidine and aspirin are approved for prevention of ischemic stroke in the United States. Clopidogrel resembles ticlopidine but may have fewer severe side effects. It is currently being studied in a large multicenter clinical trial. The therapeutic roles of dipyridamole and sulfinpyrazone have not been established. Suloctidil is no longer used because of toxic effects and will not been discussed. We will now review current information about commercially available and promising antiplatelet agents for stroke prevention.

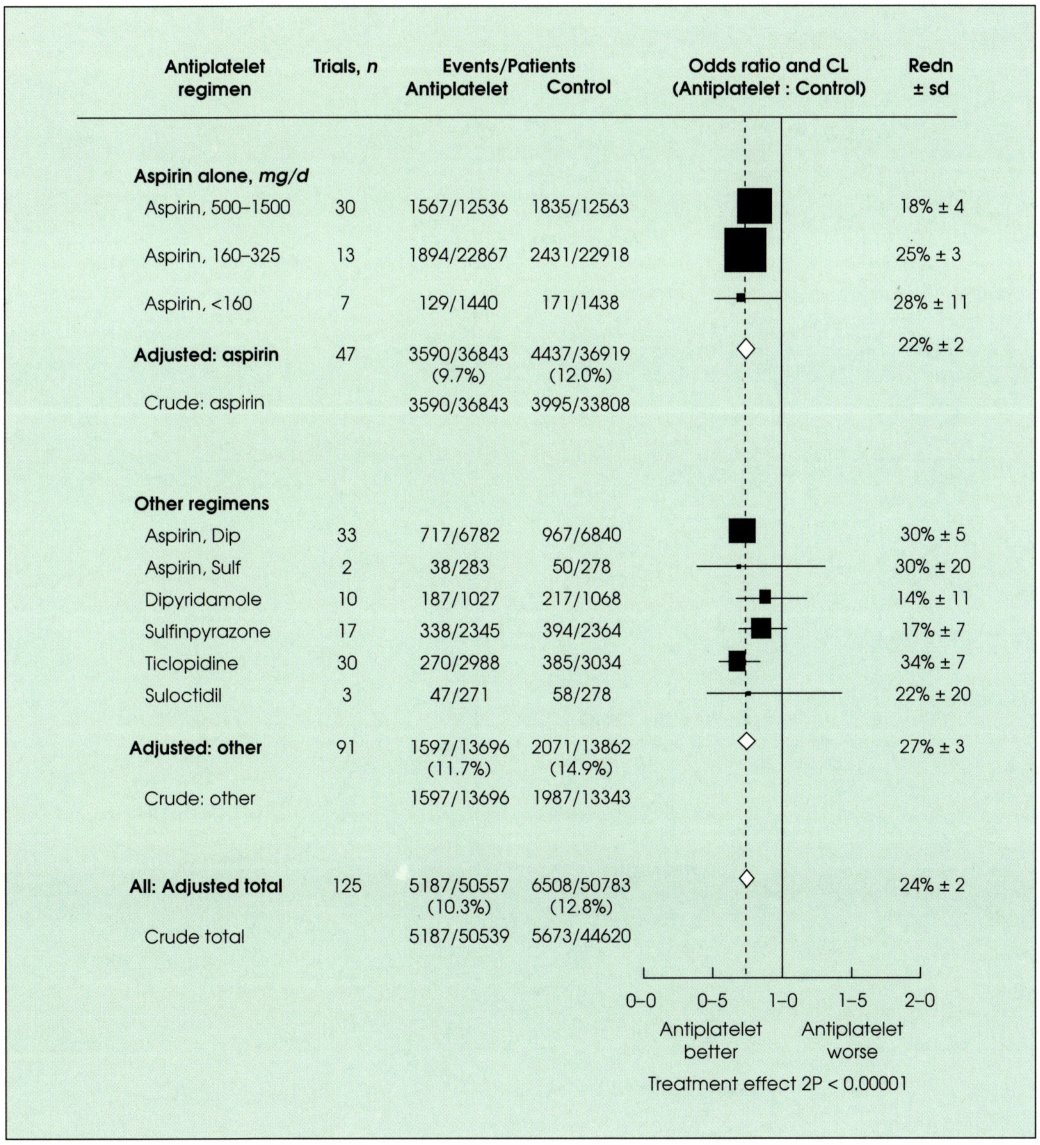

Antiplatelet regimen	Trials, *n*	Events/Patients Antiplatelet	Events/Patients Control	Redn ± sd
Aspirin alone, *mg/d*				
Aspirin, 500–1500	30	1567/12536	1835/12563	18% ± 4
Aspirin, 160–325	13	1894/22867	2431/22918	25% ± 3
Aspirin, <160	7	129/1440	171/1438	28% ± 11
Adjusted: aspirin	47	3590/36843 (9.7%)	4437/36919 (12.0%)	22% ± 2
Crude: aspirin		3590/36843	3995/33808	
Other regimens				
Aspirin, Dip	33	717/6782	967/6840	30% ± 5
Aspirin, Sulf	2	38/283	50/278	30% ± 20
Dipyridamole	10	187/1027	217/1068	14% ± 11
Sulfinpyrazone	17	338/2345	394/2364	17% ± 7
Ticlopidine	30	270/2988	385/3034	34% ± 7
Suloctidil	3	47/271	58/278	22% ± 20
Adjusted: other	91	1597/13696 (11.7%)	2071/13862 (14.9%)	27% ± 3
Crude: other		1597/13696	1987/13343	
All: Adjusted total	125	5187/50557 (10.3%)	6508/50783 (12.8%)	24% ± 2
Crude total		5187/50539	5673/44620	

FIGURE 15.4

Indirect randomized comparisons of the effects of different prolonged antiplatelet treatments on vascular death, nonfatal myocardial infarction, or nonfatal stroke; the *black squares* reflect areas proportional to the amount of information attributed. Dip—dipyridamole; Redn—odds reduction; Sulf—sulfinpyrazone. (*From* Antiplatelet Trialists Collaboration [3]; with permission.)

ASPIRIN

Clinical Pharmacology

Aspirin is the acetylated form of salicylic acid (Figure 15.6). Following oral ingestion, aspirin is rapidly absorbed. Maximal blood levels are achieved within 15 to 20 minutes [18,20]. Effects on platelet aggregation occur within 1 hour of dosing as there is competition with arachidonic acid for the active cyclooxygenase site on prostaglandin endoperoxide synthase (Figures 15.7 and 15.8) [18,21–23]. Aspirin acetylates the serine 52 g fraction of the protein prostaglandin G/H synthase and irreversibly inactivates platelet cyclooxygenase [21,22]. Suppression of platelet cyclooxygenase leads to reduction of the prostaglandin endoperoxide and thromboxane A_2, a powerful vasoconstrictor and potent stimulus for platelet aggregation (Figure 15.8). Apart from its actions on thromboxane A_2, aspirin counteracts the effects of a number of stimuli for platelet aggregation, including epinephrine, thrombin, collagen, and ADP (Figure 15.9) [24]. Aspirin does not shorten platelet survival or reduce the total platelet count [25]. Its effects persist for the life span of the platelet because the acetylation of cyclooxygenase is permanent.

APT1 vs APT2	Trials, *n*	Events/Patients APT1	Events/Patients APT2	Odds ratio and CL (APT1 : APT 2)	Redn ± sd
Asp (>325) vs Asp (325)	4	198/1278	206/1279		6% ± 11
Asp (325) vs Asp (40)	1	5/28	2/28		
Dip + Asp vs Asp	14	327/2822	330/2811		2% ± 9
Sulf vs Asp	5	102/674	89/673		22% ± 19
Ticl vs Asp	3	379/1730	414/1741		10% ± 8
Asp + Dip vs Sulf	2	20/187	14/173		35% ± 42
Asp + Sulf vs Sulf	2	38/283	71/296		71/296

0–0 0–5 1–0 1–5 2–0

APT1 better | APT2 better

FIGURE 15.5

Direct randomized comparisons of the effects of different prolonged antiplatelet treatments on vascular death, nonfatal myocardial infarction, or nonfatal stroke; the *black squares* reflect areas proportional to the amount of information attributed. APT—antiplatelet; ASP—aspirin; Dip—dipyridamole; Redn—odds reduction; Sulf—sulfinpyrazone; Ticl—ticlopidine. (*From* Antiplatelet Trialists' Collaboration [3]; with permission.)

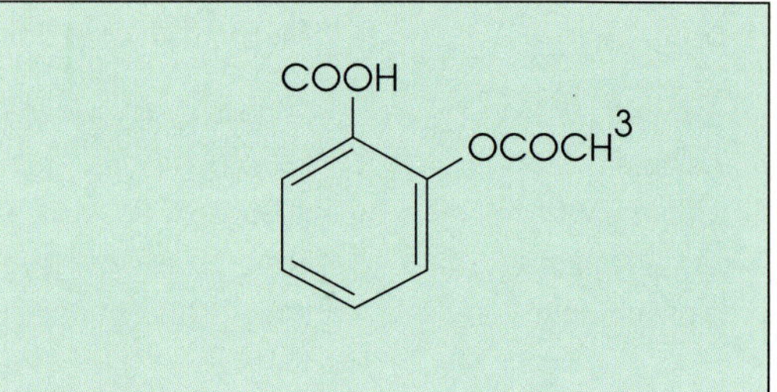

FIGURE 15.6

Chemical composition of acetylsalicylic acid.

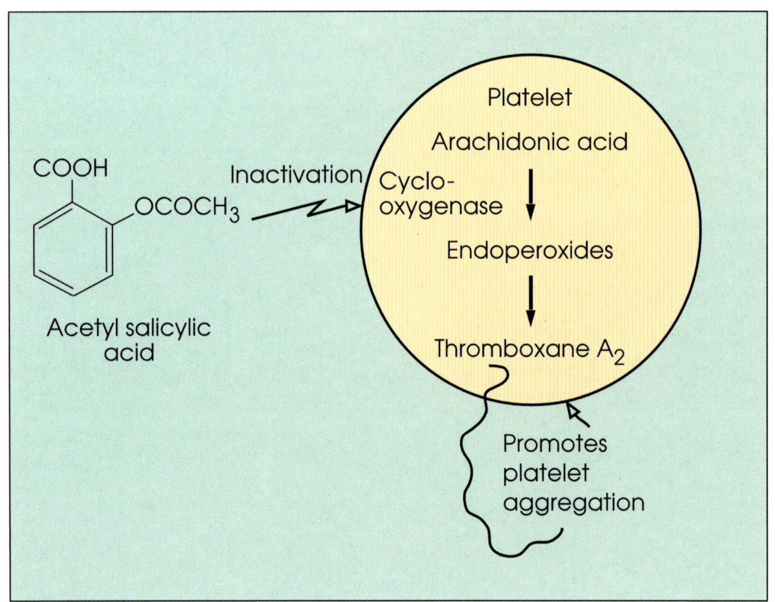

FIGURE 15.7

Inactivation of platelet cyclooxygenase by aspirin. The salicylate moiety positions the aspirin molecule in such a way that the acetyl group can irreversibly bind to the active site of the enzyme. (*From* van Gijn [90]; with permission.)

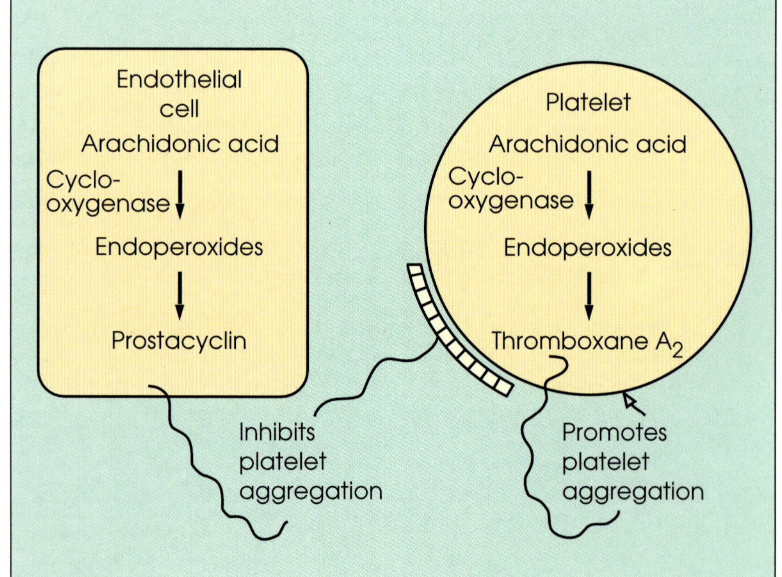

FIGURE 15.8

The antagonism between thromboxane A_2 in platelets and prostacyclin in endothelial cells. Both are synthesized from arachidonic acid, with cyclooxygenase controlling the first step. (*From* van Gijn [90]; with permission.)

Daily supplementation of aspirin is needed to acetylate newly formed platelets each day. Although aspirin's actions on platelet function are primarily mediated through its effects on cyclooxygenase, it may have other actions on coagulation such as lowering of concentrations of vitamin K–dependent clotting factors II, VII, IX, and X [26,27]. Maximal effects of aspirin are noted when platelet thromboxane A_2 production is reduced by 95% to 99% [28]. Several studies have explored the dose-response effect of aspirin on platelet function [29–31].

Aspirin in doses as low as 20 to 40 mg/day reduce thromboxane formation, lessen platelet aggregation, suppress platelet responsiveness to external stimuli, and prolong the bleeding time [21,27,32–39]. However, doses less than 20 mg/day are not effective [37]. The antiaggregating effects of low-dose aspirin may not appear until after several doses are given [26,35,39]. Following an initial dose of 100 to 300 mg, which achieves maximal blockade of cyclooxygenase, a 40 to 75 mg daily dose maintains the pharmacologic effects [34–36]. A recent report notes that individual doses of aspirin inhibit platelet aggregation variably among patients [40]. In summary, studies suggest that the antiplatelet-aggregating effects of aspirin are similar in daily doses ranging from 30 mg to 1.3 g.

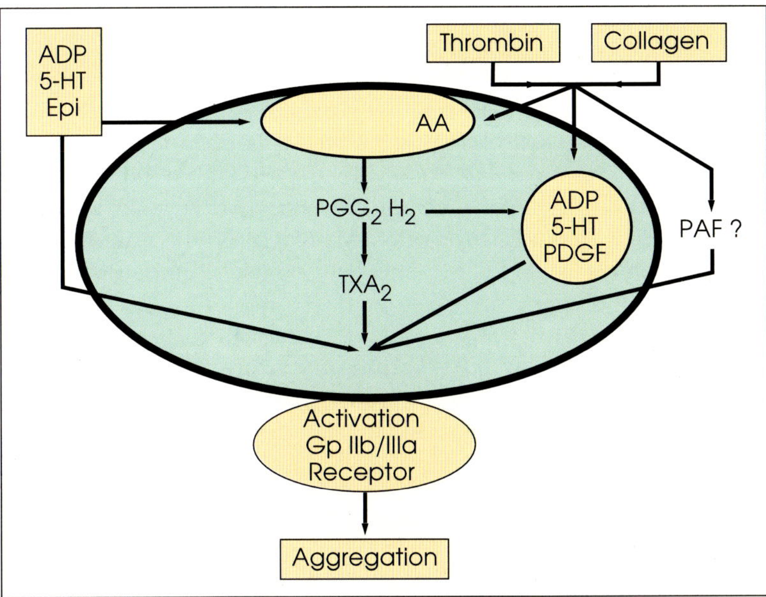

FIGURE 15.9

Different pathways that can stimulate platelet aggregation by activating glycoprotein IIb/IIIa receptor on the surface of platelets. AA—arachidonic acid; Epi—epinefrin; GP—glycoprotein; 5-HT—5-hydroxytryptamin; PAF—platelet-activating factor; PDGF—platelet-derived growth factor; PGG_2/H_2—prostaglandin-endoperoxide G_2/H_2; TXA_2—thromboxane A_2. (*From* Keyser [91]; with permission.)

Side Effects

Adverse reactions to chronic aspirin therapy are summarized in Table 15.3. Aspirin increases the risk of gastrointestinal side effects by two- to fivefold in both men and women [41]. These side effects are associated with aspirin's action on prostaglandins in the gastric mucosa [42] and are more likely in patients older than 60 years of age, after prolonged use, or among patients who have had prior epigastric complaints.

There is a clear relationship between dose and frequency of major gastrointestinal side effects in stroke prevention studies as shown in (Table 15.4). The likelihood of major adverse effects is much less among patients taking low doses [15,18,43–46]. Some clinicians advocate starting aspirin in a daily dose of 1.3 g to prevent stroke and lower the dose subsequently if gastric or other significant side effects occur [13].

Table 15.3. Adverse effects of aspirin

- Major side effects
  - Bleeding
    - Gastrointestinal
    - Cerebral
    - Abdominal aorta
- Minor side effects
  - Bleeding
    - Urogenital
    - Epistaxis
    - Skin
  - Gastric discomfort
  - Allergic reaction
    - Skin
    - Asthma

Table 15.4. Overview of adverse effects reported in recent trials testing aspirin alone after transient ischemic attack or minor stroke*†

	Dose of aspirin, *mg/d*		
	< 100	300	>1000
Adverse effect			
Gastrointestinal hemorrhage	13	27	40
Other major hemorrhage	76	75	20
Gastric discomfort	249	502	414
Minor hemorrhage	49	105	22
Other adverse effects	104	161	76
Total adverse effects	491	870	572
Total years of follow-up	5856	7322	3557
Calculated risk of any adverse effect per year	8.4	11.9	16
Calculated risk of major hemorrhage per year	0.015	0.014	0.028

**Data from* The Canadian Cooperative Study Group [7], The Dutch TIA Trial Study Group [44], The SALT Collaborative Group [45], and UK TIA Study Group [46].

†These figures represent absolute numbers, aggregated from the aforementioned studies.

Administration of a soluble form of aspirin with water may shorten contact with the gastric mucosa resulting in fewer side effects [47]. Enteric-coated aspirin causes less damage to the gastric mucosa than plain formulas [48–51]. Ancillary therapies, such as antacids, H-2 receptor antagonists, sucralfate, or misoprostol, can also reduce the risk of associated bleeding.

Because aspirin affects coagulation, bleeding is a potential complication. Common and minor hemorrhages include epistaxis, bruising, and hematuria. In the Dutch TIA trial, significantly fewer cases of minor bleeding occurred in the 30-mg group than in the 283-mg group (relative risk: 0.58; 95% CI 0.41–0.83) [44]. Aspirin may increase the risk of intracranial hemorrhage. The British study of aspirin in stroke prevention reported an increased risk of intracranial hemorrhage but diagnoses were not confirmed by computed tomography (CT) [43,46]. Another recent trial of aspirin (1300 mg/d) in patients with recent TIA or minor stroke reported seven intracranial hemorrhages among 1538 patients followed for an average of 3 years [6]. The Dutch TIA trial is the first stroke prevention study that required CT confirmation of cerebral outcome events; only 28 cerebral hemorrhages were diagnosed among 3131 patients during a mean follow-up period of 2.6 years and there was no dose-related effect [44]. The frequency of major intracranial hemorrhages that can be directly attributed to aspirin is low and is less than that of oral anticoagulants [49]. The efficacy of aspirin in preventing ischemic stroke far exceeds the risk of intracranial bleeding [15].

Efficacy

Aspirin is effective in the prevention of myocardial infarction (MI), ischemic stroke, or vascular death among patients at high risk of vascular disease (Figure 15.10). It is now recommended for patients with recent MI, unstable angina, stable angina, intermittent claudication, and ischemic cerebrovascular disease [3,18]. Aspirin has been studied for primary prevention of cardiovascular disease (Figure 15.11) [50,51], and may be useful in patients older than 40 years of age who are at increased risk of MI [2].

Aspirin is useful for secondary prevention after acute MI (Figure 15.12) (Table 15.5), although warfarin may be superior (ASPECT Collaborating Study Group, Personal communication.) The ISIS-2 Collaborative Group [52] found that 160 mg of

Trials analyzed	Trials, *n*	Events/Patients Antiplatelet	Events/Patients Control	Redn ± sd
Cerebral disease				
Prior stroke/TIA	17	1082/5803	1315/5833	
Acute stroke	1	2/15	3/14	
Vascular	3	16/373	29/374	
SAH postsurgery	3	121/429	136/436	
Cardiac disease				
Prior MI	11	1321/9877	1685/9914	
Acute MI	5	1225/9060	1588/9066	
Unstable angina	7	184/1991	285/2027	
Post CABG	16	120/2417	119/2422	
Post PTCA	3	30/609	60/616	
Stable angina/CAD	3	27/229	42/228	
Atrial fibrillation	2	82/888	113/904	
Rheumatic valve disease	1	9/78	17/76	
Valve surgery	6	46/602	79/642	
Peripheral vascular disease				
Intermittent claudication	12	151/1306	186/1327	
Noncoronary grafts	9	65/771	69/768	
Peripheral angioplasty	1	5/132	8/134	
Other high risk				
Renal dialysis	10	2/256	6/269	
Other	12	39/1116	38/1107	
Adjusted total	122	4527/35952 (12.8%)	5778/36157 (16.0%)	26% ± 2
Crude total		4527/35934	5090/31724	

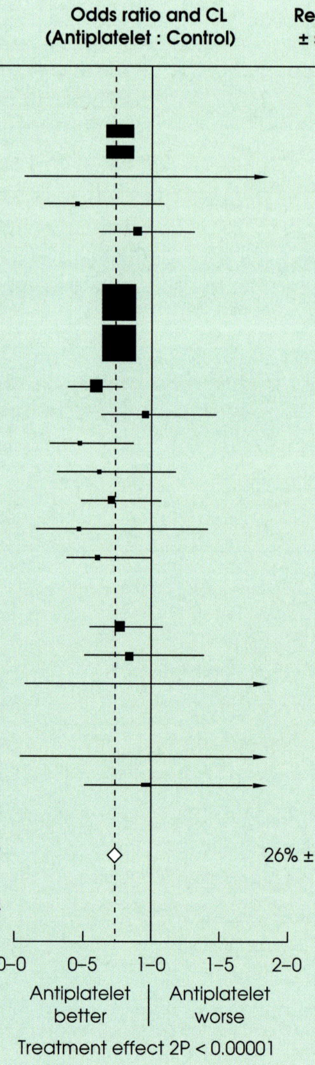

Odds ratio and CL (Antiplatelet : Control): 0–0, 0–5, 1–0, 1–5, 2–0

Antiplatelet better | Antiplatelet worse

Treatment effect 2P < 0.00001

FIGURE 15.10

Apparent effect on vascular death, nonfatal myocardial infarction (MI), or nonfatal stroke in trials of prolonged antiplatelet therapy versus control among patients at high risk of vascular disease, subdivided by type of patient; the areas of the *black squares* are proportional to the amount of information attributed. CABG—coronary artery bypass grafting; CAD—coronary artery disease; PTCA—percutaneous transluminal coronary angioplasty; Redn—odds reduction; SAH—subarachnoid hemorrhage; TIA—transient ischemic attack. (*From* Antiplatelet Trialists Collaboration [3]; with permission.)

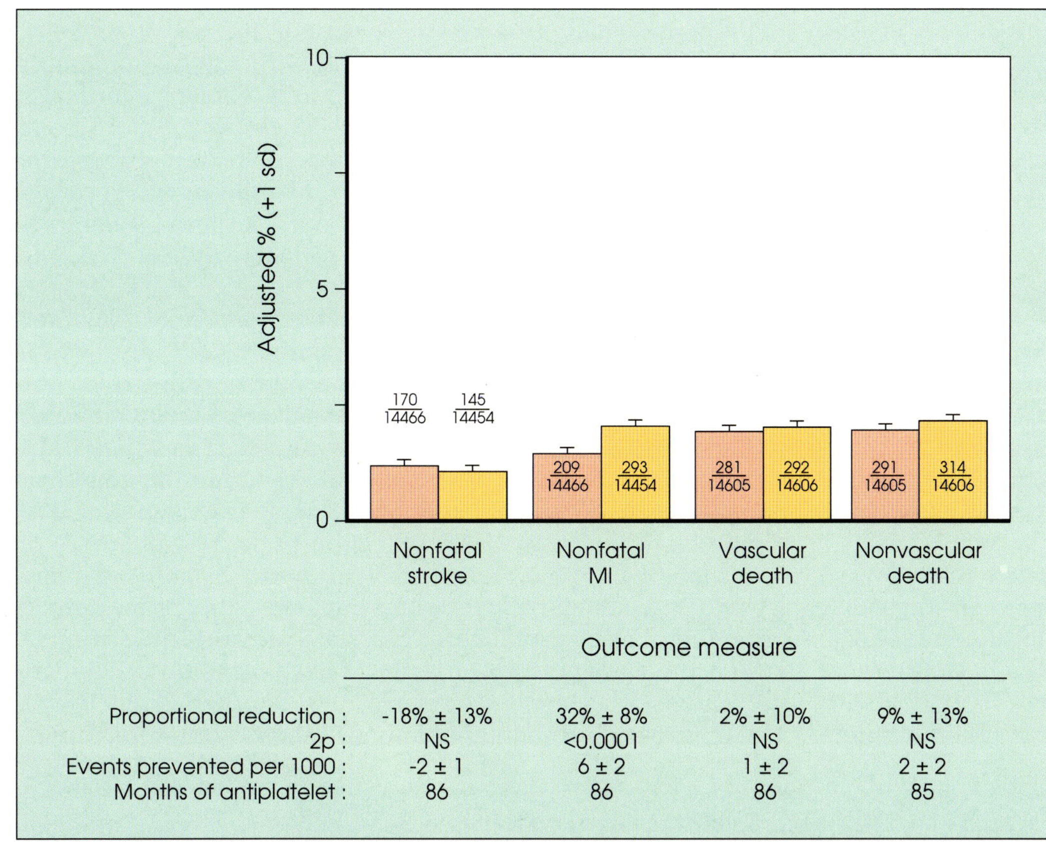

FIGURE 15.11

Absolute rates of nonfatal myocardial infarction (MI), nonfatal stroke, vascular, and nonvascular death, represented by underlined numbers on bars, in randomized trials of prolonged antiplatelet therapy versus control in primary prevention. *Orange bars* indicate treatment; *yellow bars* indicate controls. (*From* Antiplatelet Trialists Collaboration [3]; with permission.)

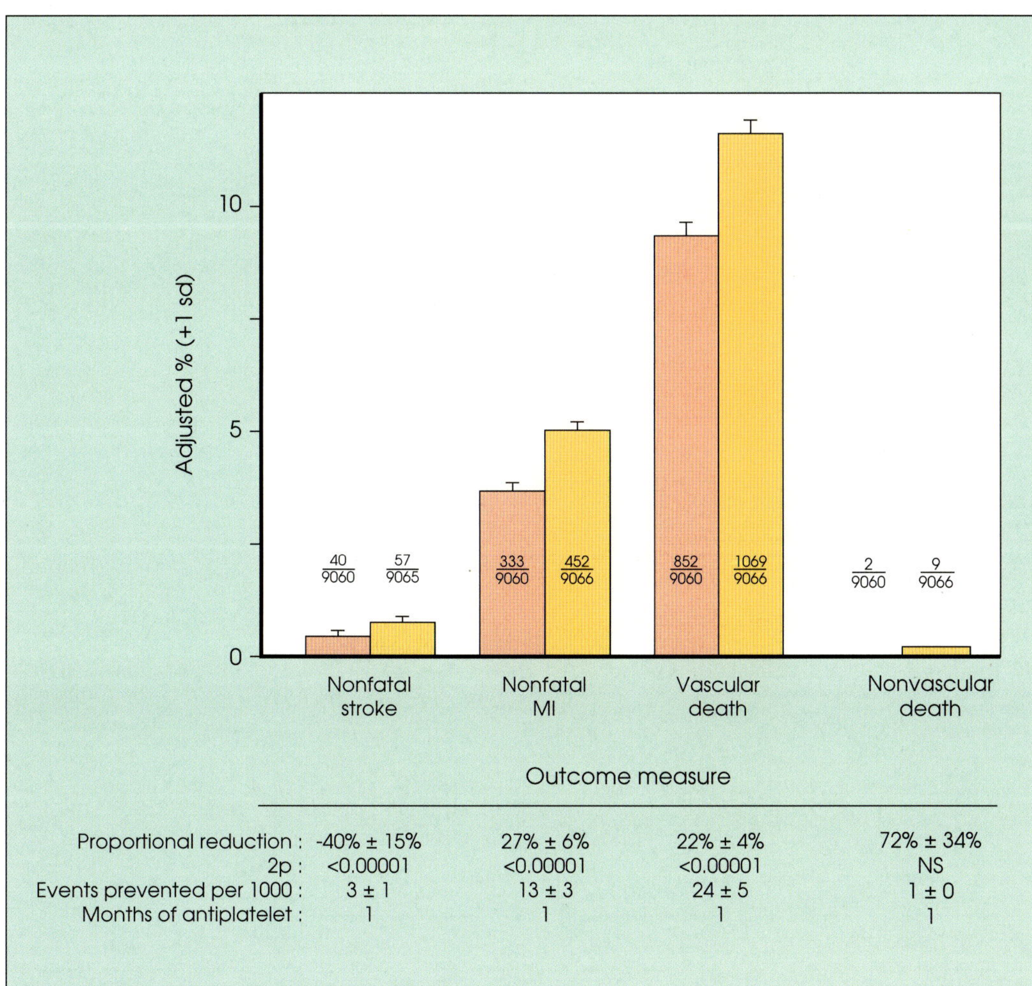

FIGURE 15.12

Absolute rates of nonfatal myocardial infarction (MI), nonfatal stroke, vascular and nonvascular death, represented by underlined numbers on bars, in randomized trials of prolonged antiplatelet therapy versus control in patients with acute MI. *Orange bars* indicate active treatment; *yellow bars* indicate controls. (*From* Antiplatelet Trialists Collaboration [3]; with permission.)

enteric-coated aspirin reduced nonfatal stroke from 0.6% to 0.3% per year in patients with recent MI. The RISC study [53] showed that aspirin (75 mg/d) reduced the risk of MI among men with unstable coronary artery disease by 57% to 69% [53]. Another trial found that aspirin (650 mg/d) was effective during the acute phase of unstable angina [54]. Ridker and coworkers [55] observed that 325 mg of aspirin every other day diminished the likelihood of MI among patients with chronic stable angina. A recent panel advised low-dose aspirin (160 mg/d) as a preventative for ischemic vascular events [18].

Aspirin's efficacy in preventing major vascular events among persons with a TIA or minor stroke has been tested in a large number of clinical trials as shown in Table 15.6. Some have tested aspirin alone while others have examined aspirin in combination with another therapy, most commonly dipyridamole. Several doses have been studied, yet only two trials have directly compared two different doses of aspirin [44,46].

In the Canadian Cooperative study, aspirin or sulfinpyrazone, alone or in combination, was compared to a placebo in patients with recent TIA or minor stroke [7]. Outcomes among the 290 patients assigned to the two groups treated with aspirin were compared with the number of events among the 295 patients assigned to one of the two groups that did not receive aspirin. In the former, there was a 31% decrease in the risk of stroke or death. Although the trial was not designed to study differences in treatment responses between men and women, men had a 50% reduction in events, whereas no benefit was noted among women. The patients who received the combination of aspirin and sulfinpyrazone did slightly better than those who received aspirin alone, but this difference was not statistically significant. Event rates were similar among the patients who received the placebo or sulfinpyrazone alone.

In a three-armed study, Bousser and coworkers [8] compared treatment with aspirin (1 g/d), dipyridamole (225 mg/d), or a placebo in 604 patients. A significant reduction in stroke was seen, but there was no benefit from treatment with dipyridamole. This trial demonstrated that aspirin was efficacious in women [8].

The European Stroke Prevention Study tested the combination of aspirin (975 mg/d) and dipyridamole (225 mg/d) against a placebo. There was a 33% reduction in the risk of stroke or death [56]. Favorable responses were noted in both men and women and among patients with symptoms either in the carotid or vertebrobasilar circulation. This trial provides the strongest evidence for the efficacy of large doses of aspirin in secondary prevention of ischemic vascular events among persons with a TIA or stroke, but the simultaneous administration of dipyri-

Table 15.5. Overview of trials in which the effects of antiplatelet treatment were studied in patients with a prior myocardial infarction*

		Events/patients		
Endpoint	**Trials, *n***	**Antiplatelet**	**Control**	**Proportional reduction, % ± *sd***
Nonvascular death	11	147/9877	135/9914	-13 ± 14
Vascular death	11	734/9877	867/9914	15 ± 5
Nonfatal stroke	11	92/8375	135/8372	35 ± 11
Vascular death, nonfatal myocardial infarction, nonfatal stroke	11	1321/9877	1685/9914	25 ± 4

**Adapted from* Fuster and coworkers [2] and Antiplatelet Trialists' Collaboration [3]; with permission.

Table 15.6. Overview of trials in which the effects of antiplatelet treatment after transient ischemic attack or stroke were studied*

		Events/patients		
Endpoint	**Trials, *n***	**Antiplatelet**	**Control**	**Proportional reduction, % ± *sd***
Nonvascular death	17	178/5803	2140/5833	18 ± 10
Vascular death	17	495/5803	551/5833	12 ± 7
Nonfatal stroke	17	474/5803	595/5833	23 ± 6
Vascular death, nonfatal myocardial infarction, nonfatal stroke	17	1082/5803	1315/5833	23 ± 4

**Adapted from* Antiplatelet Trialists' Collaboration [3].

damole weakens any conclusions about the efficacy of high-dose aspirin alone.

Two doses of aspirin (300 mg/d and 1200 mg/d) were tested against a placebo in a British trial [43,46]. Evidence in favor of either high- or low-dose aspirin when compared to the placebo was not found. However, when outcomes of controls were compared to combined results of the two-dose aspirin–treated groups, a modest reduction in stroke or death was noted. Ischemic events occurred at approximately the same rate in both aspirin-treated groups. Largely because of the lower rate of gastrointestinal side effects among patients treated with the lower aspirin dose, the investigators concluded that 300 mg/day of aspirin was superior to 1200 mg/day.

Dutch physicians compared two doses of aspirin (30 mg/d or 283 mg/d) in a study that did not include a placebo treatment group [44]. There was no significant difference between the two groups concerning the risk reduction of death, nonfatal stroke, or nonfatal MI. Low-dose aspirin after TIA or minor stroke was recommended for prevention. An initial dose of at least 120 mg of aspirin which would rapidly inhibit platelet aggregation was recommended, and then daily doses of 30 to 81 mg could be administered to maintain these effects. A major criticism of this trial is that a higher dose of aspirin was not studied in the reference group [57]. Skepticism for low-dose aspirin is supported by data demonstrating lack of substantial benefit when aspirin is administered in doses of 300 mg/day [13,14]. However, Swedish researchers recently tested the effects of 75 mg of aspirin a day and showed a statistically significant (18%) reduction in stroke or death in the aspirin as compared to the placebo group [45].

As yet, no study has compared very low dose (100 mg or less) with high dose (975 to 1300 mg/d) aspirin. Those who advocate high-dose aspirin therapy maintain that risk reduction with high doses of aspirin is greater than with lower doses [13,14]. Furthermore, they argue that lessened risk of side effects should not be a reason to favor low-dose aspirin as serious side effects are rare. Thus, high-dose aspirin would be adjusted downward only if side effects occurred. Experts who prefer low-dose aspirin argue that doses as low as 75 mg are efficacious [45]. The British and Dutch trials found that the effects of 300 and 1200 mg and of 283 mg and 30 mg were approximately equal. These data and the reduced rate of side effects would favor the use of low-dose aspirin [10–12]. This disagreement will persist until the results of a trial in which both high- and low-dose aspirin are directly compared.

Aspirin has also been studied in prevention of recurrent ischemic events among patients who underwent carotid endarterectomy, and the results are mixed [58,59]. CEA has been established as an effective intervention for reducing the likelihood of stroke among persons who have a high-grade, symptomatic, carotid stenosis [60,61]. A recent subanalysis from the North American Symptomatic Carotid Endarterectomy Trial group [13] suggested that high-dose aspirin was superior to low-dose aspirin in the prevention of ipsilateral stroke after CEA. This observation is important but must be verified in a prospective trial comparing high or low doses of aspirin in stroke prevention after CEA.

Aspirin has been studied in two trials to test its efficacy in the primary prevention of embolic events in persons with atrial fibrillation. In a Danish study, 75 mg of aspirin daily was ineffective [62]. Conversely, Stroke Prevention in Atrial Fibrillation (SPAF) investigators found that 325 mg of aspirin was useful in the prevention of thromboembolic events, although warfarin may be more effective [63,64]. In a recent analysis of the SPAF data, Miller and coworkers [65] concluded that much of the efficacy of aspirin among patients with atrial fibrillation could be attributed to prevention of noncardioembolic strokes. The differences between the two studies may, in part, be attributed to the disparity of doses, but it may also reflect older and higher risk patients enrolled in the Danish study. The European Atrial Fibrillation Trial tested 300 mg of aspirin, warfarin, and a placebo to prevent recurrent embolism in patients with atrial fibrillation who had recent TIA or minor stroke [66]. Patients who were given aspirin had a lower risk of a vascular outcome event than patients receiving the placebo, although this difference was not statistically significant (hazard ratio: 0.83; 95% CI: 0.65–1.05). Direct comparison of aspirin and warfarin showed that warfarin reduced the risk of recurrent vascular events significantly more than aspirin (hazard ratio: 0.60; 95% CI: 0.41–0.87).

Currently, warfarin is being compared with 325 mg of aspirin in a North American study of patients with recent stroke, and with 30 mg of aspirin in a Dutch trial of patients with TIA or minor stroke. In the SPAF III study very low dose warfarin is being compared to 325 mg of aspirin in patients with atrial fibrillation.

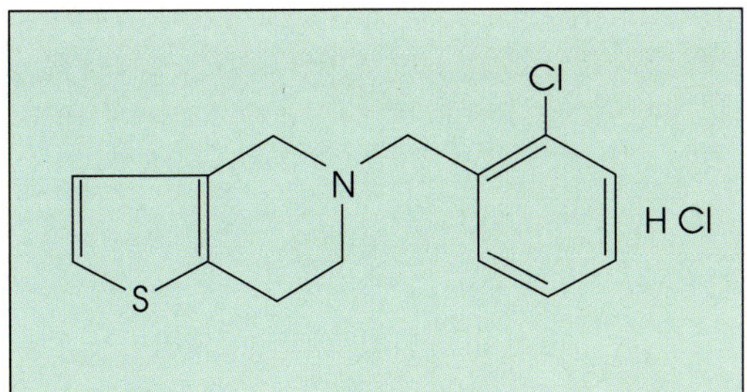

FIGURE 15.13
Chemical composition of ticlopidine hydrochloride.

TICLOPIDINE

Clinical Pharmacology

Ticlopidine hydrochloride (Figure 15.13) is the first drug developed chiefly for its antiplatelet-aggregating effects. It interferes with platelet membrane function and is a potent blocker of fibrinogen binding to platelets [67]. It causes an irreversible modification of platelets, specifically affecting ADP-dependent activation of glycoproteins 2b and 3a. Ticlopidine lessens aggregation responses induced by collagen, epinephrine, arachidonic acid, thrombin, or platelet activating factor [67,68]. It reduces the adhesion of platelets to atherosclerotic plaques [69]. Ticlopidine prolongs the bleeding time and decreases plasma levels of platelet factor 4, β-thromboglobulin, and fibrinogen [67,68,70]. The drug is rapidly absorbed after oral administration [67]. The usual dose is 250 mg twice daily given with meals. Changes in platelet function are seen within 24 to 48 hours after the first dose and will persist up to 10 days [67,71]. The effects of ticlopidine may persist longer among elderly patients.

Side Effects

The most frequent adverse experiences are abdominal pain, nausea, indigestion, or diarrhea as given in Table 15.7. These complaints appear soon after starting treatment and can be reduced if ticlopidine is taken after a meal. Lowering the dose may also allow some patients to continue the medication. Allergic reactions, including skin eruptions or urticaria, occur in approximately 10% to 15% of patients and are most likely to happen within 2 weeks of starting therapy [5,6].

Despite its prominent effect on coagulation, the use of ticlopidine has not been accompanied by a high rate of hemorrhage, including intracranial bleeding. In the Ticlopidine-Aspirin Stroke Study (TASS) the number of intracranial hemorrhages (seven) among ticlopidine-treated patients was identical to that of patients assigned to aspirin treatment (five). Thrombocytopenia is a rare complication, and the syndrome of thrombotic thrombocytopenic purpura can occur [72]. Monitoring of platelet counts during the first 3 months of treatment is recommended. A serious side effect is neutropenia. In TASS and the Canadian-American Ticlopidine Study (CATS), granulocyte counts under 1200/mm^3 were noted in 2.4% of treated patients; in 0.8%, the count was below 450/mm^3 [5,6]. The cause of neutropenia is not well established, but it appears to be an idiosyncratic reaction. The neutropenia, which can progress to agranulocytosis, is seen within the first few weeks of treatment and has a peak frequency between 30 to 60 days. Thereafter, the likelihood of this complication diminishes and the risk is low after 3 months of continuous treatment. Because the decline in neutrophils may be asymptomatic, monitoring of the leukocyte count every 2 weeks is a mandatory part of management during the first 3 months of treatment. The neutrophil count generally returns to normal within a few days after stopping ticlopidine.

Efficacy

The Canadian-American Ticlopidine Study was a placebo-controlled trial among patients with moderate-to-severe stroke [5]. An intention-to-treat analysis documented a 23% risk reduction for all events and a 20% decrement in recurrent stroke. Using an on-treatment efficacy analysis, the investigators found that ticlopidine reduced the risk of major ischemic events by 30%, a response seen in men and women. TASS directly compared ticlopidine with aspirin (1300 mg/d) among patients with recent TIA, retinal ischemia, or minor stroke [6]. With an intention-to-treat analysis, the 3-year event rates for death or nonfatal stroke were 17% for ticlopidine and 19% for aspirin (a 12% improvement with ticlopidine). There was a 21% risk reduction in fatal or nonfatal stroke with ticlopidine. Ticlopidine was better than aspirin in both men and women, although the degree of reduction was larger among women. The rates of cardiovascular events among patients taking either aspirin or ticlopidine were similar [73].

Table 15.7. Side effects among 2043 patients taking ticlopidine 500 mg/d*

Side effect	Patients, *n*
Bleeding disorders	153
Neutropenia	24
Rash	223
Diarrhea	353
Other gastrointestinal disorders	503
Urticaria	30
Total of any adverse experience	1228

*Absolute numbers aggregated from Gent and coworkers [5] and Hass and coworkers [6].

Several post-hoc subgroup analyses of the TASS data have been reported [74–76]. Grotta and coworkers [74] concluded that women, patients with vertebrobasilar TIA, those who develop recurrent symptoms despite aspirin therapy, and persons with diffuse atherosclerotic disease benefit most from ticlopidine. Conversely, patients with high-grade extracranial carotid artery stenosis may respond better to aspirin. Harbison and coworkers [75] reported that the superiority of ticlopidine was slightly greater among patients with minor strokes than among those with TIAs. A recent paper suggests that ticlopidine may be particularly effective among nonwhite patients [76].

Ticlopidine has also been studied in 30 different trials in patients with peripheral vascular disease, ischemic heart disease, TIA, or stroke [3]. The Antiplatelet Trialists' Collaboration [3] reported an overall risk reduction of major vascular events of 34% in trials testing ticlopidine versus a placebo for all types of vascular disease (Figure 15.4).

A number of experts have debated the role of ticlopidine in stroke prevention. Warlow [77] has been skeptical about the use of ticlopidine because it is only marginally more efficacious than aspirin, has more side effects, and is more expensive. Conversely, Haynes and coworkers [78] concluded that ticlopidine is an effective and important alternative to aspirin. A recently published consensus statement advises ticlopidine as an alternative to aspirin [18]. Based on an independent review, Albers [79] concludes that the risk-benefit ratio for ticlopidine is favorable and that it is a particularly valuable agent for preventing stroke among patients who cannot take aspirin.

Because aspirin and ticlopidine act independently, there is interest in the combined use of these drugs [80], yet clinical experience is limited. Uchiyama and coworkers [81] prescribed the use of 81 mg of aspirin and 100 mg of ticlopidine in 23 patients and noted marked inhibition of platelet aggregation and very prolonged bleeding times. The responses far exceeded those to either drug alone. Hemorrhagic events were more common among patients who received both drugs. Further study of the combination of aspirin and ticlopidine is needed. The simultaneous use of the two drugs should be discouraged until additional information about their safety and efficacy is known.

CLOPIDOGREL

Clopidogrel is a new thienopyridine compound that is related to ticlopidine and has similar effects on platelets [82]. It has less toxicity than ticlopidine in animal studies. Its presumed mode of action is comparable to that of ticlopidine. It also causes an irreversible modification of platelets, affecting specifically ADP-dependent activation of glycoproteins 2b and 3a [83]. The optimal dose of clopidogrel is 50 to 75 mg/day. Results of randomized clinical trials are not yet available. The drug is now being compared with aspirin in a large international study in patients with peripheral vascular disease and MI or stroke.

SULFINPYRAZONE

Sulfinpyrazone is a uricosuric agent used in the treatment of gouty arthritis. Because it can reversibly suppress cyclooxygenase, it has platelet antiaggregating activity [84]. In the Canadian Cooperative trial, investigators concluded that this drug alone was less effective than aspirin, although the combination of drugs was slightly better than treatment with aspirin alone [7]. Large trials in which sulfinpyrazone is compared with a placebo in patients with cerebral ischemia are lacking.

Sulfinpyrazone was not efficacious in reducing the incidence of MI or cardiac death in patients with unstable angina pectoris [85]. However, after MI, the drug was shown to be useful in the prevention thromboembolic events [86].

Although sulfinpyrazone is an alternative or adjunctive treatment to prevent stroke, there is limited clinical trial data [77]. Sulfinpyrazone should be considered to be of limited efficacy in persons at high risk for stroke, and more data is needed to better clarify its role [77].

DIPYRIDAMOLE

Dipyridamole is a vasodilator and an inhibitor of phosphodiesterase. It has antiplatelet-aggregating effects in high concentration, but its antithrombotic actions in humans are not well established [87]. It is relatively safe and complications are rare and usually not serious.

One small trial did not demonstrate any benefit of dipyridamole after acute MI [88]. Two larger trials compared the combination of aspirin and dipyridamole with aspirin alone and found no significant differences in outcome events [8,89]. Conversely, the European Stroke Prevention Study found that the combination of aspirin and dipyridamole was very effective in reducing the risk of stroke [56]. However, the individual contribution of dipyridamole or aspirin alone is not known. Currently, a second larger European trial is being performed to compare aspirin and dipyridamole. At present, there are no conclusive data that dipyridamole is efficacious in stroke prevention [87]. Presently, there is little evidence to support its use for this purpose.

CONCLUSIONS

At present, aspirin and ticlopidine have been shown to be efficacious in prevention of ischemic vascular disease. Both drugs have acceptable margins of safety, and both are effective in men and women. The threat of intracranial hemorrhage appears low and the value of these drugs in the prevention of brain ischemia outweighs any risk of bleeding complications. Epigastric pain, peptic ulcer disease, and gastrointestinal bleeding are known complications of aspirin. A relationship between the dose of aspirin and these adverse effects is well documented. The most common side effects of ticlopidine are skin eruptions and diarrhea. Neutropenia and thrombocytopenia are rare but reversible complications that necessitate monitoring during the first few months of treatment.

The optimal dose of aspirin is debated. Current data indicate that low doses (<100 mg/d) are effective in the prevention of ischemic events. There are no data that low doses are superior to high doses (975 to 1300 mg/d) in prevention of stroke, but low doses are safer. A study directly comparing high- and low-dose aspirin is needed.

Currently, aspirin is the drug of choice to prevent stroke after major vascular disease. Ticlopidine may be prescribed to patients who cannot tolerate aspirin or who have not had a favorable response to the drug. The combination of aspirin and ticlopidine is not recommended. Dipyridamole or sulfinpyrazone are not first choice treatments for stroke prevention.

ACKNOWLEDGMENTS

The authors thank Professor Jan van Gijn MD, FRCPE, for his useful and stimulating comments.

REFERENCES

1. Craven LL: Experiences with aspirin (acetylsalicylic acid) in the nonspecific prophylaxis of coronary thromboses. *Miss Valley Med J* 1953, 75:38–43.
2. Fuster V, Dyken M, Vokonas PS, *et al.*: Aspirin as a therapeutic agent in cardiovascular disease. *Circulation* 1993, 87:659–675.
3. Antiplatelet Trialists' Collaboration: Collaborative overview of randomized trials of antiplatelet therapy. Part I: Prevention of death, myocardial infarction, and stroke by prolonged antiplatelet therapy in various categories of patients. *BMJ* 1994, 308:81–106.
4. Sze PC, Reitman D, Pincus MM, *et al.*: Antiplatelet agents in the secondary prevention of stroke: meta-analysis of the randomized control trials. *Stroke* 1988, 19:436–442.
5. Gent M, Blakely JA, Easton JD, *et al.*: The Canadian-American ticlopidine study (CATS) in thromboembolic stroke. *Lancet* 1989, 1:1215–1220.
6. Hass WK, Easton JD, Adams HP, Jr, *et al.*: A randomized trial comparing ticlopidine hydrochloride with aspirin for the prevention of stroke in high-risk patients. *N Engl J Med* 1989, 321:501–507.
7. The Canadian Cooperative Study Group: A randomized trial of aspirin and sulfinpyrazone in threatened stroke. *N Engl J Med* 1978, 299:53–59.
8. Bousser MG, Eschwege E, Haquenau M, *et al.*: "A.I.C.L.A." controlled trial of aspirin and dipyridamole in the secondary prevention of atherothrombotic cerebral ischemia. *Stroke* 1983, 14:5–14.
9. Sivenius J, Laakso M, Penttila IM, *et al.*: The European stroke prevention study: results according to sex. *Neurology* 1991, 41:1189–1192.
10. Van Gijn J, Algra A, Kappelle LJ, *et al.*: In vivo antithrombotic effect of aspirin: dose versus nongastrointestinal bleeding. Response. *Stroke* 1993, 24:139.
11. Warlow C: Secondary prevention of stroke. *Lancet* 1992, 39:724–727.

12. van Gijn J: Aspirin: dose and indications in modern stroke prevention. *Neurol Clin* 1992, 10:193–207.
13. Dyken ML, Barnett HJM, Easton JD, *et al.*: Low-dose aspirin and stroke: "it ain't necessarily so". *Stroke* 1992, 23:195–199.
14. Barnett HJM, Hachinski V: Comment. aspirin: dose and indications in modern stroke prevention. *Neurol Clin* 1992, 10:208.
15. Barnett HJM: Aspirin in stroke prevention: an overview. *Stroke* 1990, 21(suppl IV):IV40–IV43.
16. Easton JD: Antiplatelet therapy for prevention of ischemic stroke. *Cerebrovasc Dis* 1992, 2(suppl 1):6–13.
17. Dyken ML: Meta-analysis in the assessment of therapy for stroke prevention. *Cerebrovasc Dis* 1992, 2(suppl 1):35–40.
18. Hirsh J, Dalen JE, Fuster V, *et al.*: Aspirin and other platelet active drugs: the relationship between dose, effectiveness, and side effects. *Chest* 1992, 102:327S– 336S.
19. Sherman DG, Dyken ML, Jr, Fisher M, *et al.*: Antithrombotic therapy for cerebrovascular disorders. *Chest* 1992, 102:529S–537S.
20. Pedersen AK, FitzGerald GA: The human pharmacology of platelet inhibition: pharmacokinetics relevant to drug action. *Circulation* 1985, 72:1164–1176.
21. Vane JR, Flower RJ, Botting RM: History of aspirin and its mechanism of action. *Stroke* 1990, 21(suppl IV):IV12– IV23.
22. DeGaetano G, Cerletti C, Dejana E, *et al.*: Pharmacology of platelet inhibition in humans: implications of the salicylate-aspirin interaction. *Circulation* 1985, 72:1185–1193.
23. Patrono C: Aspirin and human platelets: from clinical trials to acetylation of cyclooxygenase and back. *Trends Pharmacol Sci* 1989, 10:453–458.
24. Weksler BB, Kent JL, Rudolph D, *et al.*: Effect of low-dose aspirin on platelet function in patients with recent cerebral ischemia. *Stroke* 1985, 16:5–9.
25. Packham M, Mustard JF: Pharmacology of platelet-affecting drugs. *Circulation* 1980, 62(suppl V):V26–V41.
26. Harker LA, Fuster V: Pharmacology of platelet inhibitors. *J Am Coll Cardiol* 1986, 8:21B–32B.
27. Lekstrom JA, Bell WR: Aspirin in the prevention of thrombosis. *Medicine* 1991, 70:161–178.
28. Patrono C: Aspirin for the prevention of coronary thrombosis: current facts and perspectives. *Eur Heart J* 1986, 7:454–459.
29. Lejeune A, Fattet M, Degos JD: Aspirin dose, bleeding time, platelet adhesion and aggregation in cerebral thrombosis. *Int J Clin Pharmacol Ther Toxicol* 1988, 26:237–242.
30. Lee TK, Chen YC, Kuo TL: Comparison of the effect of acetylsalicylic acid on platelet function in male and female patients with ischemic stroke. *Thromb Res* 1987, 47:295– 304.
31. Pedersen AK, FitzGerald GA: Dose-related kinetics of aspirin: presystemic acetylation of platelet cyclooxygenase. *N Engl J Med* 1984, 311:1206–1211.
32. Boysen G, Boss AH, Odum N, *et al.*: Prolongation of bleeding time and inhibition of platelet aggregation by low-dose acetylsalicylic acid in patients with cerebrovascular disease. *Stroke* 1984, 15:241–243.
33. Jakubowski JA, Stampfer MJ, Vaillancourt R, *et al.*: Cumulative antiplatelet effect of low-dose enteric-coated aspirin. *Br J Haematol* 1985, 60:635–642.
34. DeCaterina R, Giannesi D, Bernini W, *et al.*: Selective inhibition of thromboxane-related platelet function by low-dose aspirin in patients after myocardial infarction. *Am J Cardiol* 1985, 55:589–590.
35. Tohgi H, Tamura K, Kimura B, *et al.*: Individual variation in platelet aggregability and serum thromboxane B_2 concentrations after low-dose aspirin. *Stroke* 1988, 19:700–703.
36. Patrono C, Ciabattoni G, Pinca E, *et al.*: Low-dose aspirin and inhibition of thromboxane B_2 production in healthy subjects. *Thromb Res* 1980, 17:317–327.
37. Kallmann R, Kieuwenhuis HK, de Groot PG, *et al.*: Effects of low doses of aspirin, 10 mg and 30 mg daily, on bleeding time, thromboxane production, and 6-keto-PG1 alpha excretion in healthy subjects. *Thromb Res* 1989, 45:355– 361.
38. DeCaterina R, Giannessi D, Boem A, *et al.*: Equal antiplatelet effects of aspirin 50 mg or 324 mg/day in patients after acute myocardial infarction. *Thromb Haemost* 1985, 54:528–532.
39. Patrono C, Ciabattoni G, Davi G: Thromboxane biosynthesis in cardiovascular diseases. *Stroke* 1990, 21(suppl IV):IV130–IV133.
40. Helgason CM, Tortorice KL, Winkler SR, *et al.*: Aspirin response and failure in cerebral infarction. *Stroke* 1993, 24:345–350.
41. Gabriel SE, Jaakkimainen L, Bombardier C: Risk for serious gastrointestinal complications related to use of nonsteroidal anti-inflammatory drugs: a meta-analysis. *Ann Intern Med* 1991, 115:787–796.
42. Cryer B, Feldman M: Effects of nonsteroidal anti-inflammatory drugs on endogenous gastrointestinal prostaglandins and therapeutic strategies for prevention and treatment of nonsteroidal anti-inflammatory drug-induced damage. *Arch Intern Med* 1992, 152:1145–1155.
43. UK TIA Study Group: United Kingdom transient ischemic attack (UK-TIA) trial. interim results. *BMJ* 1988, 296:316– 320.
44. The Dutch TIA Trial Study Group: A comparison of two doses of aspirin (30 mg vs 283 mg a day) in patients after a transient ischemic attack or minor ischemic stroke. *N Engl J Med* 1991, 325:1261–1266.
45. The SALT Collaborative Group: Swedish aspirin low-dose trial (SALT) of 75 mg aspirin as secondary prophylaxis after cerebrovascular ischaemic events. *Lancet* 1991, 338:1345– 1349.
46. UK TIA Study Group: The United Kingdom transient ischemic attack (UK-TIA) aspirin trial: final results. *J Neurol Neurosurg Psych* 1991, 54:1044–1054.
47. Gatti G, Barzaghi N, Attardo-Parinello G: Pharmacokinetics of salicylic acid following administration of aspirin tablets and three different forms of soluble aspirin in normal subjects. *Int J Clin Pharmacol Res* 1989, 9:385.
48. Lanza FL, Royer GL, Nelson RS: Endoscopic evaluation of the effects of aspirin, buffered aspirin, and enteric-coated aspirin on gastric and duodenal mucosa. *N Engl J Med* 1980, 303:136–138.
49. Anderson DC, Litin SC, McBride R, on behalf of the SPAF Investigators: Intracranial hemorrhage during anticoagulation for atrial fibrillation: interim results of the second-stroke prevention in atrial fibrillation (SPAF-II) trial. *Stroke* 1993, 24:187.
50. Steering Committee of the Physicians' Health Study Research Group: Final report on the aspirin component of the ongoing Physicians' Health Study. *N Engl J Med* 1989, 321:129–135.
51. Peto R, Gray R, Collins R, *et al.*: Randomised trial of prophylactic daily aspirin in British male doctors. *BMJ* 1988, 296:313–316.
52. ISIS-2 Collaborative Group: Randomised trial of intravenous streptokinase, oral aspirin, both or neither among 17,187 cases of suspected acute myocardial infarction. ISIS-2. *Lancet* 1988, 2:349–360.
53. The RISC Group: Risk of myocardial infarction and death during treatment with low-dose aspirin and intravenous heparin in men with unstable coronary artery disease. *Lancet* 1990, 336:827–830.
54. Theroux P, Ouiment H, McCans J, *et al.*: Aspirin, heparin, or both to treat acute unstable angina. *N Engl J Med* 1988, 319:1105–1111.
55. Ridker P, Manson JE, Gaziano JM, *et al.*: Low-dose aspirin therapy for chronic stable angina: a randomized, placebo-controlled clinical trial. *Ann Intern Med* 1991, 114:835–840.
56. The ESPS Group: The European stroke-prevention study (ESPS): principal endpoints. *Lancet* 1987, 2:1351–1354.
57. Sandercock P: Aspirin for strokes and transient ischemic attacks. *BMJ* 1988, 297:995–996.
58. Boysen G, Soelberg-Sorensen PS, Juhler M. Danish very-low-dose aspirin after carotid endarterectomy trial. *Stroke* 1988,19:1211-1215.
59. Kretschmer G, Pratschner T, Prager M, *et al.*: Antiplatelet treatment prolongs survival after carotid bifurcation endarterectomy. *Ann Surg* 1990, 211:317–322.

60. European Carotid Surgery Trialists' Collaborative Group: MRC European Carotid Surgery Trial: interim results for symptomatic patients with severe (70%–99%) or with mild (0%–29%) stenosis. *Lancet* 1991, 337:1235–1243.
61. North American Symptomatic Carotid Endarterectomy Trial Collaborators: Beneficial effect of carotid endarterectomy in symptomatic patients with high-grade carotid stenosis. *N Engl J Med* 1991, 325:445–453.
62. Petersen P, Boysen G, Godtfredsen J, *et al.*: Placebo-controlled randomized trial of warfarin and aspirin for prevention of thromboembolic complications in chronic atrial fibrillation: the Copenhagen AFASAK study. *Lancet* 1989, 1:175–179.
63. Stroke Prevention in Atrial Fibrillation Investigators: Preliminary report of the stroke prevention atrial fibrillation study. *N Engl J Med* 1990, 322:863–868.
64. Stroke Prevention in Atrial Fibrillation Investigators: Stroke prevention in atrial fibrillation study: final results. *Circulation* 1991, 84:527–540.
65. Miller VT, Rothrock JF, Pearce LA, *et al.*: Ischemic stroke in patients with atrial fibrillation: effect of aspirin according to stroke mechanism. *Neurology* 1993, 43:32–36.
66. European Atrial Fibrillation Trial Study Group: Secondary prevention in nonrheumatic atrial fibrillation after transient ischaemic attack or minor stroke. *Lancet* 1993, 342:1255–1262.
67. Saltiel E, Ward A. Ticlopidine: a review of its pharmacodynamic and pharmacokinetic properties, and therapeutic efficacy in platelet-dependent disease states. *Drugs* 1987, 34:222–262.
68. Hardisty RM, Powling MJ, Nokes TJC: The action of ticlopidine on human platelets: studies on aggregation, secretion, calcium mobilization, and membrane glycoproteins. *Thromb Haemost* 1990, 64:150–155.
69. Isaka Y, Kiumra K, Etani H, *et al.*: Effect of aspirin and ticlopidine on platelet deposition in carotid atherosclerosis: assessment by indium-111 platelet scintigraphy. *Stroke* 1986, 17:1215–1220.
70. Ciuffetti G, Aisa G, Mercuri M, *et al.*: Effects of ticlopidine on the neurologic outcome and the hemorrheologic pattern in the postacute phase of ischemic stroke: a pilot study. *Angiology* 1990, 41:505–511.
71. McTavish D, Faulds D, Goa KL: Ticlopidine: an updated review of its pharmacology and therapeutic use in platelet-dependent disorders. *Drugs* 1990, 9:238–259.
72. Ellie E, Durrieu C, Besse P, *et al.*: Thrombotic thrombocytopenic purpura associated with ticlopidine. *Stroke* 1992, 23:922–923.
73. Hass WK, Molony BA, Anderson A, *et al.*: Comparison of ticlopidine and aspirin for the prevention of stroke. *N Engl J Med* 1990, 322:94–95.
74. Grotta JC, Norris JW, Kamma B, and the TASS Baseline and Angiographic Data Subgroup: Prevention of stroke with ticlopidine: who benefits most? *Neurology* 1992, 42:111– 115.
75. Harbison JW, for the Ticlopidine Aspirin Stroke Study Group: Ticlopidine versus aspirin for the prevention of recurrent stroke: analysis of patients with minor stroke from the ticlopidine aspirin stroke study. *Stroke* 1992, 23:1723– 1727.
76. Weisberg LA, for the Ticlopidine Aspirin Stroke Study Group: The efficacy and safety of ticlopidine and aspirin in nonwhites: analysis of a patient subgroup from the ticlopidine aspirin stroke study. *Neurology* 1993, 43:27–31.
77. Warlow C: Ticlopidine, a new antithrombotic drug, but is it better than aspirin for long-term use? *J Neurol Neurosurg Psych* 1990, 53:185–187.
78. Haynes RB, Sandler RS, Larson EB, *et al.*: A critical appraisal of ticlopidine, a new antiplatelet agent: effectiveness and clinical indications for prophylaxis of atherosclerotic events. *Arch Intern Med* 1992, 152:1376–1380.
79. Albers GW: Role of ticlopidine in prevention of stroke. *Stroke* 1992, 23:912–916.
80. DeCaterina R, Sicari R, Bernini W, *et al.*: Benefit-risk profile of combined antiplatelet therapy with ticlopidine and aspirin. *Thromb Haemost* 1991, 65:504–510.
81. Uchiyama S, Sone R, Nagayama T, *et al.*: Combination therapy with low-dose aspirin and ticlopidine in cerebral ischemia. *Stroke* 1989, 20:1643–1647.
82. Mills DCB, Puri R, Hu CJ, *et al.*: Clopidogrel inhibits the binding of ADP analogues to the receptor-mediating inhibition of platelet adenylate cyclase. *Arterioscleros Thrombos* 1992, 12:430–436.
83. Driot F, Defreyn G, Cazenave JP, *et al.*: Ticlopidine and SR 25990C selectively suppress platelet adenylate cyclase (AC) inhibition by ADP. *Thromb Haemost* 1989, 62:99.
84. Evans G: Effects of drugs that suppress platelet surface interaction on incidence of amaurosis fugax and transient ischemic attacks. *Surg Forum* 1972, 23:240–241.
85. Cairns JA, Gent M, Singer J, *et al.*: Aspirin, sulfinpyrazone, or both in unstable angina. *N Engl J Med* 1985, 313:1369–1375.
86. Anturan Reinfarction Italian Study Group: Sulfinpyrazone in post-myocardial infarction. *Lancet* 1982, 1:237–242.
87. Fitzgerald GA: Dipyridamole. *N Engl J Med* 1987, 316:1247–1256.
88. Acheson J, Danta G, Hutchinson EC: Controlled trial of dipyridamole in cerebral vascular disease. *BMJ* 1969, 1:614–615.
89. The American-Canadian Cooperative Study Group: Persantine aspirin trial in cerebral ischemia. Part 2. Endpoint results. *Stroke* 1985, 16:406–415.
90. van Gijn J: What dose of aspirin is most likely to reduce the risk of stroke? In *More Dilemmas in the Management of the Neurological Patient.* Edited by Warlow C, Garfield J. Edinburgh: Churchill Livingstone; 1987:145–155.
91. Keyser A: Antithrombotica bij cerebrovasculaire aandoeningen. *Ned Tijdschr Chron Zieken* 1993, 3:1–5.

Chapter 16

Anticoagulation in Cerebrovascular Disease

VINCENT T. MILLER

The use of anticoagulants for cerebrovascular ischemic disease has a powerful intuitive appeal due to the key role thrombosis plays in ischemic stroke. Perhaps as a result many physicians have employed anticoagulants in this setting in spite of any sound documentation of their efficacy. Because they are unproven in most instances and have the potential for significant complications, enormous controversy has surrounded anticoagulant usage [1–5]. Physicians, faced with the urgent need to treat stroke patients, become easily entangled in the proliferation of conflicting opinions and case reports that exist [6–8]. Well-designed clinical studies, published in the late

1980s, provide the first insights that promise to guide us out of this morass.

In this chapter, the mechanisms of action, as well as common usages of anticoagulants in cerebrovascular disease are reviewed. Randomized, controlled trials are summarized and recommendations follow. In the many instances where such reliable data are not available, we take a pragmatic approach and make suggestions based on personal experience and what is considered a balanced view of the literature. These recommendations and suggestions are then incorporated into a decision analysis based on how patients actually present to the physician.

When contemplating the use of anticoagulants in patients with cerebral ischemia, the physician must ask two fundamental questions. 1) What is the present or potential stroke pathophysiologic mechanism? 2) Am I trying to halt the progression of ongoing stroke or prevent a future event?

Regarding the first question, the common ischemic stroke mechanisms include atherothrombotic, cardioembolic, and small vessel (lacunar) disease (Table 16.1). Anticoagulants are also routinely employed in less frequent stroke types such as arterial dissections, cerebral venous thrombosis, and disorders of coagulation such as the antiphospholipid antibody syndrome.

The distinction emphasized by the second question impacts on the rapidity with which anticoagulation must be achieved, the choice of agents, and the duration of therapy.

ANTICOAGULANT PHARMACOLOGY

Heparin and Heparinoids

Heparin is a mixture of glycosaminoglycans that occurs naturally in mammalian tissue and is usually prepared commercially from either porcine intestinal mucosa or bovine lungs [9,10]. The resultant heterogeneous product has molecular weights ranging from 3000 to 40,000 d. Recently, the recognition that pharmacologic activity varies with molecular weight has led to the development of low molecular weight heparin (LMWH) with distinctive properties. Standard heparin accomplishes its anticoagulant effect primarily by combining with antithrombin III (AT III) and inactivating a number of factors in the coagulation cascade, the most important of these being thrombin and Factor Xa (Figure 16.1). At higher doses, heparin also combines with heparin cofactor II to inactivate thrombin. The action of LMWH is confined primarily to potentiating AT III's inhibition of Xa leaving thrombin unaffected. There are several theories to explain this disparity in action. One proposes that thrombin is inhibited by binding to AT III with

Table 16.1. Clinical differentiation of common focal strokes

Stroke type	Onset	TIAs	Associations
Atherothrombotic	Gradual Stuttering During sleep	Common	Peripheral vascular disease Carotid bruit
Cardioembolic	Sudden	Rare	Cardiac abnormalities Previous cardioembolism
Lacunar	Gradual Stuttering Lacunar syndromes	Common	Hypertension
Intracerebral hemorrhage*	Gradual Sudden	Very rare	Hypertension

*Readily diagnosed by immediate noncontrast computed tomography scanning.
TIA—transient ischemic attack.

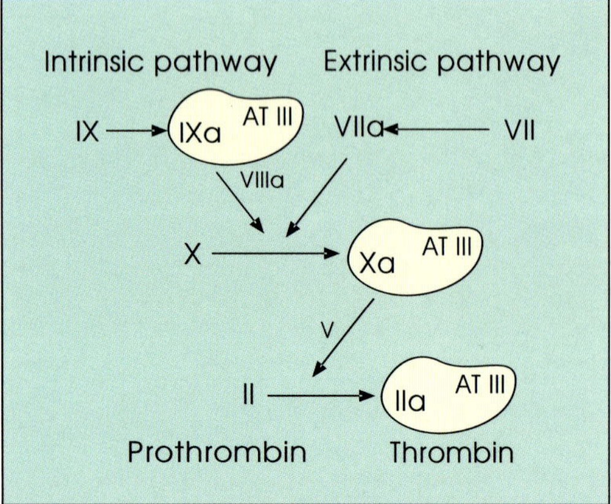

FIGURE 16.1
Heparin's principal sites of action. *Circles* indicate inactivation with antithrombin III (AT III).

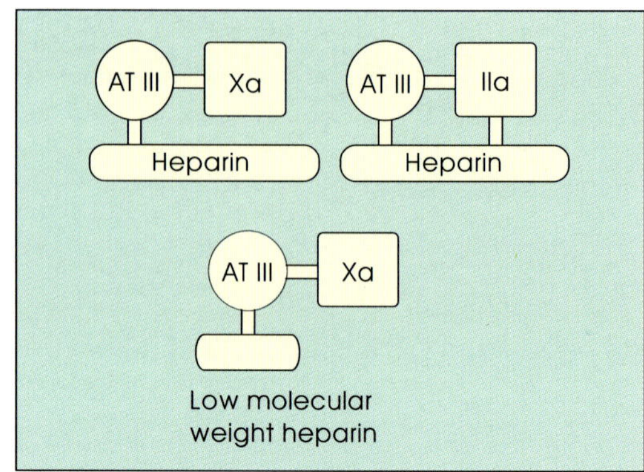

FIGURE 16.2
Heparin complexes leading to inactivation of IIa and Xa.

heparin molecules linking to both the AT III and the thrombin itself, something structurally possible only with longer heparin molecules, whereas Xa is inhibited simply by AT III that in turn is bound to the heparin (Figure 16.2).

Heparin must be administered parenterally, either subcutaneously or intravenously. Plasma half-life for standard heparin averages approximately 90 minutes but may be altered in either direction by disease states. With standard heparin, therapy is usually monitored by measuring the activated partial thromboplastin time (PTT). The therapeutic range is considered about twice that of the control or a prolongation from baseline by 20 seconds. Although standard practice in the treatment of conditions such as pulmonary embolism employs an initial bolus of 5000 to 10,000 μ of heparin followed by an adjusted continuous infusion of about 1000 μ/hr, for cerebrovascular ischemia the bolus can usually be eliminated, which presumably lessens the risk of hemorrhage [11].

The half-life for LMWH is up to twice as long after intravenous infusion. Its effect is monitored by measuring Xa activity. Thus far, it has been used successfully in stroke patients to prevent deep venous thrombosis [12,13]. A current study is comparing LMWH with placebo in terms of neurologic outcome for patients with acute stroke [14].

The main complication of heparin therapy is of course hemorrhage. The risk of hemorrhage while on heparin is influenced by factors such as the method of administration, total daily dose of heparin, underlying clinical condition of the patient, and the concurrent use of antiplatelet agents (Table 16.2) [13,15]. It is important to realize that the risk of bleeding on heparin has not been demonstrated to correlate with the activated PTT nearly as well as the risk of hemorrhage while on warfarin correlates with the prothrombin time. Protamine sulfate can reverse the anticoagulant effects of heparin. When given intravenously, 1 mg neutralizes 100 units of heparin [10].

A second less common side effect is thrombocytopenia [10,16]. Two varieties of this exist. One occurs in the first few days of therapy and is generally mild. The second, hypothesized to be immune mediated, is usually delayed until the second week of treatment, although it may occur earlier in patients exposed to heparin previously. It is severe and can be associated with both arterial and venous thrombosis. Recognition is essential given the intuitive inclination of most physicians to increase heparin dosage when thrombosis occurs. Treatment consists of immediate discontinuation of heparin and therapy with oral anticoagulants supplemented initially by antiplatelet agents.

Importantly, heparin has no significant thrombolytic effect. In the setting of cerebrovascular ischemia, it can reasonably be expected to prevent the formation or the extension of a thrombus, but not to lyse thrombi that have already developed. However, thrombus formation and lysis are dynamic, opposing processes, the relative strength of which determine whether a clot will wax or wane. By inhibiting thrombosis, the balance may be tipped in favor of clot lysis leading to resolution (Figure 16.3).

Warfarin

Warfarin is the most commonly employed coumarin derivative in the United States. Investigations into "sweet clover disease" in cattle led to the development of these orally administered agents. Warfarin exerts its anticoagulant effect by altering the production of vitamin K–dependent clotting factors II, VII, IX, and X (Figure 16.4). These altered factors do not undergo their usual conformational changes when binding calcium and are rendered inactive [17]. Warfarin additionally affects the production of proteins C and S, two antithrombotic factors. While warfarin's half-life is about 36 hours, the onset of its anticoagulant effect is dependent on the half-life of the circulating coagulation factors. Protein C has one of the shortest half-lives of these factors, and as a result, an early, transient prothrombotic state is hypothetically possible after the initiation of warfarin therapy.

Warfarin dosages are adjusted based on the measurement of the prothrombin time (PT), but the method of reporting PT results has recently been refined. A pivotal observation has been that the degree of prolongation of the prothrombin time while on warfarin therapy varies widely with the type of thromboplastin used to perform the test [18]. This has led to the recommendation that the international normalized ratio (INR), which takes into account the sensitivity of the thromboplastin employed, be used instead of simple PT ratios. Thromboplastin sensitivity is quantitated by the international sensitivity index (ISI). The INR can be calculated from the PT ratio and the ISI.

As with heparin, the main complication of warfarin therapy is hemorrhage. This correlates well with the INR, and the risk for hemorrhage can be lowered by meticulous attention to proper monitoring and dosing. Of particular note are the large number of

Table 16.2. Factors possibly increasing risk of brain hemorrhage with heparin

Concomitant thrombolytic therapy
Increasing heparin dose
Recent surgery, trauma, or hemorrhage
Concurrent aspirin usage
Early heparinization after large cerebral infarction
Hypertension (mean arterial pressure > 120 mm Hg)
Bolus heparin dosing
Age, female gender

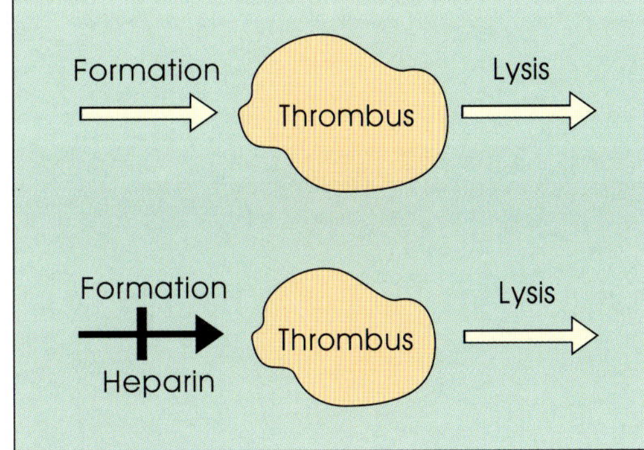

FIGURE 16.3

Heparin's effect on existing thrombi.

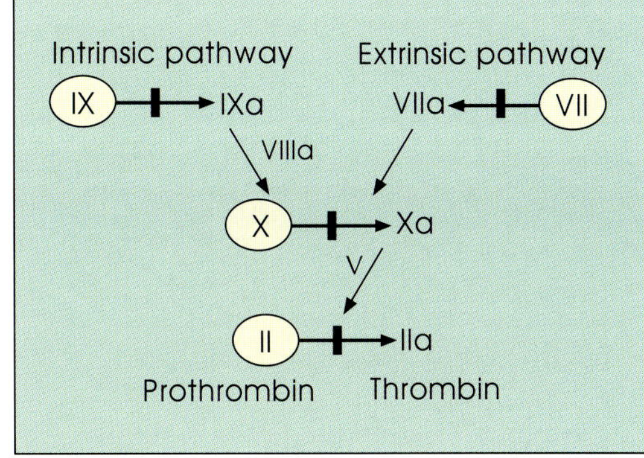

FIGURE 16.4

Warfarin's principal sites of action. *Circles* indicate structural change in molecule, impairing normal activation.

medications that can interact with warfarin and change dosage requirements (Table 16.3). Factors including advanced age, previous hemorrhage, concurrent antiplatelet therapy, prolonged duration of therapy, and underlying medical illnesses can also increase the hemorrhagic risk (Table 16.4). The anticoagulant effects of warfarin can be reversed in 6 to 10 hours by the administration of vitamin K. In more urgent situations fresh frozen plasma is used to replace defective coagulation factors [17].

Tissue necrosis is an uncommon but devastating complication of warfarin. It may result from the early inhibition of protein C activity [10]. It can be prevented in protein C–deficient individuals by first anticoagulating the patient with heparin and then switching to warfarin. Finally, warfarin has important teratogenic effects, especially during the first trimester, and is not recommended during pregnancy [17].

CARDIOEMBOLIC STROKE

The physician faces two common clinical problems in regard to cardioembolic stroke. The first of these is the primary prevention of stroke in patients with cardiac conditions increasing the risk of thrombus formation. The other involves the prevention of recurrent stroke in patients presenting with a cardioembolic stroke. In the former setting, the first and only well-conducted clinical trials of anticoagulation for cerebral ischemia allow definite recommendations to be made.

Primary Prevention

Although a number of cardiac abnormalities may predispose to clot formation, nonvalvular atrial fibrillation accounts for nearly half of cardioembolic strokes. The prevalence of atrial fibrillation increases with age and is about 5% in those aged over 70 years [19]. One to one and a half million Americans have atrial fibrillation [20]. Most of these patients carry approximately a 5% annual risk of stroke if left untreated. About 65% to 70% of these strokes are cardioembolic in origin [21].

There have now been five well designed and executed clinical trials establishing that warfarin can safely reduce the risk of stroke in those with atrial fibrillation (Table 16.5) [22–27]. The pooled data from these studies showed an incidence of 4.5% annually in control patients compared to 1.4% annually in those treated with warfarin, a 68% risk reduction (95% CI = 50%–79%) [27]. The annual risk of major hemorrhage was 1.3% for those given warfarin compared with 1.0% for those given placebo. Hence, we recommend the use of warfarin (INR = 2.0–3.0) to prevent stroke in many atrial fibrillation patients without contraindications. One clear exception, however, applies to patients with lone atrial fibrillation. These patients, who are less than 60 years of age with idiopathic atrial fibrillation and no other cardiac disease, have such a low risk of cardiac emboli that warfarin therapy is not justified [28,29].

Only two controlled studies have tested aspirin for patients with atrial fibrillation. The larger of these, the Stroke Prevention in Atrial Fibrillation (SPAF) trial, demonstrated a 44% decrease in stroke among those receiving aspirin 325/mg/day, compared with those given placebo [23]. The second study showed only an 18% decrease with aspirin 75/mg/day [22]. Combining these data results in a 36% risk reduction (P = 0.03) [27]. This figure cannot be directly compared with that for warfarin because of differences in the population of patients studied. The SPAF study initially showed that both aspirin and warfarin prevented strokes, but did

Table 16.3. Common drugs altering the effect of warfarin

Potentiating warfarin's effect		Impairing warfarin's effect
Erythromycin	Thyroxine	Penicillin
Metronidazole	Disulfiram	Griseofulvin
Ketoconazole	Amiodarone	Rifampin
Trimethoprim-sulfamethoxazole	Piroxicam	Carbamazepine
Fluconazole	Phenylbutazone	Barbiturates
Isoniazid	Tamoxifen	Alcohol
Sulfinpyrazone	Quinidine	
Clofibrate	Phenytoin	
Cimetidine	Anabolic steroids	
Omeprazole	Vitamin E	

Table 16.4. Factors increasing hemorrhagic risk with warfarin in stroke

- Increasing international normalized ratio or prothrombin time
- Age
- Past gastrointestinal bleeding
- Recent myocardial infarction, severe anemia, or renal failure
- Concurrent antiplatelet therapy

Table 16.5. Randomized primary prevention trials of warfarin in atrial fibrillation

Study	Patient-years warfarin	Patient-years control	Relative risk (95% CI)
Petersen and coworkers [22]	413	398	0.59 (0.06–0.82)
BAATAF [24]	487	435	0.86 (0.39–0.97)
Connolly and coworkers [25]	237	241	0.43(-0.07–0.81)
SPAFI[23]	263	245	0.66(0.15–0.87)
Ezekowitz and coworkers [26]	489	483	0.74(0.37–0.90)

BAATAF—Boston Area Anticoagulation Trial for Atrial Fibrillation Investigators; SPAFI—The Stroke Prevention in Atrial Fibrillation Investigators.

not compare the efficacy of the two. Recently, a follow-up study by the same investigators suggested that warfarin is somewhat more effective than aspirin in preventing ischemic strokes, but the increase in hemorrhagic complications with warfarin nullifies much of this advantage [30]. The low cost, safety, and ease of administration of aspirin also argue for its usage.

The choice between these two agents can be guided by consideration of risk factors. Within the population of atrial fibrillation patients, these risk factors segregate those at higher from those at lower risk for stroke. Clinical risk factors include past transient ischemic attack (TIA) or stroke, recent congestive heart failure, diabetes, and hypertension [27,31]. Echocardiographic risk factors have also been defined [32] (Table 16.6). In patients with risk factors, treatment with warfarin is indicated. In those without risk factors, aspirin is an acceptable alternative.

Warfarin (INR = 2.0–3.0) is recommended for 3 weeks in patients about to undergo cardioversion who have been in atrial fibrillation for more than 48 hours [29]. They are then kept on oral anticoagulation until they remain in sinus rhythm for 4 weeks.

In several settings other than nonvalvular atrial fibrillation, anticoagulants are routinely employed, although this practice is not backed up uniformly by clinical studies of similar quality. Patients with rheumatic mitral valvular disease and either atrial fibrillation, increased left atrial diameter, or a previous history of cardiac embolism should be chronically anticoagulated [33]. Patients with mechanical heart valves require anticoagulation to an INR of 2.5 to 3.5 [34]. Those with mitral bioprosthetic valves should be anticoagulated for 3 months after insertion, and chronically in some instances. However, patients in sinus rhythm with bioprosthetic values in the aortic position have a lower risk of thromboembolism and thus anticoagulation for 3 months is considered optional. Patients recovering from myocardial infarction who are at increased risk of embolization due to such factors as mural thrombus formation, severe left ventricular dysfunction, or prior embolization should also receive anticoagulants [35]. Finally, patients with infective endocarditis, mitral valve prolapse, or mitral annular calcification usually do not require anticoagulation [34].

Recurrence Prevention

After an acute cardioembolic stroke, the physician must promptly consider the risk of recurrent embolism. Estimates of this risk in untreated patients have run as high as 10% to 15% in the first 2 weeks after stroke [36]. Many of the cardiac pathologies leading to cardioembolic events are chronic and not correctable. Thus, anticoagulation becomes the mainstay of prophylactic therapy. The timing of the initiation of anticoagulation is critical.

Embolic cerebral infarctions commonly undergo a hemorrhagic conversion. The incidence of this phenomenon has been reported as high as 41% if patients are followed with computed tomography (CT) scanning for 1 month [37]. It occurs more commonly in large infarctions, especially in the first few days after the stroke [11,38]. Hemorrhage probably results from clot lysis or migration allowing reperfusion of previously ischemic tissue. Increased collateral perfusion may also contribute [39]. Weakened, necrotic vessel walls can no longer totally contain the blood, and hemorrhage follows (Figure 16.5) [40]. In many instances this is nothing more than petechial bleeding without clinical symptoms but it can become a major hemorrhage with catastrophic consequences (Figure 16.6). Anticoagulants sometimes increase the amount of bleeding [11]. Thus, while their immediate use decreases the risk of recurrent embolic stroke, it increases the chances of deterioration due to hemorrhage from the initial stroke. In a small randomized study of early versus delayed anticoagulation for these patients, those receiving early anticoagulation appeared to do better than those in whom anticoagulation was delayed 10 days, though the results were not statistically significant [41].

Table 16.6. Factors increasing risk of embolism in atrial fibrillation

Clinical factors	Echocardiographic factors
Hypertension	Left ventricular dysfunction
Previous thromboembolism	Increased left atrial diameter
Recent congestive heart failure	
Diabetes mellitus	

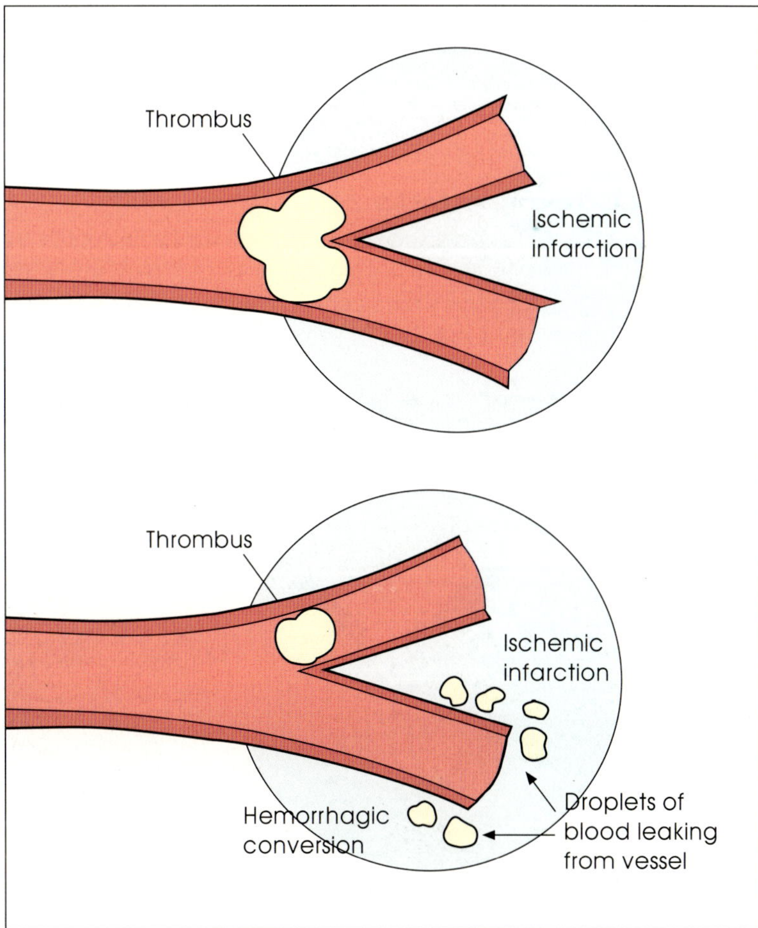

FIGURE 16.5

Hemorrhagic conversion of embolic brain infarction.

Recent studies have suggested that the risk of recurrent emboli may not be as high as previously thought, and probably varies with the cardiac pathology leading to thrombus formation [38,42]. We recommend delaying anticoagulation with heparin after acute embolic stroke for at least 48 hours in small strokes and up to 14 days in larger ones [11,43]. A CT scan without infusion is checked before the institution of heparin, and if hemorrhage has occurred, anticoagulation is further delayed. Once on heparin, most patients are then switched over to warfarin therapy after a few days. In some instances, such as the prevention of recurrent stroke in a patient with nonvalvular atrial fibrillation, simply starting warfarin several days after the first stroke without using heparin may be acceptable [43]. Again, this is predicated on the CT scan ruling out hemorrhage.

ATHEROTHROMBOTIC STROKE

The largest portion of ischemic strokes are considered to be atherothrombotic in origin. The underlying pathology is the atherosclerotic plaque. A stroke may result when thrombosis develops on the plaque causing either increased stenosis and reduced blood flow to the brain or embolization from atherosclerotic debris to a distal artery. Other mechanisms such as intraplaque hemorrhage may also be important (Figure 16.7). The natural history of atherothrombotic strokes includes both the common occurrence of TIAs and often the gradual evolution of the stroke itself over several hours. Both of these characteristics provide therapeutic windows through which the final ischemic event might be prevented if the thrombotic process could be curtailed.

Transient Ischemic Attacks

The onset of TIAs marks an increased risk of stroke, perhaps as high as 10% to 15% in the first year. Antiplatelet therapy with either aspirin or ticlopidine has been proven to reduce the risk of stroke and death in a number of controlled, randomized clinical trials [44–46]. Similarly, carotid endarterectomy reduces stroke risk in patients with TIAs due to severe carotid stenosis [47,48].

Anticoagulation has not yet been shown to be effective in similarly designed clinical trials, although such trials are currently being undertaken. One small study compared heparinization with aspirin therapy in 55 patients with the new onset of TIAs. Eight patients had further TIAs and one a stroke on heparin, compared with seven having TIAs and four developing stroke in the aspirin group, an insignificant difference [49]. For now, the value of anticoagulation in atherothrombotic cerebral ischemia either acutely or chronically for TIAs remains speculative.

We recommend antiplatelet therapy for patients with TIAs unless contraindications exist or severe side effects develop. Patients who have an appropriate severe carotid stenosis (70%–99%) and who are good surgical candidates should undergo endarterectomy. In situations where definite ischemic events continue in spite of antiplatelet therapy and surgery is not an option, we sometimes employ warfarin on empiric grounds. Similarly, we sometimes heparinize patients while they are undergoing diagnostic testing in anticipation of endarterectomy.

Progressing or Partial Stroke

The term *progressing stroke* denotes the situation in which a patient's neurologic deficits are increasing in scope or severity over a matter of hours. The process can occasionally continue for as long as 2 or 3 days, especially in the vertebrobasilar territory [1,7]. Partial strokes are those in which the deficits are mild or do not impair all of the neurologic functions commonly affected by ischemia in that vascular distribution. These are commonly encountered and sometimes become progressing strokes after a brief period of stability. Finally, by completed stroke we mean one in which the symptomatology is stable or improving. The terms provide descriptive information about stroke deficit and time course, but do not precisely define the underlying stroke pathophysiologic mechanism.

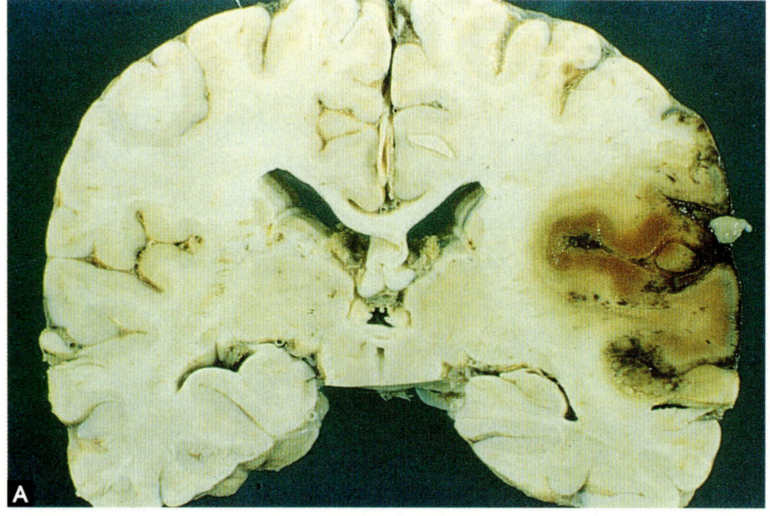

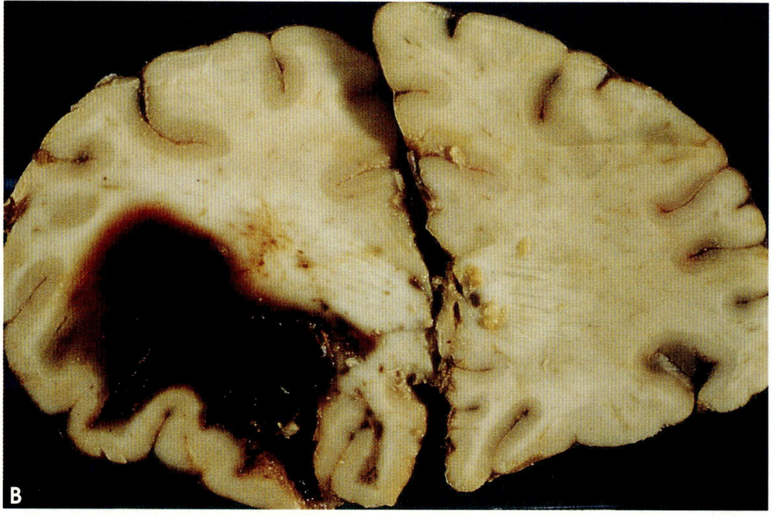

FIGURE 16.6

A, Minor asymptomatic hemorrhage in patient who died of cardiac causes. **B**, Major hemorrhage in anticoagulated patient resulting in transtentorial herniation and death.

In both progressing and partial stroke, acute anticoagulation with heparin may be used to stop further progression presumably by inhibiting further thrombosis. Whether it does so is an unsettled issue. Initial recommendations for use of heparins were derived from poorly designed trials that are unacceptable by current standards [17]. Only one study [50] focused on the issue with controlled, randomized methodology. In that study of 225 patients with acute partial stroke, 17% of patients heparinized within 48 hours of symptom onset showed progression compared with 19.5% of those not anticoagulated, an insignificant difference [50]. Even in recent uncontrolled series, the value of heparin seems questionable. Haley and coworkers [51] reported a 50% incidence of stroke progression in spite of "therapeutic" levels of anticoagulation with heparin in 36 patients [51].

Until better data are available, we recommend heparin only in instances of well-documented progressing stroke when no contraindications exist. Vascular imaging demonstrating medium or large vessel high-grade atherosclerotic stenosis in this setting further argues for the use of heparin. However, the clinician must realize that deterioration in a stroke patient may occur for many reasons other than progressive thrombosis, and in these instances anticoagulation would be inappropriate (Table 16.7) [52]. An important clinical issue is that of hypertension attending the progressing stroke. A transient, reactive increase in blood pressure is common and is probably beneficial because it increases cerebral perfusion [53]. In most instances it is better left untreated, and when present, is a relative contraindication to anticoagulation.

For completed stroke, anticoagulation is not indicated [43]. Antiplatelet therapy has been proven to prevent recurrent events and is recommended. In instances of mild completed stroke associated with severe carotid atherosclerosis, endarterectomy has proven to be efficacious.

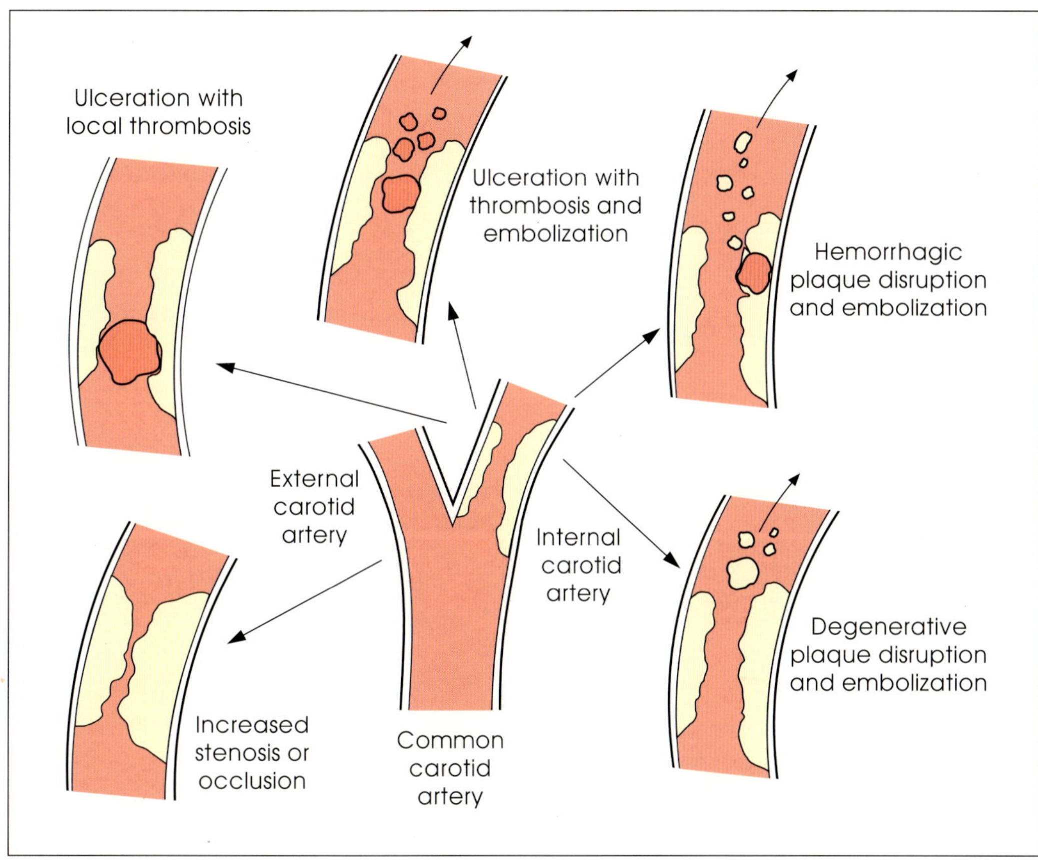

FIGURE 16.7

Possible stroke mechanisms associated with atherosclerosis.

Table 16.7. Possible causes of deterioration in acute stroke patients
Hemorrhagic conversion of infarction
Cerebral edema formation
Concurrent seizures
Intercurrent infection (pneumonia, urosepsis, and so forth)
Metabolic abnormalities (hypoglycemia, hyponatremia, and so forth)
Hypotension (including iatrogenic)

LACUNAR STROKE

Lacunar strokes are thought to occur most commonly as a result of degenerative changes in small intracranial penetrating arteries, usually less than a millimeter in diameter [54]. Thrombosis in the parent vessels near the ostia of the penetrating branches, and emboli from the heart or proximal vasculature are other causes. Lacunar strokes are sometimes preceded by TIAs and may demonstrate a progressive course. The value of heparin in their treatment has been been seriously questioned [55]. Furthermore, realization that the same degenerated vessels that account for lacunar stroke can also give rise to intracerebral hemorrhages gives pause regarding anticoagulation.

Initially, the clinical distinction between small vessel disease and atherothrombosis of larger arteries can be difficult. Clues suggesting small vessel pathology include the presentation of classic lacunar syndromes (Table 16.8), a flurry of repetitive identical TIAs over 24 to 48 hours, and the absence of appropriate larger vessel disease on vascular imaging and brain scanning [56]. We rarely use heparin in patients thought to have lacunar ischemia on the basis of small vessel disease.

Table 16.8. Classic lacunar syndromes
Pure motor hemiplegia
Pure sensory stroke
Ataxic hemiparesis
Dysarthria-clumsy hand syndrome

MISCELLANEOUS CONDITIONS

There are a variety of less common clinical conditions that may cause ischemic stroke and are sometimes treated with anticoagulants. They are summarized below.

Antiphospholipid Antibody Syndrome

In the increasingly recognized antiphospholipid antibody syndrome, various circulating coagulation inhibitors are associated with a paradoxically increased incidence of thrombotic events, including stroke [57,58]. The presence of these inhibitors may be suggested by an abnormally prolonged activated PTT, false-positive serology, or a low platelet count. Definitive screening, however, is accomplished by measuring anticardiolipin antibodies and a dilute Russel's viper venom time or

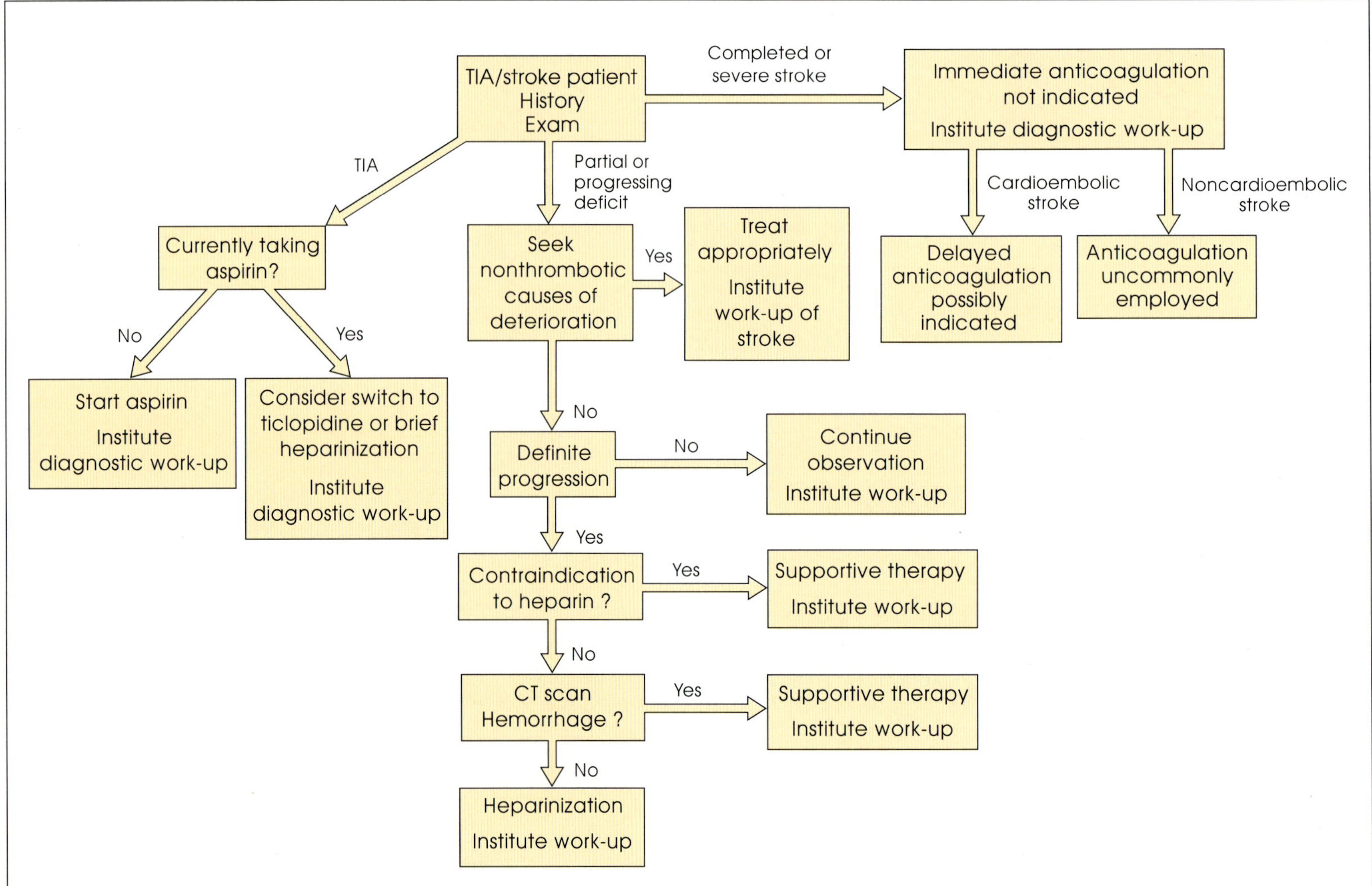

FIGURE 16.8

Decision analysis for anticoagulation of cerebrovascular patients. CT—computed tomography; TIA—transient ischemic attack.

kaolin clotting time. The natural history and the value of various therapies such as steroids, antiplatelet agents, and anticoagulants are currently being assessed [59].

Arterial Dissection

Dissection of major cerebral vessels either intracranially or extracranially can occur with minimal or no apparent trauma and lead to stroke [60]. Establishing the clinical diagnosis can be difficult but may be suggested by neck pain, headache, or a Horner's syndrome in conjunction with cerebral ischemic symptoms. The diagnosis usually requires angiography.

The mechanisms of stroke following dissection vary, but stenosis and thrombosis at the site of injury or distal embolization are considered common. As a result, many authorities recommend anticoagulation [61].

Venous Thrombosis

Cortical vein or intracranial venous sinus thromboses, while generally rare, make up a high proportion of strokes in certain patient populations such as women in the puerperium [62]. Headache, mental status changes, and seizures in addition to focal neurologic abnormalities should alert the physician to these possibilities. Currently, the diagnosis can usually be secured by magnetic resonance (MR) scanning, eliminating the need for angiography as was formerly the case.

Anticoagulants would seem a logical choice for the treatment of venous thrombosis. However, cerebral venous infarctions have a very high rate of spontaneous hemorrhagic conversion. Thus, opinions concerning treatment differ [63].

Antithrombotic Factor Deficiencies

Hereditary or acquired deficiencies of protein C, protein S, and antithrombin III have all been associated with stroke although they more commonly cause venous thrombotic events. Given the physiologic antithrombotic activity of these factors this would be expected, and these patients are sometimes treated with anticoagulants for as long as the deficiency persists [64,65].

PATIENT MANAGEMENT

Many physicians find themselves confused when treating a patient with stroke, especially concerning the need for anticoagulation. This section and the accompanying flow diagram (Figure 16.8) summarize decision analysis about the use of anticoagulants based on the recommendations outlined above.

The first step in evaluating a patient with acute stroke is to obtain a detailed history. This must sometimes be obtained from a family member because the patient is aphasic or unable to communicate. Key points include the nature of the symptoms, their temporal pattern of onset, history of previous cerebral ischemic or other vascular events, and review of risk factors and current medications. During the examination that follows, the physician documents the extent of neurologic dysfunction as well as seeks evidence of associated signs such as carotid bruits or cardiac abnormalities. When this is completed, the physician should have narrowed the range of possible pathophysiologic mechanisms responsible for the event.

Many physicians obtain an immediate CT scan of the brain in patients suspected of having a stroke. This is not always necessary and is not cost-effective because a second CT scan is often later required. While all stroke patients should have brain imaging, in situations other than those outlined, it is better to wait 48 to 72 hours before performing CT scanning, at which time an ischemic infarction is better visualized (Table 16.9).

If the stroke is severe and apparently completed, immediate anticoagulation is not indicated. If it is later determined to be cardioembolic in origin, anticoagulation might be necessary after a delay of 2 to 14 days depending on stroke severity. Completed atherothrombotic and lacunar stroke patients are not anticoagulated. When the patient's deficit is mild or partial but apparently stable, we prefer to hold off on anticoagulation. Such patients are admitted and closely monitored for signs of progression.

When the physician observes further neurologic deterioration, or when upon presentation the patient provides a compelling history thereof, progressing stroke is diagnosed. Immediate heparinization is considered. At this juncture, contraindications to heparin must be sought and nonthrombotic reasons for deterioration must be eliminated. The most obvious contraindications are a history of hemorrhage or an intolerance of heparin. Hypertension is a relative contraindication. When mean arterial pressure runs above 120 to 125 mm Hg we prefer to avoid heparinization. Starting new antihypertensive treatment at this point is not indicated unless the pressure is extremely high or other end organ damage is present. The suspicion that small vessel disease is causing a lacunar stroke also argues against the use of heparin. Nonthrombotic causes of deterioration in stroke patients have been outlined (Table 16.7).

If, after considering these factors, the decision to use heparin is made, a CT scan without infusion is obtained to rule out intracranial hemorrhage or other lesions, such as tumors that may present as stroke. Heparin is started by intravenous infusion at 1000 μ/hr without a bolus dosage. Dosing is adjusted based on subsequent activated PTT values aiming for a range of 1.5 to 2.0 times control. Patients are admitted and closely followed while their diagnostic work-up proceeds. In those patients who then stabilize, a decision about long-term oral anticoagulation must be made. Generally speaking, those with severe symptomatic arterial stenosis that is not surgically accessible, or those who have failed antiplatelet therapy are considered for long-term warfarin therapy.

Table 16.9 Indications for immediate computed tomography scanning in acute stroke

Severe hypertension (to rule out intracerebral hemorrhage)
Decreased level of consciousness (to rule out intracranial hemorrhage or other mass)
Intended immediate anticoagulation (to rule out intracranial hemorrhage)
Patients who are immunocompromised or have known malignancy (to rule out nonvascular pathology)
Possible subarachnoid hemorrhage (sudden headache, nuchal rigidity)

Patients presenting with TIAs are usually treated with antiplatelet agents while diagnostic testing is being conducted. For those who have TIAs while on low-dose aspirin (325 mg/d), several options exist. These include the following: 1) increasing the aspirin dosage up to 650 mg bid; 2) switching to ticlopidine; and 3) heparinization with the same considerations as outlined for progressing stroke. Long-term treatment will be determined by the results of thorough diagnostic testing to uncover the underlying stroke pathophysiologic mechanism.

REFERENCES

1. Miller VT, Hart RG: Heparin anticoagulation in acute brain ischemia. *Stroke* 1988, 19:403–406.
2. Phillips SJ: An alternative view of heparin anticoagulation in acute focal brain ischemia. *Stroke* 1989, 20:295–298.
3. Miller VT, Hart RG: Heparin in acute stroke [letter]. *Stroke* 1989, 20:1284–1285.
4. Scheinberg P: Heparin in acute stroke [letter]. *Stroke* 1989, 20:1285.
5. Phillips SJ: Heparin in acute stroke [letter]. *Stroke* 1989, 20:1285–1286.
6. Biller J: Medical management of acute cerebral ischemia. *Neurol Clin* 1992, 10:63–85.
7. Rothrock JF, Hart RG: Antithrombotic therapy in cerebrovascular disease. *Ann Intern Med* 1991, 115:885–895.
8. Marsh EE, Adams HP, Biller J, *et al.*: Use of antithrombotic drugs in the treatment of acute ischemic stroke: a survey of neurologists practice in the United States. *Neurology* 1989, 39:1631–1634.
9. Hirsh J, Dalen JE, Deykin D, Poller L: Heparin: mechanism of action, pharmacokinetics, dosing considerations, monitoring, efficacy and safety. *Chest* 1992, 102(suppl):337S–351S.
10. Kwaan HC, Samama MM, Kher AR: Anticoagulant therapy. In *Clinical Thrombosis.* Edited by Kwaan HC, Samama MM. Boca Raton: CRC Press; 1989:473–496.
11. Cerebral Embolism Study Group: Immediate anticoagulation of embolic stroke: brain hemorrhage and management options. *Stroke* 1984, 15:779–789.
12. Turpie AGG, Gent M, Cote R, *et al.*: A low-molecular weight heparinoid compared with unfractionated heparin in the prevention of deep vein thrombosis in patients with acute ischemic stroke. *Ann Intern Med* 1992, 117:353–357.
13. Sandercock PAG, van den Belt AGM, Lindley RI, Slattery J: Antithrombotic therapy in acute ischaemic stroke: an overview of the completed randomised trials. *J Neurol Neurosurg Psychiatry* 1993, 56:17–25.
14. Adams HP, Woolson RF, Biller J, Clark WR: Studies of ORG 10172 in patients with acute ischemic stroke: the TOAST study group. *Haemostasis* 1992, 22:99–103.
15. Levine MN, Hirsh J, Landefeld S, Raskob G: Hemorrhagic complications of anticoagulant therapy. *Chest* 1992, 102(suppl):352S–363S.
16. Becker PS, Miller VT: Heparin-induced thrombocytopenia. *Stroke* 1989, 20:1449–1459.
17. Hirsh J, Dalen JE, Deykin D, Poller L: Oral anticoagulants: mechanism of action, clinical effectiveness, and optimal therapeutic range. *Chest* 1992, 102(suppl):312S–326S.
18. Hirsh J: Is the dose of warfarin prescribed by American physicians unnecessarily high? *Arch Intern Med* 1987, 147:769–771.
19. Wolf PA, Abbott RD, Kannel WB: Atrial fibrillation as an independent risk factor for stroke: the Framingham study. *Stroke* 1991, 22:983–988.
20. Halperin JL, Hart RG: Atrial fibrillation and stroke: new ideas, persisting dilemmas. *Stroke* 1988, 19:937–941.
21. Miller VT, Rothrock JF, Pearce LA, *et al.*: Ischemic stroke in patients with atrial fibrillation: effect of aspirin according to stroke mechanism. *Neurology* 1993, 43:32–36.
22. Petersen P, Boysen G, Godtfredsen J, *et al.*: Placebo-controlled, randomized trial of warfarin and aspirin for prevention of thromboembolic consequences in chronic atrial fibrillation. *Lancet* 1989, 1:1215–1220.
23. The Stroke Prevention in Atrial Fibrillation Investigators: Stroke Prevention in Atrial Fibrillation Study: final results. *Circulation* 1991, 84:527–539.
24. Boston Area Anticoagulation Trial for Atrial Fibrillation Investigators: The effect of low-dose warfarin on the risk of stroke in nonrheumatic atrial fibrillation. *N Engl J Med* 1990, 323:1505–1511.
25. Connolly SJ, Laupacis A, Gent M, *et al.*: Canadian Atrial Fibrillation Anticoagulation (CAFA) Study. *J Am Coll Cardiol* 1991, 18:349–355.
26. Ezekowitz MD, Bridgers SL, James KE, *et al.*: Warfarin in the prevention of stroke associated with nonrheumatic atrial fibrillation. *N Engl J Med* 1992, 327:1406–1412.
27. Atrial Fibrillation Investigators Collaboration: Risk factors for stroke and efficacy of antithrombotic therapy in atrial fibrillation. *Arch Intern Med* 1994, 154:1449–1457.
28. Kopecky SJ, Gersh BJ, McGoon MD, *et al.*: The natural history of lone atrial fibrillation: a population based study over three decades. *N Engl J Med* 1987, 317:669–674.
29. Laupacis A, Albers G, Dunn MI, Feinberg WM: Antithrombotic therapy in atrial fibrillation. *Chest* 1992, 102(suppl):426S–433S.
30. Stroke Prevention in Atrial Fibrillation Investigators: Warfarin versus aspirin for prevention of thromboembolism in atrial fibrillation: Stroke Prevention in Atrial Fibrillation II Study. *Lancet* 1994, 343:687–691.
31. The Stroke Prevention in Atrial Fibrillation Investigators: Predictors of thromboembolism in atrial fibrillation: I. Clinical features of patients at risk. *Ann Intern Med* 1992, 116:1–5.
32. The Stroke Prevention in Atrial Fibrillation Investigators: Preditors of thromboembolism in atrial fibrillation: II. Echocardiographic features of patients at risk. *Ann Intern Med* 1992, 116:6–12.
33. Levine HJ, Pauker SG, Salzman EW, Eckman MH: Antithrombotic therapy in valvular heart disease. *Chest* 1992, 102(suppl):434S–444S.
34. Stein PD, Alpert JS, Copeland J, *et al.*: Antithrombotic therapy in patients with mechanical and biological prosthetic heart values. *Chest* 1992, 102(suppl):445S–455S.
35. Cairns JA, Hirsh J, Lewis HD Jr, *et al.*: Antithrombotic agents in coronary artery disease. *Chest* 1992, 102(suppl):456S–481S.
36. Cerebral Embolism Task Force: Cardiogenic brain embolism. *Arch Neurol* 1986, 43:71–84.
37. Okada Y, Yamaguchi T, Minematsu K, *et al.*: Hemorrhagic transformation in cerebral embolism. *Stroke* 1989, 20:598–603.
38. Cerebral Embolism Task Force: Cardiogenic brain embolism: the second report of the Cerebral Embolism Task Force. *Arch Neurol* 1989, 46:727–743.
39. Ogata J, Yutani C, Imakita M, *et al.*: Hemorrhagic infarct of the brain without a reopening of the occluded arteries in cardioembolic stroke. *Stroke* 1989, 20:876–883.
40. Toole JE, ed.: *Cerebrovascular Disorders.* New York: Raven Press; 1984.
41. Cerebral Embolism Study Group: Immediate anticoagulation of embolic stroke: a randomized trial. *Stroke* 1983, 14:668–676.
42. Rothrock JF, Dittrich HC, McAllen S, *et al.*: Acute anticoagulation of cardioembolic stroke and TIA. *Stroke* 1989, 20:734.
43. Sherman DG, Dyken ML Jr, Fisher M, *et al.*: Antithrombotic therapy for cerebrovascular disorders. *Chest* 1992, 102(suppl):529S–537S.
44. Antiplatelet Trialists Collaboration: Secondary prevention of vascular disease by prolonged antiplatelet treatment. *BMJ* 1990, 21:1122–1130.

45. Hass WK, Easton JD, Adams HP Jr, *et al.*: A randomized trial comparing ticlopidine hydrochloride with aspirin for the prevention of stroke in high-risk patients: Ticlopidine Study Aspirin Study Group. *N Engl J Med* 1989, 321:501–507.
46. Gent M, Blakely JA, Easton JD, *et al.*: The Canadian American Ticlopidine Study (CATS) in thromboembolic stroke. *Lancet* 1989:1215–1220.
47. North American Symptomatic Carotid Endarterectomy Trial Collaborators: Beneficial effect of carotid endarterectomy in symptomatic patients with high-grade carotid stenosis. *N Engl J Med* 1991, 325:445–453.
48. European Carotid Surgery Trialists' Collaborative Group: MRC European Carotid Surgery Trial: interim results for symptomatic patients with severe (70-99%) or with mild (0-29%) carotid stenosis. *Lancet* 1991, 337:1235–1243.
49. Biller J, Bruno A, Adams HP Jr, *et al.*: A randomized trial of aspirin or heparin in hospitalized patients with recent transient ischemic attacks. *Stroke* 1989, 20:441–447.
50. Duke RJ, Bloch RF, Turpie AG, *et al.*: Intravenous heparin for the prevention of stroke progression in acute partial stable stroke. *Ann Intern Med* 1986, 105:825–828.
51. Haley EC, Kassell NF, Torner JC: Failure of heparin to prevent progression in progressing ischemic infarction. *Stroke* 1988, 19:10–14.
52. Hachinski V, Norris JE: The deteriorating stroke. In *Cerebral Vascular Disease 3: Proceedings of the 10th Salzburg Conference.* Edited by Meyer JS, Lechner H, Reivich M, Ott EO, Aranibar A. Amsterdam: Excerpta Medica; 1981:315–318.
53. Powers WJ: Hemodynamics and metabolism in ischemic cerebrovascular disease. *Neurol Clin* 1992, 10:31–48.
54. Miller VT: Lacunar stroke, a reassessment. *Arch Neurol* 1983, 40:129–134.
55. Dobkin BH: Heparin for lacunar stroke in progression. *Stroke* 1983, 14:421–423.
56. Fisher CM: Lacunar strokes and infarcts: a review. *Neurology* 1982, 32:871–876.
57. Brey RL, Hart RG, Sherman DG, Tegeler CH: Antiphospholipid antibodies and cerebral ischemia in young people. *Neurology* 1990, 40:1190–1196.
58. Coull BM, Goodnight SH: Antiphospholipid antibodies, prothrombotic states, and stroke. *Stroke* 1990, 21:1370–1374.
59. Antiphospholipid Antibodies in Stroke Study Group (APASS): Antiphospholipid antibodies and cerebral ischemia: selected clinical and laboratory features. *Stroke* 1990, 21:1268–1273.
60. Hart RG, Easton JD: Dissections and trauma of cervicocerebral arteries. In *Stroke: Pathophysiology, Diagnosis and Management.* Edited by Barnett HJM, Stein BM, Mohr JP, Yatsu FM. New York: Churchill Livingstone; 1986:775–788.
61. Caplan LR, Stein RW: *Stroke: A Clinical Approach.* Boston: Butterworths; 1986:179–182.
62. Biller J, Adams HP Jr: Cerebrovascular disorders associated with pregnancy. *Am Fam Physic* 1986, 33:125–132.
63. Bousser MG, Chiras J, Boris J, *et al.*: Cerebral venous thrombosis: a review of 38 cases. *Stroke* 1985, 16:199–213.
64. Conrad J, Horellou MH, Samama MM: Congenital deficiency of antithrombin III and of heparin cofactor II. In *Clinical Thrombosis.* Edited by Kwaan HC, Samama MM. Boca Raton: CRC Press; 1989:235–241.
65. Green D: Protein C and protein S. In *Clinical Thrombosis.* Edited by Kwaan HC, Samama MM. Boca Raton:CRC Press; 1989:243–253.

Chapter 17

Novel Therapeutic Approaches to the Treatment of Ischemic Stroke and Transient Ischemic Attack

CATHY M. HELGASON

While new therapies are devised and tested for the treatment of acute ischemic stroke and transient ischemic attack (TIA), public and physician unfamiliarity with cerebrovascular disease remains a major challenge to this effort. Stroke is the third leading cause of death in the United States, and a major cause of long-term disability. A recent Gallup poll indicated that the majority of Americans remain unaware of the signs of impending stroke. Many physicians show a lack of rationale when caring for the stroke patient. Physicians continue to work in terms of the temporal evolution of symptoms and signs using the constructs of TIA, reversible ischemic neurologic deficit (RIND), completed stroke, and stroke in evolution as the basis for determination of diagnosis and treatment options. There is not, however, a direct correlation between symptoms or signs and degree of cerebral tissue injury from ischemia; synaptic silence will also cause symptoms. Rational treatment for any disease, stroke included, must be based on pathogenesis and pathophysiology [1]. For ischemic stroke, the aim of treatment is limitation of tissue damage and prevention of recurrence [2].

Ischemic stroke, as defined in this chapter, is due to local rather than global cerebral ischemia and localized to the vascular distribution of an occluded artery. It involves destruction of neurons, glia, and vascular elements [2]. Recent advances in basic neuroscience have led to an understanding of the mechanism of ischemic brain injury. This has allowed for the development of novel therapies for acute stroke based on the concepts of limitation of metabolic consequences of tissue ischemia, enhancement of tissue perfusion, and promotion of recovery from stroke [2]. New technologic advances in diagnosis have allowed for the identification of etiology and risk factors for the ischemic event so that preventive strategies specifically relate to pathogenesis. As a result of thorough investigation, stroke patients could have more than one potential source for thromboembolism or a combination of findings leading to new constructs in diagnosis and management. In view of the latter, as with any other symptom or sign with multiple potential etiologies, an exhaustive search for the most common causes must be made in each instance, instead of halting diagnostic procedures once one abnormality is found. This means using the most sensitive diagnostic techniques to detect vascular morphologic changes, systemic disease associated with stroke, cardiac sources for thromboembolism, and hypercoagulable states. Recent advances in technology for the coagulation laboratory, cardiac and vascular imaging, and functional physiology have made it possible to approach stroke treatment and prevention rationally, and tailor it to the individual patient.

PREVENTIVE STRATEGIES FOR RECURRENT STROKE

Atrial Fibrillation

Until recently, most preventive therapies for recurrent stroke have ignored pathogenesis. However, it is unlikely that one intervention could address all potential causes for cerebral ischemia, including thrombosis, embolism, or decreased perfusion. The first therapies designed specifically to prevent recurrent stroke by using pathophysiologic mechanisms are illustrated by those used for chronic nonvalvular atrial fibrillation (NVAF) and symptomatic carotid artery stenosis [3,4]. The Stroke Prevention in Atrial Fibrillation (SPAF) study was mainly a primary prevention trial. However, previous stroke, as long as it had occurred more than 2 years previously, was not an exclusion to patient participation. NVAF is a cardiogenic source for thromboembolism, although it may also be a marker for increased risk of ischemic stroke. The pathogenic mechanism of stroke in patients with atrial fibrillation is presumed to be an embolism of red thrombus (fibrin-erythrocyte rich), which forms in the left atrial appendage. While patients with chronic NVAF may develop red thrombi in their hearts, a large proportion will have concomitant mitral annulus calcification and aortic or carotid atheroma, which are potential sources for white thrombus (fibrin-platelet rich) formation. The effect of warfarin is to prevent red thrombus formation. The SPAF study, like its Danish counterpart, the Copenhagen AFASAK trial, tested the efficacy of two agents, warfarin or aspirin, which were expected to cover all potentially known mechanisms in these patients for thrombus formation (*ie*, red or white clot) [5]. In the SPAF, both aspirin and warfarin were found to be more effective than placebo for prevention of stroke or systemic embolism, but for those aged over 74 years, aspirin was less efficacious in reducing the risk of embolic stroke. Subgroups of patients were identified for increased embolic risk. How the clinical factors associated with increased stroke risk, *ie*, hypertension, previous thromboembolism, and recent congestive heart failure, relate to pathogenesis of systemic embolism in these patients is unclear [6,7].

Another platelet-dependent mechanism for thrombosis in patients with NVAF has been suggested by Helgason and coworkers [8] who discovered that some patients on warfarin have the previously unrecognized potential for medication failure due to the presence of hyperaggregable platelets. These authors also showed that those patients taking aspirin may not be on the biologicaly effective dosage needed to prevent aggregation of platelets [8]. The ongoing SPAF study innovatively addresses the issues of combined anticoagulant-antiplatelet therapy for stroke prevention in the population of patients at high risk for systemic embolism. Other trials that have addressed stroke prevention in patients with NVAF have compared warfarin with placebo and have confirmed the efficacy of the former. Only the Danish AFASAK study compared aspirin with placebo for prevention of systemic embolism. This study did not find aspirin to be effective [5]. However, aspirin was administered in a very low-dose regimen (75 mg/d).

Extracranial Carotid Atheroma

The North American Symptomatic Carotid Endarterectomy Trial (NASCET) addresses how to prevent stroke in the setting of internal carotid artery stenosis and absence of a cardiac source for embolism in patients with TIA and minor stroke [4]. Presumed mechanisms for ischemic stroke in this setting are arterial origin embolism or decreased perfusion. The NASCET will compare carotid endarterectomy and medical therapy or medical therapy alone in patients with 30% to 99% carotid stenosis as defined by cerebral angiography. Medical therapy includes the administration of aspirin. Both medical and surgical treatments are meant to eliminate the pathogenic source for future thromboembolic stroke. The NASCET did not study the role of endarterectomy when carotid stenosis is measured by other methodology such as magnetic resonance angiography or carotid duplex [9]. Surgical method is not dictated by protocol and the role of new surgical methods such as microendarterectomy, where endarterectomy is done with illumination and magnification of the operating microscope, remains undefined [10]. Early data from the NASCET study confirm the superiority of carotid endarterectomy over medical therapy alone for patients with high-grade (77%–99%) symptomatic extracranial carotid artery stenosis. The NASCET study continues to evaluate the role of surgery versus medical therapy for symptomatic carotid stenosis of 30% to 69%.

PREVENTION OF THROMBOEMBOLIC STROKE

Antithrombotic Therapy

Most trials of antithrombotic therapy for the prevention of recurrent stroke have not been based on a thorough analysis of the pathogenic risk for stroke recurrence. When this is done, aspirin or other substances that affect platelet function would be prescribed for prevention of white clot and anticoagulants would be administered for the prevention of red clot [1]. Arterial origin emboli may be composed of cholesterol, calcium, atheromatous plaque debris, red thrombi, or white thrombi. Red thrombi form in areas of tight stenosis or stagnation where there is reduced flow, and white thrombi form on irregular arterial surfaces exposed to moving arterial streams. Red thrombi can form over white thrombi. Cardiac origin emboli may also be composed of red thrombus, calcium, tumor, or infectious material. The significance of platelet-fibrin (white) clot in this setting is unclear. The ongoing National Institutes of Health (NIH)–funded Warfarin Aspirin Recurrent Stroke Study (WARSS) may lead to some conclusions regarding the efficacy of this approach. The significance of the findings of this trial will depend on the accuracy of patient diagnosis with regard to pathogenesis.

Unlike warfarin, the biologic effect of aspirin will not be measured in the WARSS trial. The optimal intensity of oral anticoagulant therapy by which INR-specific incidence rates of events are calculated will not be used [11]. Without assurance of the optimum biologic effect of either aspirin or warfarin, it may be that neither drug is tested at its optimum dose for efficacy. This dose may depend not only on the individual, but on the pathogenic mechanism. Apart from the dosage of warfarin used to prevent different types of cardiogenic embolism, nothing is currently known regarding the optimum intensity of warfarin or aspirin with regard to stroke mechanism [12]. Conclusions, therefore, regarding the usefulness of aspirin or warfarin in particular subtypes of stroke may be valid only for those doses of each agent used in the trial.

Although most antiplatelet trials for prevention of recurrent stroke have not specifically addressed pathogenesis or biologic effect there have been other innovations. These are twofold in type. On the one hand, new antiplatelet agents have been developed according to the knowledge of how white thrombi form and how platelets participate in thrombus formation. On the other hand, new technology allows measurement of the biologic effect of these agents. Ticlopidine inhibits ADP-stimulated platelet aggregation and may be effective under the special circumstances of platelet aggregation where the von Willebrand factor serves as a ligand and there is high shear flow. It does not inhibit cyclooxygenase-dependent pathways of platelet aggregation. It may inhibit platelet release reaction and platelet adhesion [13]. Clopidogrel, a new antiplatelet agent and a more potent ticlopidine analogue, is currently being compared with aspirin for recurrent stroke prevention. Unfortunately, a thorough, prospective, systematic attempt to categorize stroke type by mechanism is not attempted in these trials. It is tantalizing to speculate that ticlopidine or clopidogrel could be effective where thrombosis occurs in smaller intracranial vessels, where high shear stress exists and where aspirin used in low doses may not prevent platelet aggregation induced by shear stress. It is possible to measure shear-induced platelet aggregation as well as platelet aggregation dependent on cyclooxygenase or dependent on other mechanisms. The efficacy of antiplatelet agents has not been assessed in any large trial with a view to dosing for efficacy.

Combination therapy with antiplatelet agents that work by different mechanisms has been tried. The European Stroke Prevention Study (ESPS) [14] seeks to prevent thromboembolic stroke not only using aspirin that inhibits cyclooxygenase-dependent platelet aggregation, but also by using dipyridamole, a phosphodiesterase inhibitor, which counteracts platelet activation at the platelet-endothelial interface through endothelial-derived prostacyclin. In this study [14], aspirin and dipyridamole are given together and compared with placebo to prevent recurrent stroke. Combination therapy may achieve a potential additive effect against recurrent stroke. However, previous studies that have compared aspirin and dipyridamole with aspirin alone did not show an additive effect for recurrent stroke prevention.

Whether trials for stroke prevention of other antiplatelet agents that block GPIIb/IIIa receptors (monoclonal antibodies), thromboxane synthetase inhibitors (dazoxiben and pirmagrel), inhibitors of thromboxane and endoperoxide receptors, or φ-3 fatty acids will be mounted has yet to be seen [13]. Clinical investigation of prostacyclin analogues (iloprost and ciprostene, inhibitors of platelet activation) for stroke prevention may be mounted if precursor trials for prevention and treatment of coronary artery disease show promise [13]. Finally, platelet-derived growth factor inhibitors (trapidil) lower cholesterol, cause vasodilation, and inhibit smooth muscle cell and fibroblast proliferation. Such agents may prove effective in prevention of atherothrombotic stroke.

A potentially more sensitive and innovative approach to antiplatelet therapy for stroke prevention entails measuring a desired biologic effect and dosing the antiplatelet agent appropriately towards that end. The Swedish Aspirin Low Dose Trial (SALT) used low-dose aspirin, 40 mg/day, and documented the one-time effect of this dose on thromboxane B_2 levels [15]. Aspirin, however, was not purposefully dosed by protocol to achieve a particular and constant effect on thromboxane B_2 levels. Low-dose aspirin theoretically has a shorter lasting effect on vascular wall cyclooxygenase than on that of platelets, and thus may preserve vascular prostacyclin, a vasodilator and platelet antiaggregant, but inhibit platelet thromboxane B_2 production. Prostacyclin metabolites were measured by Toghi and coworkers [16] in order to gauge aspirin effect on vascular wall cyclooxygenase. A dose-dependent effect was found. Helgason and coworkers [17] in a pilot study administered aspirin in patients with stroke who were taking aspirin for recurrent stroke prevention to achieve the antithrombotic effect of inhibition of platelet aggregation. By this method, it was found that each individual requires a different dose of aspirin and that some individuals are aspirin-resistant. Preliminary results of the same trial suggest that the same individual may become resistant to the effect of a particular dose of aspirin over time [18]. Ultimately, as with warfarin, it may be that the desired antiplatelet effect must be achieved in order to counteract a certain pathogenic mechanism and that this effect must be monitored and dosage adjusted over time (Table 17.1)

Finally, it is currently being recognized that there is a uniform principle of pathogenesis of stroke for the carotid and vertebrobasilar cerebrovascular territories. Caplan [19] suggested that the double standard for vertebrobasilar disease be dropped and that the same potential etiologies, thoroughness of evaluation, and specific pathogenesis-related treatments that are applied to the carotid circulation be sought in patients with symptomatic ischemia in this vascular territory.

The advent of newer technologies such as transesophageal echocardiography and ultrafast computed tomography of the heart allows for the detection of cardiac pathologies associated with thromboembolism. The identification of left atrial stroke, atrial septal aneurysm, patent foramen ovale, or aortic arch plaque by transesophageal echocardiography is an example. The need for antiplatelet or other antithrombotic therapy is not well understood for these and other identifiable pathologies such as intracardiac thrombus, wall dyskinesis, or akinesis. Randomized trials are needed and newer technologies may help to show disappearance of active thrombus formation, embolism, or define the nature of the thrombus. These include indium platelet or other scintigraphy, and carotid or transcranial Doppler.

SURGICAL THERAPY FOR PREVENTION OF ARTERIAL THROMBOEMBOLISM

Surgical approaches other than carotid endarterectomy may apply in prevention of recurrent stroke. Despite the failure of the Extracranial Intracranial Arterial Bypass Trial (EC-ICA Bypass Trial) to demonstrate efficacy of superficial temporal to middle cerebral artery bypass in preventing stroke in patients with symptomatic carotid territory ischemia, articles continue to appear claiming efficacy of this procedure in subgroups of patients defined by various pathophysiologic parameters such as collateral circulation, quantitation of cerebrovascular reactivity, and global and regional cerebral blood flow [20]. Direct endarterectomy of the middle cerebral artery to prevent recurrent hemispheric ischemia is a treatment less well defined for middle cerebral artery high-grade stenosis due to atheromatous disease [21]. Reconstruction of the internal carotid artery at the skull base with saphenous vein graft where the petrous or cavernous portion of the artery has been injured or involved by various pathologic processes (tumor, aneurysm) may avoid the necessity for arterial ligation and cerebral ischemic complications [22]. Surgical bypass, as well as endarterectomy, may be applied to the vertebrobasilar system [23]. Vertebral artery reconstruction may be performed in its proximal portion via transubclavian endarterectomy or open endarterectomy. Transposition into the common carotid artery or subclavian may be done. Reconstruction of the distal cervical vertebral artery may be done through bypass, transposition, or decompression. Selective vertebral endarterectomy has also been performed for the treatment of stenotic lesions of the third and fourth portions of the vertebral artery [19,24].

Balloon angioplasty may be applied to symptomatic atheromatous cerebrovascular stenosis of the extracranial or intracranial carotid or vertebrobasilar circulation as well as to fibromuscular dysplasia of these arteries [25–34]. This technique may be best applied for prevention of recurrent stroke where the arterial stenosis is smooth and where brain single photon emission tomography (SPECT) with diamox identifies a critical reduction in perfusion [35]. Angioplasty of a stenotic collateral vessel may lead to neurologic improvement [34]. A microballoon technique may be feasible for use in small intracranial vessels. Laser angioplasty may prove effective when there is nonstenotic, ulcerated atheroma because this technique avoids the potential complications of balloon angioplasty—embolization and intimal splitting [36–38].

Table 17.1. Principles underlying the use of antiplatelet agents for recurrent stroke prevention

Previous studies have for the most part disregarded pathogenesis and dose-related biologic effects
Recent studies such as the SPAF [3] study have shown efficacy based on pathogenesis
Other studies—dose and individual-related biologic effect of aspirin
Future studies must address biologic effect appropriate to pathogenesis for efficacy [12]

SPAF—Stroke Prevention in Atrial Fibrillation.

TREATMENT OF ACUTE ISCHEMIC STROKE

Based on knowledge of the mechanism of ischemic brain tissue damage, once symptoms or signs have begun, the approach to treatment may be threefold: 1) interruption of the metabolic and tissue damaging consequences of ischemia; 2) increasing perfusion (interrupting "ischemia") to cerebral tissue; and 3) promotion of functional recovery after brain infarction. These therapies must be used in conjunction with vigilant prevention and treatment of the most common complications of stroke such as aspiration, urosepsis, decubiti, and deep venous thrombosis with subsequent pulmonary embolism. One, a combination, or all of these therapies may be appropriate for any given individual patient.

Repair after Brain Infarction

The most dramatic approach to enhancing recovery of ischemic or infarcted brain tissue is transplantation. Grabowski and coworkers [39] have shown that fetal cortical cells when placed in infarcted rat brain tissue survive, receive fiber input from other brain regions, and respond to somatosensory stimuli from the environment. The behavioral implications of improvement in neurologic function after fetal cell transplant into infarcted brain of human survivors of stroke remain untested. Such functional behavior in laboratory animals appears to be related to vascularization (capillarization) and the production of trophic factors [39,40].

Increased Perfusion to Ischemic Brain

There are medical and surgical approaches that aim to improve cerebral blood flow. These approaches are based on the premise that the ischemic penumbra will be salvaged and the ultimate size of brain infarction will be smaller. Therapies for the reestablishment of flow in ischemic cerebral tissue entail limitation of vascular thrombosis, prevention of immediate and ongoing recurrent thromboembolism, and the anatomic or rheologic preservation of cerebral blood flow. These therapies all are currently investigational.

Limitation of Vascular Thrombosis and Recurrent Thromboembolism

Trials of antithrombotic agents in acute stroke may suffer from the same lack of precise definition of pathophysiologic mechanisms and thrombus-dependent mechanisms. While aspirin has been shown to decrease the risk of recurrent cerebral infarct in patients with TIA or minor stroke, it has not been shown that administration of an antiplatelet agent during the acute phase (first 7 days) of cerebral infarction is effective towards this end nor towards the end of enhancing tissue perfusion [41]. Likewise, although administration of an anticoagulant such as heparin may be safe, its efficacy has not been established [42]. In a small series reported by Pessin and coworkers [43], it appeared that administration of heparin during the acute and subacute phase after stroke may be safely continued in some patients despite hemorrhagic transformation of infarction. This may be justified in the setting of high risk of recurrent thromboembolism. Heparin has several problems, however. These include a variability in dose response and resistance due to its binding to proteins other than antithrombin III (AT III), endothelial cells, macrophages, and platelets. It can inhibit platelet function and this may contribute to some hemorrhagic complications [44]. Heparin, however, carries not only the risk of hemorrhage but the risk of heparin-induced thrombocytopenia. Heparin-AT III has little or no effect on thrombin bound to fibrin and factor Xa bound in the prothrombinase complex on the platelet surface [44]. As an alternative to heparin, low molecular weight heparinoids have been devised and offer some advantage. Low molecular weight heparinoids bind less to platelets, plasma proteins, and endothelial cells. Thus, they have a more predictable dose response, dose-independent mechanism of clearance, longer plasma half-life, and fewer hemorrhagic complications than heparin for equivalent antithrombotic effect [44]. The current low molecular weight heparinoid trial of ORG10172 in acute stroke (TOAST study [45]) compares placebo with ORG10172 for determination of outcome in the first 7 days after acute stroke. Preliminary study supports the safety and efficacy of this agent in the acute ischemic stroke setting [45]. Some studies, however, suggest that thrombocytopenia may persist in patients with heparin-induced thrombocytopenia receiving low molecular weight heparinoid due to cross immunoreactivity of these two drugs [46–48]. Thus, the safety of the low molecular weight heparinoid in all patients who have the potential for heparin-induced thrombocytopenia such as in those with previous heparin exposure is uncertain.

In a unique attempt to decrease recurrent thromboembolism in patients with recent frequent TIA, prolonged englobulinlysis time (ELT), and elevated spontaneous platelet aggregation, Vinazzer [49,50] tested oral prophylaxis with pentosan polysulfate (PPS), a low molecular weight heparinoid. Prophylaxis with PPS shortened the ELT. In another cohort of patients with recurrent TIA and hypercoagulable state manifest by diminished tissue plasminogen activator (tPA) and increased platelet aggregation, those patients who received aspirin had 30% fewer vascular occlusions. Those who received PPS alone had 50% fewer vascular occlusions, and when both PPS and ASA were given together, there were 67% fewer vascular occlusive events. Vinazzer [49,50] presumed that PPS enhanced fibrinolysis in most patients by increasing tPA.

Combination antiplatelet-anticoagulant therapy offers an alternative to traditional antithrombotic treatment. Recently aspirin and heparin, when used in combination, were shown to halt the progression of acute carotid thrombosis [51]. The role of other new antithrombotic agents in the ischemic stroke setting has not yet been studied. These agents are the new AT III–independent thrombin inhibitors and the AT III–independent factor Xa inhibitors. The former are hirudin and hirulog. The latter is a tick anticoagulant protein. These agents show improved antithrombotic effects on experimental models of thrombosis [13].

Ancrod is a rapidly acting defibrinogenating agent derived from the Malayan pit viper that does not cause immune thrombocytopenia and is immunologically distinct from heparin. Ancrod may have some fibrinolytic potential as well. A recent pilot study of ancrod for acute stroke showed a trend towards efficacy and safety. Resistance to ancrod has been reported and is believed to be due to prior exposure and the presence of antiancrod antibodies. The safety and dosage of ancrod is monitored and titrated during intravenous therapy by achieving an optimal therapeutic concentration of serum fibrinogen [52–55].

While the use of antithrombotic agents for acute stroke has been predicated on the assumption that such therapy will prevent propagation of thrombosis, prevention of recurrent thromboembolism may also be important in ultimate clinical outcome. Some patients enrolled in the low molecular weight heparinoid and ancrod studies may be shown to harbor intracardiac thrombi. Yasaka and Yamaguchi [56] assessed the effect of immediate anticoagulation on intracardiac thrombus formation by serial two dimensional echocardiography in patients with acute cardioembolic stroke. After 14 days of intravenous heparin therapy, oral warfarin therapy was commenced [56]. Though this study was not randomized, recurrence or enlargement of intracardiac thrombi was not detected in those patients who received anticoagulant therapy, but was, as was systemic embolism recurrence, detected in those who did not receive anticoagulation. It is hoped that the efficacy of ancrod or ORG10172 in the setting of acute stroke with intracardiac thrombus will be studied. However, the number of such patients may be too small to draw substantial conclusions.

The role of surgical procedures such as emergency carotid endarterectomy or thromboendarterectomy to limit vascular thrombosis and embolism in the acute stroke setting is unclear at this time [57–59].

Reinstitution of Blood Flow to Cerebral Tissue

Thrombolysis with fibrinolytic agents streptokinase, recombinant tissue plasminogen activator (rtPA), urokinase, or acetylated plasminogen streptokinase activator complex (APSAC) may proceed with reconstitution of cerebral blood flow (CBF) to ischemic tissue [60–62]. Fibrinolytic drugs may be given intravenously or intra-arterially at the site of vascular thrombotic occlusion and their effect measured by angiographically demonstrable disappearance of thrombus and by clinical outcome or infarct size on neuroimaging. The intra-arterial route is accomplished by regional perfusion or local infusion. The intra-arterial route is associated with a high frequency of vascular recanalization. With intravenous administration, early intervention is more likely to result in vascular patency. Overgaard and coworkers [63] have shown a correlation between cerebral reperfusion as measured by SPECT, angiographic arterial patency after intravenous rtPA, and improved clinical outcome, even in those with severe initial clinical and reional CBF deficit when treated within 6 hours of symptom onset. Patients with severe neurologic deficit, however, are frequently excluded from acute stroke trials. Yamaguchi and coworkers [64] showed that early reperfusion after administration of rtPA within 6 hours of symptom onset of embolic stroke led to arterial reperfusion as defined by postinfusion angiography, improved clinical outcome, and absence of hemorrhagic transformation of the cerebral infarct [65].

Problems concerning hemorrhagic transformation after the use of fibrinolytic agents remain unresolved [66,67]. Hemorrhagic transformation does not always have a clinical correlate and appears to be more common when thrombolytic therapy is administered after a delay of greater than 6 hours poststroke onset or from collateral arterial sources. Parenchymatous hemorrhage often occurs at a site distant from the infarct and is more frequently associated with clinical deterioration. Parenchymatous hemorrhage may be related to dosage. Likewise, the microvascular response to reperfusion and the role of reperfusion injury and reperfusion edema that may affect clinical outcome remain undefined [68]. How or whether distal embolization of thrombus affects clinical outcome is unknown. There is some evidence that different thrombolytic agents or routes of administration may affect recanalization depending on thrombus source, size, and arterial territory.

While recanalization and clinical improvement have been documented, no prospective, controlled trial by intra-arterial infusion fibrinolysis has been undertaken in patients with acute ischemic stroke. After intravenous fibrinolysis, the presence of established patent collaterals on entry cerebral angiogram is suggested to affect neurologic outcome. Although data regarding recanalization after the intra-arterial administration of fibrinolytic agents are available for both the carotid and vertebrobasilar territories, little experience exists with intravenous fibrinolysis in the vertebrobasilar territory for either recanalization or clinical outcome. Many arterial occlusions undergo spontaneous thrombolysis with distal embolization. Current ongoing trials of the use of thrombolytic agents in acute stroke will better define their role in improving not only immediate but long-term clinical outcome. So far, no preference for the intra-arterial or intravenous administration of one thrombolytic agent over another can be stated for use in acute stroke [69]. The use of adjunctive mechanical manipulation of the thrombus, with agents such as α-2–antiplasmin monoclonal antibodies, monoclonal antibodies to platelet GIIb/IIIa receptor, or other antiplatelet or antithrombotic agents such as clopidogrel, SR46349 (a novel 5-HT2 antagonist), heparin, low molecular weight heparinoid, or hirudin are undefined [70]. Shock wave or ultrasound-assisted thrombus ablation has not yet been tried in the setting of ischemic stroke [71].

Clinical studies have not shown hypervolemic or normovolemic hemodilution to be effective for the treatment of acute stroke [72–77]. Questions still remain about methodology. Koltringer and coworkers [74] point out that the application time of this therapy may not have been sufficient to show efficacy due to the occurrence of transient potentially deleterious changes in hemorrheologic parameters such as viscoelasticity. Others have emphasized the hemodilution regimen and need for individualization of therapy to explain failures of hemodilution trials. These latter emphasize rehydration with crystalloids rather than viscosity reduction and long-acting hemodilution with albumin. Therapy as it is individualized is guided on the basis of pulmonary capillary wedge pressure [75].

Other methods to improve regional CBF under the setting of acute stroke may include angioplasty, emergency thromboendarterectomy of the extracranial internal carotid artery, and embolectomy of the middle cerebral artery. Narrow therapeutic windows probably will apply to the use of these methods. In addition, definition of collateral flow, CBF reserve, cerebral perfusion, and oxygen consumption would possibly better define those individuals in whom these or other medical methods for cerebral reperfusion will be efficacious [35,78].

Limitation of the Metabolic and Tissue Damaging Consequences of Ischemia

The aforementioned treatments are aimed at improving CBF or limiting progression of its compromise. While the ultimate goal of these methods is to limit tissue damage, they may need to be used in conjunction with therapies aimed at interruption of the metabolic consequences of the ischemia [79]. The first step in cerebral tissue ischemic injury is depolarization and presynaptic release of excitatory amino acids followed by dysfunction of ion-exchange pumps in the postsynaptic cell membrane. The latter results in a shift of sodium and calcium ions from the extracellular fluid to the intracellular fluid space. Cytotoxic edema occurs early. There is also intracellular accumulation of inositol-1-4-5-triphosphate and diacylglycerol. Following this induction phase, calcium is released from intracellular storage pools of the neuron and there is spread of excitation to other neurons. There is an enhancement of excitatory synaptic efficacy coupled with excitatory amino acid receptor stimulation. This is the amplification stage. This in turn triggers the expression stage where generation of free radicals, destruction of lipids, nuclei, acids, and protein, and the production of vasoactive substances from arachidonic acid ensue. The latter include platelet-activating factor (PAF) and eicosanoid. At the induction stage of cytotoxic edema and excess intracellular calcium, neurons become synaptically silent. At this stage the patient may be symptomatic but the neurons have not undergone irreversible structural damage. All stages of the final ischemic cascade may theoretically be addressed by therapeutic intervention [2].

Treatments may be aimed at inhibition of presynaptic release of excitatory amino acids either by altering its presynaptic synthesis or by acting on presynaptic receptors that modify calcium entry or intrasynaptic calcium release, thus altering the capacity of depolarization to release glutamate. Glutamate or excitatory amino acid clearance from the synaptic cleft may be enhanced. Postsynaptic action at excitatory amino acid receptor sites may be accomplished by interruption of glutamate receptors (such as the *N*-methyl-D-aspartate [NMDA] receptor), AMPA/kainate receptors, and quisgualate metabotrophic receptors. Events secondary to receptor activation may be targeted such as voltage-gated calcium pumps. Free radical scavengers or lipoxygenases may act at the late expression stage. These include drugs acting on the arachidonic acid cascade (Figure 17.1).

Antagonists of the glutamate receptors currently are the subject of phase I trials [80,81]. These include trials of MK-801, dextrorphan, dextromethorphan, and ketamine [82,83]. However, the potential psychomimetic properties of NMDA noncompetitive antagonists that act on the phencyclidine receptor and the potential for interference with normal NMDA-receptor function, such as long-term potentiation that would interfere with new memory formation and depression of cortical activity through blockage of fast excitatory neurotransmission, may impair the utility of these agents for the treatment of acute ischemic stroke. In addition, neurocytopathologic changes in medium- and large-sized neurons and lytic degradation of mitochondria have been described. This has been described in the limbic system, cingulate gyrus, and hippocampus and may be responsible for the psychotic side effects of these drugs. Neuroprotective effects of nitrous oxide (NO) may result from down regulation of NMDA-receptor activity by reactions with thiol groups of the receptor redox modulatory site. Nitroglycerine is an NO-generating compound that leads to a decrease in NMDA-receptor toxicity. Trials of nitroglycerin have not yet been contemplated for acute ischemic stroke. Nitric oxide itself may be neurotoxic depending on its redox state [84]. Drugs acting at other sites of the NMDA receptor are being considered for trial in cerebroprotection [2,83].

Non-NMDA excitatory amino acid receptor antagonists that include kainate, AMPA, and metabotropic antagonists such as the quinoxaline dione analogue NBQX[2-3,dihydroxy-6-nitro-7-sulfamoylbenzo(F)quinoxaline] may be candidates for use with NMDA-receptor antagonists [83]. To date, nimodipine is the only calcium channel blocker shown to be effective in reducing the incidence of cerebral ischemias, and this is in association with subarachnoid hemorrhage [85]. It is not certain whether this effect is due to metabolic protection or vasodilatation. Clinical trials of nimodipine for acute ischemic stroke treatment may not have used appropriate therapeutic windows. Antioxidant or antioxygen radical therapy is aimed toward reducing injury to lipids, proteins, and nucleic acids in the expression phase of ischemia. The 21 amino steroids are currently undergoing phase

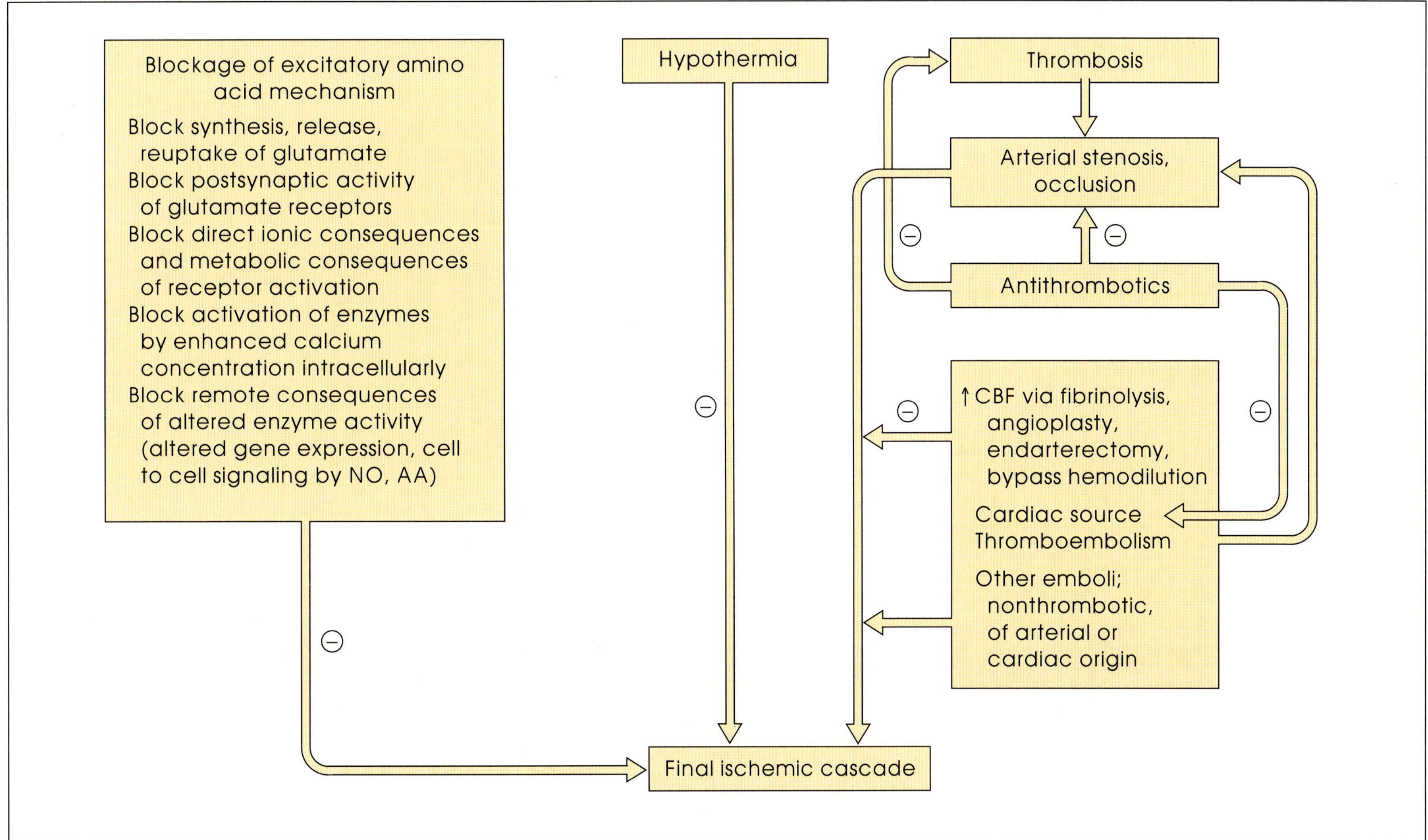

FIGURE 17.1

Drugs and therapies acting on the final ischemic cascade. AA—arachidonic acid; CBF—cerebral blood flow; NO—nitrous oxide.

I trials. Selective blockade of the prolonged action of glutamate at its receptor or "receptor dependent abuse–dependent toxicity" may be affected by gangliosides [81,83]. GMI monosialoganglioside is one such drug [86,87]. The exact mechanism of PAF in causing injury during cerebral ischemia needs to be tested. Inhibition of PAF may be linked to inhibition of phospholipase A2, improved microcirculation, reduced edema, and improved blood-brain barrier integrity [88]. Randomized double-blinded studies will be needed to assess the use of these and other therapies aimed at interrupting the final metabolic consequences of ischemia.

Hypothermia may interrupt the final ischemic cascade. There is some evidence that excitatory mechanisms of cerebral injury are interrupted during its use. A short window and difficulties in measuring brain temperature noninvasively may alter the feasibility of this treatment. Therapies designed to limit elevation in brain temperature may prove to have an effect on limiting brain damage from ischemia [89]. Anecdotal benefit of lowering core temperature in patients with multiple sclerosis by use of a body vest suggests that this might be tried for the stroke patient.

Recent studies of cerebral ischemia indicate a role for endogenous interleukin-1 [90]. Lipocortin-1 is a neuroprotective agent that under experimental conditions has been shown to halt neuronal death induced by middle cerebral artery occlusion. Lipocortin-1 is an endogenous calcium and phospholipid binding protein. Interleukin-1 is a cytokine involved in neuroimmune reactions in the brain. More research in this area may open new avenues for neuroprotection during cerebral ischemia [90].

CONCLUSIONS

The treatment of acute ischemic stroke or impending stroke consists of halting ischemic destruction set in motion and preventing recurrence (Figure 17.2). In each instance, understanding the etiology of the stroke will be important so that therapies may specifically address pathogenic mechanisms. A

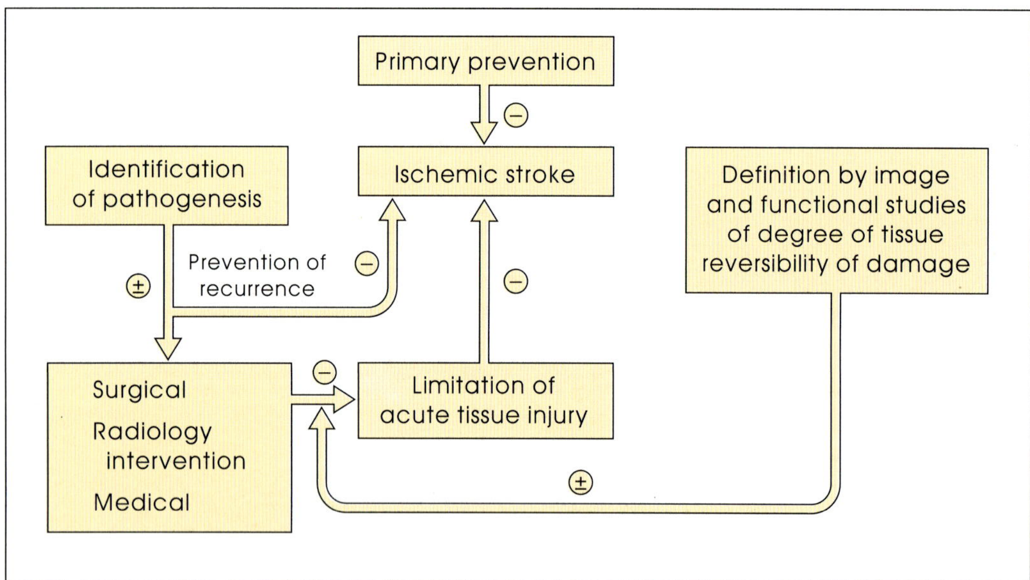

FIGURE 17.2

Scheme for the treatment of cerebral ischemia.

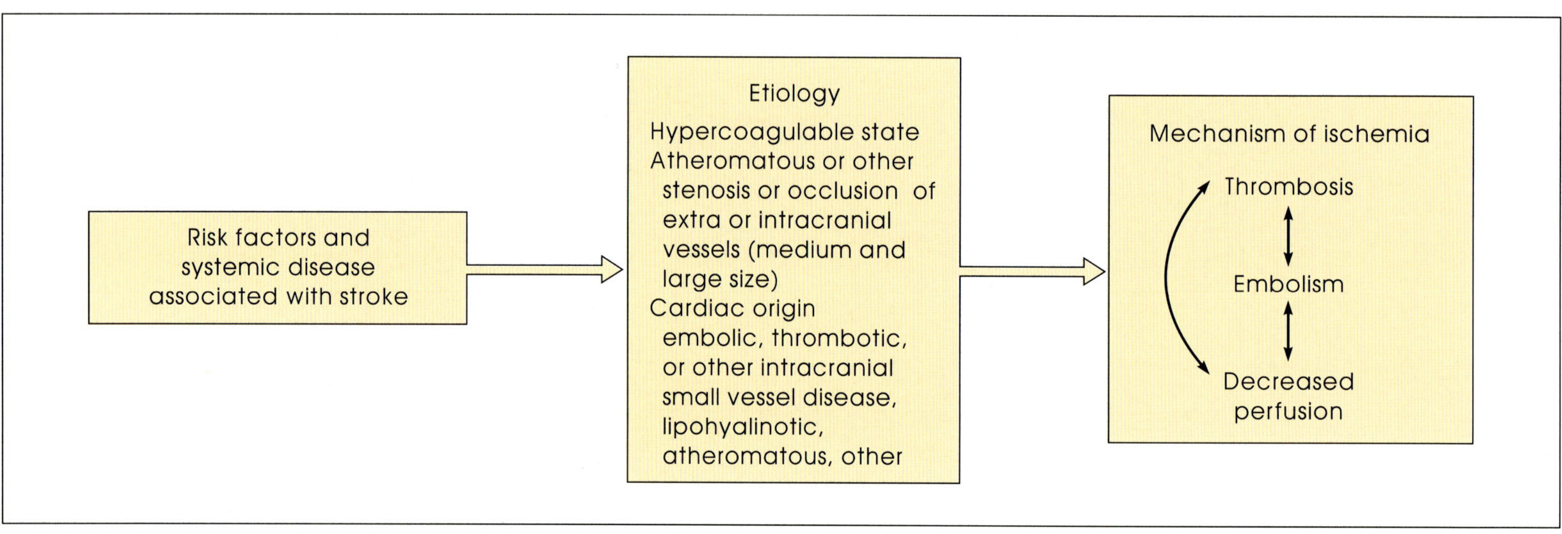

FIGURE 17.3

Scheme for the mechanism, etiology, and risk factors for stroke.

common ischemic metabolic pathway of damage may apply, and if so, treatment to limit injury may be instigated before other strategies of prevention for immediate recurrence are applied (Figure 17.3). The need to prevent immediate reoccurrence emphasizes the rapid but thorough identification of pathogenic mechanisms in each individual. While stroke outcome may ultimately be measured by neurologic deficit and infarct size when acute therapy is judged in terms of limitation of tissue damage, outcome and recurrence will also depend on the efficacy of prevention of the acute complications of stroke and a meticulous search for the pathogenic mechanism and etiology. New and better technologies will define not only the pathogenesis but also identify the state and amount of salvageable cerebral tissue at the time of stroke [35,78,91–97]. Finally, it may be ultimately possible to custom tailor therapeutic intervention to the individual both for prevention of recurrence and during the acute phase of cerebral injury. Such custom tailoring would be based on ischemic mechanism, as well as stage of injury.

REFERENCES

1. Caplan LR: *Stroke. A Clinical Approach.* Second Edition. Boston: Butterworth-Heineman.
2. Ginsberg MD: Emerging strategies for the treatment of ischemic brain injury. *The Molecular and Cellular Approaches to the Treatment of Neurological Diseases.* Edited by SG Waxman. New York: Raven Press, Ltd.; 1993:207–237.
3. Stroke Prevention in Atrial Fibrillation Investigators: Stroke Prevention in Atrial Fibrillation study—final results. *Circulation* 1991, 84:527–539.
4. North American Symptomatic Carotid Endarterectomy Trial (NASCET) Collaborators: Beneficial effects of carotid endarterectomy in symptomatic patients with high grade carotid stenosis. *N Engl J Med* 1991, 325:445–453.
5. Peterson P, Boysen G, Godfredsen J: Placebo controlled randomized trial of warfarin and aspirin for prevention of thromboembolic complications in chronic atrial fibrillation: The Copenhagen AFASAK study. *Lancet* 1989, 1:175–179.
6. The Stroke Prevention in Atrial Fibrillation Investigators: Predictors of thromboembolism in atrial fibrillation: I. Clinical features of patients at risk. *Ann Intern Med* 1992, 116:1–5.
7. The Stroke Prevention in Atrial Fibrillation Investigators: Predictors of thromboembolism in atrial fibrillation: I. Echocardiographic features of patients at risk. *Ann Intern Med* 1992, 116:6–12.
8. Helgason CM, Hoff JA, Kondos GT, Brace LD: Platelet aggregation in patients with atrial fibrillation taking aspirin or warfarin. *Stroke* 1993, 24:1458–1462.
9. Alexandrov AV, Blandin CF, Maggiasano R, Norris JW: Measuring carotid stenosis: time for a reappraisal. *Stroke* 1993, 24:1292–1296.
10. Findlay JM, Lougheed WM: Carotid microendarterectomy. *Neurosurgery* 1993, 32:792–798.
11. Rosendaal FR, Cannegieter SC, Van der neer FJM, Briet E: A method to determine the optimal intensity of oral anticoagulant therapy. *Thromb Haemost* 1993, 69:236–239.
12. Poller L, Hirsh J: Optimal therapeutic ranges for oral anticoagulation. In *Thrombosis in Cerebrovascular Diseases.* Edited by V Fuster, M Verstraete. Philadelphia: WB Saunders; 1992:161–173.
13. Becker RC: Antiplatelet therapy in coronary heart disease: emerging strategies for the treatment and prevention of acute myocardial infarction. *Arch Pathol Lab Med* 1993, 117:89–96.
14. ESPS Group: European stroke prevention study. *Stroke* 1990, 21:1122–1130.
15. The SALT Collaborative Group: Swedish aspirin low-dose trial (SALT) of 75 mg aspirin as secondary prophylaxis after cerebrovascular ischemic events. *Lancet* 1991, 338:1345–1349.
16. Toghi H, Konno S, Tamura K, Kimura B, Kawano K: Effects of low to high doses of aspirin on platelet aggregability and metabolites of thromboxane A_2 and prostacyclin. *Stroke* 1992, 23:1400–1404.
17. Helgason CM, Tortice KL, Winkler SR, *et al.*: Aspirin response and failure in cerebral infarction. *Stroke* 1993, 24:345–350.
18. Helgason CM, Hoff JA, Winkler SR, Brace LD: Increased dosage requirement and development of aspirin resistance over time in patients with previous stroke [abstract]. *Stroke* 1994, 25:in press.
19. Caplan LR: Vertebrobasilar disease: should we continue the double standard of patients with brain ischemia? *Heart Dis Stroke* 1993, 2:377–381.
20. Anderson DE, McLane MP, Reichman OH, Origitano TC: Improved cerebral blood flow and CO_2 reactivity after microvascular anastomosis in patients at high risk for recurrent stroke. *Neurosurgery* 1992, 31:26–34.
21. de los Reyes RA, Bederson JB, Germano IM: Direct endarterectomy of the middle cerebral artery for treatment of symptomatic stenosis: case report. *Neurosurgery* 1993, 32:464–468.
22. Sen C, Sekhar LN: Direct vein graft reconstruction of the cavernous, petrous, and upper cervical internal carotid artery: lessons learned from 30 cases. *Neurosurgery* 1992, 30:732–743.
23. Diaz FG, Ausman JI: Cerebral revascularization of the vertebrobasilar circulation. In *Vertebrobasilar Arterial Disease.* Edited by R Berguer, LR Caplan. St. Louis: Quality Medical Publishing, Inc.; 1992:290–291.
24. Berguer R, Caplan LR, eds: *Vertebrobasilar Arterial Disease.* St. Louis: Quality Medical Publishers, Inc.; 1992.
25. Konishi Y, Maemura E, Shiota M, *et al.*: Treatment of vasospasm by balloon angioplasty: experimental studies and clinical experiences. *Neurol Res* 1992, 14:271–279.
26. Brown MM: Balloon angioplasty in cerebrovascular disease. *Neurol Res* 1992, 14:159–163.
27. Lewis DH, Eskridge JM, Newell DM, *et al.*: Brain SPECT and the effect of cerebral angioplasty in delayed ischemia due to vasospasm. *J Nucl Med* 1992, 33:1789–1796.
28. Yamamoto Y, Smith RR, Bernanke DH: Mechanism of action of balloon angioplasty in cerebral vasospasm. *Neurosurgery* 1992, 30:1–6.
29. Theron J, Courtheoux P, Alachkar F, *et al.*: New triple coaxial catheter system for carotid angioplasty with cerebral protection. *AJNR* 1990, 11:869–874.
30. Ahuja A, Guterman LR, Hopkins LN: Angioplasty for basilar artery atherosclerosis. *J Neurosurg* 1992, 77:941–944.
31. Terada T, Nakamura Y, Yoshida N, *et al.*: Percutaneous transluminal angioplasty for the M_2 portion vasospasm following SAH: development of the new microballoon and report of cases. *Surg Neurol* 1993, 39:13–17.
32. Rostomily RC, Mayberg MR, Eskridge JM, *et al.*: Resolution of petrous internal carotid artery stenosis after transluminal angioplasty. *J Neurosurg* 1992, 76:520–523.
33. Purdy PD, Devous MD Sr, Unwin DH, *et al.*: Angioplasty of an atherosclerotic middle cerebral artery associated with improvement in regional cererbral blood flow. *AJNR* 1990, 11:878–880.
34. Troughton AH, Morgan RA, Paxton RM, Wells IP: External carotid angioplasty in the treatment of developing stroke. *Br J Radiol* 1992, 65:825–827.
35. Rosenkranz K, Hierholzer J, Langer R, *et al.*: Acetazolamide stimulation test in patients with unilateral internal carotid artery obstructions using transcranial Doppler and 99M TC-HM-PAO-SPECT. *Neurol Res* 1992, 14:135–138.

36. Turnbull IW, Bannister CM: Can laser angioplasty replace carotid endarterectomy in the management of nonstenotic atheromatous disease of the carotid bifurcation? *Surg Neurol* 1992, 38:73–76.
37. Isner JM, Rosenfield K, White CJ, *et al.*: In vivo assessment of vascular pathology resulting from laser irradiation. *Circulation* 1992, 85:2185–2196.
38. Mohan SR, Hawker RJ, Wolinski AP, *et al.*: Platelet accumulation after laser angioplasty: a scintigraphic assessment. *Angiology* 1992, 1:11–21.
39. Grabowski M, Brundin P, Johansson BB: Functional integration of cortical grafts placed in brain infarcts of rats. *Ann Neurol* 1993, 34:362–368.
40. Sharp FR: Transplants for stroke patients? *Ann Neurol* 1993, 34:322–323.
41. Lindley RI, Sandercock AG: Why test antiplatelet therapy in acute ischemic stroke and how can this be done? *Prostgrad Med J* 1992, 68(suppl 2):S14–S19.
42. Korczyn AD: Heparin in the treatment of acute stroke. *Neurol Clin North Am* 1992, 10:209–217.
43. Pessin MS, Estol CJ, LaFranchise F, Caplan LR: Safety of anticoagulation after hemorrhagic infarction. *Neurology* 1993, 43:1298–1303.
44. Hirsh J: Sol Sherry lecture in thrombosis: the limitations of heparin and potential advantages of new anticoagulants. *Circulation* 1993, 88(suppl):I-C–I-D.
45. Adams HP, Woolson RF, Biller J, *et al.*: Studies of ORG10172 in patients with acute ischemic stroke. *Haemostasis* 1992, 22:99–103.
46. Ortel TL, Gockerman JP, Califf RM, *et al.*: Parenteral angicoagulation with the heparinoid lomoparan (ORG10172) in patients with heparin induced thrombocytopenia and thrombosis. *Thromb Haemost* 1992, 67:292–296.
47. Leroy J, Leclerc MH, Delahousse B, *et al.*: Treatment of heparin associated thrombocytopenia and thrombosis with low molecular weight heparinoid (Cy216). *Semin Thromb Haemost* 1985, 11:326–329.
48. Gouault-Heilmann M, Huet Y, Adnot S, *et al.*: Low molecular weight heparin fractions as an alternative therapy in heparin induced thrombocytopenia. *Hemostasis* 1987, 17:134–140.
49. Vinazzer H: Effect of pentosan polysulfate on fibrinolysis: basic tests and clinical applications. *Semin Thromb Haemost* 1991, 17:375–378.
50. Vinazzer H, Stemberger A, Haas S, Blumel G: Influence of heparin, of different heparin fractions and of a low molecular weight heparin-like substance on the mechanism of fibrinolysis. *Thromb Res* 1982, 27:341–352.
51. Huaug Z-S, Teng C-M, Lee T-K, *et al.*: Combined use of aspirin and heparin inhibits in vivo acute carotid thrombosis. *Stroke* 1993, 24:829–839.
52. Bell WR, Pitney WR, Goodwin JF: Therapeutic defibrination in the treatment of thrombotic disease. *Lancet* 1968, 1:490–493.
53. Sharp AA, Warren BA, Paxton AM, Allington MJ: Anticoagulant therapy with a purified fraction of Malayan pit viper venom. *Lancet* 1968, 1:493–499.
54. Cole CW, Bormanis J: Ancrod: a practical alternative to heparin. *J Vasc Surg* 1988, 8:59–63.
55. Olinger CP, Brott TG, Barsen WG, *et al.*: Use of ancrod in acute or progressing ischemic cerebral infarction. *Ann Emerg Med* 1988, 17:1208–1209.
56. Yasaka M, Yamaguchi T: Immediate anticoagulation for intracardiac thrombus in acute cardioembolic stroke. *Angiology* 1992, 11:886–892.
57. McCormick PW, Spetzler RF, Bailes JE: Thromboendarterectomy of the symptomatic occluded internal carotid artery. *J Neurosurg* 1992, 76:752–758.
58. Meyer FB, Sundt TM Jr, Piepgras G: Emergency carotid endarterectomy for patients with acute carotid occlusion and profound neurological deficits. *Ann Surg* 1986, 203:82–89.
59. Walters BB, Ojemann RG, Heros RC: Emergency carotid endarterectomy. *J Neurosurg* 1984, 66:817–823.
60. del Zoppo GJ: Thrombolytic therapy in acute stroke: recent experience. *Cerebrovasc Dis* 1993, 3:256–263.
61. Brott T: Thrombolytic therapy. *Neurol Clin North Am* 1992, 10:219–232.
62. Brott T: Thrombolytic therapy for stroke. *Cerebrovasc Brain Metab Rev* 1991, 3:91–113.
63. Overgaard K, Sperling B, Boysen G, *et al.*: Thrombolytic therapy in acute ischemic stroke: a Danish pilot. *Stroke* 1993, 24:1939–1947.
64. Yamaguchi T, Hayakawa T, Kiuchi H, for the Japanese Thrombolysis Study Group: Intravenous tissue plasminogen activator ameliorates the outcome of hyperacute embolic stroke. *Cerebrovasc Dis* 1993, 3:269–272.
65. Wolpert SM, Bruckmann H, Greenlee R, *et al.*: Neuroradiologic evaluation of patients with acute stroke treated with recombinant tissue plasminogen activator. *AJNR* 1993, 14:3–13.
66. Lyden PD, Zivin JA: Hemorrhagic transformation after cerebral ischemia: mechanisms and incidence. *Cerebrovasc Brain Metab Rev* 1993, 5:1–16.
67. Okada Y, Sadoshima S, Saku Y, *et al.*: Influence of hemorrhagic transformation on the outcome of thrombolytic therapy for patients with acute brain embolism. *Neurol Res* 1992, 14(suppl):167–169.
68. Von Kummer R, Forstring M: Effects of recanalization and collateral blood supply on infarct extent and brain edema after middle cerebral artery occlusion. *Cerebrovasc Dis* 1993, 3:252–255.
69. Mori D: Safety and efficacy of fibrinolytic agents in acute ischemic stroke. *Cerebrovasc Dis* 1993, 3:264–268.
70. Herbert JM, Bernat A, Sainte-Marie M, *et al.*: Potentiating effect of clopidrogel and SR 46349, a novel 5-HT_2 antagonist, on streptokinase-induced thrombolysis in the rabbit. *Thromb Haemost* 1993, 69:268–271.
71. Rosenschein U, Yakuboo SU, Guberiainich D, *et al.*: Shock wave thrombus ablation, a new method for non-invasive mechanical thrombolysis. *Am J Cardiol* 1992, 70:1358–1361.
72. Italian Acute Stroke Study Group: Haemodilution in acute stroke: results of the Italian haemodilution trial. *Lancet* 1988, 1:318–321.
73. Scandinavian Stroke Study Group: Multicenter trial of haemodilution in acute ischemic stroke. I. Results in the total patient population. *Stroke* 1987, 18:691–697.
74. Kortringer P, Langsteger W, Reisecker F, Eber O: Hypervolemic haemodilution and completed stroke: how important is the application time for its effect? *Neurol Res* 1992, 4.
75. Goslinga H, Eijzenbach V, Heuvelmans BS, *et al.*: Custom-tailored haemodilution with albumin and crystalloids in acute ischemic stroke. *Stroke* 1992, 23:181–188.
76. Haemodilution in Stroke Study Group: Hypervolemic hemodilution treatment of acute stroke: results of a randomized multicenter trial using pentastarch. *Stroke* 1989, 20:317–323.
77. Asplund K: Haemodilution in acute stroke. *Cerebrovasc Dis* 1991, (suppl 1):129–138.
78. Marchal G, Serrati C, Rioux P, *et al.*: PET imaging of cerebral perfusion and oxygen consumption in acute ischemic stroke: relation to outcome. *Lancet* 1993, 341:925–927.
79. Zivin JA, Choi DW: Stroke therapy. *Sci Am* 1991, 7:56–63.
80. Buchan AM: Do NMDA antagonists protect against cerebral ischemia? Are clinical trials warranted? *Cerebrovasc Brain Metab Rev* 1990, 2:1–26.
81. Meldrum B: Protection against ischemic neuronal damage by drugs acting on excitatory neurotransmission. *Cerebrovasc Brain Metab Rev* 1990, 2:27–57.
82. Albers GW, Saenz RE, Moses JA Jr, Choi DW: Safety and tolerance of oral dextromethorphan in patients at risk for brain ischemia. *Stroke* 1991, 22:1075–1077.
83. Choi DW: Methods for antagonizing glutamate neurotoxicity. *Cerebrovasc Brain Metab Rev* 1990, 2:105–147.

84. Lipton SA, Choi Y-B, Pan ZH, *et al.*: A redox-based mechanism for the neuroprotective and neurodestructive effects of nitric oxide and related nitroso-compounds. *Nature* 1993, 364:626–631.

85. Robinson MJ, Teasdale GM: Calcium antagonists in the management of subarachnoid hemorrhage. *Cerebrovasc Brain Metab Rev* 1993, 5:205–227.

86. Carolei A, Fieschi C, Bruno R, Toffano: Monosialoganglioside GM1 in cerebral ischemia. *Cerebrovasc Brain Metab Rev* 1991, 3:134–187.

87. Baume S: Is ganglioside GM1 effective in the treatment of stroke? *Drugs and Aging* 1991, 1:57–66.

88. Frerichs KU, Feuestein GZ: Platelet activating factor—key mediator in neuro injury? *Cerebrovasc Brain Metab Rev* 1990, 2:148–161.

89. Ginsberg MD, Sternau LL, Globus MJ, *et al.*: Therapeutic modulation of brain temperature: relevance to ischemic brain injury. *Cerebrovasc Brain Metab Rev* 1992, 4:189–224.

90. Rothwell NJ, Relton JK: Involvement of interleukin-1 and lipocortin-1 in ischemic brain damage. *Cerebrovasc Brain Metab Rev* 1993, 5:178–199.

91. Newell DW, Aaslid R: Transcranial Doppler: clinical and experimental uses. *Cerebrovasc Brain Metab Rev* 1992, 4:122–144.

92. Knight LC: Scintigraphic methods for detecting vascular thrombosis. *J Nucl Med* 1993, 34:554–561.

93. Wyper DJ: Functional neuroimaging with single photon emission computed tomography (SPECT). *Cerebrovasc Brain Metab Rev* 1993, 5:199–218.

94. Waxman SG, ed: *The Molecular and Cellular Approaches to the Treatment of Neurological Disease.* New York: Raven Press, Ltd.; 1993.

95. Anson JA, Heiserman JE, Drayer BP, Spetzler RF: Surgical decisions on the basis of magnetic resonance angiography of the carotid arteries. *Neurosurgery* 1993, 32:335–343.

96. Marangos PJ, Lal H, eds: *Emerging Strategies in Neuroprotection.* Boston: Binkhauser; 1992.

97. Edelman RR, Warach S: Magnetic resonance imaging. *N Engl J Med* 1993, 328:708–715.

Chapter 18

Carotid Endarterectomy and Novel Surgical Therapies for Cerebral Ischemia

ROBERT M. CROWELL
CHRISTOPHER S. OGILVY

The decision to proceed with carotid endarterectomy in a patient with extracranial atherosclerotic disease is based on the belief that transient ischemic attacks and cerebral strokes are caused by the disease process at the carotid bifurcation. Whether neurologic symptoms are caused by reduced flow and associated ischemia or whether they are caused by small embolic events remains a topic of some controversy. Some recent information from randomized, double-blind studies comparing surgery with medical therapy has shed light on the management of patients with symptomatic stenosis. A brief review of the indications for carotid endarterectomy will be provided, followed by a more detailed description of the exact techniques and the subsequent results expected.

CAROTID ENDARTERECTOMY

Indications

Specific, commonly encountered conditions associated with extracranial atherosclerotic disease will be covered. The general patterns of presentation have been outlined elsewhere [1].

Transient Ischemic Attacks with Unilateral Carotid Stenosis or Ulceration

Carotid endarterectomy is often indicated for patients with transient ischemic attacks (TIAs) and severe stenosis or ulceration in the common carotid bifurcation or proximal internal carotid artery (ICA). These attacks are signals of the potential for significant stroke. The North American Symptomatic Carotid Endarterectomy Trial (NASCET) [2] demonstrated that carotid endarterectomy is highly beneficial to patients with recent hemispheric and retinal TIAs or nondisabling strokes and ipsilateral high-grade stenosis (70%–99%) of the ICA (Figure 18.1). Similar results have been reported from a Veteran's Administration–based study [3] and a European study [4]. In addition to attacks ipsilateral to severe stenosis, other conditions may well respond favorably to endarterectomy.

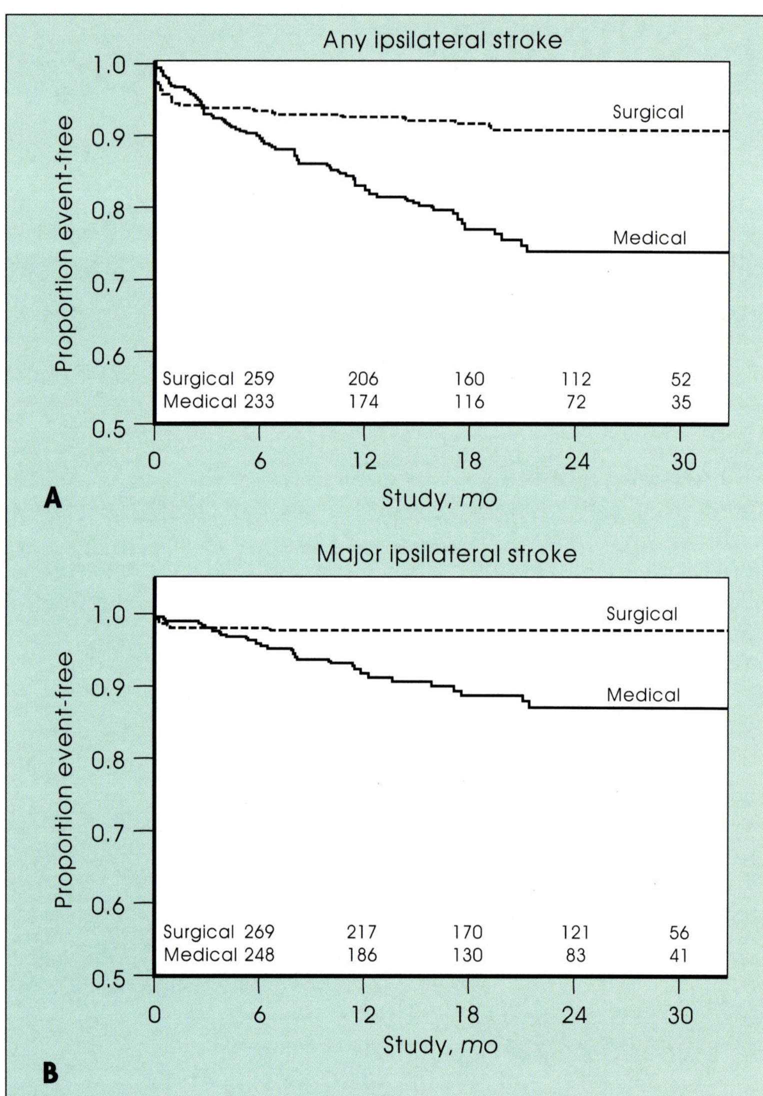

FIGURE 18.1

A and **B**, Results of the North American Symptomatic Carotid Endarterectomy Trial (NASCET) study comparing surgical versus medical (four aspirin a day) treatment in patients with unilateral transient ischemic attacks or transient monocular attacks. The number of patients in each cohort are shown for each group. As can be seen, although there is a higher risk in the perioperative interval, the long-term results favor surgical management of critical (70%–99%) stenosis.

Transient Ischemic Attacks with Bilateral Carotid Stenosis

When a patient presents with TIA, bilateral stenosis can sometimes be identified (Figure 18.2). There may be bilateral carotid bruits. Noninvasive flow studies and magnetic resonance (MR) imaging/MR angiography may be necessary to help determine the hemodynamic significance of the lesions. Carotid endarterectomy is indicated for the hemodynamically significant lesions. When only one side is symptomatic it is generally treated first unless the asymptomatic side has a tighter stenosis with a more severe hemodynamic lesion. If both sides are symptomatic, the side with the most severe hemodynamic lesion is operated first. The second side is usually done within 7 to 14 days unless there is a neurologic complication. During the interval of waiting the patient is maintained on intravenous heparin.

Transient Ischemic Attacks with Ipsilateral Carotid Stenosis and Contralateral Carotid Occlusion

In patients with this combination of lesions, TIA usually relates to the ICA stenosis. Occasionally, patients will have neurologic symptoms related to the contralateral ICA occlusion. There may be a bruit present on the side of the tight stenosis. The indications for surgery in this condition are the same as for TIAs associated with unilateral ICA stenosis. A patient with a contralateral ICA occlusion is more likely to have an electroencephalography (EEG) change during the procedure and need a shunt placed at the time of carotid cross clamping for the endarterectomy. There appears to be no increase in neurologic complications in patients with contralateral ICA occlusion or stenosis [5].

Transient Ischemic Attacks with Internal Carotid Stenosis in the Neck and in the Siphon (Tandem Lesion)

The clinical features of a patient with tandem stenoses are identical to those with a single lesion. MR imaging studies are less sensitive in delineating the anatomy of siphon stenosis and a true cerebral angiogram may be necessary. Increasingly, however, we use MR imaging combined with MR angiography studies in conjunction with carotid noninvasive flow studies to define carotid disease prior to surgery. This avoids the risk of cerebral angiography.

If tandem stenosis is present, it is often the case that the stenosis in the neck is more severe than the distal lesion in the siphon [6]. If the residual lumen in the neck is less than 1.5 mm, carotid endarterectomy is indicated for TIAs even if the distal lesion is also significantly stenotic. This maintains perfusion in an effort to prevent thrombosis. Postoperatively, a decision is made between anticoagulation and antiplatelet therapy.

Transient Ischemic Attacks with Ipsilateral Carotid Occlusion

Transient ischemic attacks can occur in the territory normally supplied by a completely occluded ICA (Figure 18.3). The cause of these symptoms may be an embolus from the distal end of a thrombus in the occluded ICA or an embolus passing through the external carotid artery circulation from atheromatous stenosis of the external or distal common carotid artery or from the stump proximal to the occlusion in the ICA. Alternatively, a reduction in flow to the eye or cerebral hemisphere may occur as a result of the occlusion. If low flow is the etiology of the symptoms, patients may describe symptoms accentuated when they initially rise to a standing position.

If an angiogram is done, complete evaluation of the collateral circulation from the opposite carotid artery is necessary. In addition, the vertebrobasilar circulation must be well studied. One question to determine in evaluating patients with unilateral occlusion is how far down the ICA the dye flows. This is important in deciding the etiology of the symptoms and the probability of reopening the complete occlusion with a surgical exploration of the ICA. In one report, the chance of opening an occluded ICA was correlated with the degree of thrombosis. If thrombosis was present to the intracranial carotid bifurcation, it was impossible to open the vessel in these patients. At the other extreme, in patients with retrograde flow down into the skull base portion of the carotid artery, it was often possible to open the occlusion [7]. Of interest was the fact that in this study, in patients with retrograde flow into the carotid canal near the base of the skull who underwent endarterectomy, it was possible to open the vessel regardless of the time of occlusion.

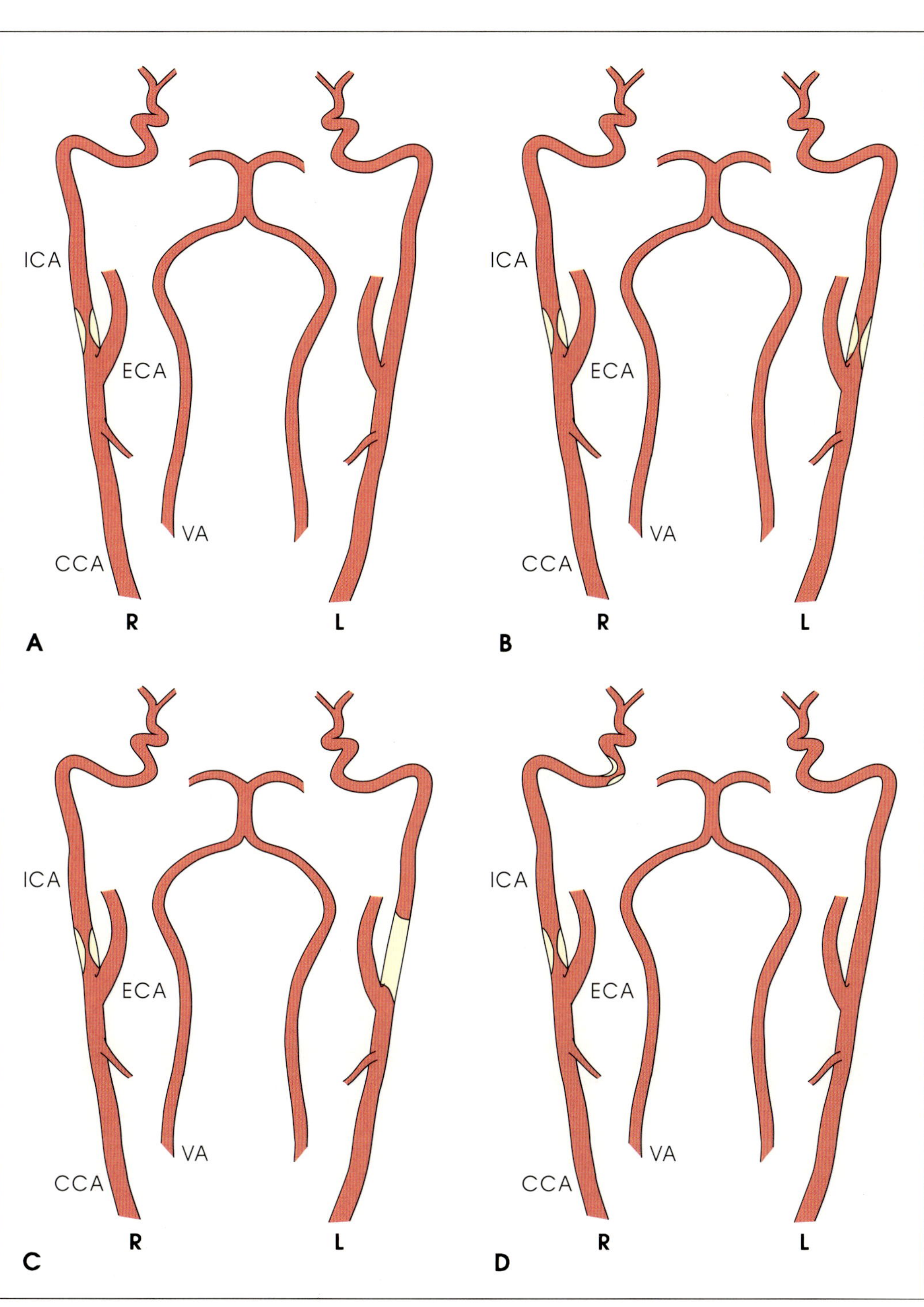

FIGURE 18.2

Schematic diagrams of conditions described in the text for extracranial atherosclerotic disease. **A**, Transient ischemic attack (TIA) with unilateral carotid stenosis and ulceration. **B**, TIA with bilateral carotid stenosis. **C**, TIA with ipsilateral carotid stenosis and contralateral carotid occlusion. **D**, TIA with internal carotid artery (ICA) stenosis in the neck and in the siphon (tandem stenosis). CCA—common carotid artery; ECA—external carotic artery; VA—vertebral artery.

Transient Ischemic Attacks with External Carotid Stenosis or Occlusion

The external carotid artery can supply significant collateral flow to intracranial circulation. This occurs through the ophthalmic system or the corticotympanic branches or meningeal branches of the ICA. When the ICA is occluded, stenosis at the origin of the external carotid artery may be associated with TIAs. When this is the case, external endarterectomy may be considered in an effort to alleviate symptoms of TIA. At times, opening of a severely stenotic external carotid artery may stop the progression of ischemic retinopathy. When an ICA is opened, external carotid artery stenosis or occlusion is usually not associated with significant clinical symptoms. An isolated occluded external carotid artery can be the source of stump embolus into the ICA.

Posterior Circulation Transient Ischemic Attacks with Carotid Stenosis

At times, patients may present with symptoms consistent with posterior circulation TIAs as the result of carotid stenosis. The most characteristic symptoms of TIA in the vertebrobasilar circulation are ataxia, diplopia, dysarthria, dizziness, and weakness or numbness of part or all of both sides of the body [8]. At times headache or staggering gait may be the presenting symptoms. In addition, blindness or ptosis as well as dysphagia, confusion,

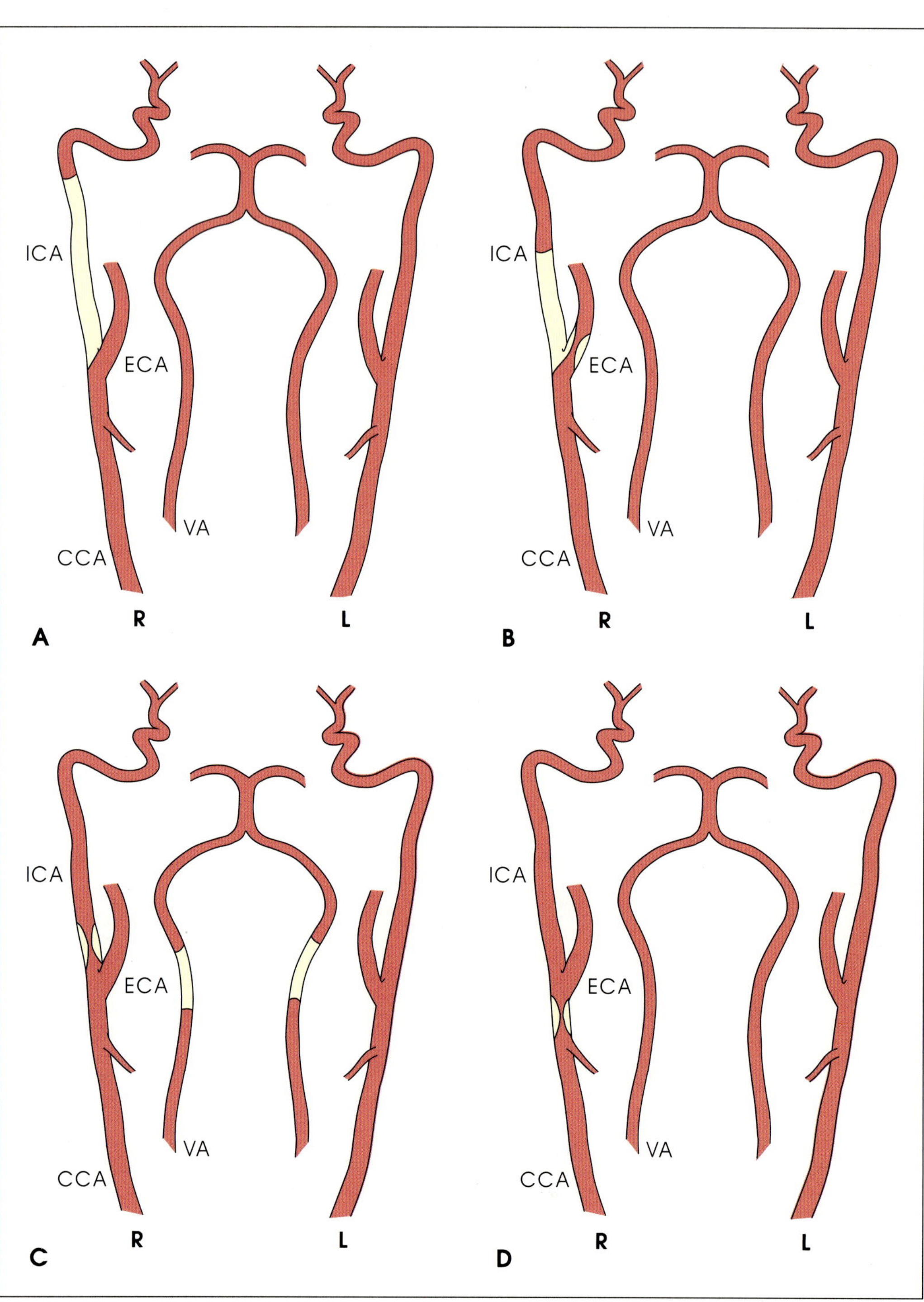

FIGURE 18.3

Schematic diagrams of extracranial atherosclerotic disease as described in the text. **A**, Transient ischemic attack (TIA) with ipsilateral carotid occlusion. **B**, TIA with external carotid stenosis or occlusion. **C**, Posterior circulation TIA with carotid stenosis. **D**, TIA with common carotid stenosis or occlusion.

and memory lapse can occur. When there is evidence of carotid artery disease, a complete angiography should be carried out to evaluate the vertebrobasilar as well as the carotid system. Carotid endarterectomy may be indicated if the angiogram shows filling of the posterior cerebral artery via the stenotic ICA or filling of the posterior circulation from the ICA because of vertebral artery occlusive disease. Alternatively, a persistent hypoglossal or trigeminal artery may give rise to posterior circulation TIAs from carotid artery stenosis. If severe carotid stenosis is present with no filling of the posterior circulation from the stenotic artery, the condition should be considered as an asymptomatic carotid stenosis.

Transient Ischemic Attacks with Common Carotid Stenosis or Occlusion

Isolated stenosis or occlusion of the common carotid artery without involvement of the internal vessel is rare. More likely it is a situation where the distal common carotid artery is involved at the bifurcation. At times a stenosis may involve the midportion of the common carotid artery. Occlusion of the common carotid artery may be due to a retrograde thrombosis from the ICA disease. If indeed the common carotid artery is occluded, a reconstructive procedure to restore anterograde flow to the ICA is almost always possible when the ICA is open distal to the occlusion.

Technique

Once the decision has been made to proceed with carotid endarterectomy, great care must be taken in the preparation of the patient for surgery as well as the sequence of events that transpire during the operation. Once the patient is positioned for surgery and the EEG leads are applied, an arterial catheter is placed in the radial artery. Careful blood pressure regulation is an absolute essential during this procedure. The region of the distal saphenous vein in the leg is usually prepped in the event that a saphenous vein patch is necessary during the procedure. Once the patient is positioned, an incision is made on the anterior border of the sternocleidomastoid muscle (Figure 18.4).

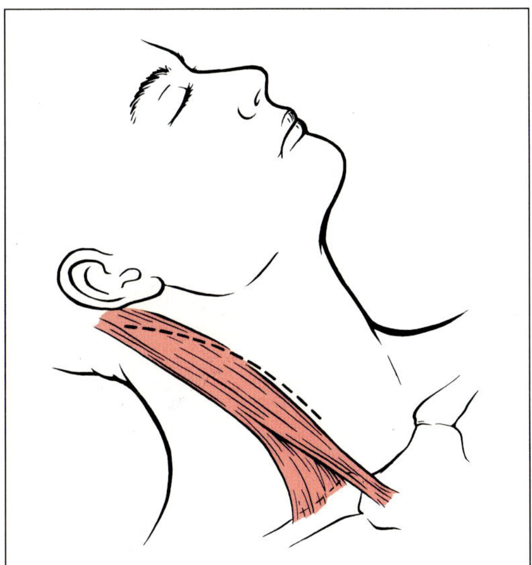

FIGURE 18.4

General positioning of patient and location of incision used by carotid endarterectomy.

Dissection is then undertaken to identify the great auricular nerve superiorly in the wound (Figure 18.5A). Retractors are deepened and the sternocleidomastoid muscle is retracted laterally, exposing the descending hypoglossal nerve medially and the ansa cervicalis medially. The internal jugular vein is identified and retracted laterally beneath the sternocleidomastoid muscle (Figures 18.5A and 18.5B).

The common carotid artery is then isolated proximally (Figure 18.5B). The carotid artery bifurcation is blocked using a local anesthetic in order to minimize or avoid any change in heart rate during the remainder of the dissection. A solution of 0.5% xylocaine without epinephrine is used and injected with a 25-gauge needle into the carotid body (Figure 18.5B). Once this step is complete, continued dissection of the ICA and external carotid artery is undertaken. Great care is taken to identify the hypoglossal nerve, and this is isolated with a small tape so that

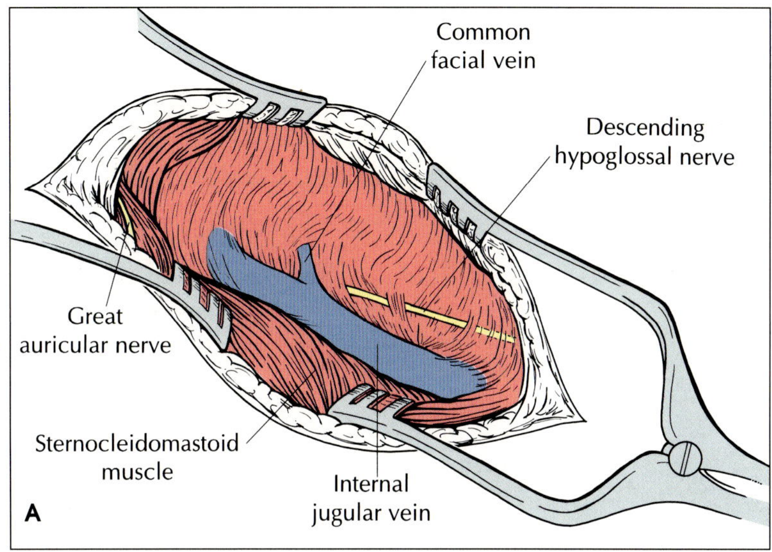

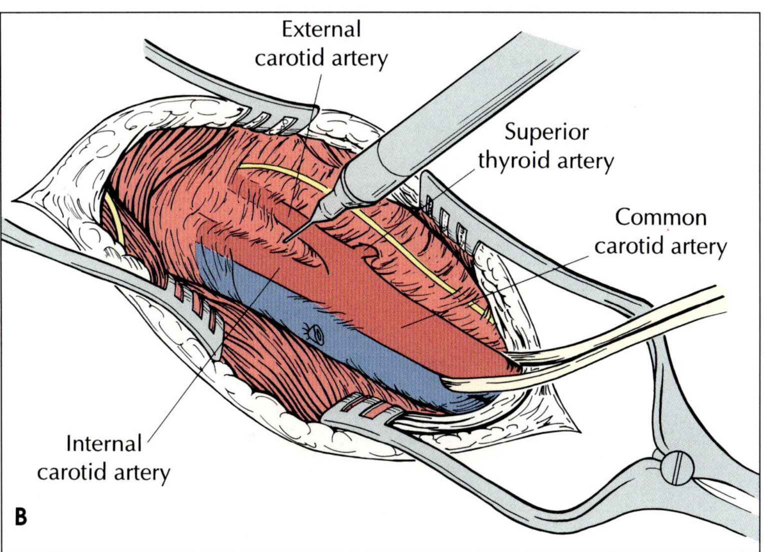

FIGURE 18.5

A, Surgical exposure of the carotid artery involves lateral retraction of the sternocleidomastoid muscle and internal jugular vein. The great auricular nerve is identified in the superior extent of the incision. **B**, Once the carotid artery is exposed, the carotid bifurcation is blocked with local anesthetic.

the surgeon can avoid any retraction or dissection of this nerve (Figure 18.6A). The vessels are then occluded by clamping first the internal and subsequently the common and external branches of the carotid artery. A separate clip is placed on the superior thyroid artery (Figure 18.6A). Prior to cross clamping the vessels, 5000 units of USP heparin is administered intravenously. The endarterectomy is then begun by creating a linear incision with a number 15 scalpel blade. The vessel is opened with a Potts scissors (Figure 18.6B). The plane between the carotid artery plaque and the normal vessel wall is dissected free and this plane is opened in order to make it possible to dissect out and remove the plaque itself (Fig. 18.7A). Once the

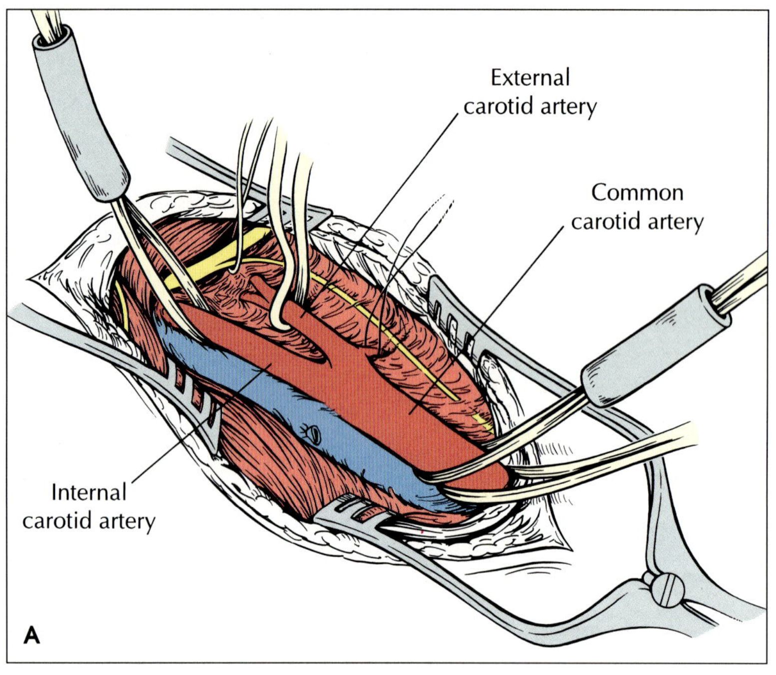

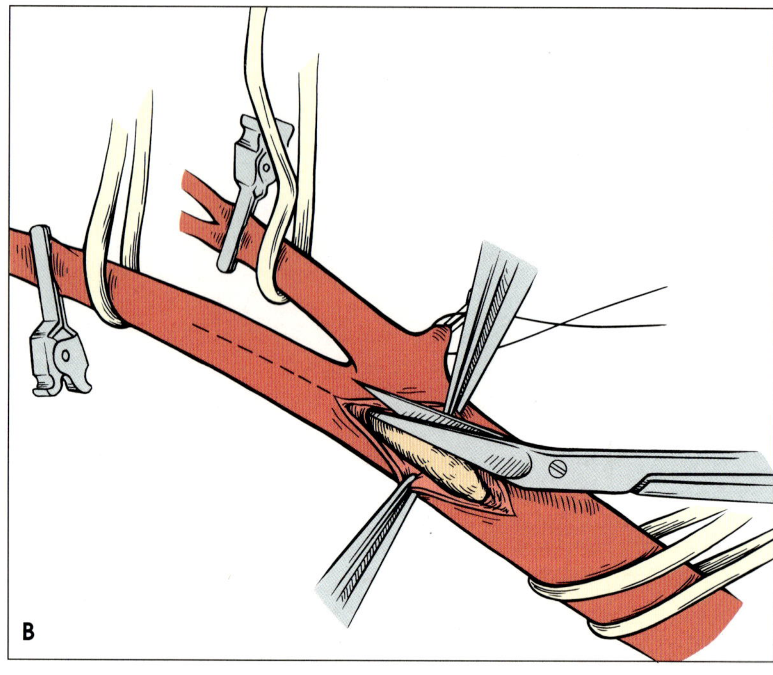

FIGURE 18.6

A, Carotid artery with vessels clamped immediately prior to endarterectomy. As can be seen, the hypoglossal nerve is identified superiorly in the wound. Pump tourniquets are in place in the event that a shunt should become necessary during the initial phase of endarterectomy. **B**, Opening the endarterectomy site with a Potts scissors.

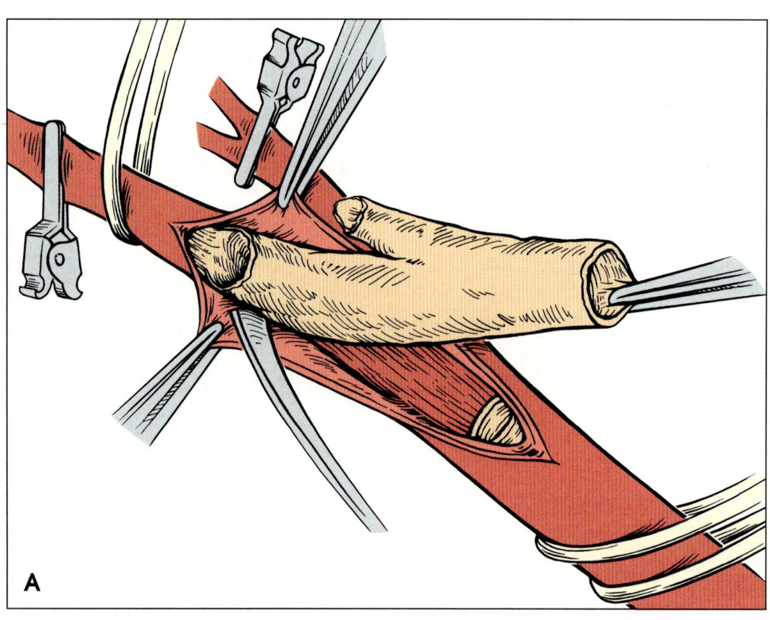

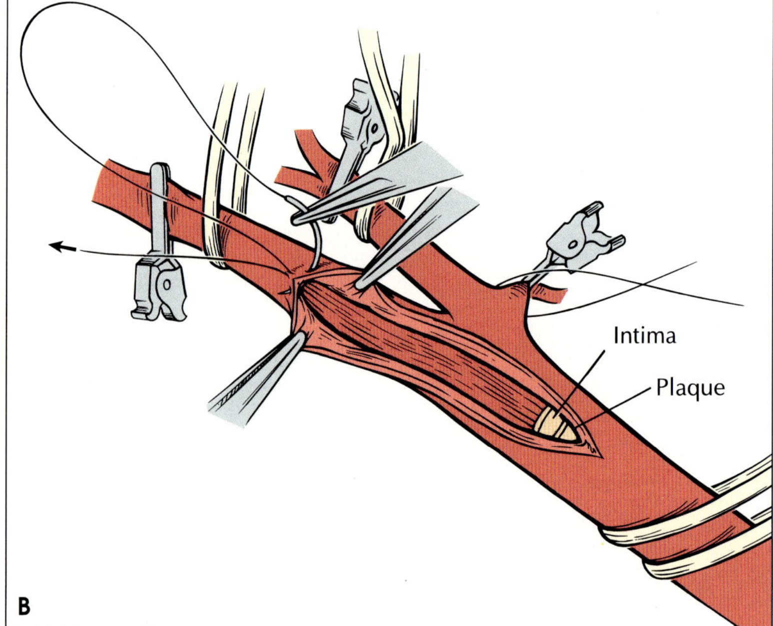

FIGURE 18.7

A, Diagrammatic representation of removing the carotid atherosclerotic plaque from the external and internal vessels. **B**, The closure on the endarterectomy site is started distally with a running 6-0 or 5-0 prolene suture. The endarterectomy site has been cleaned of all plaque material.

plaque is removed, the walls of the endarterectomy site are carefully inspected using loupe magnification. Any small bits of plaque are then removed with a fine instrument so that a smooth wall is present. In addition, great care is taken to establish a smooth transition between the area of the endarterectomy and the normal vessel wall distally.

Once the plaque is completely removed, endarterectomy closure is begun. A 5-0 or 6-0 prolene suture is used and started at the distal end of the endarterectomy (Figure 18.7B). The suture is then run proximally two thirds of the distance of the closure. A second suture is started in the proximal vessel and run distally to meet the initial suture, whereupon both are tightly secured (Figure 18.8A).

At our institution, EEG is used in all operations for carotid endarterectomy. At the time of cross clamp, any significant change in the EEG pattern is noted and the determination of whether or not to use a shunt during the procedure is made based on the EEG record.

When EEG changes are encountered during initial cross clamping, we proceed with placement of a shunt. The shunt is inserted by completely opening the endarterectomy and its plaque and inserting the shunt first distally into the ICA and securing a pump tourniquet around the shunt itself (Figure 18.8B). The proximal end of the shunt is then inserted into the common carotid artery after a clamp on the shunt tubing has been opened, allowing for back flow of blood to occur from the internal carotid vessel. The proximal end of the tubing is then inserted into the common carotid artery and a pump tourniquet is placed around the tubing (Figure 18.8B). The clamp is then removed from the shunt tubing and circulation is allowed around the endarterectomy site through the shunt tubing itself.

Once a shunt is in place, the endarterectomy proceeds as without a shunt and the plaque is removed from the vessel itself. The vessel is then closed, and prior to the last two or three sutures being placed, the shunt tubing is removed. There is then 3 or 4 minutes of ischemia while the final sutures are placed in the endarterectomy closure site. Once the endarterectomy is completely closed, clamps are removed and flow is reestablished.

At times the distal ICA vessel is small and a graft is placed. Some surgeons place a graft in every endarterectomy. We prefer to make a judgement at the time of the surgery regarding the distal vessel size, and if the diameter is less than 5 mm, a graft is placed. If the vessel lumen is larger than 5 mm, usually no graft is necessary. This size cutoff was defined by the group at the Mayo Clinic and helps prevent postoperative thrombosis. The graft material used can be a synthetic material such as dacron or a patch can be fashioned from a piece of saphenous vein. We prefer to use saphenous vein patch grafts. The dacron material can provide a stiff surface against which to suture into the endarterectomy site.

A graft is fashioned from the saphenous vein in an ellipse shape (Figure 18.9A). To do this, the saphenous vein is opened longitudinally, providing a flat surface. Care is taken to be sure there are no venous valves present in the segment of vessel to be used for the endarterectomy patch. The edges of the graft are trimmed to form an elliptical shape and placed into the apex of the endarterectomy closure (Figure 18.9A). Once the graft is started at the apex, the remainder of the suturing is performed as described above (Figure 18.9B). With the endarterectomy site closed, all clamps are removed and the distal and external carotid arteries are palpated in order to be certain there is no thrill or turbulent flow present. If a pulse is not palpable in the external vessel, we proceed with an external carotid endarterectomy to look for a flap or thrombus. We have found this in four or five cases in the past 120 operations. The external endarterectomy is carried out identically to the internal endarterectomy through a 1-cm incision in the external vessel. The vessel is then sutured closed using a 5-0 or 6-0 prolene suture.

Once excellent flow is documented in both internal or external vessels, a drain is placed adjacent to the endarterectomy closure

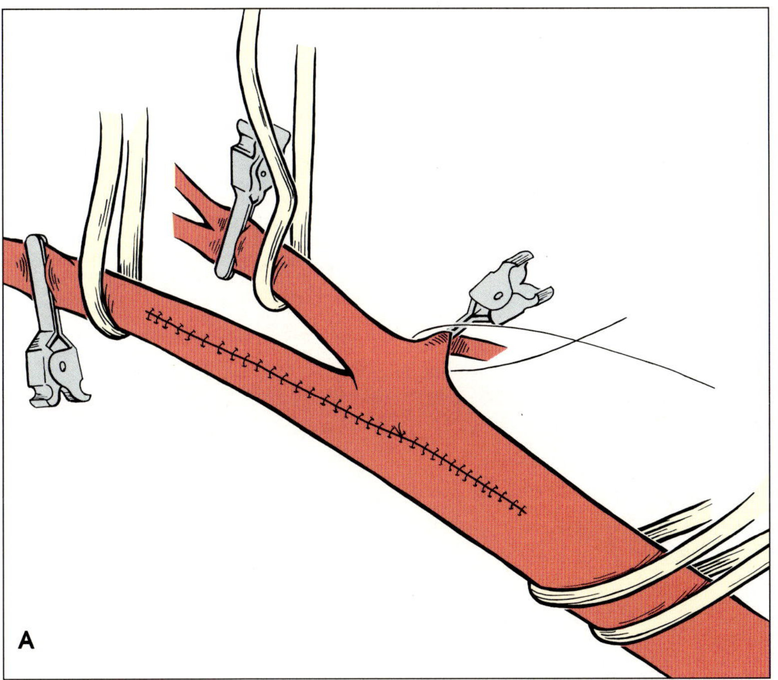

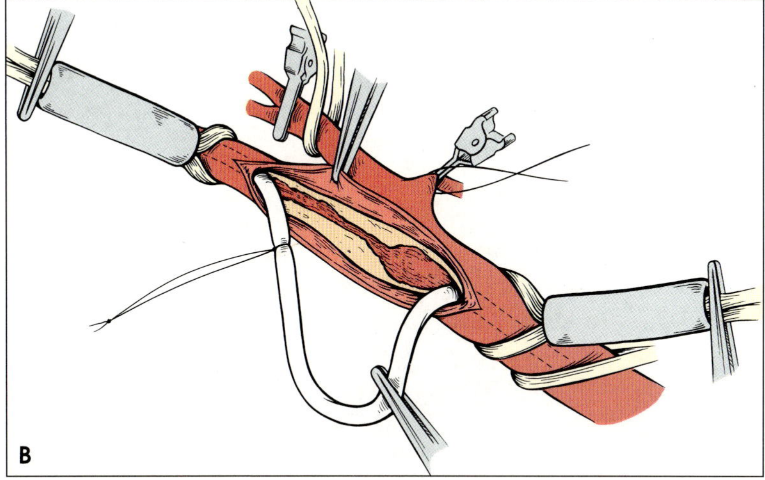

FIGURE 18.8

A, Finished product with primary closure of the endarterectomy site. **B**, Representation of a shunt in place during carotid endarterectomy. Pump tourniquets are used proximally and distally to secure the shunt into position allowing for the endarterectomy to be performed while blood flow in the internal vessel is maintained.

site. This drain is led from the wound through a separate stab incision. The layers of the wound are then closed using absorbable suture and reapproximating the platysma muscle as well as the subcutaneous tissue. The skin is often closed with a subcuticular stitch of absorbable suture and benzoin and steristrips are used to hold the skin edges together. The patient is observed in the intensive care unit postoperatively and routinely we rule out the possibility of a myocardial infarction by obtaining serial electrocardiograms and serial MB isoenzymes.

Results

Reviewing a series of 120 consecutive endarterectomy operations performed by the neurosurgical service at Massachusetts General Hospital between 1989 and 1992 revealed that 79 of the patients presented with TIA or minor stroke. Operation was performed for asymptomatic but progressive stenosis in 41 patients, for a total of 120 patients (Table 18.1). The age range was between 44 and 83 years. There were 55 women and 65 men. All patients were monitored with EEG recordings during the procedure. The need for a shunt during endarterectomy occurred in 12 patients (10%). As noted above, the decision to place a shunt was based on changes in EEG recordings. Forty-three patients required placement of a saphenous vein patch graft (36%). In these patients the distal ICA diameter was less than 5 mm. All patients were maintained on postoperative heparin at 500 units per hour that was started in the recovery room after inspecting the wound to be sure there was no postoperative hematoma. A drain was placed in the wound of all patients, as noted above (Table 18.2).

The majority of patients undergoing the operation did well (Table 18.3). There was a cerebral hemorrhage 6 days postoper-

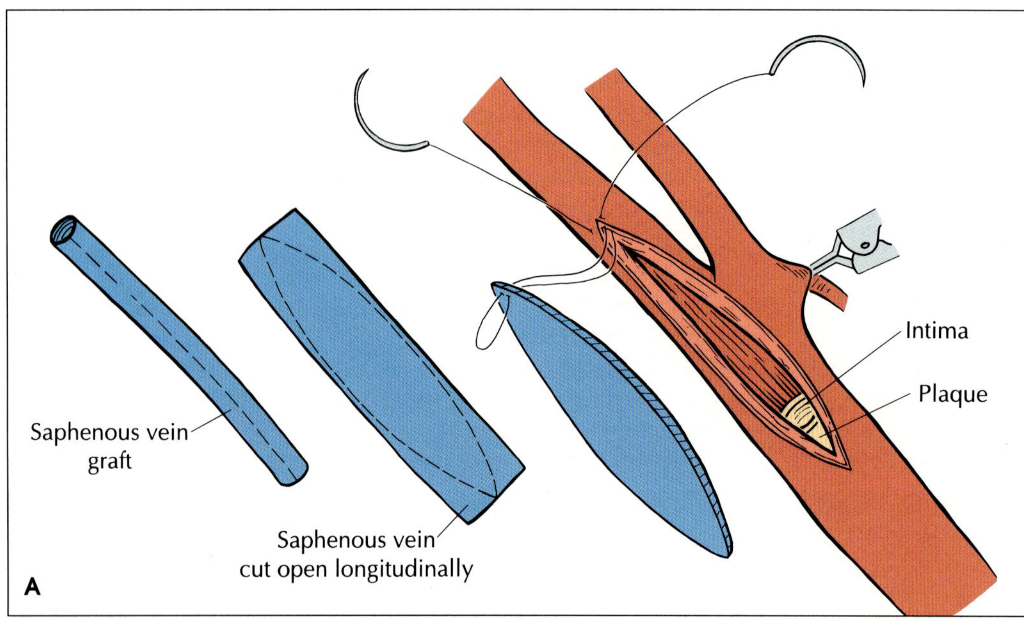

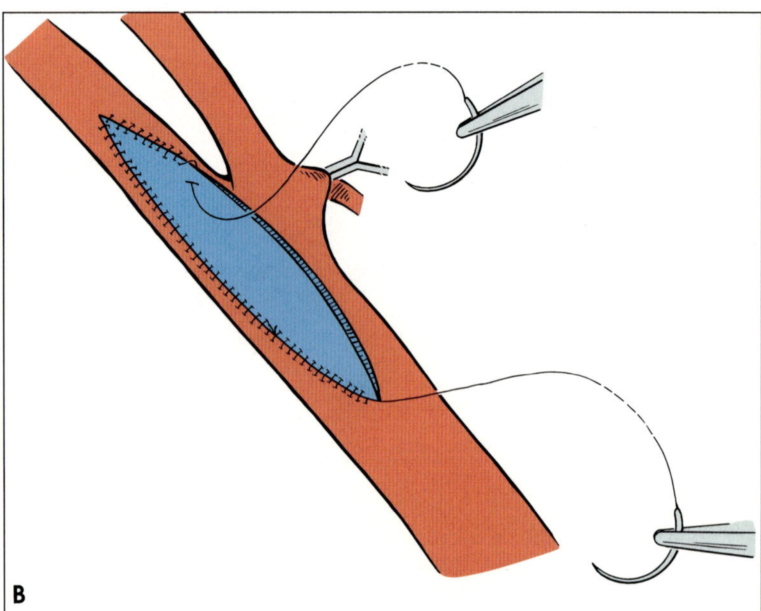

FIGURE 18.9

A, A patch graft for endarterectomy is fashioned from a segment of distal saphenous vein. The vein is opened longitudinally, trimmed in an ellipse shape, and sutured into position. **B**, The graft is sutured laterally and then medially in order to secure it into position.

atively in one patient (0.8% of the total). This hemorrhage was removed surgically and proved to have evidence of cerebral amyloid angiopathy present. Two patients had minor infarctions. One patient had a weak hand immediately after surgery and a second patient had a hemianopsia that took several days to clear. Both of these patients awoke neurologically intact and developed their deficits in the recovery room. Inspection of the carotid bifurcation with noninvasive studies (done emergently) demonstrated excellent flow in the bifurcation itself. We believe that both instances represent small emboli following endarterectomy. These two patients represent 1.6% of the total number of patients operated on. There was transient dysphagia present in two patients after endarterectomy (1.6%). Myocardial infarction occurred in two patients (1.6%). In one of these patients the myocardial infarction was silent and detected only by routine monitoring for electrocardiogram and enzyme changes; in a second patient chest pain heralded the onset of myocardial infarction 48 hours after surgery. This was managed medically and the patient did well. There were no deaths following endarterectomy in this series of patients (Table 18.3).

Carotid endarterectomy is an effective way of avoiding permanent disabling stroke in patients who present with TIA or transient monocular blindness. Current randomized control studies are in progress to evaluate the effectiveness of endarterectomy versus medical management in patients with asymptomatic yet tight carotid stenosis and in patients with symptomatic yet noncritical (30%–70%) stenosis. Results of these studies will help us further define the appropriate management for patients with carotid artery stenosis. Preliminary results suggest benefit in stroke reduction with carotid endarterectomy.

NOVEL SURGICAL THERAPIES FOR CEREBRAL ISCHEMIA

Bypass Grafting

Background

Cerebrovascular occlusive disease leads to impaired blood flow to the brain and subsequent brain infarction. Thus, it is logical to suspect that improvement in brain blood flow might reduce the likelihood of stroke. This logic applied to inaccessible intracranial occlusive disease led to the concept of direct brain revascularization.

This concept was developed and implemented with microsurgical techniques in the 1960s. The operation of superficial temporal artery (STA) to middle cerebral artery (MCA) bypass was developed and used widely with excellent patency rates and low morbidity and mortality (Figure 18.10) [9–13]. However, there were doubts regarding clinical benefit. Does STA-MCA bypass actually reduce the risk of stroke? This question was addressed with a modern randomized controlled trial known as the Extracranial-Intracranial (EC-IC) Bypass Study [14]. In this landmark study, patients were included for investigation with MCA stenosis or occlusion or ICA stenosis above C2 in the setting of TIA or minor stroke. One thousand four hundred ninety-five patients of this type were randomized to best medical therapy or best medical therapy plus EC-IC bypass. Ninety-six percent patency was demonstrated with a surgical risk of 3%. Over an average follow-up of 55.8 months, EC-IC bypass conferred no benefit regarding diminished risk of stroke (Figure 18.11).

The impact of the EC-IC bypass study has been dramatic. The number of patients referred for bypass to prevent stroke has been reduced almost to none.

Table 18.1. Presentation, age, and sex distribution for 120 consecutive endarterectomies at the Massachusetts General Hospital, 1989 through 1992

Presentation	Number
Transient ischemic attack or minor stroke	79
Asymptomatic stenosis	41
Total	120
Age, *y*	
44–83	
Sex	**Number**
Women	55
Men	65

Table 18.2. Results of 120 consecutive endarterectomies at the Massachusetts General Hospital, 1989 through 1992

Results	Patients, *n*(%)
Need for shunt during endarterectomy (based on electroencephalography changes)	12(10)
Need for saphenous vein patch	43(36)
Postoperative heparin 500 U/h	120(100)
Drain placed in wound	115(96)

Table 18.3. Complications in 120 endarterectomy patients at the Massachusetts General Hospital 1989 through 1992

Complication	Patients, *n*(%)
Cerebral hemorrhage postoperatively from cerebral amyloid angiopathy	1(0.8)
Minor infarction with complete recovery	2(1.6)
Transient dysphagia	2(1.6)
Myocardial infarction	2(1.6)
Death	0(0)

Indications

A number of possible indications have not been excluded, principally because they were not directly addressed in the EC-IC bypass study. Some authors have argued that ICA or MCA stenosis refractory to medical therapy may be a potential indication [15]. Other possible indications include low-flow syndromes and "slow stroke," ocular ischemia [16], vasospasm [17], and moyamoya syndrome [18]. Other potential indications include amaurosis fugax after demonstrated ICA occlusion, chronic cerebral ischemia, and multiinfarct dementia. Bypass might be also considered in selected cases of cerebral ischemia related to inaccessible ICA dissection.

More solidly established indications relate principally to planned ICA occlusion for cerebral aneurysm (or rarely tumor) in the setting of inadequate cerebral collateral circulation. This is the strategy of "Hunterian ligation" which Drake has recommended in the treatment of inoperable (often giant) intracranial aneurysms [19]. The method may be applied to both the anterior and posterior circulations. By far the most common application is in reference to occlusion of the ICA for ICA aneurysms. In the setting of anticipated cerebral ischemia following arterial occlusion, bypass grafting has been performed with very good results [11,20–24].

However, many patients will tolerate arterial occlusion (particularly ICA occlusion) without clinical symptoms. Thus, the need for bypass appears to involve only a minority of patients, those with inadequate collateral reserve. Patients with poor collateral circulation may be identified by tolerance test occlusion of the

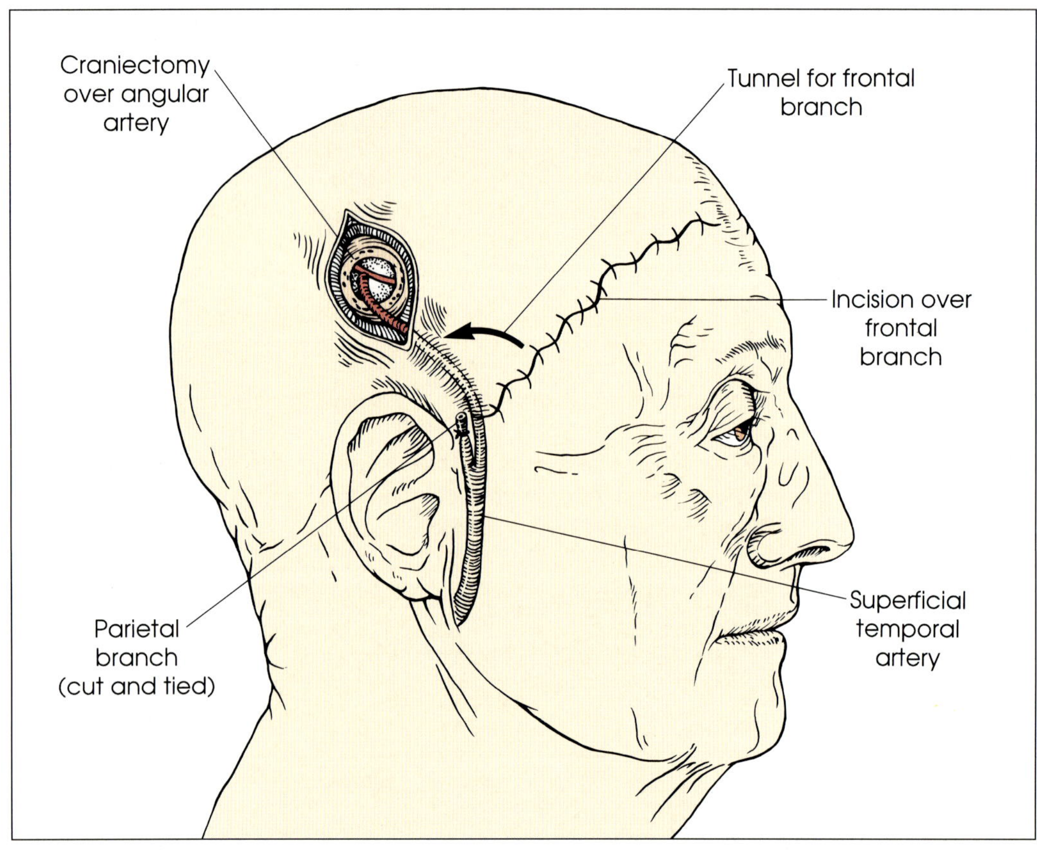

FIGURE 18.10

Superficial temporal artery–middle cerebral artery bypass graft. The first practical direct revascularization of the brain with a bypass, introduced by Donaghy and Yasargil in 1967.

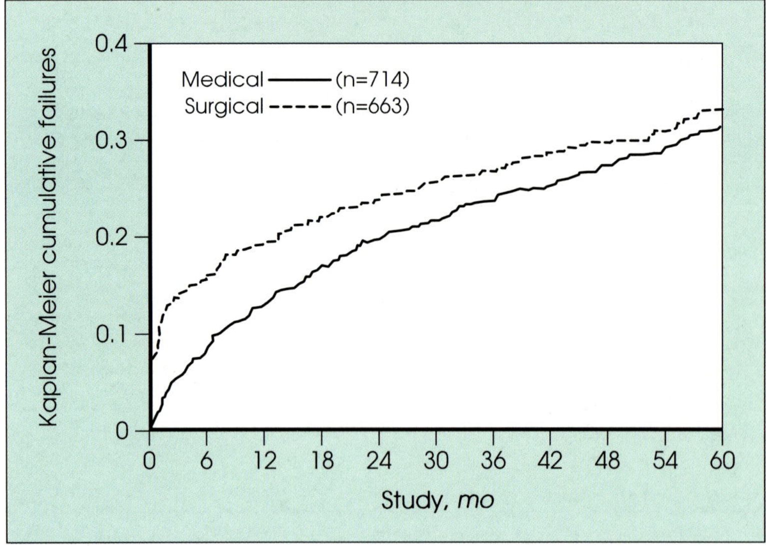

FIGURE 18.11

The Extracranial-Intracranial (EC-IC) Bypass Study. Over a 5-year follow-up period, bypass failed to confer protection against stroke as compared with medical therapy.

vessel to be permanently occluded. Clinical effects of test occlusion may be supplemented by cerebral blood flow studies or clinical evaluation during induced hypotension [25,26].

Occasionally, revascularization may be appropriate prior to intracranial tumor surgery. When an intracranial tumor causes severe narrowing of an intracranial artery (ICA, MCA, posterior cerebral artery [PCA], or anterior cerebral artery [ACA]), direct attack on the tumor for excision may lead to vascular occlusion with possible stroke and neurologic deficit. In practice the intraoperative findings usually lead the surgeon to carefully dissect the tumor off the affected artery with its preservation or leave a small rim of tumor attached to the vessel. Only rarely have we been persuaded that preoperative short vein bypass grafting to the MCA is warranted.

Evaluation

Clinical examination is of course needed, including careful neurologic assessment. Palpation of the cranial arteries and assessment of saphenous veins for bypass are also appropriate. Consultations with cardiologists and anesthesiologists are usually indicated in these complex cases. Four-vessel cerebral angiographic study is essential. This identifies intracranial aneurysms, occlusive disease, and collateral circulation. Computed tomography (CT) scanning is routine with and without contrast to demonstrate the aneurysm or tumor and possible areas of cerebral infarction and edema. In some cases MR imaging may be useful. The most direct test in the adequacy of collateral circulation is the method of tolerance test occlusion [25]. In this examination the interventional neuroradiologist introduces a transfemoral catheter with balloon into the artery that is to be occluded therapeutically. Under full heparinization the balloon is blown up to the point of occlusion of the vessel. Careful clinical evaluation of the patient's neurologic performance is assessed. In our institution we have routinely challenged the collateral circulation by the induction of hypotension, reducing the systolic blood pressure 20 to 30 mm Hg below the usual for that patient. If the patient develops no symptoms in 20 minutes, we conclude that the collateral circulation is suitable for permanent occlusion. Others have used positron emission tomography (PET) or single photon emission computed tomography (SPECT) to assess collateral circulation during test occlusion [26].

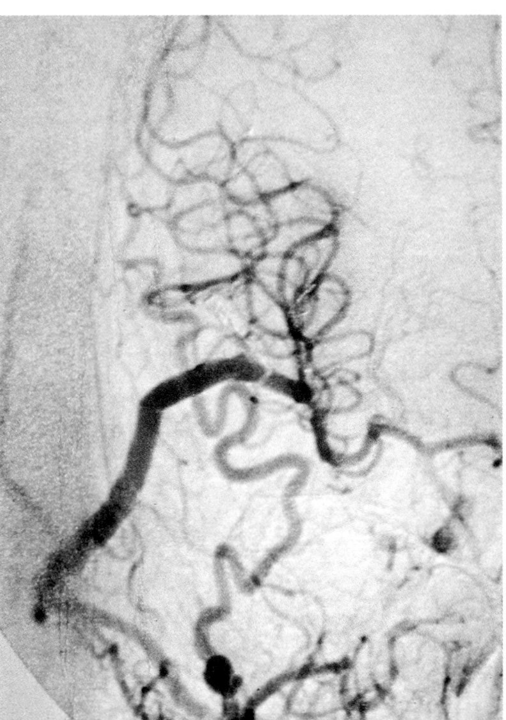

FIGURE 18.12

Superficial temporal artery (STA)–saphenous vein–middle cerebral artery (MCA) bypass (short-vein bypass) popularized by Little [27]. A practical operation to provide high flow promptly. Here an AP right carotid study shows filling of the entire right internal carotid artery territory via the bypass.

Surgical Protocol

While a variety of revascularization techniques and parent vessel occlusions may be used, a basic plan of treatment has been established in our institution. Anticoagulants are used to reduce thromboembolic complications. Since anticoagulants cannot be used immediately following intracranial revascularization, a delay of 5 days after revascularization is employed to prevent hemorrhagic complications. Therefore, parent artery occlusion is carried out by balloon catheter technique 6 days after revascularization, immediately followed by anticoagulation, first with heparin then with coumadin. To be sure the bypass is adequate, intraoperative angiography is done after bypass. This enables the surgeon to estimate the likelihood of aneurysmal blow-out induced by revascularization. In the case of vigorous aneurysm filling via the bypass, consideration is given to immediate parent vessel occlusion. Following balloon occlusion of the parent vessel, careful monitoring in the neurological intensive care unit is carried out. Angiography is used to check aneurysm status and bypass filling.

Anterior Circulation Revascularization

To provide flow in the territory of the ICA, STA–saphenous vein–MCA bypass (STA-MCA "short-vein graft") has emerged as an excellent technique to achieve prompt increase in blood flow (Figure 18.12) [27]. STA-MCA short-vein graft is currently our preferred technique for anterior circulation revascularization. The procedure is convenient, relatively rapid, and involves low risk of intraoperative ischemia or delayed thromboembolism.

The operation is a microsurgical procedure carried out by two surgeons. While one operator prepares the STA and performs a small craniotomy, the other harvests the saphenous vein graft from the calf. Then the MCA is prepared and the distal anastomosis is carried out. Finally, after trimming of the saphenous vein, the proximal end of the vein is anastomosed to the superficial temporal artery just above the zygoma. The ACA can also be revascularized by a short vein from the STA.

Results of short-vein bypass have been gratifying with patency rates of 95% and toleration of ICA occlusion in virtually all cases. When the aneurysm is at the anterior clinoid process or below, thrombosis of the aneurysm can be expected in virtually all cases.

Other vessels may be used as in STA to MCA bypass, *eg*, occipital artery–MCA bypass, external carotid saphenous (ECA)–MCA bypass (ECA-MCA "long-vein graft") [28], and subclavian-saphenous–MCA bypass (when the carotid circulation is unavailable). These techniques are much less commonly used, but may have their place in individual specialized cases.

Posterior circulation revascularization is occasionally used when the vertebral or basilar artery is to be sacrificed for aneurysm treatment [24,29–31]. Recurrent ischemic episodes in the posterior circulation related to bilateral vertebral occlusive disease or basilar occlusive disease rarely justify revascularization of the posterior circulation. In our institution, the operation of choice in this setting is STA–saphenous-PCA bypass (P2 "short-vein" bypass) (Figure 18.13). Relatively high patency rates have been achieved. The first surgeon performs a posterior temporal craniotomy and frees the STA while the second surgeon harvests the vein graft. After elevation of the temporal lobe, the P2 PCA is identified and freed up. Anastomosis of the distal saphenous vein to the P2 cerebral artery is carried out. After appropriate trimming of the length, the saphenous vein is anastomosed to the STA just above the zygoma. Intraoperative angiography is carried out to determine whether delayed parent vessel occlusion may be performed as planned, or whether immediate proximal occlusion must be carried out to avoid aneurysm rupture by the newly implanted graft.

Less commonly, other techniques of posterior circulation revascularization may be carried out such as external carotid artery–saphenous PCA bypass, or occipital artery–posterior inferior cerebellar artery bypass [24, 29–31].

Results

For the experienced neurovascular surgeon, patencies of 90% to 95% or greater can be achieved for the procedures discussed [9–13]. For the STA–saphenous-P2 bypass, because of the depth of the anastomosis and the size of the vessels, somewhat lower patencies may be expected. STA grafts with short-vein graft may provide 50 to 150 cc per minute. Aneurysm occlusion is another common measure of successful application of this combined treatment method. When the aneurysm is in the carotid circulation at the anterior clinoid process or below, rates close to 100% can be achieved [19]. The likelihood of late symptoms or rupture is greatly reduced with total obliteration. Direct brain revascularization is subject to the usual problems with intracranial surgery including meningitis, seizures, and hemorrhage, as well as systemic complications such as myocardial infarction and pulmonary embolus. Special complications of revascularization include infarction, hemorrhage, and aneurysm rupture. The overall complication rate for this sequence in our hands has been 10% or less.

Vertebral Artery Revascularization

Extracranial procedures are occasionally justified for vertebral basilar ischemia. In the setting of occlusion of one vertebral artery and substantial stenosis of the remaining vessel, direct surgery may be appropriate. In general the vertebral artery is more fragile and difficult for direct surgery as compared with the carotid artery. Nonetheless, vertebral endarterectomy at the origin of the vertebral artery has been successfully carried out by performing an arteriotomy in the subclavian artery and removing the plaque at the origin through the subclavian vessel, with final closure of the subclavian arteriotomy. Another procedure for atherosclerosis at the origin of the vertebral artery is vertebral artery replantation, with end-to-side anastomosis of the mobilized proximal vertebral artery into the side of the common carotid artery in the neck (Figure 18.14). Patency rates of 90% or greater have been achieved for the latter procedure.

Intracranial vertebral endarterectomy has been carried out occasionally (Figure 18.15) [32]. High patency rates have been obtained, but experience is quite limited and the indications are uncertain.

Other Revascularization Procedures

Arterial replantation techniques are sometimes valuable during intracranial aneurysm surgery (Figure 18.16) [33]. For complex, giant aneurysms, clipping of an important vessel may be needed, for example a division of the MCA may require occlusion. In order to maintain perfusion to the distal territory of this branch, end-to-end anastomosis of this division into the other MCA division may avert ischemia. Obviously brain protection techniques are needed during cross-clamping, such as barbiturates, mannitol, and hypothermia. Results of this type of revascularization have been quite gratifying.

Middle cerebral artery embolectomy may occasionally reverse acute stroke clot, or balloon should be extracted emergently (Figure 18.17).

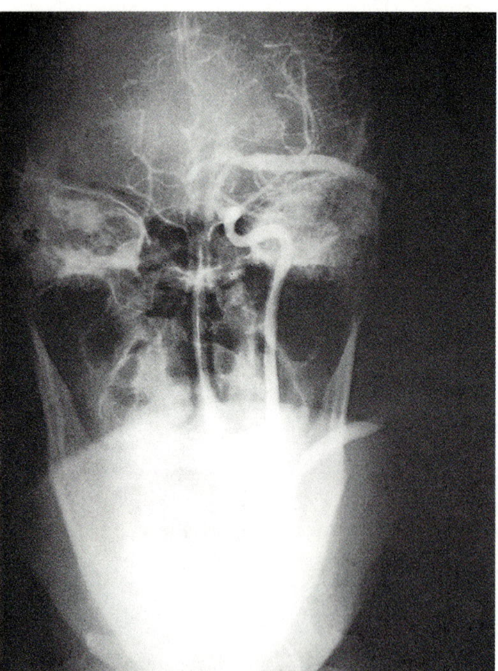

FIGURE 18.13

Short-vein posterior cerebral artery bypass. Left AP carotid angiogram shows posterior circulation filling from bypass despite (virtual) basilar occlusion.

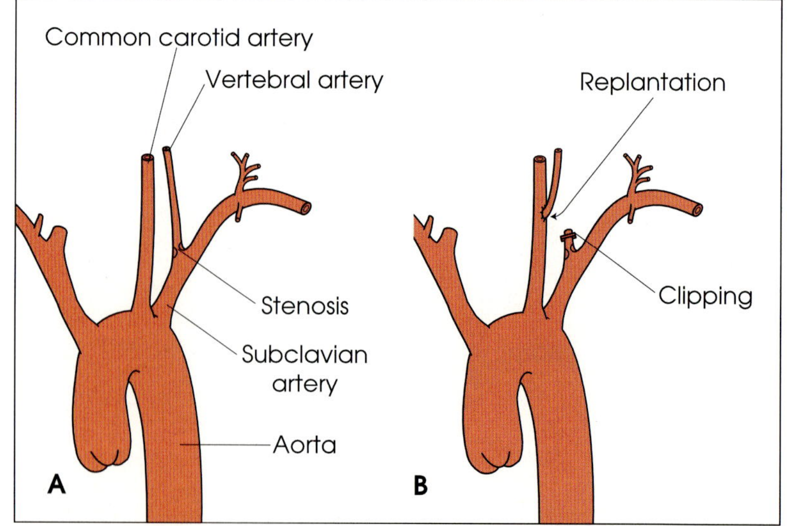

FIGURE 18.14

Vertebral–common carotid artery anastomoses. **A**, Vertebral artery origin stenosis. **B**, Vertebral artery replanked into common carotid artery to restore vertebral artery flow.

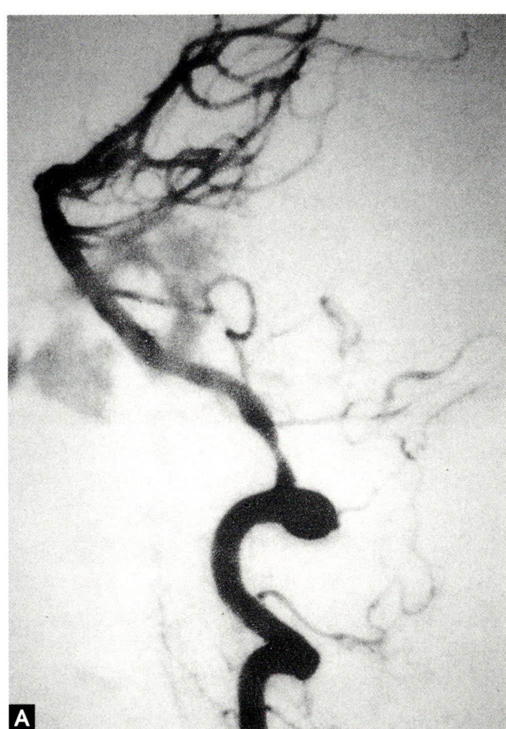

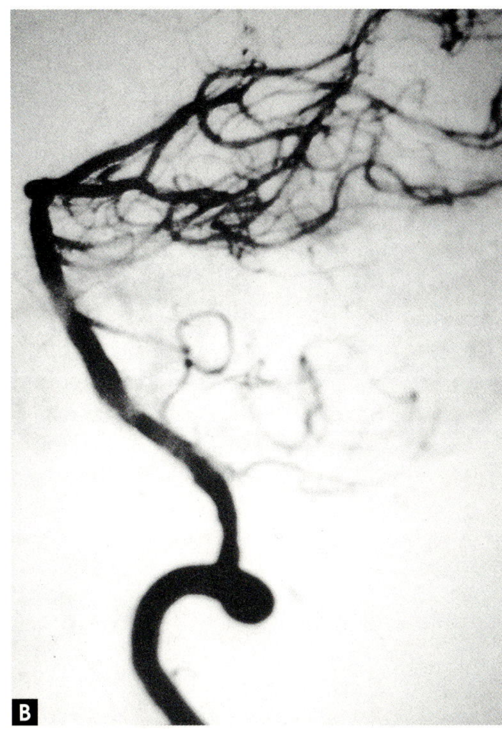

FIGURE 18.15

Intracranial vertebral endarterectomy. **A**, Preoperative vertebral artery angiogram shows severe intracranial vertebral stenosis. **B**, Postoperative angiogram shows wide-open endarterectomy site. No further transient ischemic attacks. (*From* Allen and coworkers [32]; with permission.)

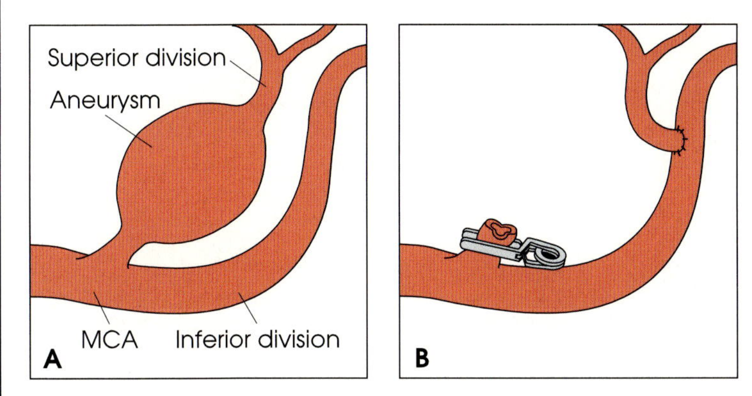

FIGURE 18.16

Intracranial arterial replantation for aneurysm surgery. **A**, AP sketch of left middle cerebral artery (MCA) superior division fusiform aneurysm. **B**, Excision of aneurysm with microsurgical replantation of superior division of MCA into inferior division.

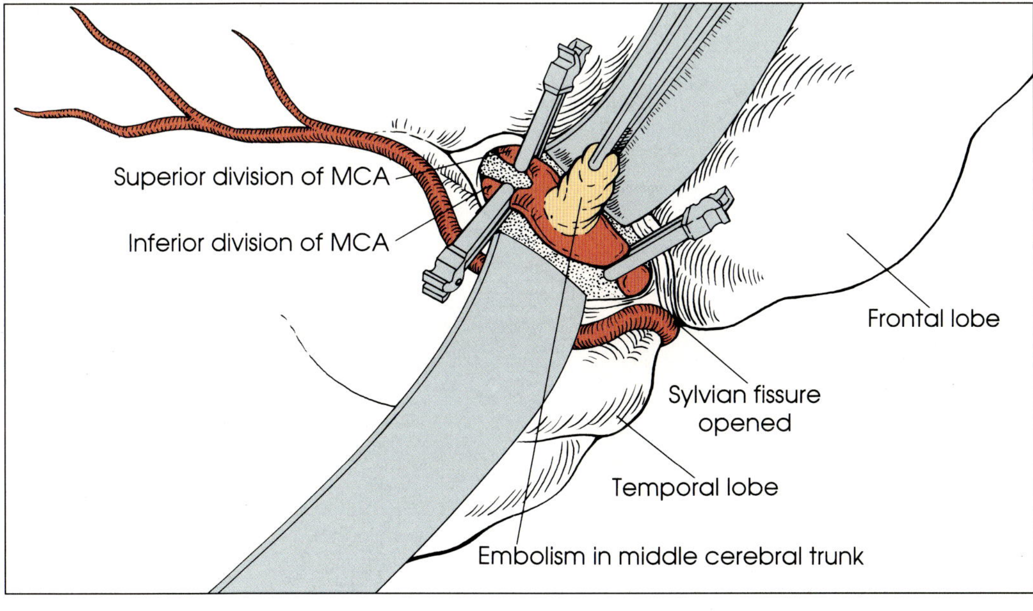

FIGURE 18.17

Middle cerebral artery (MCA) embolectomy. Microsurgical procedure can reopen occluded MCA due to thromboembolism or balloon catheter embolism.

Encephalo-duro-arterio-synangiosis (EDAS) is a revascularization procedure developed in Japan to provide new brain collateral supply without anastomosis. Most commonly a soft tissue pedicle of STA is developed and placed directly on the cortex. The method is low risk, can establish in time a wealth of tiny branches into the brain, and has been recommended for childhood moyamoya syndrome [34].

Omental grafting, like EDAS, is based on revascularization without anastomosis [35–37]. In essence, an abdominal approach frees up an omental pedicle that is brought subcutaneously to the cranium, and via craniotomy the graft is placed on the brain. Over time, vascular branches enter the brain, and improved circulation can be demonstrated. There are scattered reports of protection against subsequent stroke and even improvement of fixed deficits, but confirmation is lacking.

Direct repair of cavernous ICA dissection has been reported as successful, but this rare problem has usually been treated nonsurgically.

Venus reconstruction of the great intracranial venous sinus has been sporadically reported. Indications have not been established [38].

Endovascular Therapy

Thrombolysis with streptokinase, urokinase, or tissue plasmogen activator has been applied to intracranial arterial thrombotic occlusion with intra-arterial administration of the agent (Figure 18.18). Opening of occluded arteries by thrombolysis has been followed by remarkable neurologic recovery. On the other hand, the proportion of failures has been substantial, and

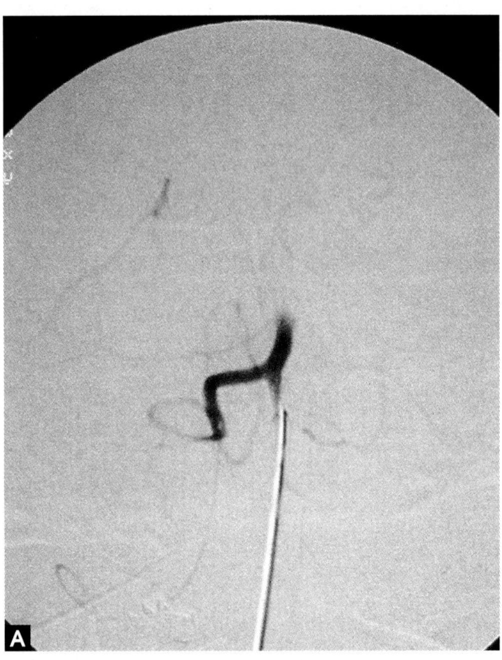

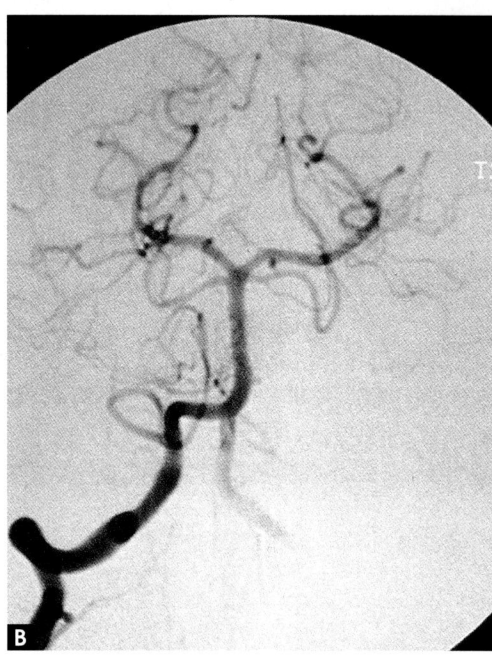

FIGURE 18.18

Thrombolysis. **A**, AP vertebral angiogram shows (virtual) basilar occlusion. **B**, After intra-arterial thrombolytic therapy, angiogram shows wide-open basilar artery. (*Courtesy of* Daryl Gress, MD.)

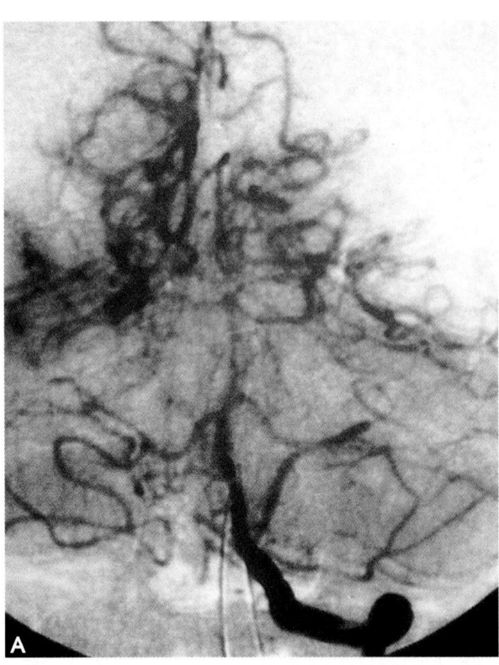

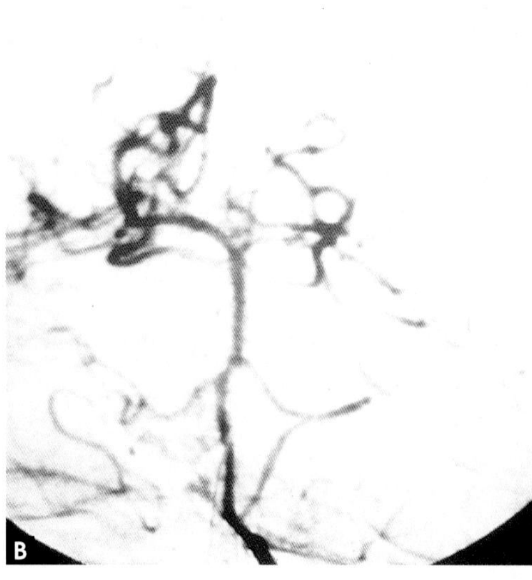

FIGURE 18.19

Angioplasty. **A**, AP vertebral angiogram shows severe basilar spasm after subarachnoid hemorrhage. **B**, After balloon angioplasty of basilar artery, flow is much improved on angiography.

control data have not yet been presented to establish indications for this promising form of treatment.

Angioplasty by use of transvascular balloon catheters has been used to expand stenotic segments of cerebral vascular arteries. Angioplasty has sometimes been used effectively in the setting of cerebrovascular vasospasm following subarachnoid hemorrhage (Figure 18.19). Good results have been reported, but the procedure must be instituted quickly following the onset of severe symptomatology to obtain significant clinical benefit.

REFERENCES

1. Ojemann RG, Heros RC, Crowell RM: Atherosclerosis of the carotid circulation: evaluation and management. In *Surgical Management of Cerebrovascular Disease*, 2nd ed. Edited by Ojemann RG, Heros RC, Crowell RM. Baltimore: Williams & Wilkins; 1988:1–34.
2. North American Symptomatic Carotid Endarterectomy Trial Collaborators: Beneficial effect of carotid endarterectomy in symptomatic patients with high-grade carotid stenosis. *N Engl J Med* 1991, 325:445–453.
3. Mayberg MR, Wilson E, Yatsu F, *et al.*: Carotid endarterectomy and prevention of cerebral ischemia in symptomatic carotid stenosis. *JAMA* 1991, 266:3289–3294.
4. European Carotid Surgery Trialists' Collaborative Group: MRC European Carotid Surgery Trial: interim results for symptomatic patients with severe (70-99%) or with mild (0-29%) carotid stenosis. *Lancet* 1991, 337:1235–1243.
5. Moore DJ, Mody JR, Finch WT, Sumner DS: Influence of the contralateral carotid artery on neurologic complications following carotid endarterectomy. *J Vasc Surg* 1984, 1:409–414.
6. Roederer GO, Langlois YE, Tan AR, *et al.*: Is siphon disease important in predicting outcome of carotid endarterectomy? *Arch Surg* 1983, 118:1177–1181.
7. Huggenholtz H, Leelgie RG: Carotid thromboendarterectomy: a reappraisal: criteria for patient selection. *J Neurosurg* 1980, 53:776–783.
8. Adams RD, Victor M: Cerebrovascular diseases. In *Principles of Neurology*, 2nd ed. Edited by Adams RD, Victor M. New York: McGraw-Hill; 1981:529–593.
9. Crowell RM: Emergency STA-MCA bypass for acute focal cerebral ischemia. In *Microneurosurgical Anastomoses for Cerebral Ischemia*. Edited by Schmidek P, *et al.* Berlin: Springer-Verlag; 1977.
10. Diaz FG, Ausman JL, Mehta B, *et al.*: Acute cerebral revascularization. *J Neurosurg* 1985, 63:200–209.
11. Ojemann RG, Heros RC, Crowell RM, eds.: *Surgical Management of Cerebrovascular Disease*. Baltimore: Williams and Wilkins; 1987.
12. Reichman OH: Complications of cerebral revascularization. *Clin Neurosurg* 1976, 23:318–335.
13. Yasargil MG, Krayenbuhl HA, Jacobson JH: Microneurosurgical arterial reconstruction. *Surgery* 1970, 67:221–233.
14. The EC-IC Bypass Study Group: Failure of extracranial-intracranial arterial bypass to reduce the risk of ischemic stroke: results of an international randomized trial. *N Engl J Med* 1985, 313:1191–1200.
15. McCormick PW, Tomecek FJ, McKinney J, Ausman JI: Disabling cerebral transient ischemic attacks. *J Neurosurg* 1991, 75(6):891–901.
16. Kearns TP, Siekert RG, Sundt TM Jr: The ocular aspects of bypass surgery of the carotid artery. *Mayo Clin Proc* 1979, 54:3–11.
17. Benzel EC, Kesterson L: Extracranial-intracranial bypass surgery for the management of vasospasm after subarachnoid hemorrhage. *Surg Neurol* 1988, 30:231–234.
18. Karasawa J, Kikuchi H, Furuso S, *et al.*: Treatment of moyamoya disease with STA-MCA anastomosis. *J Neurosurg* 1978, 49:679–688.
19. Fox AJ, Vinuela F, Pelz DM, *et al.*: Use of detachable balloons for proximal artery occlusion in the treatment of unclippable aneurysms. *J Neurosurg* 1987, 66:40–46.
20. Gelber BR, Sundt TM JR: Treatment of intracavernous and giant carotid aneurysms by combined internal carotid ligation and extra-to intracranial bypass. *J Neurosurg* 1980, 52:1–10.
21. Iwabuchi T, Kudo T, Hatanaka M, *et al.*: Vein graft bypass in treatment of giant aneurysms. *Surg Neurol* 1979, 12:463–466.
22. Serbinenko FA, Filatov JM, Spallone A, *et al.*: Management of giant intracranial ICA aneurysms with combined extracranial-intracranial anastomosis and endovascular occlusion. *J Neurosurg* 1990, 73(1):57–63.
23. Spetzler RF, Shuster H, Roski RA: Elective extracranial-intracranial arterial bypass in the treatment of inoperable giant internal carotid artery aneurysms. *J Neurosurg* 1980, 53:22–27.
24. Sundt TM JR, Piepgras DG, Houser OW, Campbell JK: Interposition saphenous vein grafts for advanced occlusive disease and large aneurysms in the posterior circulation. *J Neurosurg* 1982, 56:205–215.
25. Morioka T, Matsushima T, Fujii K, *et al.*: Balloon test occlusion of the internal carotid artery with monitoring of compressed spectral arrays (CSAs) of electroencephalogram. *Acta Neurochir (Wien)* 1989, 101:29–34.
26. Powers WJ, Martin WR, Herscovitch P, *et al.*: Extracranial-intracranial bypass surgery: hemodynamic and metabolic effects. *Neurology* 1984, 34:1168–1174.
27. Little JR, Furlan AJ, Bryerton B: Short vein grafts for cerebral revascularization. *J Neurosurg* 1983, 59:384–388.
28. Samson DS, Gerwertz BL, Beyer CW Jr, Hodosh RM: Saphenous vein interposition grafts in the microsurgical treatment of cerebral ischemia. *Arch Surg* 1981, 116:1578–1582.
29. Ausman JI, Diaz FG, de los Reyes RA, *et al.*: Superficial temporal to proximal superior cerebellar artery anastomosis for basilar artery stenosis. *Neurosurgery* 1981, 9:56–59.
30. Ausman JI, Diaz FG, de los Reyes RA, *et al.*: Extracranial-intracranial anastomoses in the posterior circulation. In *Vertebrobasilar Arterial Occlusive Disease*. Edited by Berguer R, Bauer BB. New York: Raven Press; 1984:313–319.
31. Hopkins LN, Martin NA, Hadley MN, *et al.*: Vertebrobasilar insufficiency. Part 2. Microsurgical treatment of intracranial vertebrobasilar disease. *J Neurosurg* 1987, 66(5):662–674.
32. Allen G, Cohen R, Preziosi T: Microsurgical endarterectomy of the intracranial vertebral artery for vertebrobasilar TIA. *J Neurosurg* 1981, 9:56–59.
33. Ausman JI, Diaz FG, Sadasivan B, *et al.*: Giant intracranial aneurysm surgery: the role of microvascular reconstruction. *Surg Neurol* 1990, 34:8–15.
34. Matsushima T, Fujiwara S, Nagata S, *et al.*: Surgical treatment for paediatric patients with moyamoya disease by indirect revascularization procedures (EDAS, EMS, EMAS). *Acta Neurochir (Wien)* 1989, 98:135–140.
35. Goldsmith HS, Duckett S, Chen WF: Prevention of cerebral infarction in the monkey by omental transposition to the brain. *Stroke* 1978, 9:224–229.
36. Havlik RJ, Fried I, Chyatte D, Modlin IM: Encephalo-omental synangiosis in the management of moyamoya disease. *Surgery* 1992, 111(2):156–162.
37. Yonekawa Y, Yasargil MG: Brain revascularization by transplanted omentum: a possible treatment of cerebral ischemia. *Neurosurgery* 1977, 1:256–259.
38. Niwa J, Ohtaki M, Morimoto S, *et al.*: Reconstruction of the venous outflow using a vein graft in dural arteriovenous malformation associated with sinus occlusion. *No Shinkei Geka* 1988, 16:1273–1280.

Chapter 19

Treatment of Aneurysmal Subarachnoid Hemorrhage

THOMAS C. ORIGITANO

Rupture of an intracranial aneurysm is a catastrophic central nervous system event. It begins a pathologic cascade with broad central nervous system and systemic effects. Management of this crisis has evolved over the past 30 years as many of the old myths and legends about patient management have been dispelled. This chapter represents a colloquium on the management of aneurysmal subarachnoid hemorrhage in the 1990s.

Approximately 5 million North Americans harbor intracranial aneurysms [1,2]. Twenty-eight thousand rupture each year, causing subarachnoid hemorrhage, for an incidence of 10 per 100,000 population [3]. The rupture of an intracranial aneurysm initiates a pathologic cascade affecting both systemic and central nervous system function. Overall morbidity and mortality may approximate 60% at 3 months [4]. Modern treatment of aneurysmal subarachnoid hemorrhage has evolved based on an understanding of the natural history and interdiction of the pathologic cascade [5–9]. Table 19.1 illustrates the spectrum of the natural history of patients with aneurysmal subarachnoid hemorrhage and emphasizes the complexity of the problem.

DIAGNOSIS

A major area of interdiction in treating aneurysmal subarachnoid hemorrhage is prompt diagnosis and treatment. Of the 10,000 patients who die or are disabled as a result of their initial hemorrhage (Table 19.1), clearly 70% are lost as warning symptoms are ignored or there is late referral or misdiagnosis. Therefore, community and physician education may have a major impact on treatment of aneurysmal subarachnoid hemorrhage.

The impact of education on patient outcome has been proven in the case of myocardial infarction. Community education about the warning signs of cardiac ischemia (chest pain, jaw-arm pain, and so forth), training in cardiopulmonary resuscitation, and rapid transport to specialized centers have improved patient outcome.

Rapid diagnosis demands a high index of suspicion, beginning with a thoughtful history. Patients with a new onset of severe headache, often described as "the worst headache of my life," should be considered to have a ruptured aneurysm until proven otherwise. The signs and symptoms of aneurysmal subarachnoid hemorrhage are listed in Table 19.2. Level of physical activity does not appear to have an influence. An equal number of patients are participating in strenuous and nonstrenuous activities when aneurysms rupture [10].

Aneurysm should also be considered in patients presenting with acute unexplained coma. A computed tomography (CT) scan of the head is often diagnostic (Figure 19.1), and the amount of subarachnoid hemorrhage prognosticates the likelihood of subsequent ischemic complication (Table 19.3) [11,12]. The greater the amount of subarachnoid hemorrhage, the higher the probability of delayed ischemic complications. A standard clinical grading scale is applied to patients on presentation and

Table 19.1. Total ruptured intracranial aneurysms, 28,000

	n	%
Dead or disabled from initial hemorrhage	10,000	36
No warning	3000	
Warning	7000	
Survive hemorrhage treatable	18,000	64
Dead or disabled from:		
Rebleeding	3000	
Ischemia	3000	
Medical complication	1000	
Surgical complication	1000	
Functional survivors	10,000	36

Adapted from Kassell and Drake [3]; with permission.

Table 19.2. Signs and symptoms of aneurysmal subarachnoid hemorrhage

- Headache
  - Acute onset
  - Worst headache of their life
- Stiff neck/meningismus
- Coma
- Nausea, vomiting
- Photophobia
- Seizure

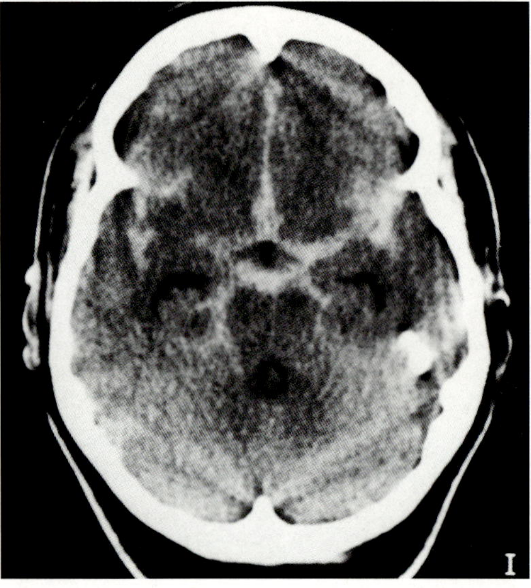

FIGURE 19.1

Computed tomography scan of head demonstrating diffuse aneurysmal subarachnoid hemorrhage.

Table 19.3 CM Fischer computed tomography subarachnoid hemorrhage scale

Group	
I	No detectable blood on computed tomography, no severe spasm predicted
II	Diffuse blood, thin, nonhomogeneous clot, no severe spasm predicted
III	Dense collection of blood greater than 1-mm thick in vertical plane or less than 5 x 3 mm in longitudinal and transverse dimension in horizontal plane, severe spasm predicted
IV	Intracerebral/intraventricular, diffuse thin or no blood in cisterns, no severe spasm predicted

Adapted from Kistler and coworkers [12]; with permission.

can also be used for prognostication (Table 19.4) [7,13]. Patients may move up and down the scale during the 2-week period following subarachnoid hemorrhage.

If the CT scan is equivocal and the history or physical examination provocative, a lumbar puncture should be performed. Experienced hands should perform this procedure and the sample observed for fresh blood or xanthochromia, which represents a recent bleed.

Transarterial 4-vessel angiography remains the gold standard for diagnosis and road mapping for aneurysmal identification and obliteration. Newer technologies such as digital angiography or MRA are not sufficiently sensitive. However, 15% to 20% of the time the primary angiogram may be negative, necessitating a second study 7 to 10 days later. All four vessels must be studied because of the 15% to 20% incidence of multiple aneurysms (Figure 19.2) [14]. A review of recommended work-up for aneurysmal subarachnoid hemorrhage is found in Table 19.5.

Table 19.4. Hunt/Hess grading scale of clinical status

Category	Criteria
I	Asymptomatic, or minimal headache and slight nuchal rigidity
II	Moderate to severe headache, nuchal rigidity, no neurologic deficit other than cranial nerve palsy
III	Drowsiness, confusion, or mild focal deficit
IV	Stupor, moderate to severe hemiparesis, possibly early decerebrate rigidity and vegetative disturbances
V	Deep coma, decerebrate rigidity, moribund appearance

Adapted from Hunt and Hess [13]; with permission.

PATHOLOGIC PROCESS

The rupture of an intracranial aneurysm is a catastrophic event [15]. The initial insult is direct injury to brain parenchyma, as blood at systolic pressure comes in contact with brain tissue. Intracranial pressure rises rapidly until diastolic levels are reached. At that point, intracranial circulatory arrest occurs and the patient loses consciousness. This rise in pressure may indeed tamponade the rupture. Failure to dissipate pressure can lead to ischemia. If left unchecked, a vicious cycle of increasing ischemia and pressure results in irreversible injury and death.

Aneurysmal rupture can present with varying amounts of subarachnoid hemorrhage, intraparenchymal hemorrhage, intraventricular hemorrhage, or a combination of all three (Figure 19.3). Clinical and neuroradiologic presentation directs therapy. Patients with intraparenchymal hemorrhage will require emergent operation for relief of the mass lesions. Those with intraventricular hemorrhage or severe hydrocephalus require external ventricular drainage.

A trial of external ventricular drainage may be considered in patients who present as grade IV or V. More aggressive approaches may be taken in these high-grade patients if improvement is noted after ventricular decompression.

SYSTEMIC EFFECTS

Subarachnoid hemorrhage often is associated with systemic involvement [16]. Massive sympathetic outflow can result in cardiac arrhythmia, myocardial infarction, and hypertension [17,18]. These are best treated with labetalol hydrochloride given as a continuous intravenous infusion. Care should be taken not to excessively lower the blood pressure. Secondary loss of autoregulation in affected vascular territories can lead to hypoperfusion and ischemia. Effects on hypothalamic function lead to the volume contraction observed [19].

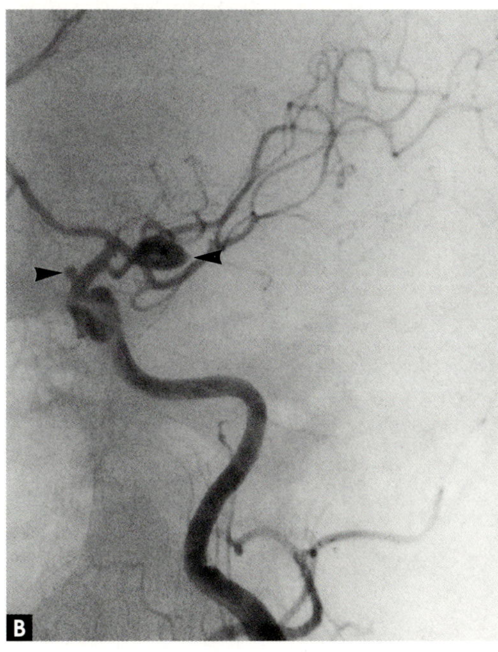

FIGURE 19.2

Cerebral angiogram demonstrating multiple aneurysms (*arrows*) including left middle cerebral (**A**) and right middle cerebral (**B**) and ophthalmic artery aneurysms in the same patient.

Table 19.5 Work-up for aneurysmal subarachnoid hemorrhage

- Careful history
- Physical evaluation
- CT scan
- Lumbar puncture if CT equivocal
- 4-Vessel angiogram
- Repeat 4-vessel angiogram 7–10 days later if negative in the face of clinical diagnosis of SAH

Monitoring of fluid and electrolyte status is mandatory. Severe sympathetic overdrive can progress to changes in pulmonary permeability that resemble respiratory distress syndrome. Ileus is common. Nasogastric tube drainage may be necessary. The use of H_2-blockers will minimize gastric oversecretion and elevate gastric pH, thus decreasing the risk of gastric ulceration. Seizures after subarachnoid hemorrhage occur in approximately 10% of patients. Prophylactic treatment with anticonvulsants such as phenytoin is advocated for all patients, especially in the perihemorrhage period.

SECONDARY INTRACRANIAL COMPLICATIONS

The triad of rebleeding, hydrocephalus, and delayed ischemia constitute the major causes of death and disability in individuals who survive the initial hemorrhage (Figure 19.4) [3,20,21].

Hydrocephalus

Ventricular dilatation after aneurysmal subarachnoid hemorrhage is seen in approximately 67% of patients after subarachnoid hemorrhage [22]. Those who present with significant hydrocephalus and a decreased neurologic grade, or whose condition deteriorates acutely, are candidates for emergent external ventricular drainage. Approximately 14% of patients will require permanent shunts. Any neurologic deterioration should prompt a repeat CT scan.

Rebleeding

The highest incidence of aneurysmal rebleeding (4.5%) occurs the day of the initial hemorrhage, with a 1.5% incidence every day afterward for approximately 2 weeks. This constitutes a 20% incidence over the 2-week period. Rebleeding is catastrophic, with a morbidity and mortality exceeding 48% to 78% [20,21]. Initial enthusiasm for the use of antifibrinolytic agents such as aminocaproic acid and tranexamic acid was quelled when ischemic complication that led to stroke obviated the benefits of a decrease in rebleeding [23]. No role for these agents as part of current subarachnoid hemorrhage management is advocated.

SURGICAL INTERVENTION

Early surgical intervention is advocated for all Hunt Hess grades except grade V and the medically unstable, *ie*, acute MI patients. Direct surgical intervention with clip obliteration remains the primary mode of treatment (Figure 19.5). Past concerns about higher morbidity and mortality with early surgery have not been proven [24,25]. Prompt surgery (within 24 hours of diagnosis) reduces rebleeding and permits a more aggressive approach to ischemic complications should they occur. Novel endovascular approaches to aneurysm obliteration using transarterially placed coils and balloons are currently under investigation (Figure 19.4) [26–30]. Their application and impact on the surgical treatment of intracranial aneurysms may revolutionize treatment. However, sufficient data to justify their replacement of standard surgical approaches is still lacking at this date.

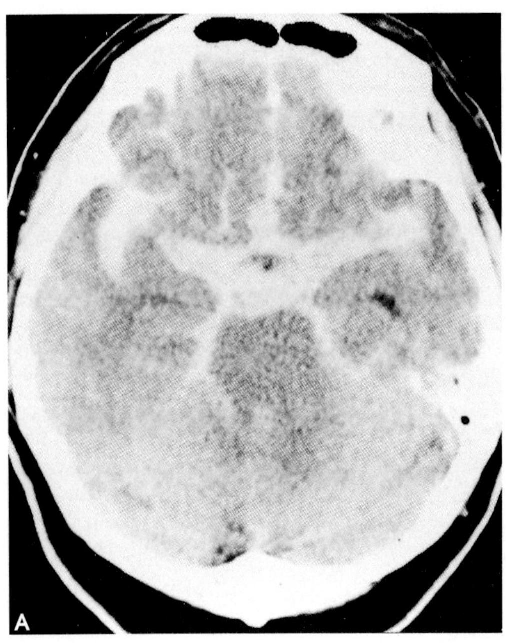

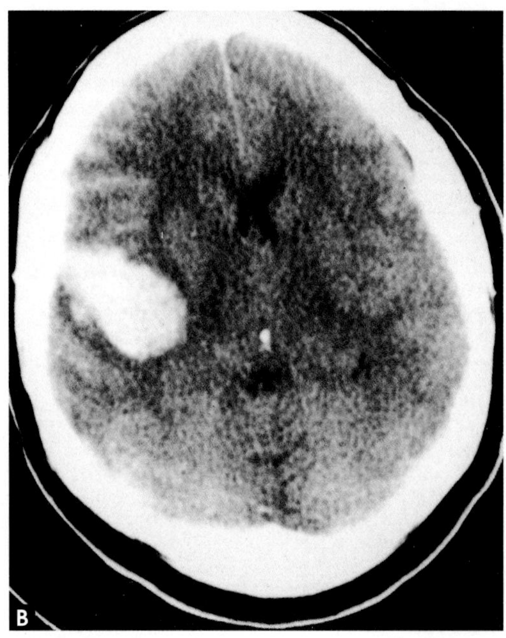

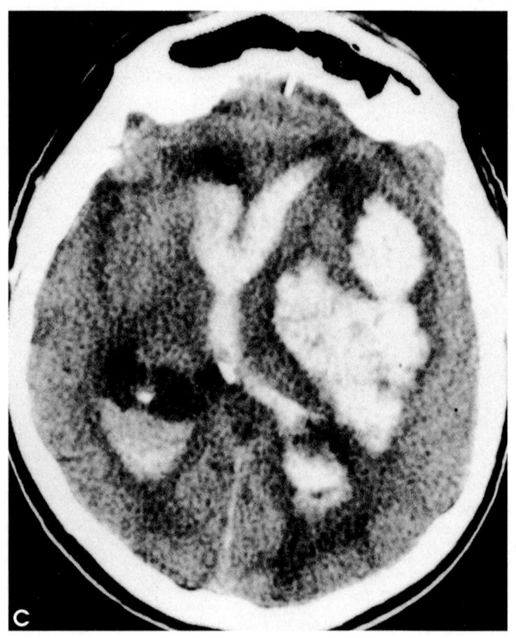

FIGURE 19.3

Intracranial aneurysms can present as subarachnoid hemorrhage (**A**), intraparenchymal hemorrhage (**B**), intraventricular hemorrhage (**C**), or in combination.

TREATMENT OF DELAYED ISCHEMIA

The major cause of death and disability in individuals who survive their initial subarachnoid hemorrhage is delayed cerebral ischemia (DCI), and it affects 25% to 37% of patients [31]. Vasospasm develops between days 4 and 14 after hemorrhage with a peak incidence between days 6 and 8, and maximal luminal narrowing between days 10 and 17 (Figure 19.6) [32]. Delayed cerebral ischemia involves a pathologic cascade initiated by hemoglobin release and breakdown [33,34], propagated by free radical lipid perioxidation [35,36], that results in pathologic calcium metabolism [37–40], which leads to a decrease in luminal diameter (Figure 19.7). The pathophysiology associated with these changes involves a decline in cerebral blood flow over the 2-week period following subarachnoid hemorrhage, reaching a nadir at day 12 (Figure 19.8) [41–44]. It is this decline in cerebral blood flow below a critical ischemic threshold that results in the delayed neurologic deficits. If this flow is not promptly restored, infarction ultimately occurs.

Numerous pharmacologic and physiologic modifiers have been investigated in an effort to improve the outcome of patients after aneurysmal subarachnoid hemorrhage [45,46]. To date, only two treatments have demonstrated an impact on patient outcome after subarachnoid hemorrhage: physiologic modification of cerebral blood flow with hypertension, volume expansion, and hemodilution [42,47–52], and utilization of the calcium channel blocking agents [53–56].

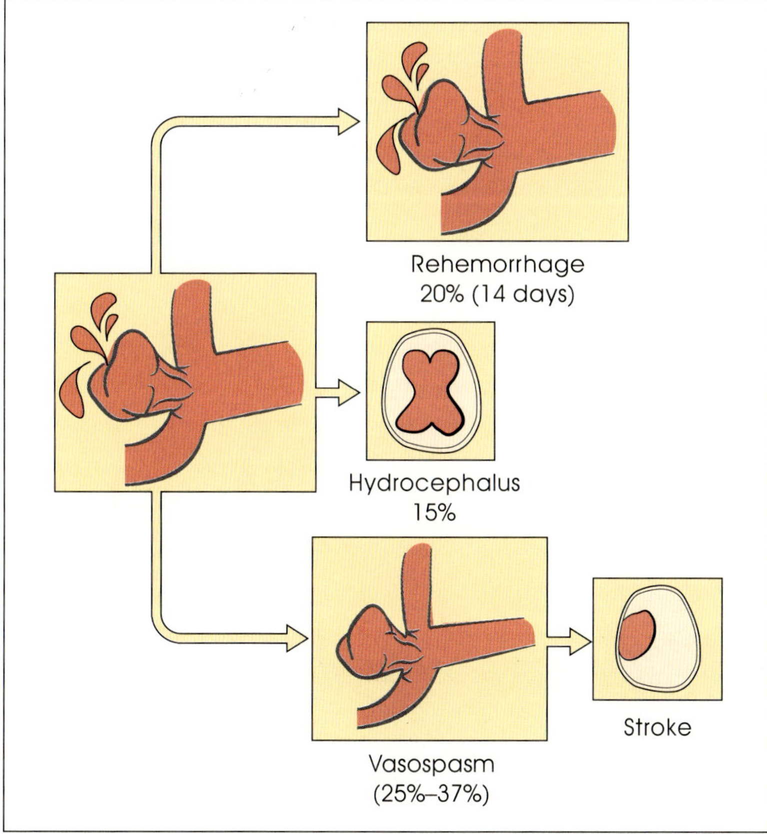

FIGURE 19.4

Rerupture, hydrocephalus, and vasospasm constitute the malignant triad responsible for the majority of morbidity and morality in patients surviving their initial hemorrhage.

The calcium channel blocking agents nimodipine and its intravenous analogue nicardipine are the agents that have been studied most. There has been an overall decrease in cerebral infarction and death in the nimodipine-treated patients in the United States and United Kingdom [53,54]. The stroke rate in the British study was 33% in the control group and 22% in the nimodipine group, with a poor outcome seen in 33% of the control and 20% of the experimental group [53].

In the American study, 121 patients were randomized into a placebo group (63 patients) and nimodipine group (58 patients) [54]. Thirteen patients in the nimodipine group developed severe neurologic deficit (22%), with one death. In the comparable placebo group, 16 patients developed severe deficits (25%); however, eight died.

The mechanism by which nimodipine exerts its beneficial effects is unknown. Originally it was hoped that it would reduce cerebral vasospasm. However, this has not been demonstrated. Human studies have shown that the incidence of chronic vasospasm is unchanged by nimodipine use [53–55]. Nimodipine failed to increase or affect the decline in cerebral blood flow after subarachnoid hemorrhage [56]. To be beneficial, it must be given in a prophylactic fashion within 96 hours. These observations have prompted speculation that nimodipine may act as a cytoprotective agent augmenting pathologic calcium influx and thereby allowing the patient to tolerate ischemia better.

More recently, the randomized control trial of the intravenous calcium blocking agent nicardipine was published [57,58]. In the randomly divided group of 906 patients, 46% of the control group and 32% of the nicardipine group developed symptomatic vasospasm. However, the overall outcome at 3 months was similar between the two groups. Good recovery was seen in 55% of the nicardipine group with deaths in 17%, as compared with a 56% good outcome in the control group and deaths in 18%, demonstrating no significant difference. The control group was treated with hypervolemia and induced hypertension for symptomatic spasm. The author's summary of these results suggests that while nicardipine prevents vasospasm, hypertensive hypervolemic therapy may be effective in reversing ischemic deficits from vasospasm once they occur [57,58].

Physiologic modulation using hypervolemic hemodilution with induced hypertension provides conditions that are physiologically optimal for improved cerebral perfusion, resulting in improved clinical grade [42,47–52]. Our results in 100 patients with a graded prophylactic protocol of hypervolemic hemodilution, augmented if necessary by induced hypertension (triple-H therapy), in combination with prompt surgery (within 24 hours of admission), demonstrate an overall stroke rate of 10%, with a 2.2% ischemic death rate (Hunt Hess Grades I–IV only) [42,57]. Chronic angiographic spasm was seen in at least 46% of all patients. Despite the presence of angiographic arterial narrowing, cerebral blood flow improved. These results are similar to those of Solomon and coworkers [50,51] in his subgroup of 56 early operated patients. Triple H therapy effectively minimizes delayed cerebral ischemia by increasing cerebral blood flow during the critical period when delayed cerebral ischemia is known to occur. It can be applied to all patients regardless of grade on admission or interval after subarachnoid

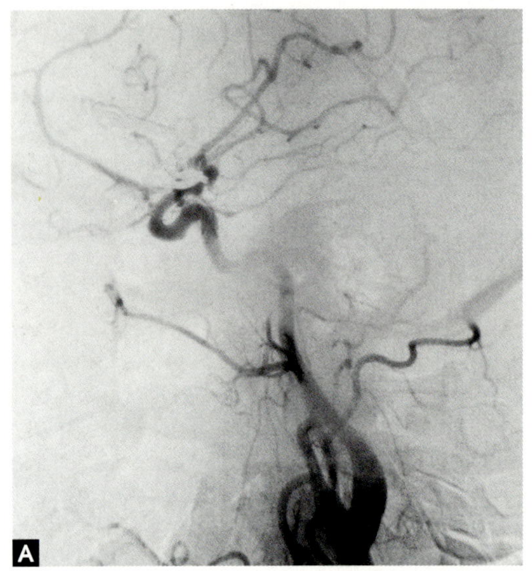

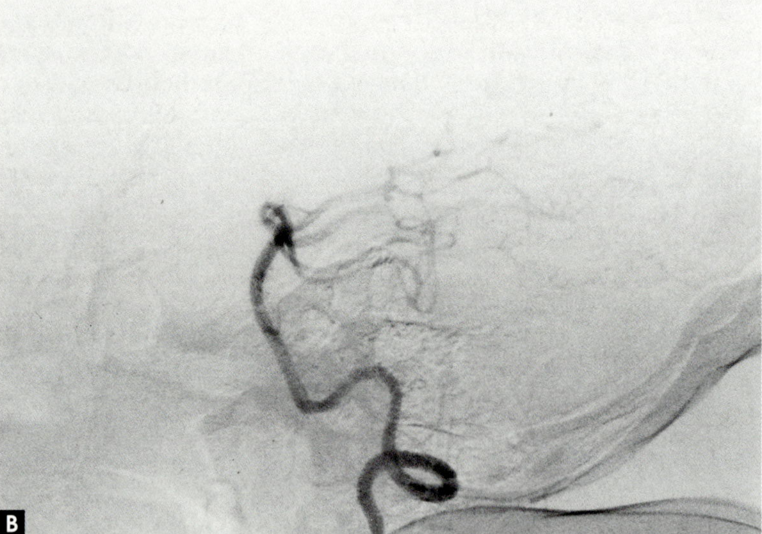

FIGURE 19.5

Angiographic arterial narrowing in a patient after subarachnoid hemorrhage. Initial postoperative angiogram (**A**) demonstrates obliteration of aneurysms. Repeat angiogram (**B**) 10 days later demonstrates diffuse spasm involving the carotid (**C**) (*arrowheads*) and basilar (**D**) (*arrowheads*) arteries.

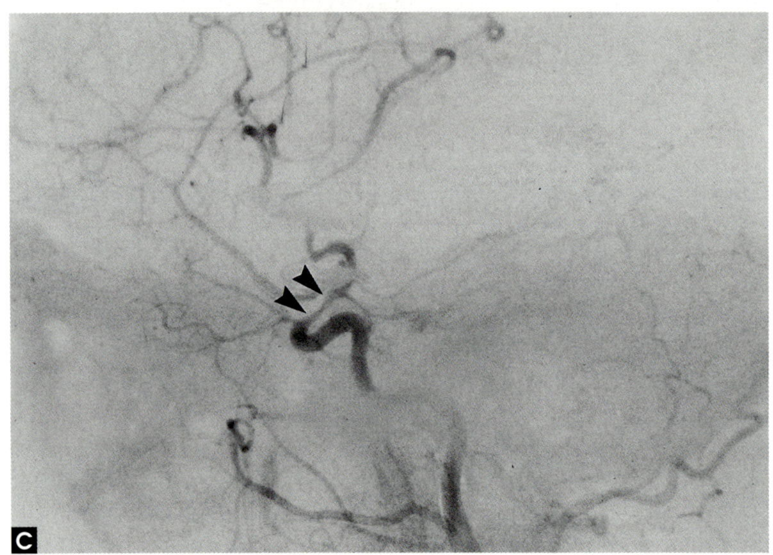

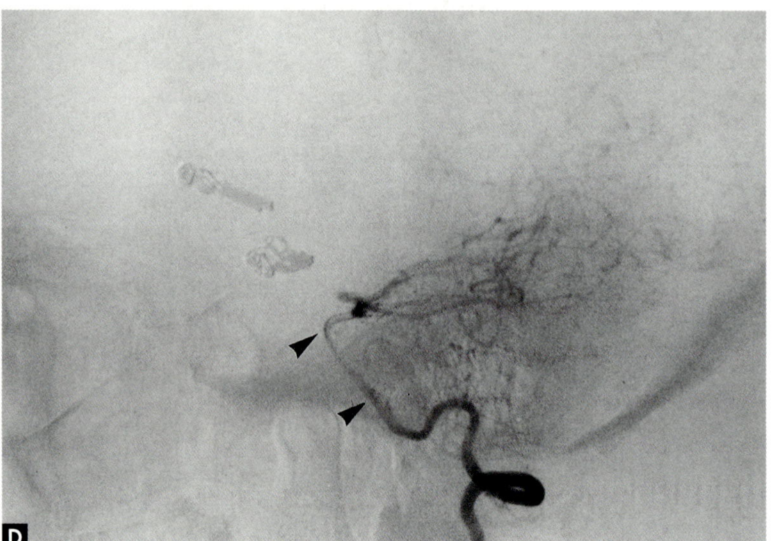

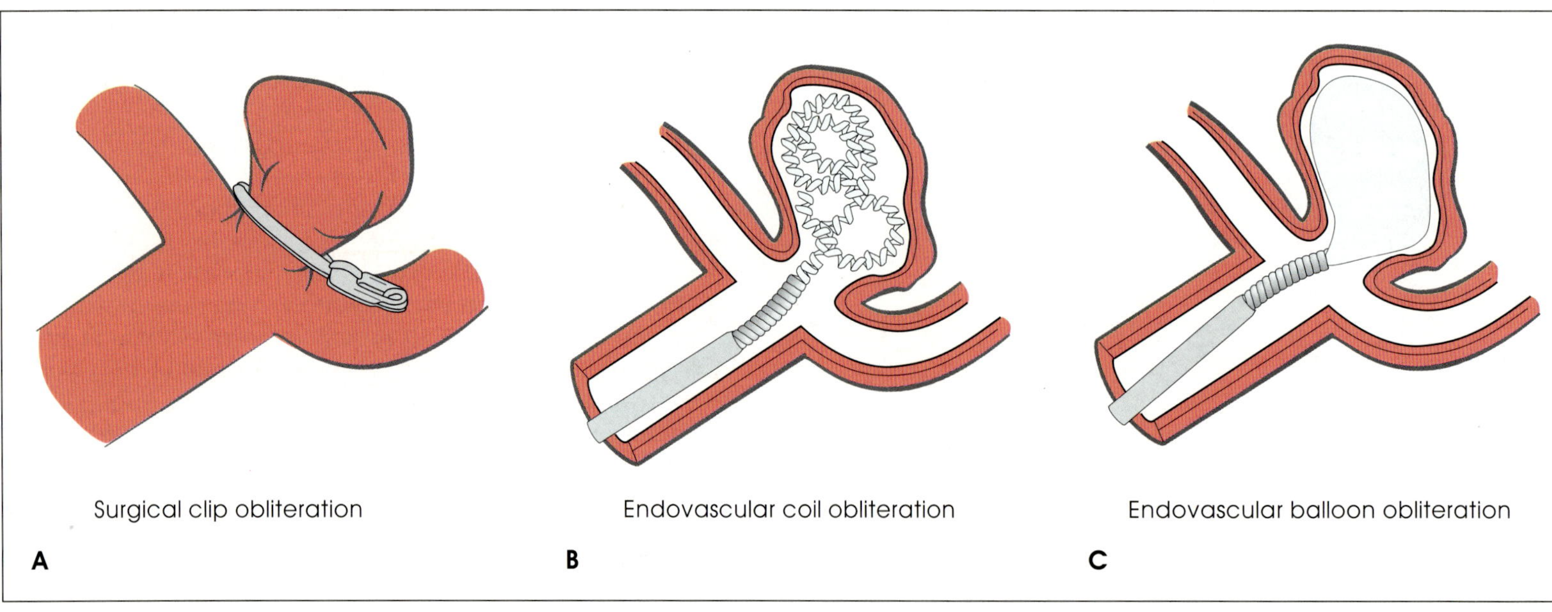

FIGURE 19.6

Obliteration of aneurysms can be carried out by direct surgical approach and clip application (**A**) by endovascular coil (**B**) or balloon occlusion (**C**). Direct surgical approach represents the gold standard in the 1990s.

hemorrhage. It causes rapid elevation in cerebral blood flow and it can reverse neurologic deficit and sustain cerebral blood flow during the period before definitive surgery. Physiologic modulation does not, however, impact on the underlying mechanisms causing vascular narrowing.

To optimize this therapy safely, the aneurysm should be secured promptly. Doing so permits a more aggressive approach and increases treatment options should ischemia occur. The question of whether this type of treatment should be employed prophylactically or after symptoms have occurred is open for debate. An ongoing randomized trial to answer this question scientifically is underway (Solomon, Personal communication). What has been demonstrated is that hypovolemia should be avoided.

PROMISING NOVEL APPROACHES

The 21-aminosteroid, U74006F, is a potent inhibitor of iron-dependent lipid perioxidation and has been shown in previous experimental studies to block development of chronic vasospasm [35,36,60–62]. This agent is currently under clinical trials in Europe and North America. Its mechanism of action involves interdiction of free radical driven lipid perioxidation reactions.

The best treatment for vasospasm is to avoid its occurrence. Mechanical removal of cisternal clot can be performed, but it is limited and hazardous. Several investigations have found that injecting recombinant tissue plasminogen activator (rt-PA) into the basal cisterns has shown promise for virtually eliminating vasospasm [9,63–66]. This agent works by allowing rapid clearance of blood from the subarachnoid space. The major potential complication is hemorrhage. A randomized trial is currently underway to establish efficacy and safety of this treatment.

In the presence of intense symptomatic, life-threatening spasm that is refractory to physiologic augmentation, a number of investigators have turned to endovascular cerebral angioplasty (Figure 19.9) [67,68]. This technique involves transarterial endovascular balloon dilatation. Criteria for patient selection and large series outcomes are forthcoming. However, preliminary results are promising, and the utilization of this technique as a heroic maneuver in the face of an acute refractory ischemia secondary to vasospasm should be considered.

OVERALL MANAGEMENT

Acute, accurate diagnoses based on a high index of suspicion and a careful history are paramount (Figure 19.10). A noncontrast CT scan should be performed; lumbar puncture is indicated if the CT is negative and the clinical impression warrants. Cerebral angiography should be performed in a timely fashion to allow for prompt surgery. Angiographic subtraction films of all four cerebral vessels must be obtained to rule out multiple aneurysms. We advocate baseline cerebral blood flow studies

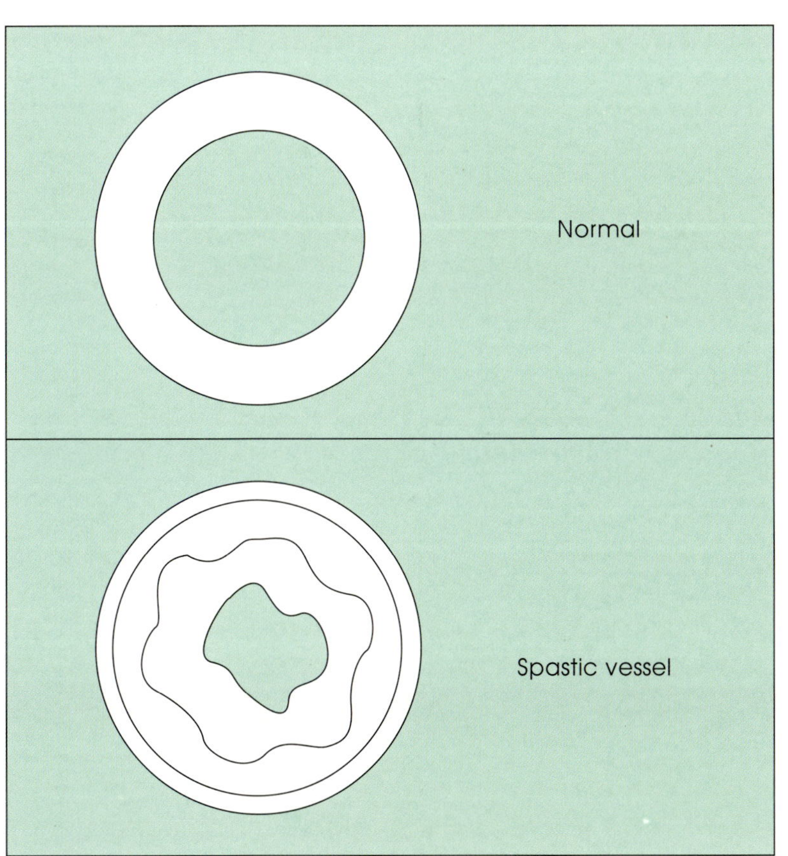

FIGURE 19.7

Illustration of normal (*top*) and vasospastic vessel (*bottom*). Note the decrease in luminal diameter resulting in decreased cerebral blood flow. (*Adapted from* Nosko and coworkers [70]; with permission.)

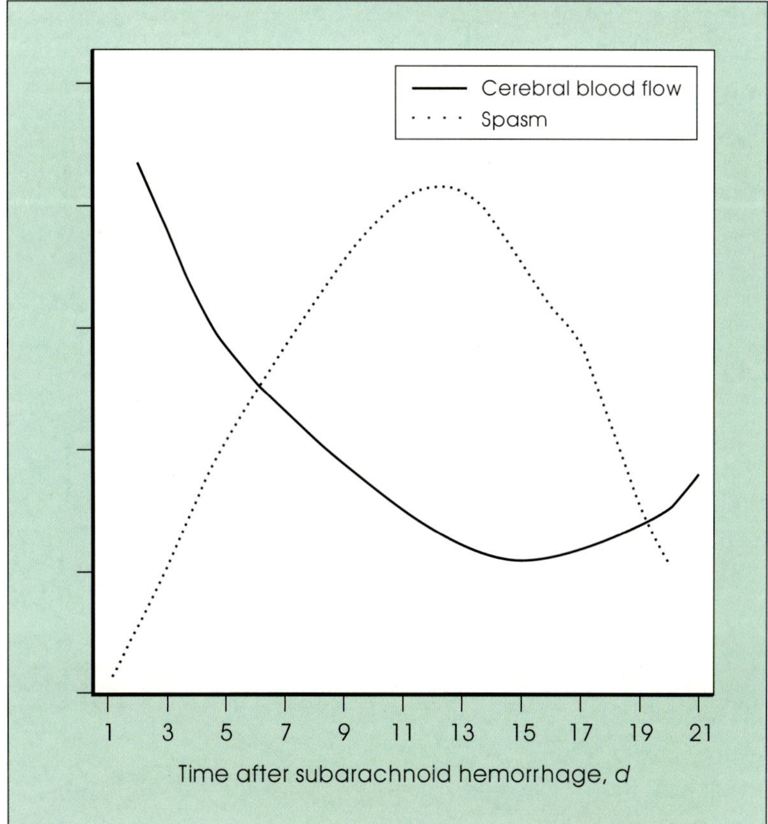

FIGURE 19.8

Graphic representation of increase in arterial narrowing and decrease in cerebral blood flow occurring after subarachnoid hemorrhage (*Adapted from* Kwak and coworkers [71] and Meyer and coworkers [41]; with permission.).

and transcranial Doppler to aid in managing these complex cases. Prompt surgery (within 24 hours of admission) virtually eliminates the risk of rehemorrhage. We then proceed with prophylactic hypervolemic hemodilution. Calcium channel blocking agents are a hedge against delayed ischemia. Serial cerebral blood flow/transcranial Doppler monitoring provides valuable information about end-organ response to these therapies, and aids in the prediction of impending ischemia. A decrease in cerebral blood flow occurs prior to changes in neurologic status and anticipates the clinical change [42,59]. Transcranial Doppler velocities are also predictive [69]. However, when physiologic augmentation is given, interpretation can be difficult. Direct cerebral blood flow measurements are confirmatory.

Neurologic deterioration during the postoperative period should prompt a repeat CT scan (to rule out hydrocephalus, rebleeding, or ischemia), metabolic work-up (for electrolyte abnormalities or infection), and cerebral blood flow studies. In the face of declining cerebral blood flow or clinical condition, hypertensive augmentation should be implemented. Serial cerebral blood flow measurements and clinical status guide the intensity and duration of therapy. Failure of these treatments would prompt reangiography and consideration of cerebral angioplasty.

We do repeat angiography routinely 10 to 12 days post–subarachnoid hemorrhage to confirm clip placement in our patients, monitor angiographic arterial narrowing, and as a reevaluation for multiple aneurysms. Patients are generally discharged 14 to 21 days post–subarachnoid hemorrhage.

Today, early diagnosis, prompt surgery, and aggressive physiologic management are having an impact on the historically poor outcome of patients with aneurysmal subarachnoid hemorrhage. Ongoing investigations are yielding promising new treatments that will further improve outcome. A vital part of any future changes will be community and physician education about the diagnosis and early treatment of this devastating disease.

ACKNOWLEDGMENT

The author thanks Jill Wallock and Virginia Cowart for editorial and graphics assistance.

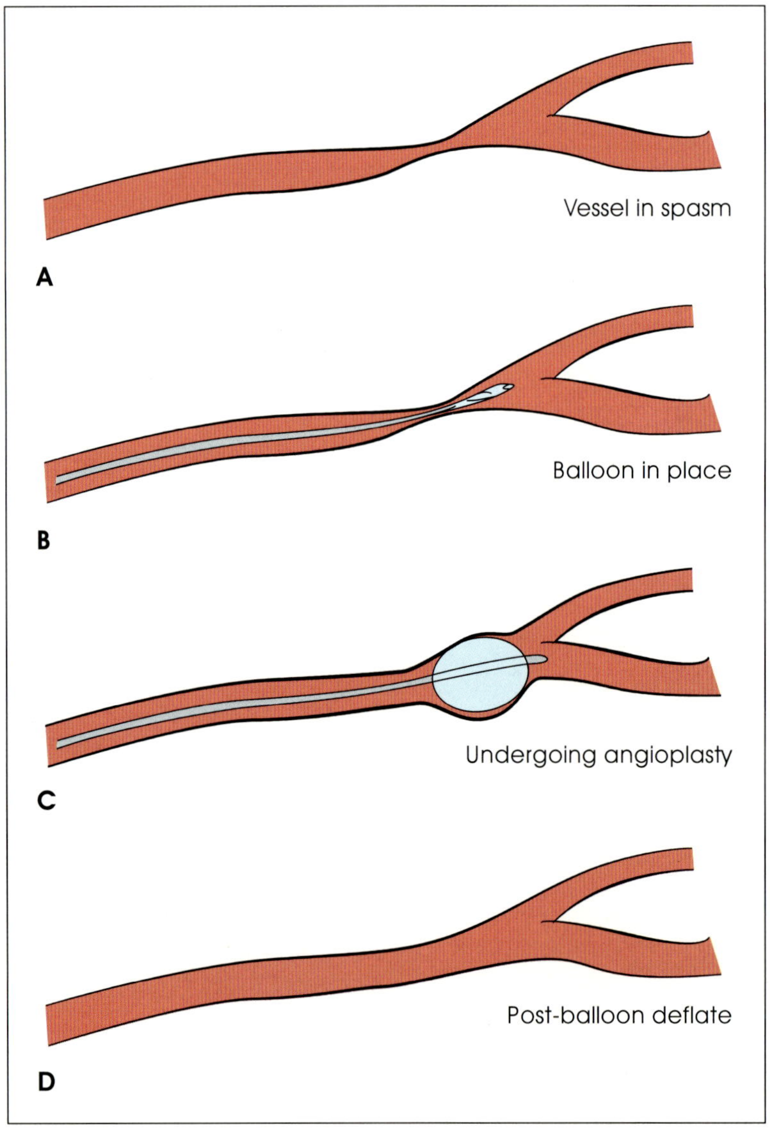

FIGURE 19.9

A–D, Angioplasty for refractory spasm. Direct balloon dilatation of constricted vessels.

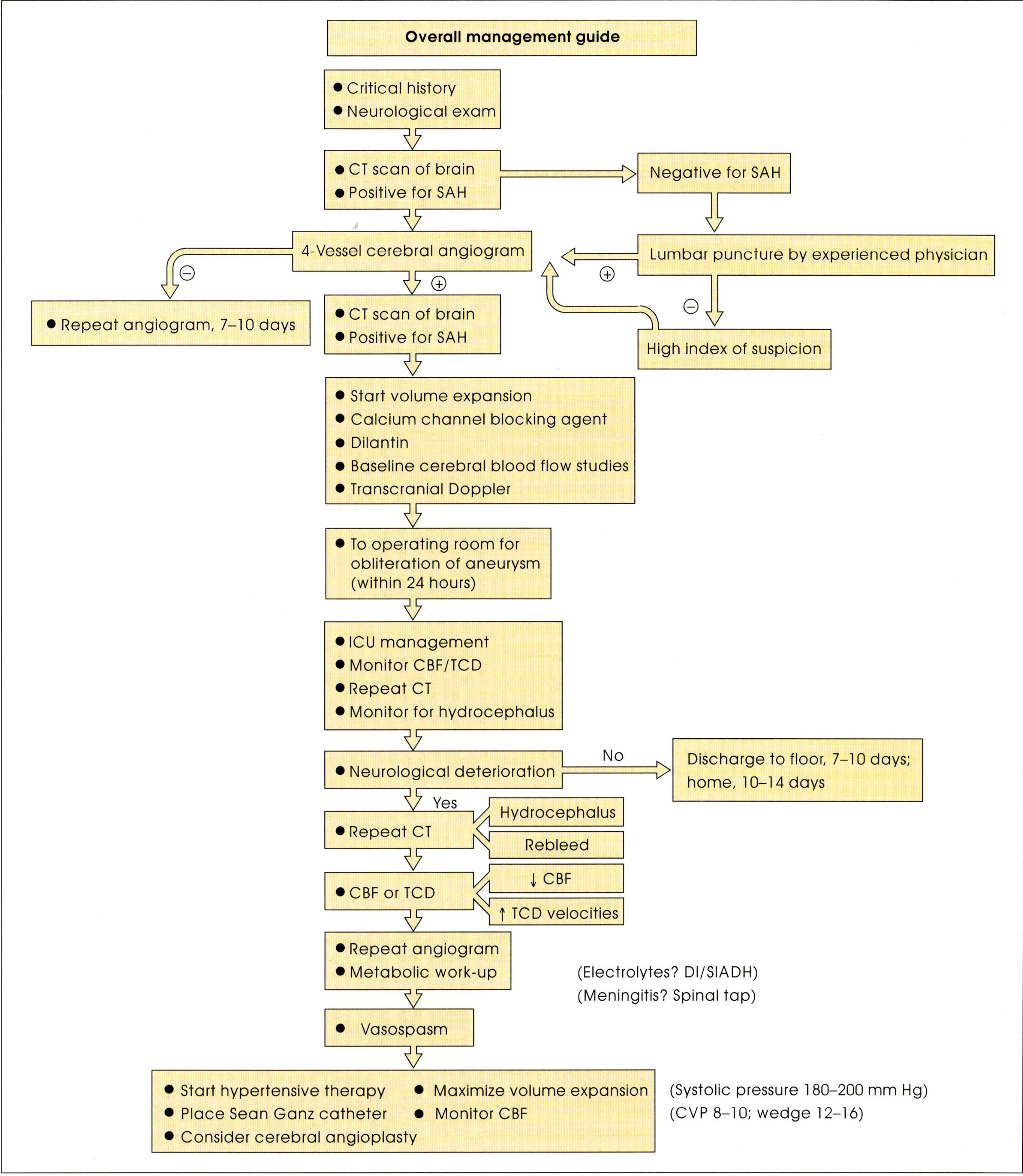

FIGURE 19.10

Overall management guide for patients with aneurysmal subarachnoid hemorrhage (SAH). CBF—cerebral blood flow; CT—computed tomography; CVP—central venous pressure; DI—diabetes insipidus; ICU—intensive care unit; SIADH—syndrome of inappropriate antidiuretic hormone; TCD—transcranial Doppler.

REFERENCES

1. Sahs AL, Nibbleunk DW, Torner JC, eds.: *Aneurysmal Subarachnoid Hemorrhage: Report of the Cooperative Study.* Baltimore:Urban and Schwarzenberg; 1981.
2. Inagawa T, Hirano A: Autopsy study of unruptured incidental intracranial aneurysms. *Surg Neurol* 1990, 34:361–365.
3. Kassell NF, Darke CG: Timing of aneurysm surgery. *Neurosurgery* 1982, 10:515–519.
4. Graf CJ, Torner JC, Penet GE, Nibbelunk DW: Cooperative aneurysm study: long term follow-up evaluation of randomized study. In *Aneurysmal Subarachnoid Hemorrhage: Report of the Cooperative Study.* Edited by Sahs AL, Nibbelunk DW, Torner JC. Baltimore: Urban and Schwarzenberg; 1981:203–248.
5. Ausman JI, Diaz FG, Malik GM, *et al.*: Current management of cerebral aneurysms: is it based on facts or fiction? *Surg Neurol* 1985, 24:625–635.
6. Ausman JI, Diaz FG, Malik GM, *et al.*: Management of cerebral aneurysms: further facts and additional myths. *Surg Neurol* 1989, 32:21–35.
7. Billér J, Godersky JC, Adams HP Jr.: Management of aneurysmal subarachnoid hemorrhage. *Stroke* 1988, 19:1300–1305.
8. Espinosa F, Weir B, Noseworthy T: Nonoperative treatment of subarachnoid hemorrhage. In *Neurological Surgery,* 3rd ed. Edited by Youmons JR. Philadelphia: WB Saunders Co; 1990:1661–1688.
9. Findlay JM, Macdonald RL, Weir BKA: Current concepts of pathophysiology and management of cerebral vasospasm following aneurysmal subarachnoid hemorrhage. In *Cerebrovascular and Brain Metabolism Reviews.* Edited by Harper AM. New York: Raven Press, Ltd; 1991:336–361.
10. Schievurk WI, Karemaker JM, Hageman LM, Van der Wef DJM: Circumstances surrounding aneurysmal subarachnoid hemorrhage. *Surg Neurol* 1989, 32:266–272.
11. Fisher CM, Kistler JP, Davis JM: Relation of cerebral vasospasm to subarachnoid hemorrhage visualized by computerized tomographic scanning. *Neurosurgery* 1980, 6:1–9.
12. Kistler JP, Crowell RM, Davis KR, *et al.*: The relation of cerebral vasospasm to the extent and location of subarachnoid blood visualized by CT scan: a prospective study. *Neurology* 1983, 33:424–436.
13. Hunt WE, Hess RM: Surgical risk as related to time of intervention in the repair of intracranial aneurysms. *J Neurosurg* 1968, 28:14–19.
14. Weir B: Intracranial aneurysms and subarachnoid hemorrhage: an overview. In *Neurosurgery.* Edited by Wilkins RH, Rengachary SS. New York: McGraw-Hill Book Company; 1985:1308–1329.
15. Grote E, Hassler W: The critical first minutes after subarachnoid hemorrhage. *Neurosurgery* 1988, 22:654–661.
16. Barker FG, Heros RC: Clinical aspects of vasospasm. *Neurosurg Clin North Am* 1990, 1:227–228.
17. Dilraj A, Botha JH, Rambiritch V, *et al.*: Levels of catecholamine in plasma and cerebrospinal fluid in aneurysmal subarachnoid hemorrhage. *Neurosurgery* 1992, 31:42–51.
18. Marion DW, Segal RS, Thompson ME: Subarachnoid hemorrhage and the heart. *Neurosurgery* 1986, 18:101–106.
19. Solomon RA, Post KD, McMurtry JG: Depression of circulating blood volume in patients after subarachnoid hemorrhage: implications for the management of symptomatic vasospasm. *Neurosurgery* 1984, 15:354–361.
20. Nishioka H, Torner JC, Graf CJ, *et al.*: Cooperative study of intracranial aneurysms and subarachnoid hemorrhage: a long-term prognostic study. II: Ruptured intracranial aneurysms managed conservatively. *Arch Neurol* 1984, 41:1142–1146.
21. Kassell NF, Torner JC: Aneurysmal rebleeding: a preliminary report of the cooperative aneurysm study. *Neurosurgery* 1983, 13:479–481.
22. Black PM: Hydrocephalus and vasospasm after subarachnoid hemorrhage from ruptured intracranial aneurysms. *Neurosurgery* 1986, 18:12–16.
23. Kassell NF, Torner JC, Adams HP: Antifibrinolytic therapy in the acute period following aneurysmal subarachnoid hemorrhage; preliminary observation from the cooperative aneurysm study. *J Neurosurg* 1984, 61:225–230.
24. Disney L, Weir B, Petruk K: Effect on management mortality of a deliberate policy of early operation on supratentorial aneurysms. *Neurosurgery* 1987, 20:695–701.
25. Kassell NF, Boarini DJ, Adams HP Jr, *et al.*: Overall management of ruptured aneurysms: comparison of early and late operation. *Neurosurgery* 1981, 9:120–128.
26. Guglielmi G, Viñuela F, Duckwiler G, *et al.*: Endovascular treatment of posterior circulation aneurysms by electrothromboses using electrically detachable coils. *J Neurosurg* 1992, 77:515–524.
27. Higashida RT, Halbach VV, Dowd CF, *et al.*: Intracranial aneurysms: interventional neurovascular treatment with detachable balloons–results in 215 cases. *Radiology* 1991, 178:663–670.
28. Taki W, Nishi S, Yamashita K, *et al.*: Selection and combination of various endovascular techniques in the treatment of giant aneurysms. *J Neurosurg* 1992, 77:37–42.
29. Heilman CB, Kan ESK, Wu JK: Aneurysm recurrence following endovascular balloon occlusion. *J Neurosurg* 1992, 77:260–264.
30. Casasco AE, Aymard A, Gobin YP, *et al.*: Selective endovascular treatment of 71 intracranial aneurysms with platinum coils. *J Neurosurg* 1993, 79:3–10.
31. Kassel NF, Sasaki T, Colohan AR, Nazar G: Cerebral vasospasm following aneurysmal subarachnoid hemorrhage. *Stroke* 1985, 16:562–572.
32. Weir B, Grace M, Hansen J, Rothberg C: Time course of vasospasm in man. *J Neurosurg* 1978, 48:173–178.
33. Macdonald RL, Weir BKA: A review of hemoglobin and the pathogenesis of cerebral vasospasm. *Stroke* 1991, 22:971–982.
34. Macdonald RL, Weir BKA, Runzer TD, *et al.*:Etiology of cerebral vasospasm in primates. *J Neurosurg* 1992, 76:725–726.
35. Kanamaru K, Weir BKA, Findlay JM, *et al.*: A dosage study of the effect of the 21-aminosteroid U74006F on chronic cerebral vasospasm in a primate model. *Neurosurgery* 1990, 27:29–38.
36. Steinke DE, Weir BKA, Findlay JM, *et al.*: A trial of the 21-aminosteroid U74006F in a primate model of chronic cerebral vasospasm. *Neurosurgery* 1989, 24:179–186.
37. Allen GS, Bahr AL: Cerebral arterial spasm: part 10. reversal of acute and chronic spasm in dogs with orally administered nifedipine. *Neurosurgery* 1979, 4:43–47.
38. Tararewicz JW, Pluta R, Salinska E, Puka M: Beneficial effect of nimodipine on metabolic and function disturbances in rabbit hippocampus following complete cerebral ischemia. *Stroke* 1989, 20:70–77.
39. Seijo BK: Pathophysiology and treatment of focal cerebral ischemia. Part I: Pathophysiology. *J Neurosurg* 1992, 77:169–187.
40. Seijo BK: Pathophysiology and treatment of focal cerebral ischemia. *J Neurosurg* 1992, 77:337–354.
41. Meyer CH, Lowe D, Meyer M, *et al.*: Progressive change in cerebral blood flow during the first three weeks after subarachnoid hemorrhage. *Neurosurgery* 1983, 12:58–76.
42. Origitano TC, Wascher TM, Reichman OH, Anderson DE: Sustained increased cerebral blood flow with prophylactic hypertensive hypervolemic hemodilution ("Triple-H" therapy) after subarachnoid hemorrhage. *Neurosurgery* 1990, 27:729–740.
43. Rosenstein J, Suzuki M, Symon L, Redmond S: Clinical use of a portable bedside cerebral blood flow machine in the management of aneurysmal subarachnoid hemorrhage. *Neurosurgery* 1984, 15:519–525.
44. Géraud G, Tremoulet M, Guell A, Bes A: The prognostic value of noninvasive CBF measurement in subarachnoid hemorrhage. *Stroke* 1984, 15:301–305.

45. Wilkins RH: Attempts at prevention or treatment of intracranial arterial spasm: an update. *Neurosurgery* 1986, 18:808–825.
46. Wilkins RH: Attempted prevention or treatment of intracranial arterial spasm: a survey. *Neurosurgery* 1980, 6:198–210.
47. Kassell NF, Peerless SS, Durward QJ, *et al.*: Treatment of ischemic deficits from vasospasm with intravascular volume expansion and induced arterial hypertension. *Neurosurgery* 1982, 11:337–343.
48. Muizelaar JP, Becker DP: Induced hypertension for the treatment of cerebral ischemia after subarachnoid hemorrhage: direct effect on cerebral blood flow. *Surg Neurol* 1986, 25:317–325.
49. Awad IA, Carter LP, Spetzler RF, *et al.*: Clinical vasospasm after subarachnoid hemorrhage: response to hypervolemic hemodilution and arterial hypertension. *Stroke* 1987, 18:365–372.
50. Solomon RA, Fink ME, Lennihan L: Prophylactic volume expansion therapy for the prevention of delayed cerebral ischemia after early aneurysm surgery. *Arch Neurol* 1988, 45:325–332.
51. Solomon RA, Fink ME, Lennihan L: Early aneurysm surgery and prophylactic hypervolemic hypertensive therapy for the treatment of aneurysmal subarachnoid hemorrhage. *Neurosurgery* 1988, 23:699–704.
52. Levy ML, Giannotta SL: Cardiac performance indices during hypervolemic therapy for cerebral vasospasm. *J Neurosurg* 1991, 75:27–31.
53. Pickard JD, Murray GD, Illingworth R, *et al.*: Effect of oral nimodipine on cerebral infarction and outcome after subarachnoid haemorrhage: British aneurysm nimodipine trial. *BMJ* 1989, 298:636–642.
54. Allen GS, Ahn HS, Preziosi TJ, *et al.*: Cerebral arterial spasm: a controlled trial of nimodipine in patients with subarachnoid hemorrhage. *N Engl J Med* 1983, 308:619–624.
55. Petruk KC, West M, Mohr G, *et al.*: Nimodipine treatment in poor-grade aneurysm patients: results of a multicenter, double-blind placebo-controlled trial. *J Neurosurg* 1988, 68:505–517.
56. Neil-Dwyer G, Mee E, Dorrance D, Lowe D: Early intervention with nimodipine in subarachnoid hemorrhage. *Eur Heart J* (suppl K) 1987, 8:41–47.
57. Haley EC, Kassell NF, Torner JC, *et al.*: A randomized controlled trial of high-dose intravenous nicardipine in aneurysmal subarachnoid hemorrhage. *J Neurosurg* 1993, 78:537–547.
58. Haley EC, Kassell NF, Torner JC, *et al.*:A randomized trial of nicardipine in subarachnoid hemorrhage: angiographic and transcranial Doppler ultrasound results. *J Neurosurg* 1993, 78:548–553.
59. Origitano TC, Wascher TM, Reichman OH, Anderson DE: Cerebral blood flow patterns in patients with aneurysmal subarachnoid hemorrhage treated with "Triple-H" therapy. *Neurosurgery.*
60. Zuccarello M, Marsch JT, Schmit G, *et al.*: Effect of the 21 aminosteroid U-74006F on cerebral vasospasm following subarachnoid hemorrhage. *J Neurosurg* 1989, 71:98–104.
61. Zuccarello M, Anderson DK: Protective effect of a 21-amminosteroid on the blood-brain barrier following subarachnoid hemorrhage in rats. *Stroke* 1989, 20:367–371.
62. Vollmer DG, Kassell NF, Hongo K, *et al.*: Effect of the nonglucocorticoid 21-aminosteroid U74006F on experimental cerebral vasospasm. *Surg Neurol* 1989, 31:190–194.
63. Findlay JM, Weir BK, Gordon P, *et al.*: Safety and efficacy of intrathecal thrombolytic therapy in a primate model of cerebral vasospasm. *Neurosurgery* 1989, 24:491–498.
64. Findlay JM, Weir BKA, Steinke D, *et al.*: Effect of intrathecal thrombolytic therapy on subarachnoid clot and chronic vasospasm in a primate model of SAH. *J Neurosurg* 1988, 69:723–735.
65. Findlay JM, Weir BK, Kanamura K, *et al.*: The effect of timing of intrathecal fibrinolytic therapy on cerebral vasospasm in a primate subarachnoid hemorrhage. *Neurosurgery* 1990, 26:201–206
66. Mizoi K, Yoshimoto T, Takahashi A, *et al.*: Prospective study on the prevention of cerebral vasospasm by intrathecal fibrinolytic therapy with tissue-type plasminogen activator. *J Neurosurg* 1993, 78:430–437.
67. Newell DW, Eskridge JM, Mayberg MR, *et al.*: Angioplasty for the treatment of symptomatic vasospasm following subarachnoid hemorrhage. *J Neurosurg* 1989, 71:654–660.
68. Higashida RT, Halbach VV, Cahan LD, *et al.*: Transluminal angioplasty for treatment of intracranial arterial vasospasm. *J Neurosurg* 1989, 71:648–653.
69. Grosset DG, Straiton J, McDonald I, *et al.*: Use os transcranial Doppler sonography to predict development of a delayed ischemic deficit after subarachnoid hemorrhage. *J Neurosurg* 1993, 78:183–187.
70. Nosko M, Weir B, Krueger C, Cook D, *et al.*: Nimodipine and chronic vasospasm in monkeys: Part I. Clinical and radiological findings. *Neurosurgery* 1985, 16:129–136.
71. Kwak R, Niizuma H, Ohit Suzuki J: Angiographic study of cerebral vasospasm following rupture of intracranial aneurysms: Part I. Time of the appearance. *Surg Neurol* 1979, 11:257–262.

Chapter 20

Management of Intracerebral Hemorrhage

MICHAEL A. KELLY

The treatment of intraparenchymal brain hemorrhage is largely determined by several characteristics of the hemorrhage: size, location and etiology, neurologic status, and the overall medical condition of the patient. For many patients, skilled nursing care is the cornerstone of therapy. Others will need correction of hypertension or bleeding diathesis. For still others, most critical is the proper management of intracranial pressure, pulmonary function, and fluid status. Surgical evacuation is life-saving in selected patients. Meticulous care is warranted (although the mortality rate is high), because those patients who survive may do well.

CLINICAL PRESENTATION

Initial presentation of intracerebral hemorrhage (ICH) is often dramatic, the seriousness of the illness evident to both patient and physician. Treatment begins with recognition of the clinical syndromes of ICH [1]. The symptoms and signs of ICH are dependent on the location of the hematoma (Table 20.1). The most common location is within the basal ganglia, followed by cerebral cortex and subcortical white matter, thalamus, cerebellum, and pons as indicated in Figure 20.1. Computed tomography (CT) scan images of representative spontaneous ICHs are seen in Figure 20.2.

Hemiparesis results from hemorrhage within the frontal lobe, the basal ganglia, thalamus when there is involvement of the adjacent internal capsule, or the basis pontis. Quadriplegia is seen in large bilateral hemorrhage within the basis pontis. If the pontine tegmentum is involved there is absence of lateral eye movements, small reactive pupils, and coma. Depressed consciousness and coma are also seen in large putaminal, thalamic hemorrhage with midline shift, and cerebellar hemorrhages that compress brainstem structures.

Drowsiness, confusion, and impaired memory may be seen in thalamic hemorrhage. Intraventricular hemorrhage may be nonfocal and manifest only as headache and confusion. Difficulty with gait is characteristic of cerebellar hemorrhage, often with complaints of nausea, vomiting, and headache. Visual loss is seen in occipital lobe hemorrhage. Aphasia, sensory loss, and neglect accompany hemorrhage in frontal and parietal lobes. Gaze deviation is common in putaminal hemorrhage and may be seen in brainstem or cerebellar hemorrhage. Thalamic hemorrhage is notable for downward and inward deviation of the eyes.

Table 20.1. Localization of signs of intracerebral hemorrhage

Sign	Location
Weakness	Frontal lobe, putamen/internal capsule, basis pontis
Depressed consciousness	Large lesions of lobes, putamen, thalamus, mesencephalic and pontine tegmentum
Confusion	Caudate, thalamus.
Gaze palsy	Frontal lobe, putamen, thalamus, mesencephalic and pontine tegmentum
Gait disorder	Cerebellum

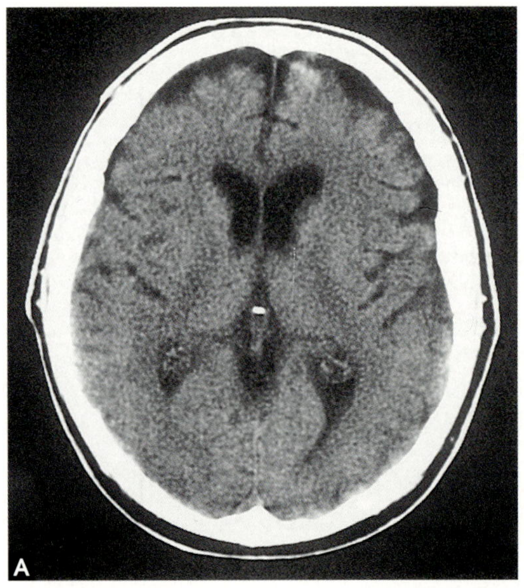

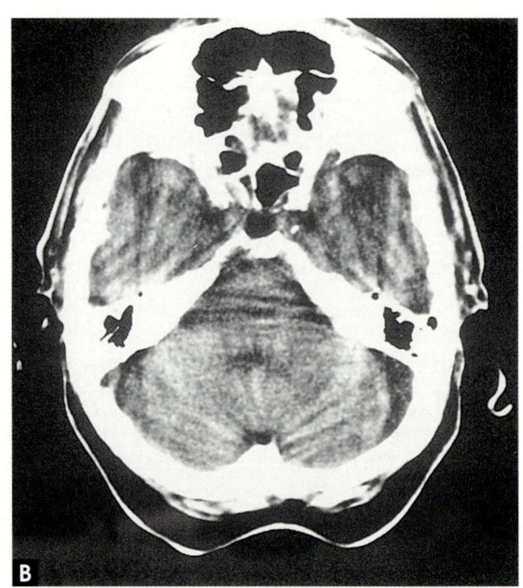

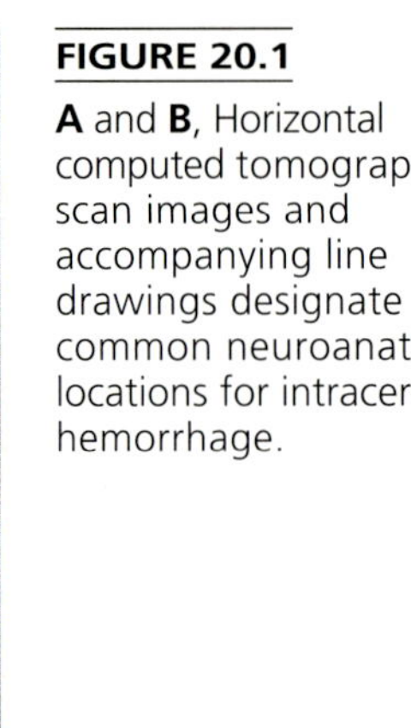

FIGURE 20.1

A and **B**, Horizontal computed tomography scan images and accompanying line drawings designate the common neuroanatomic locations for intracerebral hemorrhage.

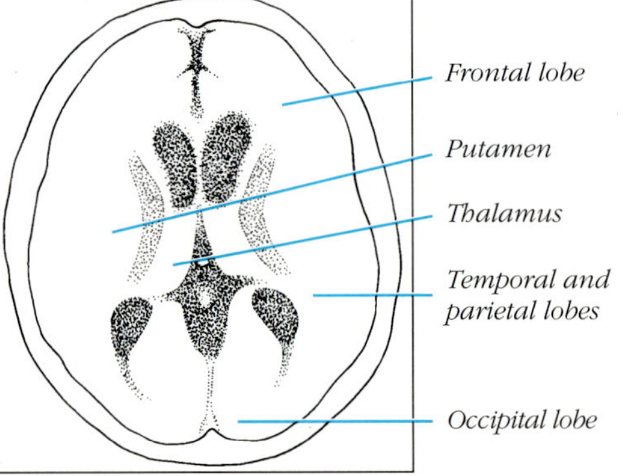

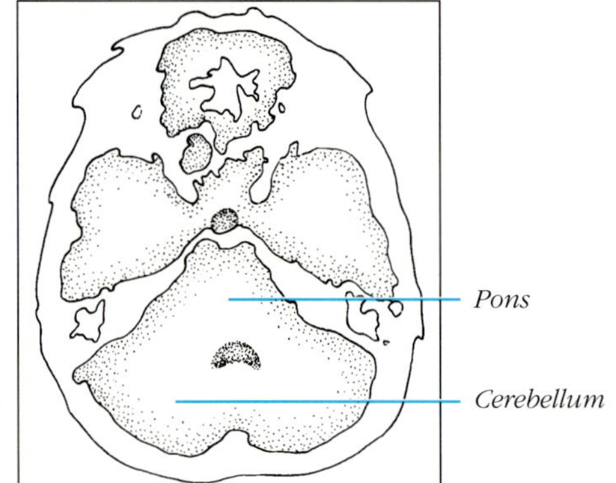

PREDICTORS OF OUTCOME

Predictors of outcome after ICH (Table 20.2) include clinical features, primarily level of consciousness, and the size, location, and extent of hemorrhage on CT scan. Blood pressure, level of consciousness, eye findings, and motor weakness are independent predictors of outcome [2–5]. Supratentorial hemorrhage volume of greater than 50 cm^3 is a poor prognostic sign [2,3,6,7].

Intraventricular extension of hemorrhage is a predictor of poor outcome, independent of size or location of parenchymal hemorrhage [3]. Cerebellar hemorrhages large enough to compress brainstem structures are associated with a poor prognosis [8,9]. Using the Glasgow Coma Scale and volume of ICH on CT scan, Broderick and coworkers [2] were able to predict mortality with an accuracy of greater than 95%.

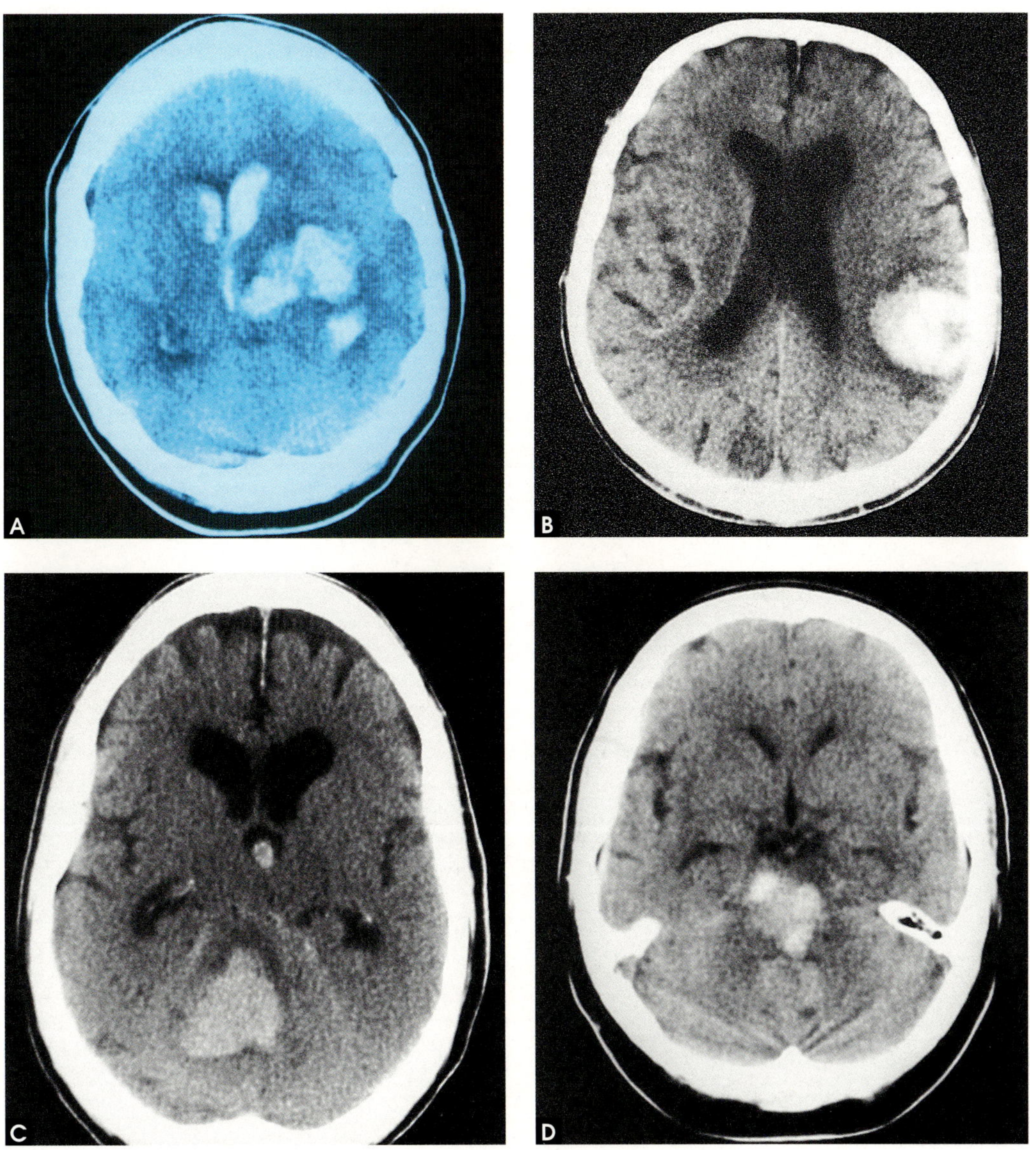

FIGURE 20.2

Computed tomography scan images depict intracerebral hemorrhage within brain structures. **A**, Basal ganglion extending into the ventricles. **B**, Parietal lobe. **C**, Cerebellum. **D**, Pons.

Table 20.2. Predictors of outcome in intracerebral hemorrhage

Age	Strength (motor power)	Hemorrhage volume*
Glasgow coma scale*	Systolic blood pressure	Intraventricular blood*
Consciousness*	Arterial pulse pressure	Midline shift
Eye movements	Hemorrhage location	Intracranial pressure

*More powerful predictors.

ETIOLOGY

Hypertension, both chronic and acute, is responsible for the majority of spontaneous ICH, although amyloid angiopathy is a frequent cause of lober hemorrhage in the elderly [10,11]. Chronic hypertension predisposes to hemorrhage by inducing degenerative changes in intracranial vessels [12] and microaneurysm formation. Sudden and severe hypertension, as may be seen in antihypertensive medication withdrawal or noncompliance, kidney disease, or following ingestion of drugs such as cocaine or amphetamines, may cause ICH directly by rupture of otherwise normal blood vessels [13]. Blood pressure is often elevated as a consequence of the hemorrhage itself regardless of cause. Management requires careful blood pressure control both short and long term.

Following hypertension, other causes of ICH are many and include vascular malformations, aneurysms and other angiopathies, disorders of coagulation, and trauma (Table 20.3) [14]. Arteriovenous malformation (AVM) is a common cause of hemorrhage after hypertension (Figure 20.3). Patients may report a premorbid history of headache or seizures. Initial CT or subsequent magnetic resonance (MR) imaging or angiography will demonstrate most AVMs unless small or obliterated by the hematoma. Cryptic AVMs not evident on these examinations may be responsible for hemorrhages in nonhypertensive patients as well as for some in patients with hypertension [14–16]. Unless surgically resected or otherwise obliterated, the risk of recurrent hemorrhage remains [17].

Arterial aneurysms may cause ICH by rupturing into the brain substance [18]. If minimal subarachnoid hemorrhage is present, the diagnosis of aneurysm may not be immediately apparent. CT or MR imaging may visualize the aneurysm in some cases. Basal location of the hemorrhage, particularly if interhemispheric or adjacent to the sylvian fissure, suggests an aneurysmal origin. Conventional angiography will usually demonstrate the aneurysm if present. Mycotic aneurysm and arteritis are rare causes of ICH.

Cerebral amyloid angiopathy [19] is increasingly recognized as a cause of ICH in the elderly, particularly if normotensive or demented. Multiple or recurrent lobar hemorrhages are characteristic. Surgical evacuation of ICH may be complicated by difficulties with hemostasis resulting from fragility of blood vessels [20,21].

Table 20.3. Etiologies of intracerebral hemorrhage

Hypertension (chronic, acute, and severe)	Coagulation disorders	Warfarin
Arteriovenous malformation	Platelet disorders	Aspirin, ticlopidine
Cerebral amyloid angiopathy	Thrombocytopenia	Thrombolytics
Aneurysm	Factor deficiencies	Hemorrhagic infarction
Arteritis	Hemophilia	Tumor
	Liver disease	Trauma (direct, delayed)

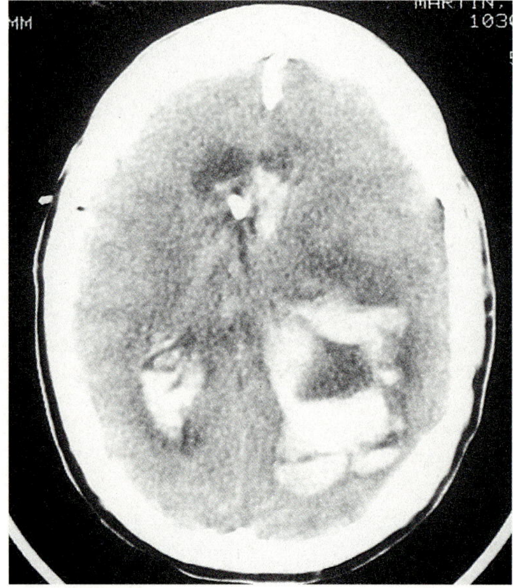

FIGURE 20.3

Computed tomography scan image of lobar hemorrhage with intraventricular extension arising from a cortical arteriovenous malformation.

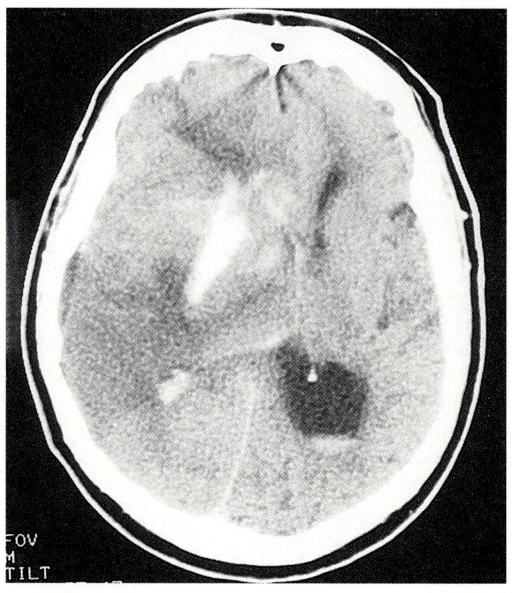

FIGURE 20.4

Computed tomography scan image of a large hemispheric infarction with hemorrhagic transformation and hematoma formation.

Intracerebral hemorrhage is a well known complication of anticoagulant therapy with heparin or warfarin [22,23]. Protamine will reverse the effect of heparin. Intravenous vitamin K administration will correct warfarin-induced prolongation of clotting time. Immediate reversal of warfarin anticoagulation can be accomplished by administering whole blood, fresh frozen plasma, or prothrombin complex concentrate [24]. More recently, ICH has been associated with fibrinolytic therapy for acute myocardial infarction occurring in approximately 0.5% of cases [25]. Immediate administration of cryoprecipitate and fresh frozen plasma may be helpful [26]. Hematologic disorders such as leukemia, thrombocytopenia, and deficiencies of coagulation factors may be responsible for ICH. Antineoplastic agents and liver disease may predispose to these hemorrhagic conditions.

Underlying brain tumor, either primary or metastatic, may cause ICH. Potential mechanisms include spontaneous rupture of surrounding abnormal capillaries, invasion of vessels by tumor, or vessel destruction within areas of tumor necrosis. Neuroradiologic appearance and evidence of systemic neoplasm may provide the diagnosis, although at times it can only be made on pathologic examination of the evacuated hematoma. Hemorrhagic transformation of bland infarction is a frequent occurrence [27], usually little more than a coalescence of petechial hemorrhage. Occasionally frank hematoma develops, at times associated with clinical decline (Figure 20.4). Thrombosis of dural sinuses or cerebral veins, often associated with hypercoagulable states, may result in cortical hemorrhage.

Table 20.4. Pertinent medical history in intracerebral hemorrhage

Hypertension (duration, severity, medications)	Headaches
Drug use (warfarin, aspirin, ticlopidine, cocaine, amphetamines, other sympathomimetics)	Seizures
Neurologic illness	Prior stroke
	Dementia
	Medical illness (coagulation disorder, liver disease, malignancy, trauma)

Table 20.5. Key elements of the neurologic examination in intracerebral hemorrhage

Mental status	Papilledema
Level of consciousness	Extremity weakness
Aphasia or neglect	Extensor plantar response
Eye deviation	Gait ataxia
Pupillary asymmetry	Abnormal respiratory pattern
Hemianopia	

TREATMENT

General Measures

The first hours of treatment are often the most critical. The medical history, examination, and initial diagnostic tests must be performed quickly and accurately. Table 20.4 notes important areas of concern in the medical history. Report of stroke, seizure, headache, or dementia suggests the possibility of underlying cerebral pathology. The general physical examination is directed at potential causes of hemorrhage to include hypertension, bleeding disorder, liver disease, or malignancy. The neurologic examination (Table 20.5) must carefully document the patient's impairments with particular attention to level of consciousness as well as disturbances of gaze, pupil size, and reactivity, respiratory pattern, extremity strength, and gait. Frequent neurologic reevaluation must be performed to detect evidence of neurologic worsening resulting from continued bleeding or the development of edema. Respiratory function and blood pressure must be closely monitored.

Computed tomography scan should be performed promptly. Blood is clearly evident on CT scan (Figure 20.2), and determination can be made of hematoma size and location and of intraventricular extension and edema. CT may provide a clue to etiology by suggesting tumor, aneurysm, or vascular malformation. Appropriate blood tests include complete blood count with platelet count, electrolytes, blood urea nitrogen, creatinine, serum glucose, liver enzymes, prothrombin time, and partial thromboplastin time. Electrocardiography and chest x-ray should be performed. MR imaging and angiography may be necessary in selected cases. Table 20.6 lists basic laboratory tests for patients with ICH.

A treatment algorithm for management of intraparenchymal hemorrhage allows visualization of the sequence of events following initial diagnosis (Figure 20.5). For most, admission to an intensive care unit is necessary to closely monitor blood pressure, respiratory and cardiac function, and neurologic status. Neurologic checks by the nursing staff should be initially performed and documented, at minimum, each hour and the frequency reduced thereafter only if the patient is stable. Management should be directed by physicians with experience in stroke and the management of elevated intracranial pressure. Neurosurgical consultation should be obtained in all patients who might need evacuation or ventricular shunt placement.

Table 20.6. Basic laboratory tests in intracerebral hemorrhage

Complete blood count, platelet count	Electrocardiogram
Prothrombin time, partial thromboplastin time	Chest X-ray
Liver enzymes	Computed tomography scan
Drug screen	Magnetic resonance imaging*
	Angiography*

*In selected cases.

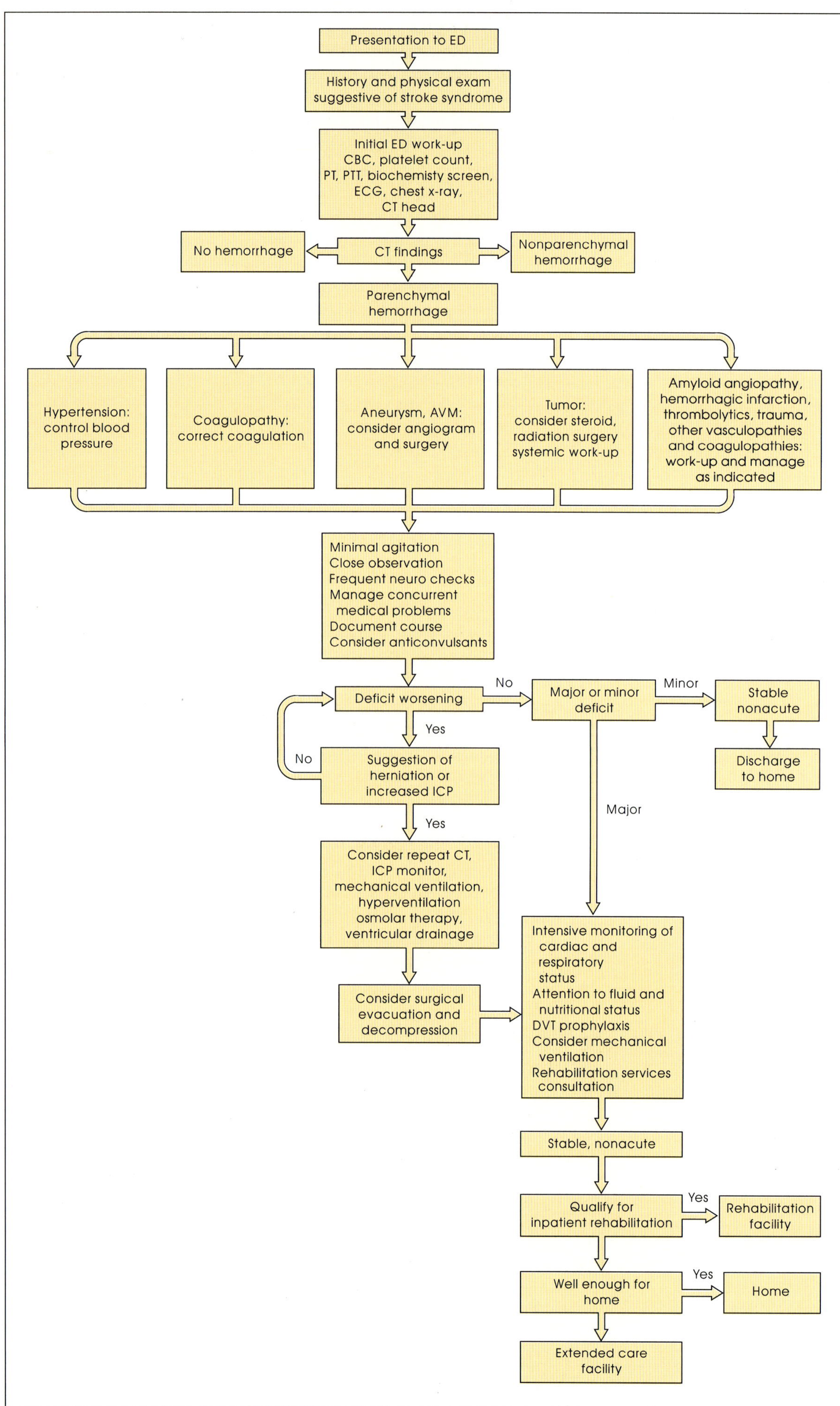

FIGURE 20.5

Treatment algorithm for management of intraparenchymal hemorrhage. AVM—arteriovenous malformation; CBC—complete blood count; CT—computed tomography; DVT—deep vein thrombosis; ECG—electrocardiogram; ED—emergency department; ICP— intracranial pressure; PT—prothrombin time; PTT—partial thromboplastin time.

Most patients will require cardiac monitoring to detect arrhythmias associated with brain hemorrhage. Pain from any procedures such as bladder catheterization, intravenous line placement, and arterial blood gases should be minimized to prevent patient discomfort and agitation that may increase blood pressure and intracranial pressure. A quiet room with a minimal number of visitors is appropriate

Deep vein thrombosis is frequent after stroke of all types, including patients with ICH [28,29]. Antithrombotic stockings and physical therapy appear to reduce the incidence of thrombosis. Pneumatic compression devices reduce the incidence of deep vein thrombosis and are useful, although they limit spontaneous movement in awake patients. Subcutaneous heparin therapy is a more difficult issue in the setting of intracranial hemorrhage, although the risk of worsening the hemorrhage is likely to be small [29]. In general, subcutaneous heparin should be instituted subacutely, well after patient stabilization.

Seizures accompanied the onset of ICH in 4.9% of 1402 patients reported by Sung and Chu [30], 2.5% of whom went on to have epilepsy. The large majority of hemorrhages associated with seizure were lobar in location. Phenytoin is most commonly used because it is effective and can be given either orally or intravenously in loading doses. Anticonvulsants may be given prophylactically in lobar hemorrhages, but are not recommended for hemorrhages in other locations.

Blood Pressure

For many patients with a history of hypertension, blood pressure should be maintained in the moderately hypertensive range of 160 to 180 mm Hg systolic, avoiding pressures above 200 mm Hg [31–33]. To lower it further may impair blood flow to compressed brain adjacent to the hematoma that may be ischemic [34], or to other areas of the brain long adapted to higher pressures. Patients with no history of hypertension may best be managed with blood pressures substantially lower. In the presence of intracranial pressure (ICP) greater than 20 mm Hg, higher blood pressures may be required to maintain cerebral perfusion pressure, the difference between mean arterial pressure and intracranial pressure. Cerebral perfusion pressure should generally be greater than 70 mm Hg. Excessively high blood pressure may promote additional bleeding and may aggravate intracranial hypertension.

In ICH, immediate control of severe hypertension can be obtained with the adrenergic-receptor antagonist labetalol adjusted according to blood pressure response [32,33,35]. As a cerebral vasodilator, sodium nitroprusside may increase ICP and has the potential to cause thiocyanate toxicity. Onset of action is immediate and duration of action only 2 to 3 minutes. Beta-blockers produce less cerebral vasodilatation and have little effect on ICP. Onset of action of labetalol is several minutes and duration of action 3 to 6 hours.

Fluids and Osmolality

Fluids should meet the systemic needs of the patient. Patients able to take fluids by mouth only need to be monitored with measured intake and output. For those requiring intravenous fluids, normal saline at replacement volumes is usually adequate. Restriction of fluids and use of loop diuretics such as furosemide are usually sufficient to achieve and maintain plasma hyperosmolality (300–310 mOsm/L) which may reduce cerebral edema by drawing free water from injured brain. Furosemide in addition reduces cerebrospinal fluid formation.

Patients with markedly elevated ICP or impending herniation may need more substantial and immediate reduction in ICP by infusion of mannitol. At doses of 0.25 to 1.0 g/kg, the plasma immediately becomes hyperosmolar, drawing water from edematous tissue. The maximal reduction in ICP occurs between 20 and 60 minutes after administration. Electrolyte imbalance (hypokalemia) and volume depletion are the major complications of the use of mannitol. The hyperosmolar state can be maintained by continued limitation of fluids, use of diuretics, and intermittent dosing with mannitol as needed.

Steroids may reduce the fraction of edema that is vasogenic in origin, but no clinical benefit was demonstrated in a prospective randomized trial of dexamethasone in 93 patients with ICH [36]. In addition, the rate of infection and complications of diabetes mellitus were higher in the treated group.

Ventilation

Patients need to be observed for respiratory rate, pattern of breathing, and the development of stridor. Unresponsive patients or others who are at high risk of aspiration may require endotracheal intubation for airway protection, pulmonary toilet, or mechanical ventilation. Respiratory failure may occur in brainstem hemorrhage or in supratentorial hemorrhage with hydrocephalus or herniation that disables brainstem respiratory centers. Intubation should be accomplished with as little patient distress as possible making use of topical anesthetics and sedative medications as needed. Coughing and resistance to passive ventilation will increase intrathoracic pressure and as a result ICP as well and should be controlled. Tracheostomy is a consideration if prolonged intubation is anticipated.

Hyperventilation ($PaCO_2$ 25–30 mm Hg) reduces ICP as reflex vasoconstriction reduces the volume of intravascular blood. The effect is immediate in onset, maximizing in approximately 30 minutes. Hyperventilation, however, has some negative aspects as well. Central venous pressure increases in hyperventilation and intracranial pressure may increase as a result. Marked hypocarbia and vasoconstriction may potentially induce ischemia in compressed, poorly perfused tissue surrounding the area of hemorrhage. The effect of hyperventilation is transient, likely less than 24 hours, as initial alkalosis is corrected by reduction in serum bicarbonate concentration and restoration of normal pH. Unless accomplished very slowly, return to normal ventilation will result in rebound vasodilatation and increased ICP. Hyperventilation is one aspect of the management of increased intracranial pressure, and should be used in conjunction with other modalities of longer duration of effect [37,38].

Ventricular Catheters and Intracranial Pressure Monitoring

Intraventricular extension of ICH may result in obstruction by clotted blood within cerebrospinal fluid pathways and subsequent hydrocephalus. Cerebellar hemorrhage may cause hydrocephalus by compression of the fourth ventricle or cerebral aqueduct. Drainage of cerebrospinal fluid by an intraventricular catheter will relieve symptomatic hydrocephalus and may assist in control of elevated ICP. With a ventricular catheter in place ICP may be monitored by connection to a transducer. Despite these benefits, intraventricular drains may introduce infection, become occluded by clotted blood, or in their placement cause additional hemorrhage. Drainage of lateral ventricles may cause a shift of intracranial contents, either from side to side in large hemispheric hemorrhages or upward in posterior fossa hemorrhages.

Intracranial pressure can be monitored with the less invasive subarachnoid bolt, but with some loss of reliability. Closed-system devices are in common use and have little risk of complication [39]. Ropper and King [40] argued for ICP monitoring to guide timely medical and surgical intervention in comatose patients with ICH, although improvement in patient outcome with this measure is difficult to demonstrate.

SURGICAL EVACUATION

Small hematomas, not likely to compress vital structures or cause hydrocephalus, do well when managed medically. Comatose patients with large ICHs have a poor prognosis regardless of treatment. Indications for surgical treatment of ICH between these extremes are controversial [34,41]. Like the 1961 study by McKissock and coworkers [42], subsequent studies have yielded equivocal results [43–47]. Most interest has been in the medical and surgical treatment of patients with lobar or basal ganglion hemorrhages of moderate size (Table 20.7). Two recent randomized studies address these groups [48,49].

Juvela and coworkers [48] prospectively randomized 52 patients with spontaneous supratentorial hemorrhages to surgical or medical treatment. All patients had depressed levels of consciousness or severe hemiparesis or aphasia. Mortality was not significantly different between the treatment groups. Surgery appeared to reduce mortality in semicomatose or stuporous patients but all remained severely disabled. More favorable results were obtained by Auer and coworkers [49] using an endoscopic technique in a randomized trial of surgical versus medical treatment of 100 patients with supratentorial hemorrhage. Surgery improved function but not mortality in patients who were awake, less than 60 years of age, and had subcortical (lobar) hemorrhages less than 50 mL in volume. For patients with hemorrhages greater than 50 mL, mortality was improved in the operated group but no difference was noted in functional recovery. No benefit in favor of surgery was found in putaminal or thalamic hemorrhages. It appears that mortality may be improved by surgical treatment of lobar and putaminal hemorrhage, but it is not clear that this is true of functional recovery.

Table 20.7. Outcome in recent studies comparing surgical and medical management of spontaneous supratentorial intracerebral hemorrhage

	Medically managed patients				Surgically managed patients			
		Independence in activities†, *n*(%)				Independence in activities, *n*(%)		
Study*	Survival, *n/n*(%)	Poor	Fair	Good	Survival, *n/n*(%)	Poor	Fair	Good
Juvela and coworkers [48]	16/26(62)	11(69)		5(31)	14/26(54)	13(93)		1(7)
Auer and coworkers [49]	15/50(30)	6(40)	4(27)	5(33)	29/50(58)	13(45)	3(10)	13(45)
Waga and coworkers [45]	95/138(69)	11(12)	19(20)	65(68)	26/44(59)	6(23)	11(42)	9(35)

*Outcome at 6 months in references 48 and 49 and 4 years in reference 45.
†Independence in activities: poor, vegetative or totally dependent; fair, partial disability: good, independent in activities of daily living.

Table 20.8. Candidates for surgical intervention in spontaneous intracerebral hemorrhage (ICH)

Candidates with good potential	Candidates with poor potential
Younger patients, good general health, noncomatose, signs of progression, hemorrhage under 50 mL	Older patients, depressed level of consciousness, large hemorrhage with intraventricular blood
Cerebellar ICH with progressive symptoms, evidence of brainstem compression, acute hydrocephalus	Putaminal ICH (generally as a life-saving measure only)
Lobar ICH with progressive symptoms, especially nondominant hemisphere	Thalamus and brainstem ICH, no benefit expected

Although studies have been limited, cerebellar hemorrhage may be the clearest indication for surgical intervention [50–52]. Patients with hemorrhage sufficiently large to put them at risk for brainstem compression or hydrocephalus should be considered for surgical decompression. Medically managed patients must be watched closely for development of these conditions. General recommendations for possible surgical intervention in ICH are outlined in Table 20.8.

OUTCOME OF INTRACEREBRAL HEMORRHAGE

Thirty-day mortality from ICH ranges from 31% to 58% as seen in recent studies (Table 20.9) [2,3,5–7,53–55], much of which occurs in the first 2 days [2]. A recent prospective study [6] of 157 patients with nonaneurysmal supratentorial hemorrhage (none operated) found that death from transtentorial herniation occurred in 37 (24%) by 2 days, most on day 1. Death occurred in 68 (43%) by 30 days and 83 (53%) by 1 year. Following herniation, common causes of death included infection, heart disease, recurrent stroke, and pulmonary embolism. After the second day, mortality was little different from brain infarction of similar severity. For survivors of spontaneous intracerebral hemorrhage, functional recovery is often good, with independent function in 43% to 75% of survivors and partial disability in 13% to 39% (Table 20.9).

In a recent series of 61 patients with pontine hemorrhages, overall mortality was 61% [56]. Prognosis was particularly poor if the hemorrhage was large and extending into adjacent structures, and best if limited to the area of the lateral tegmentum. In hemorrhages of limited size, good outcome has been reported in cases of spontaneous midbrain, pontine, and medullary hemorrhages [56–58].

Table 20.9. Outcome in medically managed spontaneous intracerebral hemorrhage (ICH)

			Mortality, %			Function in survivors, %		
Study	**ICH type**	**Patients, *n***	**30 d**	**6 mo**	**1 y**	**Dep**	**Part dep**	**Indep**
Broderick and coworkers [2]	All	188	44					
Franke and coworkers [6]	Supra	157	43		53			58
Daverat and coworkers [3]	All	166	31	43		28	29	43
Kreel and coworkers [53]	All	120	53			13	13	75
Liu and coworkers [54]	Putam	80				12	39	49
Bamford and coworkers [55]	All	66	50		62			68
Portenoy and coworkers [5]	Supra	112	58			15		
Helweg-Larson and coworkers [7]	All	53	27			21	24	55

All—all hemorrhage locations; Dep—dependent; Indep—independent; Part dep—partially dependent; Putam—putaminal location; Supra—supratentorial location.

REFERENCES

1. Caplan LR: Intracerebral hemorrhage. *Lancet* 1992, 1:656–658.
2. Broderick JP, Brott TG, Duldner JE, *et al.*: Volume of intracerebral hemorrhage: a powerful and easy-to-use predictor of 30-day mortality. *Stroke* 1993, 24:987–993.
3. Daverat P, Castel JP, Dartigues JF, Orgogozo JM: Death and functional outcome after spontaneous intracerebral hemorrhage: a prospective study of 166 cases using multivariate analysis. *Stroke* 1991, 22:1–6.
4. Tuhrim S, Dambrosia JM, Price TR, *et al.*: Prediction of intracerebral hemorrhage survival. *Ann Neurol* 1988, 24:258–263.
5. Portenoy RK, Lipton RB, Berger AR, *et al.*: Intracerebral hemorrhage: a model for the prediction of outcome. *J Neurol Neurosurg Psychiatry* 1987, 50:976–979.
6. Franke CL, van Swieten JC, Algra A, van Gijn J: Prognostic factors in patients with intracerebral hematoma. *J Neurol Neurosurg Psychiatry* 1992, 55:653–657.
7. Helweg-Larsen S, Sommer W, Strange P, *et al.*: Prognosis for patients treated conservatively for spontaneous intracerebral hematomas. *Stroke* 1984, 15:1045–1048.
8. Dunne JW, Chalzera T, Kermode S: Cerebellar hemorrhage-diagnosis and treatment: a study of 75 consecutive cases. *Q J Med* 1987, 64:739–754.
9. Taneda M, Hayalzawa T, Mogami H: Primary intracerebral hemorrhage: quadrigeminal cistern obliteration on CT scans as a predictor of outcome. *J Neurosurg* 1987, 67:545–552.
10. Mohr JP, Caplan LR, Melski JW, *et al.*: The Harvard Cooperative Stroke Registry: a prospective registry. *Neurology* 1978, 28:754–762.
11. Broderick JP, Brott TG, Tomsick T, Leach A: Lobar hemorrhage in the elderly; the undiminishing importance of hypertension. *Stroke* 1993, 24:49–51.
12. Fisher CM: Pathologic observations in hypertensive cerebral hemorrhage. *J Neuropathol Exp Neurol* 1971, 24:536–550.
13. Caplan L: Intracerebral hemorrhage revisited. *Neurology* 1988, 38:624–627.
14. Kase CS: Intracerebral hemorrhage: non-hypertensive causes. *Stroke* 1986, 17:590–595.
15. Kurata A, Miyasaka Y, Kitahara T, *et al.*: Subcortical cerebral hemorrhage with reference to vascular malformations and hypertension as causes of hemorrhage. *Neurosurgery* 1993, 32:505–511.
16. Wakai S, Kumakara N, Nagai M: Lobar intracerebral hemorrhage. *J Neurosurg* 1992, 76:231–238.
17. Graf CJ, Perret GE, Torner JC: Bleeding from arteriovenous malformations as part of their natural history. *J Neurosurg* 1983, 58:331–337.

18. Pasqualin A, Bazzan A, Cavazzani P, *et al.*: Intracranial hematomas following aneurysm rupture: experience with 309 cases. *Surg Neurol* 1986, 25:6–17.
19. Vinters HV: Cerebral amyloid angiopathy: a critical review. *Stroke* 1987, 18:311–324.
20. LeBlanc R, Preul M, Robitaille Y, *et al.*: Surgical considerations in cerebral amyloid angiopathy. *Neurosurgery* 1991, 29:712–719.
21. Greene GM, Godersky JC, Biller J, *et al.*: Surgical experience with cerebral amyloid angiopathy. *Stroke* 1990, 21:1545–1549.
22. Kase CS, Robinson RK, Stein RW, *et al.*: Anticoagulant-related intracerebral hemorrhage. *Neurology* 1985, 35:943–948.
23. Franke CL, de Jonge J, van Swieten JC, *et al.*: Intracerebral hematomas during anticoagulant treatment. *Stroke* 1990, 21:726–730.
24. Fredericksson K, Norrving B, Stromblad L-G: Emergency reversal of anticoagulation after intracerebral hemorrhage. *Stroke* 1992, 23:972–977.
25. Kase CS, Pessin MS, Zivin JA, *et al.*: Intracranial hemorrhage after coronary thrombolysis with tissue plasminogen activator. *Am J Med* 1992, 92:384–390.
26. Levine MN, Goldhaber SZ, Califf, *et al.*: Hemorrhagic complications of thrombolytic therapy in the treatment of myocardial infarction and venous thromboembolism. *Chest* 1992, 102(suppl 4):364S–373S.
27. Hornig CR, Bauer T, Simon C, *et al.*: Hemorrhagic transformation in cardioembolic cerebral infarction. *Stroke* 1993, 24:465–468.
28. Warlow C, Ogston D, Dougla AS: Venous thrombosis following stroke. *Lancet* 1972, 1:1305–1306.
29. Dickmann U, Voth E, Schicha H, *et al.*: Heparin therapy, deep vein thrombosis and pulmonary embolism after intracerebral hemorrhage. *Klin Wochenschrift* 1988, 66:1182–1183.
30. Sung CV, Chu NS: Epileptic seizures in intracerebral hemorrhage. *J Neurol Neurosurg Psychiatry* 1989, 52:1273–1276.
31. Calhoun DA, Oparil S. Treatment of hypertensive crisis. *N Engl J Med* 1990, 323:1177–1183.
32. Garcia JY, Vidt DG: Current management of hypertensive emergencies. *Drugs* 1987, 34:263–278.
33. Lavin P: Management of hypertension in patients with acute stroke. *Arch Intern Med* 1986, 146:66–68.
34. Mendelow AD: Spontaneous intracerebral hemorrhage. *J Neurol Neurosurg Psychiatry* 1991, 54:193–195.
35. Borges LF: Management of non-traumatic brain hemorrhage. In *Neurological and Neurosurgical Intensive Care, 3rd ed.* Edited by Ropper AH. New York: Raven Press; 1993:279–289.
36. Poungvarin N, Bhoopat W, Viriyavejakui A, *et al.*: Effects of dexamethasone in primary supratentorial intracerebral hemorrhage. *N Engl J Med* 1987, 316:1229–1233.
37. Williams MA, Hanley DF: Intracranial pressure monitoring and cerebral resuscitation. In *Management of the Acutely Ill Neurological Patient.* Edited by Grotta JC. New York: Churchill Livingstone; 1993:49–74.
38. Frank JI: Management of intracranial hypertension. *Med Clin North Am* 1993, 77:61–76.
39. Barnett GH: Intracranial pressure monitoring devices: principles, insertion, and care. In *Neurological and Neurosurgical Intensive Care, 3rd ed.* Edited by Ropper AH. New York: Raven Press; 1993:53–68.
40. Ropper AH, King RB: Intracranial pressure monitoring in comatose patients with cerebral hemorrhage. *Arch Neurol* 1984, 41:725–728.
41. Ojemann RG, Heros RC: Spontaneous brain hemorrhage. *Stroke* 1983, 14:468–475.
42. McKissock W, Richardson A, Taylor J: Primary intracerebral hemorrhage: a controlled trial of surgical and conservative treatments in 180 unselected cases. *Lancet* 1961, 2:221–226.
43. Batjer HH, Reisch JS, Allen BC, *et al.*: Failure of surgery to improve outcome in hypertensive putaminal hemorrhage. *Arch Neurol* 1990, 47:1103–1106.
44. Sakas DE, Singounas EG, Karvounis PC: Spontaneous intracerebral hematomas: surgical versus conservative treatment based on Glasgow Coma Scale score and computer tomography data. *J Neurosurg Sci* 1989, 33:165–172.
45. Waga S, Miyazaki M, Okada M, *et al.*: Hypertensive putaminal hemorrhage: analysis of 182 patients. *Surg Neurol* 1986, 26:159–166.
46. Volpin L, Cervellini P, Colombo F, *et al.*: Spontaneous intracerebral hematomas: a new proposal about the usefulness and limits of surgical treatment. *Neurosurgery* 1984, 15:663–666.
47. Kanno T, Sanno H, Shinomiya Y, *et al.*: Role of surgery in intracerebral hematoma. *J Neurosurg* 1984, 61:1091–1099.
48. Juvela S, Heiskanen O, Poranen A, *et al.*: The treatment of spontaneous intracerebral hemorrhage: a prospective, randomized trial of surgical and conservative treatment. *J Neurosurg* 1989, 70:755–758.
49. Auer LM, Deinsberger W, Neiderkorn K, *et al.*: Endoscopic surgery versus medical treatment for spontaneous intracerebral hematoma: a randomized study. *J Neurosurg* 1989, 70:530–535.
50. Van der Hoop RG, Vermeulen M, van Gijn J: Cerebellar hemorrhage: diagnosis and treatment. *Surg Neurol* 1988, 29:6–10.
51. Little JR, Tubman DE, Ethier R: Cerebellar hemorrhage in adults: diagnosis by computerized tomography. *J Neurosurg* 1978, 48:575–579.
52. Fisher CM, Picard EH, Polak A: Acute hypertensive cerebellar hemorrhage: diagnosis and surgical treatment. *J Nerv Ment Dis* 1965, 140:38–57.
53. Kreel L, Kay R, Woo J, *et al.*: The radiological (CT) and clinical sequelae of primary intracerebral hemorrhage. *Br J Radiol* 1991, 64:1096–1100.
54. Liu C-W, Chu N-S, Ryu S-J: CT, somatosensory and brainstem auditory evoked potentials in the early prediction of functional outcome in putaminal hemorrhage. *Acta Neurol Scand* 1991, 84:28–32.
55. Bamford J, Sandercock P, Dennis M, *et al.*: A prospective study of acute cerebrovascular disease in the community: the Oxfordshire community stroke project 1981-86, 2. Incidence, case fatality rates and overall outcome at one year of cerebral infarction, primary intracerebral hemorrhage and subarachnoid hemorrhage. *J Neurol Neurosurg Psychiatry* 1990, 53:16–22.
56. Chung C-S, Park C-H: Primary pontine hemorrhage: a new CT classification. *Neurology* 1992, 42:830–834.
57. Lancman M, Norscini J, Mesropian H, *et al.*: Tegmental pontine hemorrhages: clinical features and prognostic features. *Can J Neurol Sci* 1992, 19:236–238.
58. Shuaib A: Benign brainstem hemorrhage. *Can J Neurol Sci* 1991, 18:356–357.

Chapter 21

Basic Principles and Strategies of Rehabilitation in Cerebrovascular Disease

DAVID C. GOOD

Rehabilitation is a process through which a disabled person reaches the maximum physical, functional, and psychosocial recovery possible within the limits of his or her disability. An optimal rehabilitation program, while including specific treatment modalities, must be holistic in approach, addressing all of the physical, psychological, and social needs of the patient and family. In this respect rehabilitation is less "disease oriented" than other medical disciplines that focus primarily on diagnosis and treatment. In 1980, The World Health Organization (WHO) proposed definitions for the terms impairment, disability, and handicap as delineated in Table 21.1 [1]. In the context of these definitions, most medical disciplines address impairment, whereas rehabilitation is much more concerned with disability and handicap. A major goal of rehabilitation programs is to promote maximum function within the home and community. This mission is enhanced by the multidisciplinary approach of traditional rehabilitation, which uses the training and talents of a variety of professionals in a coordinated setting for the best interests of the patient. Although rehabilitation has traditionally been provided in a rehabilitation ward or hospital, other sites of care (*eg*, subacute or skilled nursing facilities, outpatient or day hospital programs, and home health agencies) have found increasing popularity as appropriate cost-effective alternatives for many patients.

Rehabilitation efforts are often classified as either "compensatory" or "restorative." The value of teaching compensatory techniques to patients or caregivers in order to minimize disability has been widely accepted. In motivated patients, training often permits independence in personal care and community activities, which may otherwise be impossible. For appropriate patients, specialized adaptive equipment, orthoses, or environmental alteration also improve functional abilities and quality of life. Whether rehabilitation is truly restorative, in the sense of promoting enduring beneficial reorganization of neural networks, is still a matter of debate. Considerable spontaneous recovery occurs following stroke, which makes the effect of rehabilitation efforts difficult to judge. Experimental models demonstrate tremendous fluidity and adaptability of neuronal networks in the normal adult nervous system in response to a variety of stimuli, including training programs (Figure 21.1) [2,3]. Functional mapping of the human cortex is now available in vivo through the use of the positron-emission tomography scan, the single photon emission tomography scan, biomagnetometry, and functional magnetic resonance imaging. These techniques are providing evidence of neuronal reorganization after stroke (Figure 21.2) [4,5]. A challenge for those interested in rehabilitation is the demonstration that treatment paradigms effectively alter these patterns.

EFFECTIVENESS OF STROKE REHABILITATION

Whether or not rehabilitation definitively alters neural networks, the basic question of whether a formal stroke rehabilitation program results in better functional status should be addressed.

Table 21.1. World Health Organization definitions of impairments, disabilities, and handicaps*

	Definition	Characteristics	Examples
Impairment	Loss or abnormality of structure or function	Reflects disturbances at the level of the organ	Aphasia, paraplegia, incontinence
Disability	Restriction or lack of ability to perform an activity in the manner considered normal	Reflects disturbances at the level of the person	Inability to ambulate, bathe, or communicate
Handicap	Inability to fullfill a role normal for a specific individual	Represents the socialization of an impairment or disability	Inability regarding occupation, social integration, economic self sufficiency

**From* Good [21]; with permission.

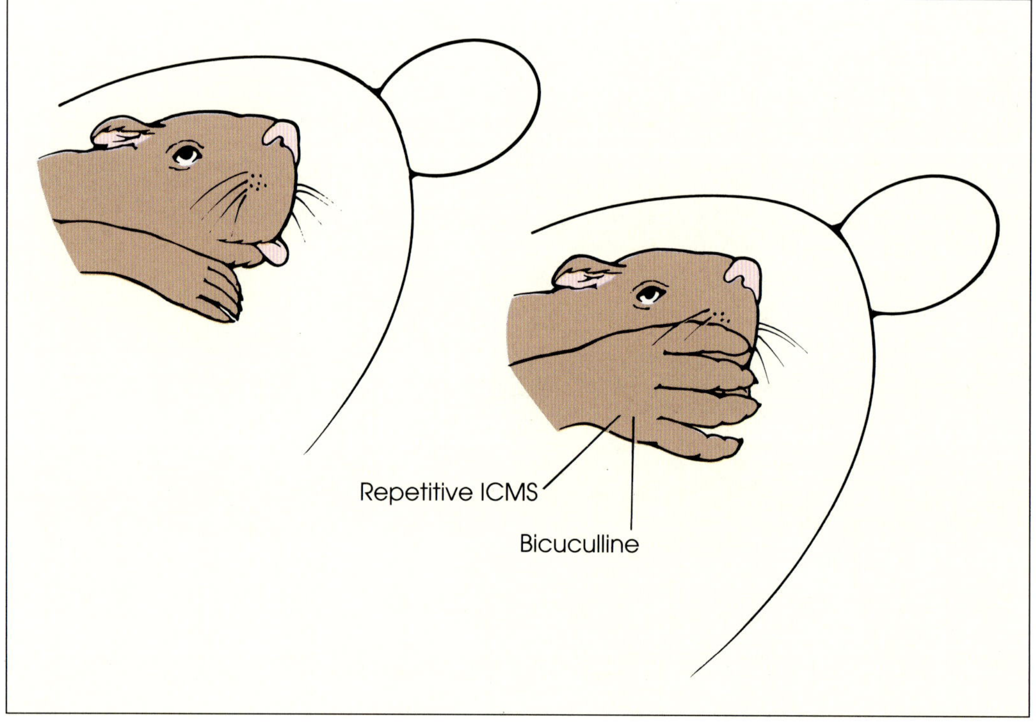

FIGURE 21.1

Changes in map of an adult rat's motor cortex resulting from repetitive intracortical microstimulation (ICMS) applied for 1 to 3 hours. Note enlargement of forelimb representation. A similar shift follows applications of the gamma–amino butyric acid antagonist bicuculline into the same zone of the rat's motor cortex. (*From* Asanuma [2]; with permission.)

Randomized studies are difficult because of the complex interaction of variables that contribute to stroke outcome, including the magnitude of neurologic deficit (Figure 21.3) [6], concurrent medical illnesses [7], and psychosocial factors [7,8]. Several attempts at randomized studies have resulted in inconclusive results [9–13]. Furthermore, all studies have various degrees of methodologic flaws, and some treatment models combined acute care on a "stroke unit" with comprehensive rehabilitation. Nonetheless, the results of many studies suggest that when compared with control patients, patients undergoing comprehensive rehabilitation are more proficient at self-care activities and more likely to live at home 1 year after stroke (Figure 21.4). The importance of the timing for initiating rehabilitation efforts is also a matter of controversy [14,15]. Two critical reviews of the literature since 1990 suggest that stroke rehabilitation programs are beneficial [16,17], whereas a third was more cautious in suggesting efficacy [18].

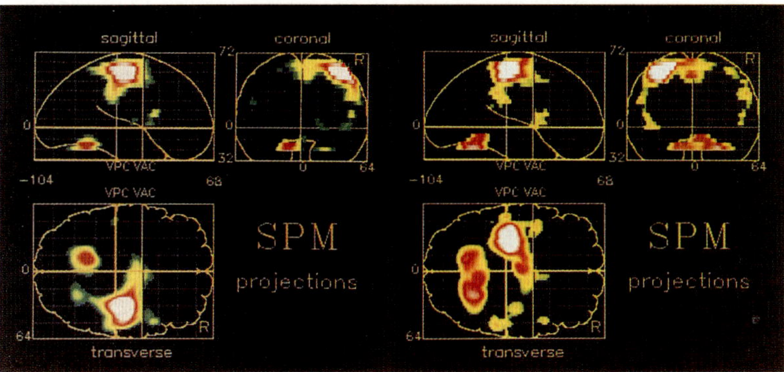

FIGURE 21.2

Comparison of mean regional cerebral blood flow (rCBF) during movement of normal fingers (*left*) versus recovered fingers (*right*) in six patients with previous stroke. Note activation of contralateral sensorimotor cortex and ipsilateral cerebellum when normal fingers are moved, but significant activation also in the ipsilateral sensorimotor cortex and both cerebellar hemispheres when the recovered fingers are moved. (*From* Chollet and coworkers [4]; with permission.)

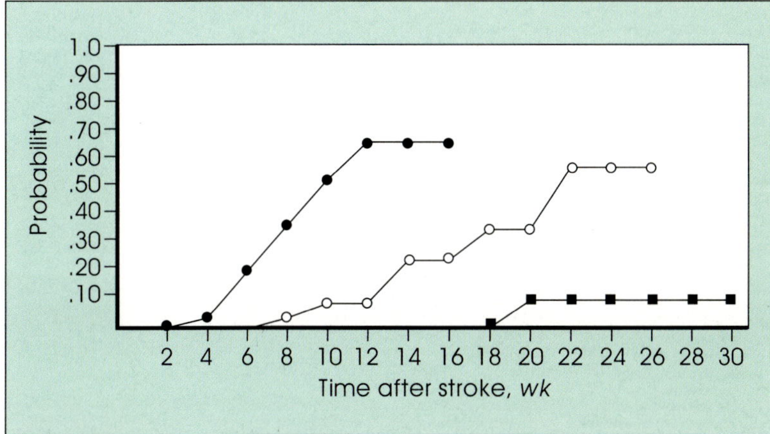

FIGURE 21.3

Life table analysis of probability of reaching Barthel Index score of ≥ 95, which correlates with ability to live independently. *Closed circles*, patients with motor deficit only (*n* = 27); *open circles*, patients with motor deficit plus somatic sensory deficit (*n* = 32); *closed squares*, patients with motor deficit plus somatic sensory deficit plus homonymous visual deficit (*n* = 32). (*From* Reding and Potes [6]; with permission.)

MEASURING OUTCOME

There is no single correct measurement of outcome for stroke. The importance of outcomes such as returning home or returning to work is self-evident, and they are easily measured. For the purpose of rehabilitation from stroke, outcome measures that provide special insight into adaptation to disability are also very useful, especially those related to functional abilities. The most commonly used measures are multifaceted assessment scales that evaluate mobility skills and ability to perform activities of daily living (ADLs). Many such scales have been devised, but the most commonly used are the Barthel Index (BI) as shown in Table 21.2 and its revised and expanded version, the Functional Independence Measure. Both scales have been rigorously evaluated for reliability and validity for stroke rehabilitation.

A BI score over 95 (a perfect score is 100) correlates strongly with ability to function independently and return home [6]. A score over 60 correlates with ambulation and care with assistance and, as delineated in Table 21.3, is generally the cut-off point at which a patient with stroke can function at home with the reasonable assistance of a spouse or caregiver [19,20].

The heavy emphasis on independence in ADLs as a major goal of rehabilitation has resulted in the use of these scales for purposes as diverse as tracking individual patient progress, assessing effectiveness of therapeutic trials, and evaluating institutional programs [21]. Other outcome measures used for stroke rehabilitation include measures of ambulation (*eg*, the ability to walk unassisted for 150 ft), comprehensive measures of motor abilities (*eg*, the Fugl-Meyer motor assessment scale [22]), and measures of overall quality of life [23]. Whenever a scale is chosen

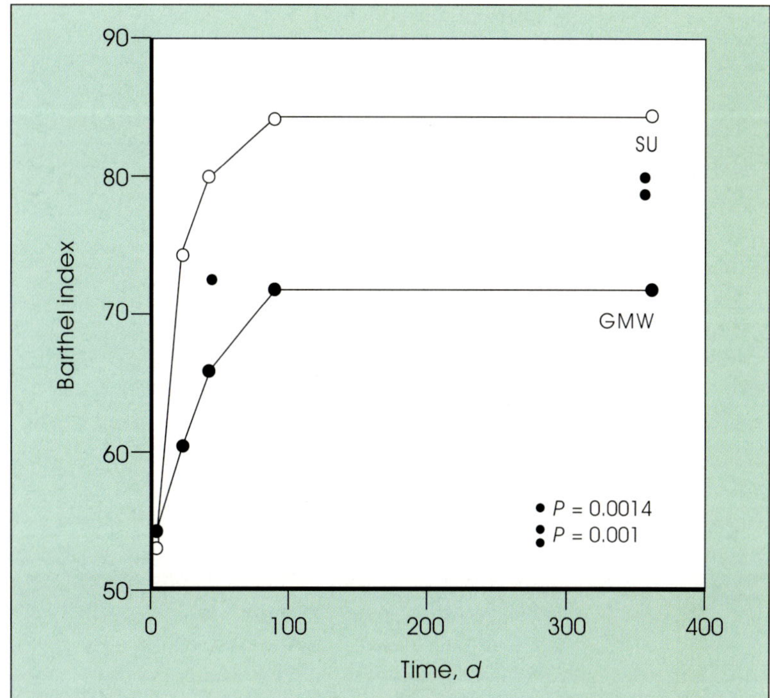

FIGURE 21.4

Graph of score on Barthel Index from 1 to 365 days. Comparison of mean scores for 77 patients in stroke unit (SU) who received intensive rehabilitation with 71 patients in general medical wards (GMW) alive after 1 year. (*From* Indredavik and coworkers [13]; with permission.)

as an outcome measure, it must be applied appropriately. In other words, the criteria used in the development of the scale must match the user's purpose. The choice of the wrong scale can lead to misleading information. Detailed discussions of measurement in neurologic rehabilitation have been published recently [21,24,25].

REHABILITATION TREATMENT STRATEGIES

Motor Function

Attempts to facilitate recovery of motor function are a major part of traditional rehabilitation programs for stroke. Approximately 70% to 88% of patients with ischemic stroke have some degree of motor impairment [7,26,27], but the severity of weakness and rate of recovery show considerable individual variation. Return of motor function generally follows a recovery curve similar to that of other impairments (Figure 21.5) [28–30]. Overall, long-term stroke survivors have a good prognosis for motor recovery. Of 148 persons in the Framingham study who survived at least 6 months, 52% had no residual weakness [31]. As shown in Table 21.4, most patients follow a typical pattern of motor recovery. Although these stages represent a continuum of recovery, many patients do not progress beyond a certain point. A few never progress beyond the flaccid stage, and many others continue to have severe spasticity and never get beyond synergistic movement.

The most widely practiced attempts at improving motor function are through programs of physical therapy. Various therapy philosophies and techniques have been developed [32], many based on concepts developed in the 1950s and 1960s.

Table 21.2. Barthel Index assessment scale*

Category	Evaluation	Score
Feeding	Totally dependent	0
	Needs help (*ie*, for cutting)	5
	Independent	10
Bathing	Cannot perform without assistance	0
	Performs without assistance	5
Grooming	Needs assistance	0
	Washes face, combs hair, brushes teeth	5
Dressing	Totally dependent	0
	Needs help but does at least half of task within reasonable period of time	5
	Independent: ties shoes, fastens fasteners, applies braces	10
Bowel control	Frequent accidents	0
	Occasional accidents or needs help with enema or suppository	5
	No accidents, able to use enema or suppository if needed	10
Bladder control	Incontinent or needs indwelling catheter	0
	Occasional accidents or needs help with device	5
	No accidents, able to care for collecting device, if used	10
Toilet transfers	No use of toilet, bedridden	0
	Needs help for balance, handling clothes, or toilet paper	5
	Independent with toilet or bedpan	10
Chair-bed transfers	Completely bedridden, use of chair not possible	0
	Able to sit, but needs maximum assistance to transfer	5
	Minimum assistance or supervision	10
	Independent, including locks of wheelchair and lifting footrests	15
Ambulation/ mobility	Sits on wheelchair, but cannot wheel self	0
	Independent with wheelchair 50 yards, only if unable to walk	5
	Ambulates with help for 50 yards	10
	Independent for 50 yards, may use assistive devices, except for rolling walker	15
Stair-climbing	Cannot climb stairs	0
	Needs help or supervision	5
	Independent; may use assistive devices	10
		Total score = (100 maximum)

**From* Good [21]; with permission.

Table 21.3. Percentage of stroke patients living in the community versus in a long-term care facility (LTCF) or dead at follow-up (according to Barthel Index scores at discharge from rehabilitation)*

Rehabilitation discharge Barthel score	0–40	41–60	61–80	81–100
Number	117	89	127	206
Follow-up status 6 months later, %				
Community	30	55	71	94
LTCF or dead	70	45	29	6

**From* Granger and coworkers [19]; with permission.

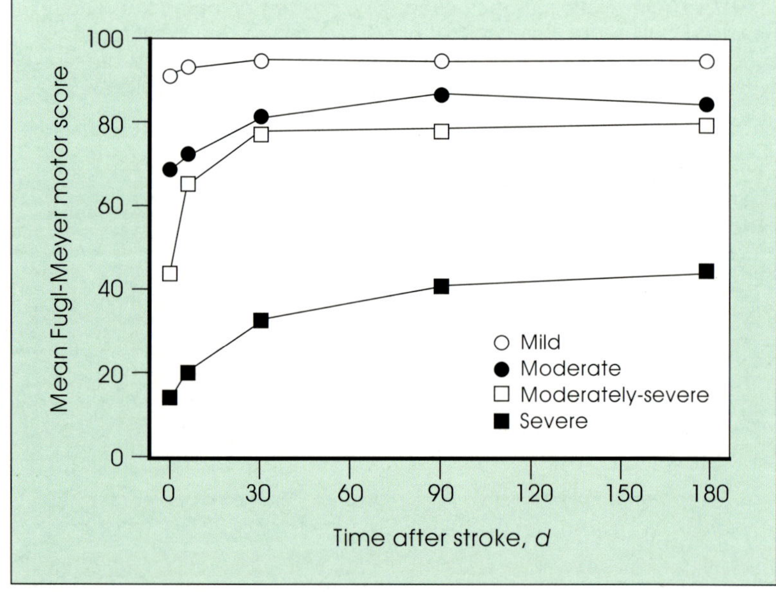

FIGURE 21.5

Graph showing recovery of motor function after stroke based on the Fugl-Meyer motor scores. Patients are stratified into groups based on the initial severity of motor deficit measured with Fugl-Meyer assessment. Regardless of the initial severity of stroke, the most dramatic recovery occurs within the first 30 days. Moderate and severe stroke patients continue to experience some recovery for 90 days. Graph represents mean Fugl-Meyer scores. (*From* Duncan and coworkers [28]; with permission.)

The technique of proprioceptive neuromuscular facilitation was developed in the 1950s by Knott and Voss [33]. It is essentially a technique of muscle strengthening using spiral and diagonal patterns and does not employ functional activities.

The neurodevelopmental treatment approach developed by Bobath [34] was perceived as a program to assist patients through a so called normal sequence of developmental motor milestones. A key principle of the Bobath approach is the facilitation of normal patterns of motor movements, and inhibition of spasticity and pathologic reflexes or synergy movements. Patients are taught to use reflex-inhibiting movement patterns, as shown in the "Bobath transfer" depicted in Figure 21.6. Ambulation is usually delayed until there is adequate weight bearing through the involved leg, and quality of gait is encouraged without the use devices.

The therapy approach of Brunnstrom [35], on the other hand, encourages synergistic motor movements. In contradiction to the Bobath philosophy, synergistic movements are viewed as a necessary normal intermediate stage for further recovery (Table 21.4).

A more recent approach to physical therapy was formulated by Carr and Shepherd [36] and stresses the practice of motor activities in association with specific functional skills. Unnecessary muscle activity is discouraged and activity is "task-specific."

Table 21.4. Brunnstrom's stages of recovery

Stage	Degree of recovery
Stage 1	Flaccid paralysis
Stage 2	Movements in synergy pattern, emergence of spasticity
Stage 3	Voluntary synergy movements, producing movement across joints, increased spasticity
Stage 4	Voluntary movements outside of synergy patterns, decreasing spasticity
Stage 5	Developing control of individual or isolated movements
Stage 6	Return to near normal motor control

Unfortunately, the underlying principles of most schools of physical therapy lack sound scientific proof, and there is no compelling evidence that one approach is superior to the others [16,32]. Nevertheless, there is consensus that, at the very least, physical therapy programs in patients with stroke reduce disability through instruction in compensatory techniques. In general, motor-retraining programs should focus on functional activities. Early mobility activities should begin as soon as the patient is medically stable.

Recently, a different approach to motor retraining that does not depend on any specific theory of physical therapy has been proposed [37]. This entails the forced use of a hemiparetic extremity by restraining the normal limb, and is based on the theory that learned nonuse of a paretic limb contributes to lack of return of motor function. In patients with partial recovery of arm movement, this treatment approach has resulted in sustained improvements in arm function, even when treatment was initiated many months after stroke (Figure 21.7).

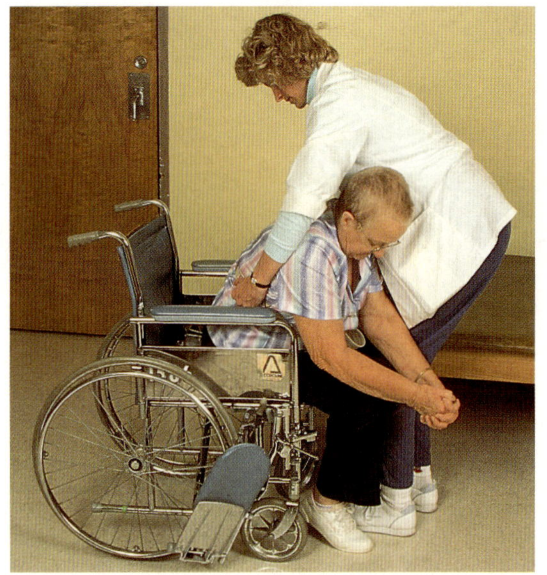

FIGURE 21.6

Physical therapist assisting a patient in a Bobath transfer from a wheelchair to a mat. The patient is asked to assume a "tone-inhibiting posture" by leaning forward and grasping the paretic limb as shown. The transfer is physically guided by the therapist from a proximal "point of control."

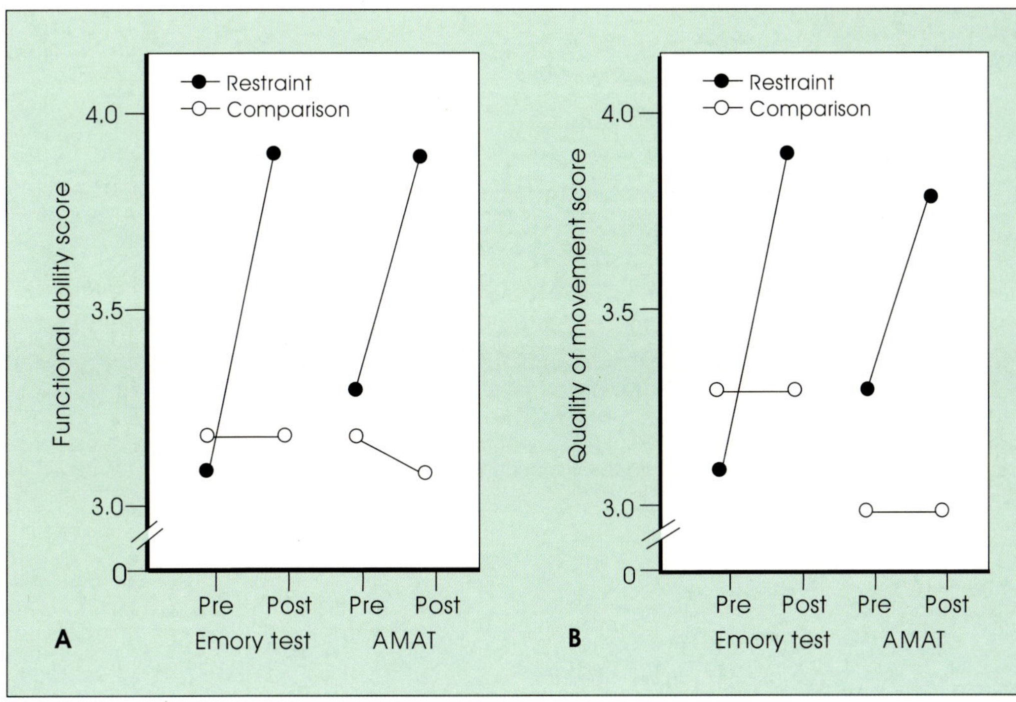

FIGURE 21.7

Patients with partial arm paresis after stroke. Results of restraining unaffected limb versus control patients. Mean functional ability (**A**) and quality of movement (**B**) on two motor ability tests, the Emory Motor Function Test and the Arm Motor Activity Test (AMAT). (*From* Taub and coworkers [37]; with permission.)

Other strategies to improve motor function include functional electrical stimulation, biofeedback, and various physical modalities [38]. In general, the use of these treatments remains controversial, and they are not used routinely for the rehabilitation of stroke in most clinical centers.

Although they do not enhance motor recovery, the importance of assistive devices and orthoses for enhancing motor function of the lower extremity and improving mobility should be stressed. Assistive devices make walking safer by increasing the base of support and redistributing weight from the legs to the arms [39]. In stroke rehabilitation, canes are the most appropriate device and are usually prescribed for leg weakness and impaired balance. Many varieties with an increasing base of support are available, ranging from a simple standard cane to a walker cane (Figure 21.8). Regardless of type, the proper height for a cane is the level of the wrist crease with the patient upright and arm extended. To ensure that the most appropriate device is prescribed and to facilitate compliance, each patient should be evaluated by an experienced physical therapist.

The most common orthosis used in stroke is the ankle-foot orthosis (AFO) (Figure 21.9) [40]. Orthoses are basically biomechanical force systems that may have one or more functions: protection, correction, assistance, and substitution. An AFO may substitute for dorsiflexion weakness, thus improving toe clear-

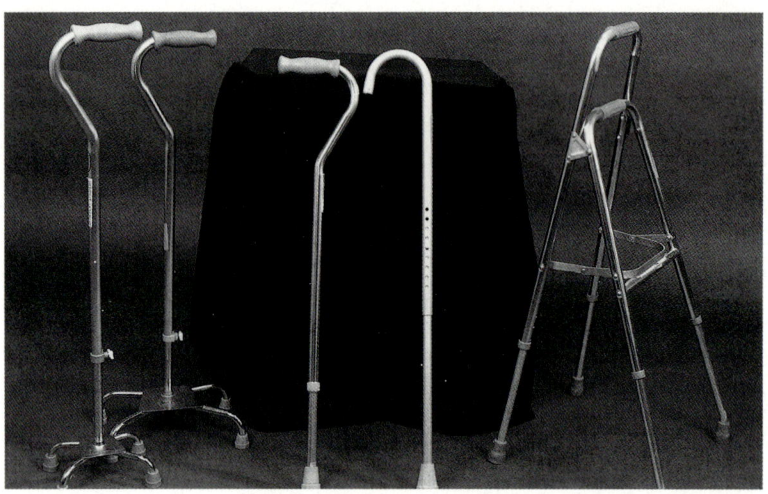

FIGURE 21.8

Left to right: narrow- and wide-based quad canes, bent cane, J cane, and walker cane. (*From* Laven [39]; with permission.)

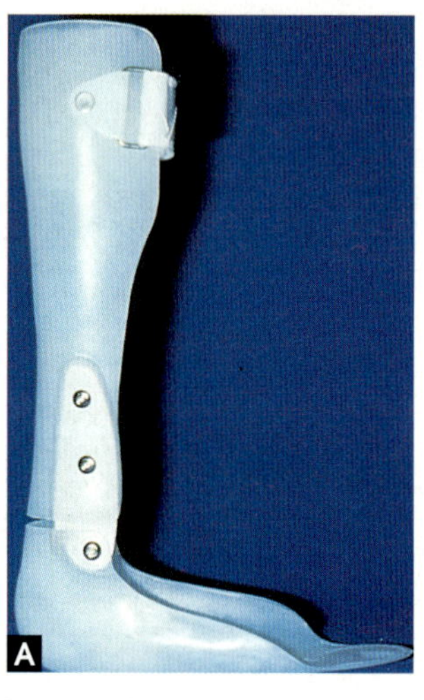

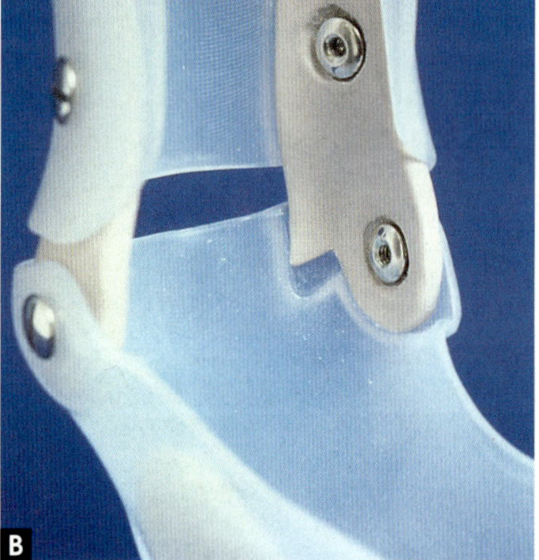

FIGURE 21.9

Custom-made plastic ankle-foot orthosis incorporating a joint with plantar flexion stop. **A**, Lateral view. **B**, Close-up view of joint with stop.

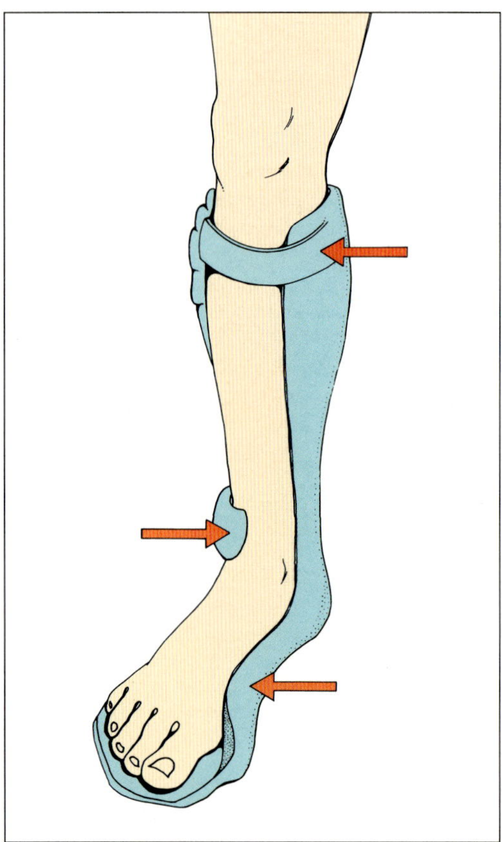

FIGURE 21.10

Biomechanical "three-point" force system to provide control of ankle inversion in spastic hemiparesis. (*Adapted from* Good and Supan [40]; with permission.)

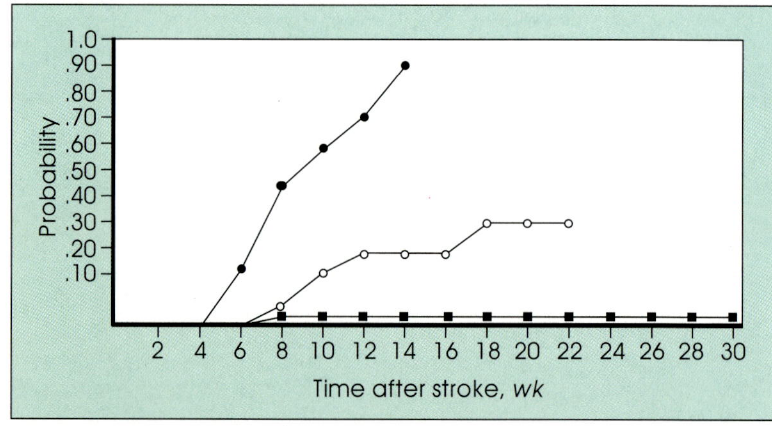

FIGURE 21.11

Life table analysis of probability of walking 150 ft or more without assistance. *Closed circles*, patients with motor deficit only ($n = 27$); *open circles*, patients with motor deficit plus somatic sensory deficit ($n = 32$); *closed squares*, patients with motor deficit plus somatic sensory deficit plus homonymous visual deficit ($n = 32$). (*From* Reding and Potes [6]; with permission.)

ance in the swing-phase of gait. An AFO may also be designed to correct excessive plantar flexion tone, allowing a more normal heel stroke, or to correct ankle inversion (Figure 21.10). By limiting ankle movement, an AFO may also be designed to alter force moments at the knee, thereby correcting gait deviations such as recurvation in some patients. Most orthoses are now plastic and are custom designed for the unique needs of the individual patient. Special adaptations include joints, stops, and flanges (Figures 21.9 and 21.10). Orthoses also have disadvantages [40]. Although an orthosis may greatly assist with one motor function, it may also resist other desirable movements. In addition, orthoses must be designed carefully to prevent skin breakdown, and can be expensive. An orthosis should not be prescribed for a patient with adequate natural muscle substitution patterns that allow the safe execution of functional tasks. One should not have unrealistic expectations regarding an orthosis. For example, an AFO will not improve ambulation in a patient whose most critical deficit is severe neglect or balance impairment, nor will it improve the gait's swing-phase in a patient whose hip flexors are too weak to advance the leg.

Approximately 80% of persons with stroke will eventually regain the ability to ambulate [41], but the time required varies with the severity of the neurologic deficit (Fig. 21.11) [6] and some will never regain independent ambulation. For those temporarily or permanently unable to walk, an appropriate wheelchair can greatly enhance mobility. Persons with hemiparesis generally require a hemichair that has a seat height 1.5 to 2 inches lower than a standard adult wheelchair and a detachable foot plate to allow propulsion of the chair with the strong arm and leg. Brake extenders on the hemiparetic side allow that side of the chair to be locked by reaching across with the strong hand. For comfort and proper functioning, the back, depth, and angle of the seat must all be considered [39]. In hemiplegic patients, seat boards and backboards often improve posture (Figures 21.12 and 21.13).

Spasticity is a frequent feature of hemiparesis, but seldom is the limiting factor in motor recovery. Muscle weakness and other features of the "upper motor neuron syndrome" including abnormal patterns of movement (*ie*, synergistic movements, cocontraction of agonists and antagonists) are much more likely to result in functional disability [38,42,43]. A common clinical misconception is the idea that treating spasticity will result in dramatic improvement in function. Nevertheless, treatment is certainly justified when spasticity is a causative factor in fixed contractures or is accompanied by mass spasms, severe clonus, or pain. Simple physical measures, such as range-of-motion exercise or prolonged static stretching, should always be used first [38,43,44], even though the therapeutic benefit is transient. Systemic pharmacologic management is sometimes necessary in patients with severe spasticity or mass spasms. Dantrolene is the drug of choice [44]. However, because its therapeutic effect occurs directly on muscle contractile mechanisms, it may cause generalized muscle weakness resulting in decreased functional abilities. Although baclofen and diazepam are well established

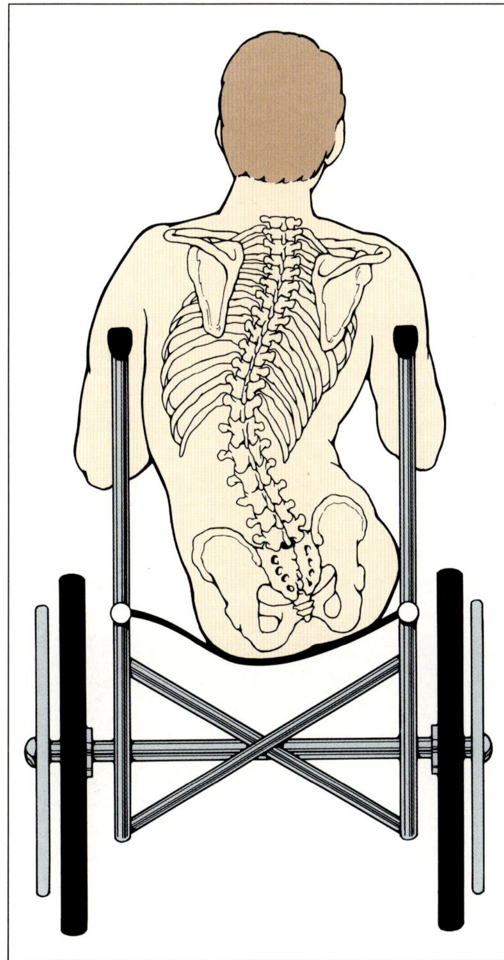

FIGURE 21.12

Hammock effect of sling seats results in asymmetrical pressure and can lead to scoliosis. (*Adapted from* Laven [39]; with permission.)

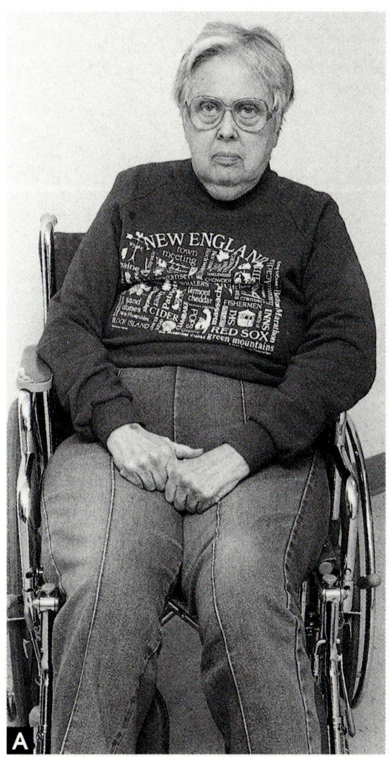

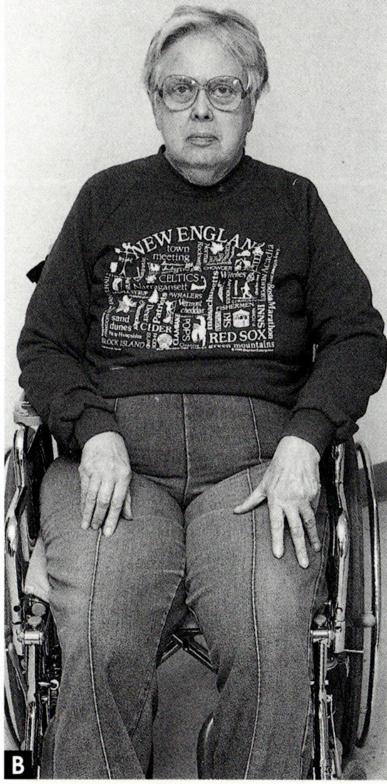

FIGURE 21.13

A, Poor posture in patient with left hemiparesis seated in wheelchair with sling seat and back. **B**, Correction of seating deviations with use of solid seat and backboard. (*From* Laven [39]; with permission.)

Table 21.5. The aphasis classification of subtypes*

Function	Broca's	Transcortical motor	Transcortical mixed	Global	Anomic	Wernicke's	Transcortical sensory	Thalamic	Conduction
Spontaneous speech	Nonfluent	Nonfluent	Nonfluent	Nonfluent	Fluent	Fluent or hyperfluent	Fluent or hyperfluent	Fluent	Fluent or impaired
Verbal output	Impaired	Impaired	Impaired	Impaired	Normal	Normal	Normal to impaired	Normal to impaired	Normal
Auditory comprehension	Normal	Normal	Impaired	Impaired	Normal	Impaired	Impaired	Normal to impaired	Impaired
Naming	Normal	Normal	Impaired	Impaired	Impaired	Impaired	Impaired	Normal	Normal
Reading	Normal	Normal	Impaired	Impaired	Normal	Impaired	Impaired	Normal	Normal
Writing	Impaired	Impaired	Impaired	Impaired	Normal	Impaired	Impaired	Normal	Normal
Repetition	Impaired	Normal	Normal	Impaired	Normal	Impaired	Normal	Normal	Impaired

**Adapted from* Lazar and Rubin [46]; with permission.

Card 2	IDENTIFICATION					Card 3	IDENTIFICATION				
	Under 5 seconds	Over 5 seconds	Category	Cue	Fail		Under 5 seconds	Over 5 seconds	Category	Cue	Fail
OBJECTS:	2 points	1 point	1/2 point	1/2 point	0	ACTIONS:	2 points	1 point	1/2 point	1/2 point	0
Chair						Smoking					
Key						Drinking					
Glove						Running					
Feather						Sleeping					
Hammock						Falling					
Cactus						Dripping					
LETTERS:						COLORS:					
L						Blue					
H						Brown					
R						Red					
T						Pink					
S						Gray					
G						Purple					
FORMS:						NUMBERS:					
Circle						7					
Spiral						42					
Square						700					
Triangle						1936					
Cone						15					
Star						7000					

Raw score:

FIGURE 21.14

Small portion of the Boston Diagnostic Aphasia Examination dealing with word discrimination. (*From* Goodglass and Kaplan [130]; with permission.)

in the treatment of spasticity of spinal cord etiology, neither plays a major role in the treatment of spasticity following stroke [44]. In addition to a usual lack of clinical response, both may cause decreased attention and memory in stroke patients.

The treatment of focal spasticity is sometimes indicated when a specific motor task is impaired (such as excessive hip adduction affecting ambulation) or when focal spasticity is contributing to a contracture. Traditionally, permanent surgical procedures (neurectomy, rhizotomy, tenotomy) or temporary "motor point blocks" using phenol or ethyl alcohol have been used in these patients [43,44]. Recently, local injection of botulinum toxin has been shown to reduce focal spasticity in multiple sclerosis and is currently under investigation for spasticity accompanying stroke [45].

Speech and Language Disorders

Aphasia occurs in approximately 23% of patients following stroke [41]. The most common scheme for organizing aphasia subtypes uses fluency and repetition difficulties for classifying clinical syndromes (Table 21.5). Precise classification is impossible in some patients. For the most part, there is consistent association between aphasia subtypes and specific anatomical lesions [46], but exceptions may occur.

A great deal of information regarding the language abilities of a patient may be obtained from a bedside or clinic examination. Because social skills and automatic responses are often preserved, the examination should rigorously evaluate comprehension, repetition, naming abilities, reading, and writing.

Many aphasia batteries are available to quantify formal language ability and to assist in planning therapeutic intervention. A small portion of the Boston Diagnostic Aphasia Examination dealing with word discrimination is illustrated in Figure 21.14. The patient is asked to point to pictures or symbols on a card and a raw score is generated.

Fortunately, many patients with aphasia after stroke improve with time, even without treatment (Figure 21.15) [47]. Recovery from aphasia is idiosyncratic, but some rough generalizations can be made. Degree of recovery correlates with the initial severity of aphasia and with the size of the lesion, particularly in Broca's aphasia [47]. Patients with Broca's aphasia tend to recover most, but even patients with global aphasia show improvement, especially in receptive abilities [47].

Although most clinicians agree that educating patients and families about aphasia and providing compensatory strategies is a valuable endeavor, the effectiveness of formal speech therapy remains controversial [46,48,49]. Although studies of speech therapy for stroke are difficult to design, several randomized trials have been attempted [50–53]. Results of many of these studies fail to provide clear evidence of benefit. Despite no consistent proof of efficacy, specific treatment techniques occasionally seem useful for individual patients [46]. In general, treatment techniques are more useful for patients with expressive aphasias than those with receptive problems. Melodic intonation therapy uses melodies or rhythmic tapping to facilitate verbal output. Sign language is occasionally helpful.

Another common problem following stroke is dysarthria, which can occur in patients with either hemispheric or brainstem infarcts. The precise incidence is difficult to ascertain because aphasia and apraxia often coexist with dysarthria and because dysarthria is often transient [54]. Since comprehension is often preserved in dysarthric patients, compensatory techniques may be taught. Cuing the patient to slow the rate of speech and teaching breath support may be rewarding in selected cases [54].

In patients with extreme dysarthria and in patients with some forms of aphasia, alternative or augmentative communication devices are available, ranging in sophistication from simple communication boards (Figure 21.16) to electronic communication prostheses, which generate synthesized or digitized speech or printed messages (Figure 21.17). Simple inexpensive systems are frequently helpful in expressing functional needs early after stroke. Because of the complexity and expense of some electronic systems, a careful assessment is needed before one is recommended [55]. This is best accomplished through an interdisciplinary evaluation that should address the patient's specific abilities, overall cognitive status, preferences, motivation, and cost, as well as how long the device will be needed [46].

Other disorders related to speech and language function may accompany stroke. While lesions involving the dominant hemisphere result in aphasia, lesions of the nondominant hemisphere may result in aprosody, or lack of emotional content of speech. This may be expressive, with intonation inaccurately reflecting mood or meaning, or receptive, with the patient failing to appreciate the emotional intonation of others.

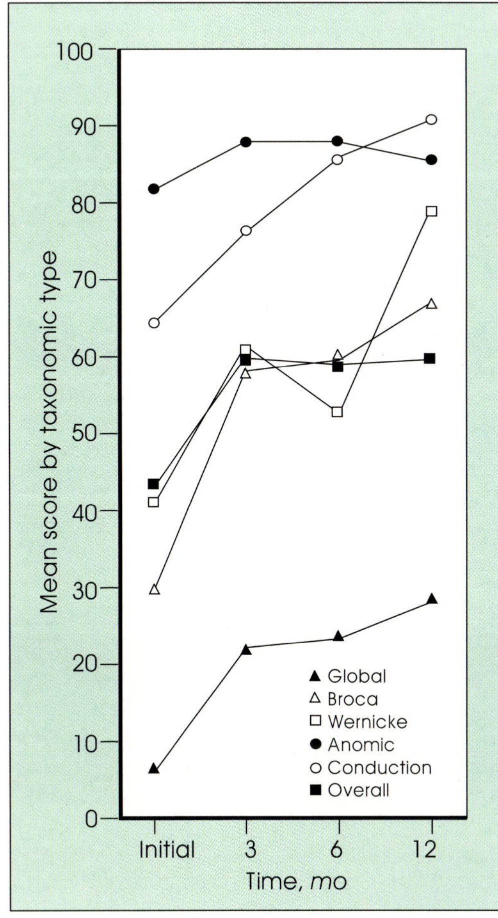

FIGURE 21.15
Recovery of comprehension in aphasic groups. (*From* Lincoln and coworkers [53]; with permission.)

Occasionally, patients with brain stem stroke may have hoarseness related to vocal cord paralysis or velopharyngeal incompetence with hypernasal speech. The latter may be treated surgically or with a palatal prosthesis.

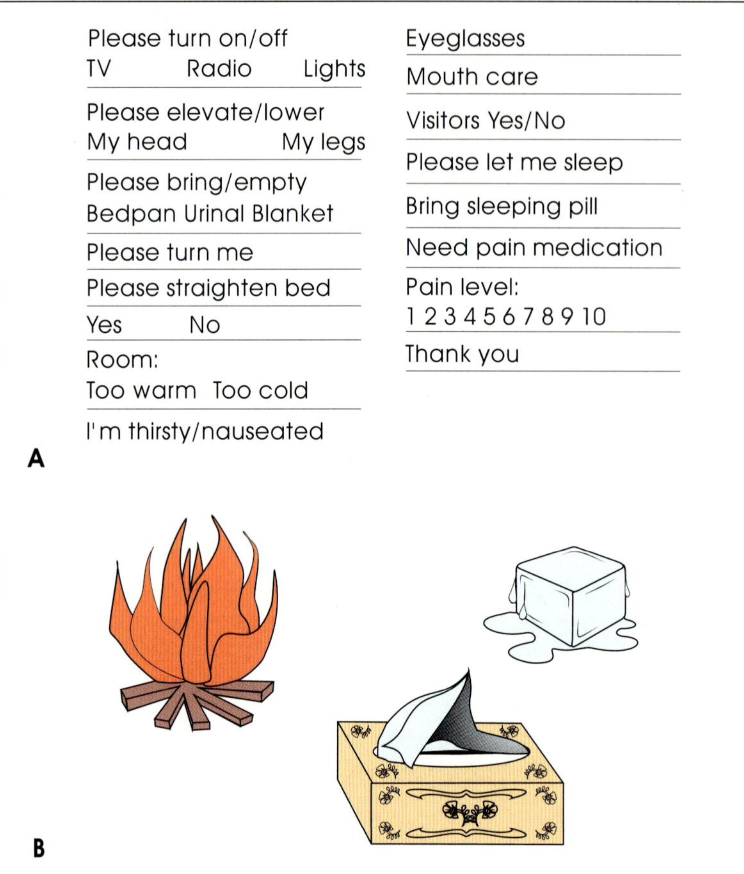

FIGURE 21.16

A, Simple communication board which might be appropriate for a patient with severe dysarthria but good comprehension. **B**, Portion of a communication board with symbols for hot, cold, and tissue.

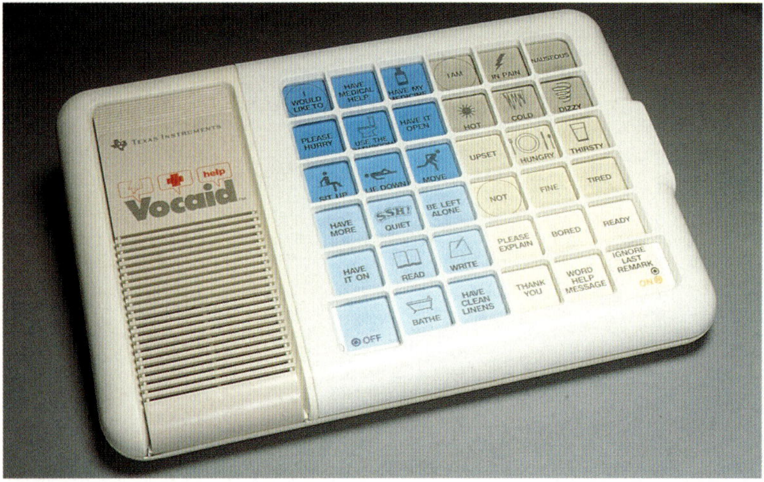

FIGURE 21.17

Simple communication prosthesis with limited options; it produces digitized speech, generated by pushing buttons.

Cognitive Disorders

A variety of cognitive disorders occur after stroke. These include global dementia as well as more discrete disorders of memory and attention. Lesions affecting the nondominant hemisphere may result in visual-spatial dysfunction and neglect. While many cognitive disorders are evident to professional staff and families, formal neuropsychologic testing is useful in quantifying deficits and for discovering subtle, but functionally important deficits.

Both dementia and stroke are common in elderly patients, and frequently occur in the same patient. The prevalence of dementia in a large cohort of stroke patients ranges from 10% at age 60 years to 25% at age 80 years (Figure 21.18) [56]. History from friends and family sometimes suggests a preexistent degenerative dementia, but vascular dementia is the second most frequent etiology of dementia in elderly patients and may be the cause of preexisting cognitive impairment in many patients with acute stroke. Whether or not dementia was present before stroke, it is clear from population-based studies that cognitive abilities decline further following stroke [57]. The presence of dementia is strongly associated with poor functional outcome after stroke [7,8,11,15]. Decreased attention span and inability to learn new tasks may accompany dementia and preclude participation in a comprehensive rehabilitation program or shift the emphasis of the program toward caregiver education and training.

Patients with mild dementia may be trained to compensate for memory loss by using written and visual reminders. For example, memory notebooks in which important information is systematically entered can be used [58]. Visual images can be taught in an attempt to recall specific items. Unfortunately, unless the individual can generate his or her own internal cues to actually use these reminders, they are of little practical value in everyday life

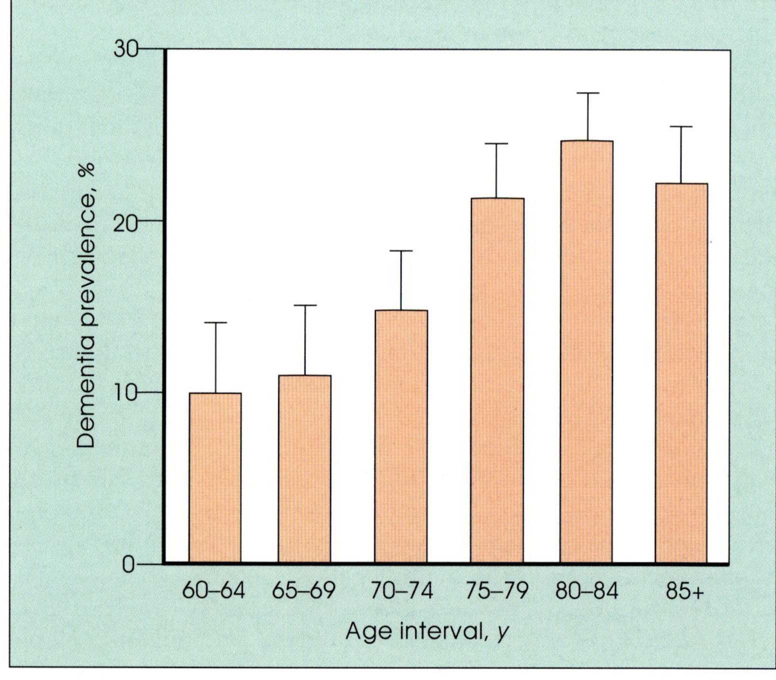

FIGURE 21.18

Bar graph. Mean ± SEM prevalence of dementia by age at stroke onset among 726 testable patients 60 years of age or older with ischemic stroke in the Stroke Data Bank. (*From* Tatemichi and coworkers [56]; with permission.)

[59]. The problem is compounded by the apathy and lack of insight which usually accompany significant dementia.

Attentional deficits that prevent encoding of new material are sometimes the primary cause of inability to learn. Different forms of attention are defined in Table 21.6. Training programs that address attentional disturbances have been devised with various degrees of success [60]. Whether such training generalizes to events of everyday life is unclear. From a practical perspective, patients with attentional deficits, but intact memory, should receive therapy under controlled circumstances. For example, a patient deficient in selective or divided attention may progress more quickly in all therapy disciplines if treatment sessions are held in a quiet secluded room.

Another very common set of cognitive deficits following stroke is associated with lesions of the nondominant hemisphere. The deficits most likely to result in functional disturbance are neglect and visual-perceptual disturbances. Profound disability may result, and some studies have suggested worse functional outcome in persons with nondominant hemisphere stroke [61,62]. It has been estimated that neglect deficit occurs in 20% to 31% of patients with stroke [63]. Inattention to the affected side during reading or eating, difficulty dressing, and difficulty finding one's way around may all be noted. Safety may become an issue, the patient catching the fingers of the affected hand in wheelchair spokes or bumping into environmental hazards on the affected side while ambulating, propelling a wheelchair, or driving. Many patients with neglect lack insight into their limitations, making it more difficult to devise a treatment program. Nevertheless, a number of treatments have been attempted, including visual and verbal cues to attend to the affected side, visual scanning and somatosensory awareness training [64,65], video feedback [66], and computerized scanning and attention training [67]. Although improvement in individual tasks has been demonstrated, evidence for generalization to ADLs and other practical tasks has been mixed [66,68,69]. Novel attempts at treating neglect have included the use of Fresnel prisms [68], eye patching (Figure 21.19) [69], and pharmacologic treatment with bromocriptine [70]. Fortunately, neglect resolves in many patients within 3 months of stroke [67]. From a practical perspective, demonstration of the problem to the patient and family and discussion of possible safety consequences is very important. Caregivers can be taught to cue the patient during specific tasks.

Apraxia is a final common cognitive impairment affecting stroke and may affect a host of tasks including those requiring linguistic and motor skills. For motor tasks, therapy should focus on spontaneous activities, which are often performed better than skilled volitional activities.

Table 21.6. Different forms of attention*

Focused attention: the ability to respond discretely to specific visual, auditory, or tactile stimuli

Sustained attention: the ability to maintain a consistent behavioral response during continuous or repetitive activity

Selective attention: the ability to maintain a cognitive set that requires activation and inhibition of responses dependent upon discrimination of stimuli

Alternating attention: the capacity for mental flexability that allows one to move between tasks having different cognitive requirements

Divided attention: the ability to respond simultaneously to multiple tasks

*From Raskin and Mateer [60]; with permission.

Activities of Daily Living

Perhaps the most rewarding strategy of rehabilitation for stroke patients is training for independence in ADLs. While this strategy is clearly compensatory and might appear to have a rather narrow focus, there is excellent correlation with performance in ADLs and ability to return home [19,21]. In addition, ability to care for one's personal needs often engenders a sense of pride and independence. Independence in ADLs is a major component of overall satisfaction with the quality of one's life following stroke [21,72]. The generally accepted basic ADLs include feeding, dressing, bathing, grooming, toileting, transfers, and ambulation or mobility. Each skill is first broken down into its component parts. After each component has been addressed, the integrated task is practiced. In situations where total independence is impossible, the patient should be taught to assist as much as possible, and a caregiver instructed to provide the remainder of the activity.

Many types of adaptive equipment are available to facilitate the performance of ADLs [39]. While too numerous to list here, these include specially designed eating utensils (Figure 21.20), dressing hooks, and other dressing adaptations (Figures 21.21 and 21.22), one-handed denture brushes (Figure 21.23), and various types of commodes (Figure 21.24).

SPECIAL PROBLEMS FOLLOWING STROKE

During the course of recovery from stroke, a variety of clinical problems may arise that complicate rehabilitation efforts. These range

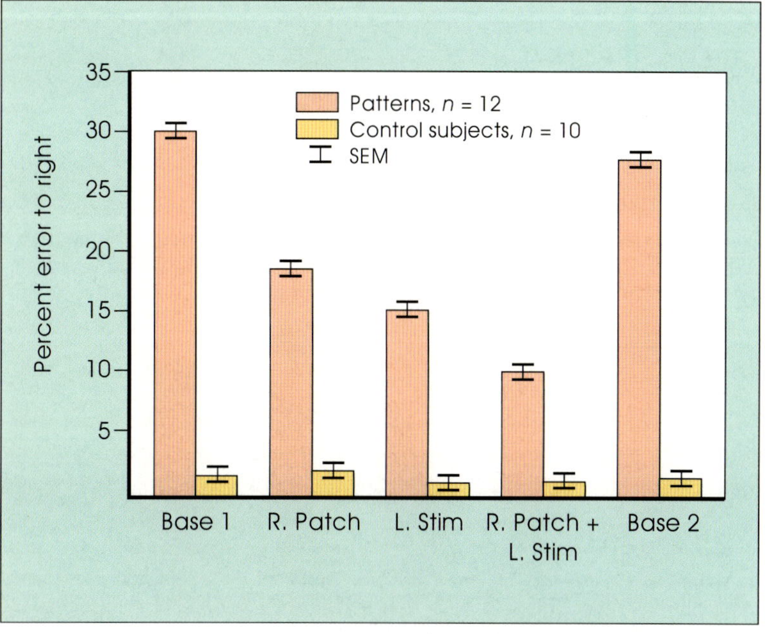

FIGURE 21.19

Transient improvement in treatment of neglect. Mean percent error to the right side of patients who received monocular patching (R. patch) and lateralized stimulation (L. stim) compared with normal control subjects in the line-bisection test. Note the transient beneficial effect during treatment and return to baseline scores after treatment ended. (*From* Butter and Kirsch [69]; with permission.)

from serious life-threatening medical illnesses to more benign clinical problems that are nonetheless bothersome to the patient and family.

Medical Complications

Patients with stroke undergoing rehabilitation are subject to a variety of medical conditions that may interfere with rehabilitation [73,74]. Many of these ailments are those expected in an elderly population and include conditions that preceded the stroke, including diabetes, hypertension, peripheral vascular disease, and degenerative arthritis. Cardiac disease deserves special mention, if only because it is the most common cause of death in stroke survivors [75,76]. From a practical perspective, angina or dyspnea related to congestive heart failure is the limiting factor in the physical rehabilitation of a few patients.

In other patients, chronic pulmonary disease or significant anemia may result in a decreased metabolic reserve, with satisfactory tissue oxygenation at rest, but decompensation with physical exertion [74].

Probably the most feared complication of stroke rehabilitation is pulmonary embolism associated with deep venous thrombosis (DVT). The risk of DVT is greatest in the paretic leg and increases substantially in nonambulatory patients (Figure 21.25). In patients undergoing rehabilitation for stroke, the incidence of pulmonary embolism has been estimated at 1% to 3% [77–79] and may present with atypical symptoms, including change in facial skin color and chest or back pain exacerbated by change in position [78]. Sudden, unexpected death on the rehabilitation ward is often due to pulmonary embolism.

Careful observation for signs and symptoms of DVT and pulmonary embolism in patients undergoing rehabilitation for stroke is imperative, and prophylactic treatment should be undertaken in patients with severe paresis or those who are bed bound. The most effective form of prophylaxis is uncertain [77,80]. Knee-high, graded elastic stockings increase blood flow in the femoral and popliteal veins of hemiplegic patients [81] and were still considered the first-line prophylaxis against pulmonary embolism by a recent international task force [82]. External pneumatic calf compression reduces the risk of DVT in patients undergoing general surgery but has not been adequately studied in patients with stroke [77]. There is also excellent evidence that low-dose subcutaneous heparin or a low-molecular-weight heparinoid are effective in preventing DVT in stroke patients [83-86].

Nutrition and Swallowing

Poor nutritional status on admission is present in 16% of patients with acute stroke and may reflect the prevalence of malnutrition in a general medical population (Figure 21.26) [87]. The nutritional status in a significant proportion of stroke patients actually deterio-

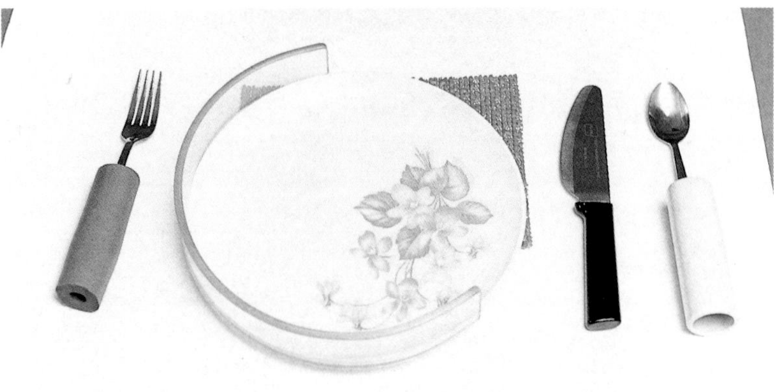

FIGURE 21.20

Commonly used adaptive eating equipment including foam utensil handles, plate guard, rocker knife for one-handed cutting, and material to prevent the plate from slipping. (*From* Laven [39]; with permission.)

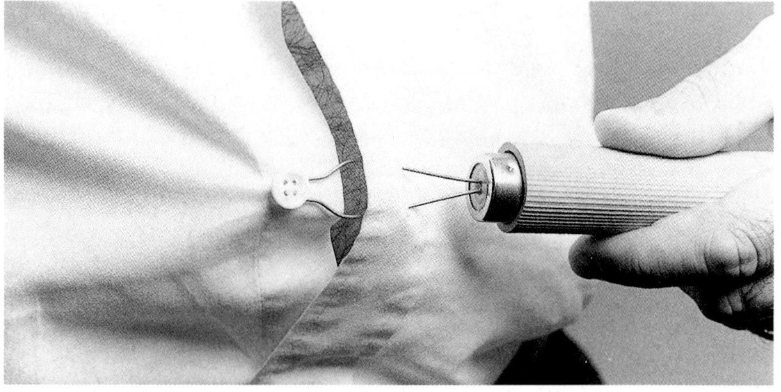

FIGURE 21.21

Button hook.

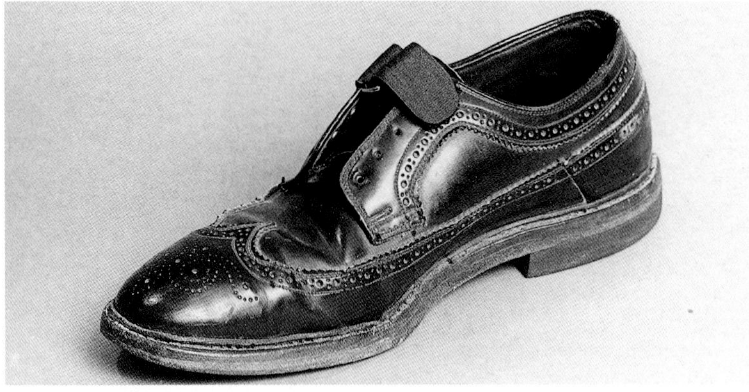

FIGURE 21.22

Shoe with velcro closure.

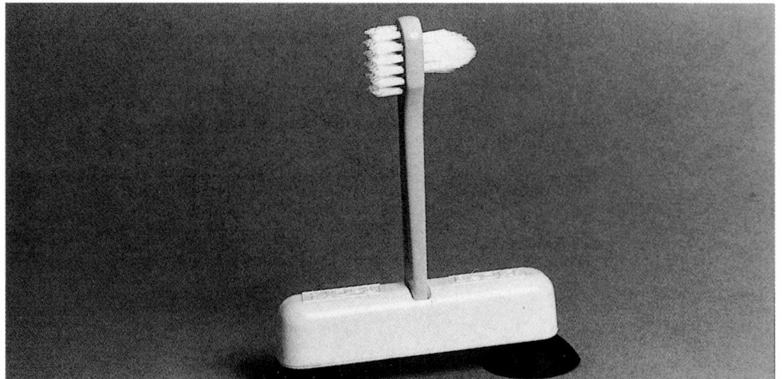

FIGURE 21.23

One-handed denture brush with suction-cup base.

rates after admission [87]. This appears to correlate with age and the frequency of medical complications, especially infection.

Another reason for poor nutrition following stroke is dysphagia, which may also result in aspiration. Although the exact incidence of swallowing disorders after stroke is unknown, almost 30% of conscious patients with acute unilateral hemisphere strokes demonstrate clinical evidence of disturbed swallowing when asked to swallow 10 mL of water [88]. Bedside examination of swallowing identifies 42% to 80% of patients subsequently determined to aspirate on videofluoroscopy [89–91], the rest having clinically "silent" aspiration. Although patients with brain stem or bilateral hemisphere strokes have a higher risk of aspiration, aspiration is not uncommon in patients with unilateral hemispheric strokes [91]. Videofluoroscopy allows much better visualization of the degree of aspiration than a bedside swallowing examination and provides insight into the specific nature of the dysphagia.

Although about one third of stroke patients develop respiratory infections [92], and pneumonia is a leading cause of death following stroke [93], the causative role of aspiration is often unclear. Oral feeding should not be attempted in patients with obvious clinical aspiration or in those with decreased level of consciousness. The nutritional needs of these patients should be promptly addressed through an enteral feeding tube, usually a nasogastric tube, until improvement occurs, or a decision about a more permanent feeding tube can be made. Although the significance of minor subclinical aspiration is unclear, experience suggests that these patients seldom develop clinical pulmonary infections.

Swallowing disorders in stroke patients often improve quickly [88], but in patients with mild-to-moderate dysphagia, compensatory techniques may permit oral feeding as improvement occurs and, occasionally, may be necessary indefinitely. All patients should eat in a sitting position. A diet consisting of thick liquids and soft solids, without thin liquids that are easily aspirated, may be all that is required. Commercially available thickeners may be added to liquids to create a jellylike consistency. The size of the bolus may also be altered. The effectiveness of these techniques is usually monitored at the bedside by nursing staff or trained therapists, but videofluoroscopy may also be used to determine the consistency and size of the bolus that facilitates optimal swal-

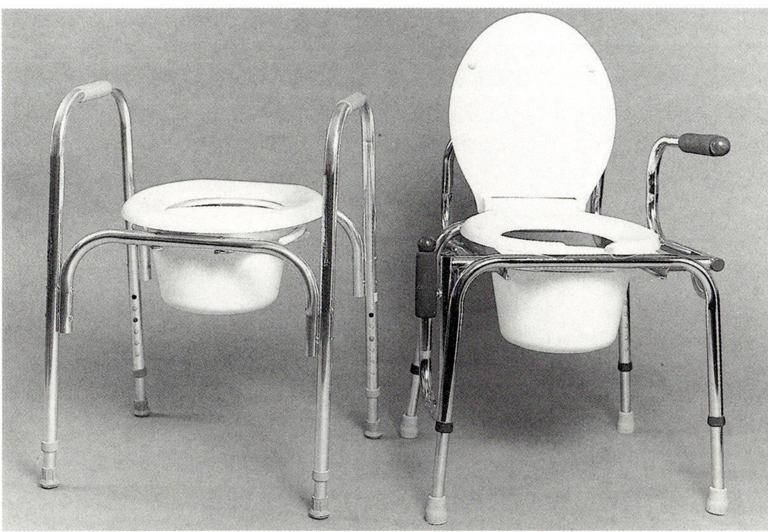

FIGURE 21.24

A three-in-one commode (*left*) may be used at bedside or over the toilet to provide arm support. A drop-arm commode (*right*) is used for patients who perform sliding board transfers or who require moderate to maximum assistance of another person for transfers. (*From* Laven [39]; with permission.)

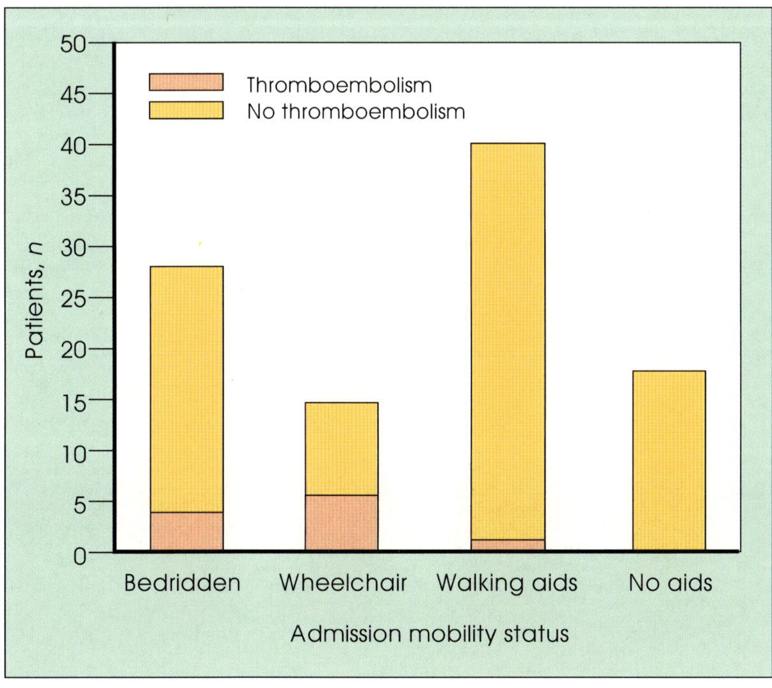

FIGURE 21.25

Distribution of mobility at the time of admission in patients with and without venous thromboembolism. (*From* Oczkowski and coworkers [79]; with permission.)

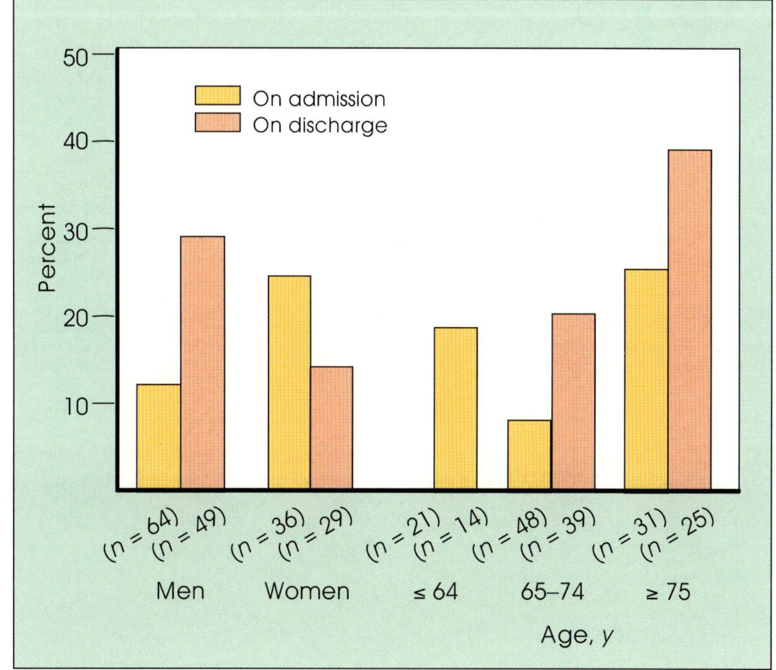

FIGURE 21.26

Proportion of patients with two or more of six chemical and physical nutritional indicators below the reference interval, divided into sex and age groups, on admission and at discharge. (*From* Axelsson and coworkers [87]; with permission.)

lowing. The effectiveness of a variety of compensatory swallowing techniques, which may be taught to patients by speech or language pathologists, can also be evaluated on videofluoroscopy. These include swallowing during a "chin-down" posture [94] or while rotating the head toward one side [95]. The supraglottic swallow (swallowing while voluntarily holding one's breath), Mendelsohn's maneuver (prolonging the period of maximal laryngeal elevation that occurs midswallow), and multiple swallows or cough and swallow sequences may be helpful in some patients [95,96].

Dehydration may occur insidiously in stroke patients with dysphagia despite adequate nutrition because of difficulty swallowing thin liquids. Careful attention to nursing intake and output reports is warranted.

Urinary Dysfunction

Urinary incontinence is a common sequela of acute stroke, with an incidence ranging from 38% to 60% in the early recovery period [97–100]. The presence of incontinence is strongly associated with worse outcome from stroke [101,102]; it is often a practical issue that families must deal with as they decide whether they can care for a stroke victim at home.

Incontinence is correlated with the size of stroke [100], degree of neurologic impairment [97], presence of aphasia [97,100], presence of dementia [100], and low Barthel Index (even when modified by removal of bladder subscores) (Table 21.7). Incontinence is not correlated with location of stroke [97,98,103]. The most common urodynamic finding associated with incontinence is detrusor hyperreflexia with a coordinated sphincter [97,98,103], while a few patients have detrusor hyporeflexia, usually associated with diabetic neuropathy or anticholinergic medications [100]. A surprising number of patients have normal urodynamic studies (Figure 21.27) [100]. Most of these patients are aphasic or have cognitive deficits and may not be able to communicate the need to void. Table 21.8 shows that incontinence following stroke improves with time [97,98]. The best treatment is a rigorous scheduled voiding program. Pharmacologic treatment of bladder hyperreflexia does not seem to improve outcome and may cause side effects.

Urinary retention, as measured by elevated postvoid residual urine, occurs frequently early after stroke, with an incidence of 36% to 53% [104,105], and also improves slowly with time. Urodynamic studies combined with cystoscopy reveal a wide variety of findings [105].

Because of the variation in bladder function following stroke, postvoid residual urine should be measured on all patients before starting an intensive rehabilitation program. A practical flow diagram based on postvoid residual urine results is shown in Figure 21.28. A conservative approach is warranted in all patients without

Table 21.7. Neurologic deficits and functional status scores in incontinent and continent patient groups*†

	Group		
	Incontinent	Continent	*P*
Aphasia			0.003‡
Present	14	10	
Absent	5	22	
Mini mental state score	24.0 ± 1.2	26.7 ± 0.6	0.041§
Barthel Index score			
Admission	21.8 ± 2.1	44.2 ± 3.1	0.0001§
Discharge	42.9 ± 4.1	73.0 ± 3.4	0.0001§
Modified Barthel Index score			
Admission	20.8 ± 1.7	38.0 ± 2.6	0.0001§
Discharge	38.7 ± 3.4	63.4 ± 3.1	0.0001§

**From* Gelber and coworkers [100]; with permission.
†Data are mean ± SEM.
‡Association of aphasia with incontinence by 2 X 2 chi^2 analysis.
§By student's t test.

Table 21.8. Prestroke and poststroke state of continence*

		Poststroke, *n(%)*		
	Prestroke continence, *n(%)*	1 week	4 weeks	12 weeks
Continent	119(77)	56(36)	70(46)	79(51)
Incontinent	26(17)	84(55)	49(32)	32(21)
Dead		14(9)	35(23)	43(28)
Unknown	9(6)			
Total	154(100)	154(100)	154(100)	154(100)

**From* Borrie and coworkers [98]; with permission.

Table 21.9. Causes of painful shoulder

Contracture or adhesive capsulitis
Rotator cuff injuries
Plexus or nerve injury (brachial nerve)
Tendonitis (long head of biceps, supraspinatus)
Subdeltoid bursitis
Sympathetically mediated pain (reflex sympathetic dystrophy)

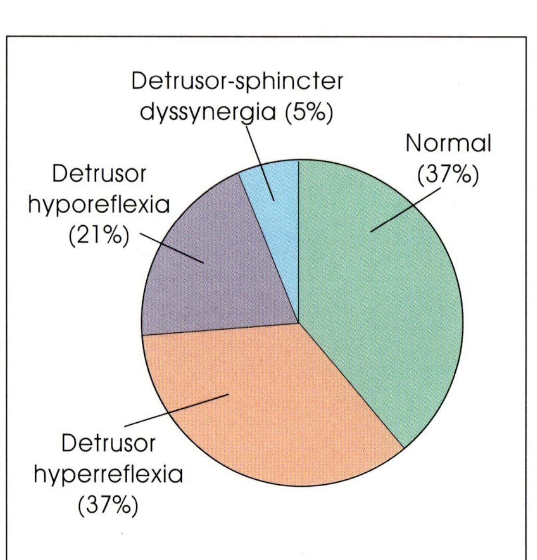

FIGURE 21.27 Graph showing results of urodynamic studies performed on a consecutive series of stroke patients with urinary incontinence (n = 19). (*From* Gelber and coworkers [100]; with permission.)

significant bladder outlet obstruction. Appropriate management includes a rigorous scheduled voiding program for incontinent patients with normal or hyperreflexic bladders, and intermittent catheterization for those with large postvoid residuals, whether or not they are incontinent. Indwelling catheters and pharmacologic management should be avoided, except in unusual circumstances.

Pain Syndromes Complicating Stroke Rehabilitation

Pain syndromes complicating stroke rehabilitation can be distracting at best and debilitating at worst. Fortunately, the most severe syndrome is the most uncommon. Infarcts or hemorrhages involving the posterolateral thalamus (Figure 21.29) may result in the thalamic pain syndrome of Dejerine-Roussy. The characteristic mild hypesthesia, accompanied by dysesthetic pain and misperception of minor sensory stimuli as excruciatingly painful, is difficult to treat, although a trial of pharmacologic management with antidepressants or anticonvulsants is warranted. A similar syndrome may be seen in lesions of the deep parietal white matter, probably due to a thalamocortical disconnection syndrome (Figure 21.30) [106].

A much more common problem is a painful shoulder, which may occur in as many as 70% to 80% of persons with hemiplegia [107,108]. Despite much study, no uniform hypothesis explaining shoulder pain has emerged, and many different etiologies have been proposed (Table 21.9), several of which may coexist in the same patient. The shoulder is a highly mobile and poorly balanced joint that is highly susceptible to trauma. The rotator cuff contributes considerably to shoulder stability, and muscle weakness results in glenohumeral subluxation (Figure 21.31). Theoretically,

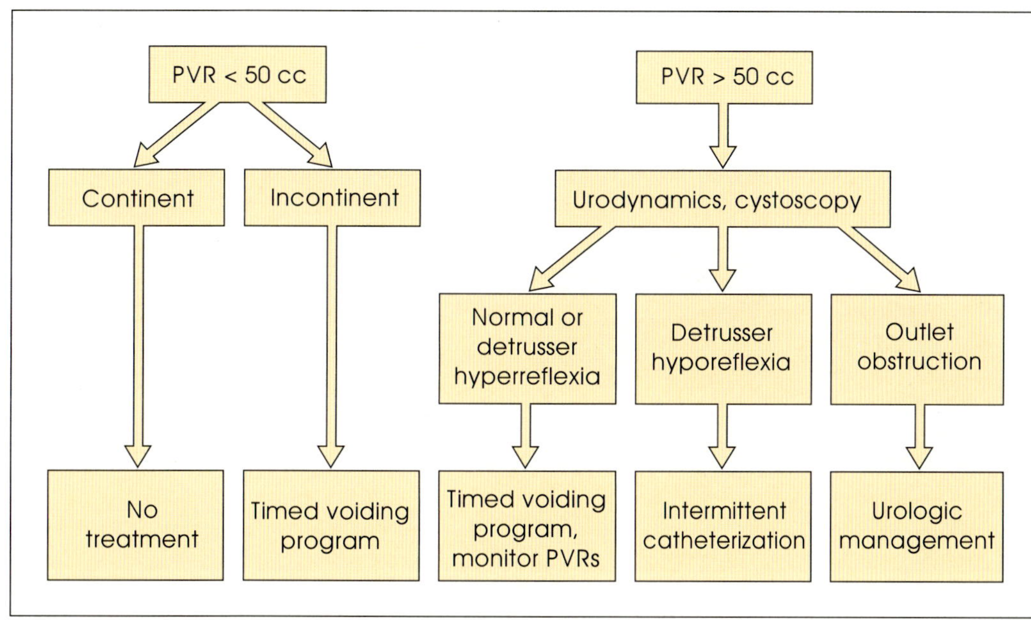

FIGURE 21.28

Algorithm for bladder management after stroke. PVR—postvoid residual urine.

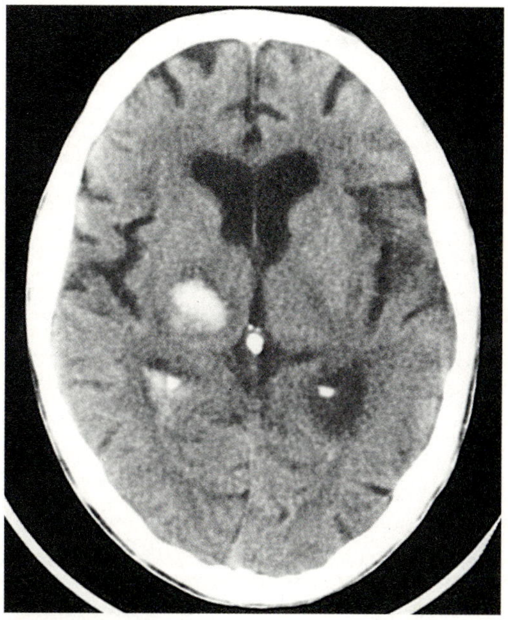

FIGURE 21.29

Right thalamic hemorrhage that resulted in a thalamic pain syndrome.

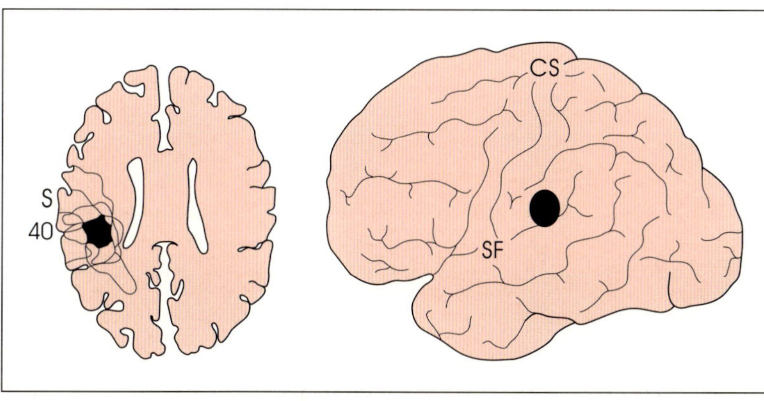

FIGURE 21.30

The sites of left parietal white matter lesions in six patients with a "pseudo-thalamic" pain syndrome. The lesion common to all cases is shown by the blackened area. CS—central sulcus; S—primary somatosensory cortex; SF—sylvian fissure; 40—area 40 in the inferior parietal lobe. (*From* Schmahmann and Leifer [106]; with permission.)

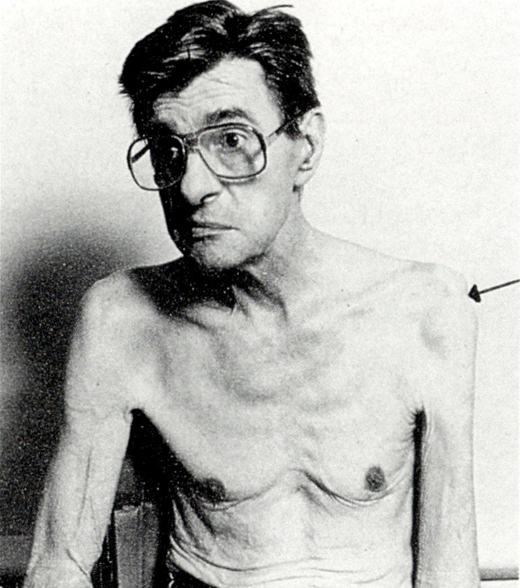

FIGURE 21.31

Subluxation of left shoulder. (*From* Lal [131]; with permission.)

gravitational pull on the upper extremity could result in painful stretching of the superior joint capsule and supraspinatus muscle. Although some studies have shown an association between subluxation and shoulder pain [107,109], others have produced contradictory results [110,111].

Rotator-cuff tears have been documented in arthrography studies of hemiplegic shoulders in some studies [112,113], while another study failed to find rotator cuff injury, but did find evidence of adhesive capsulitis [114]. Evidence of denervation found on electromyography in a small number of patients has suggested the possibility of nerve injury involving the brachial plexus or suprascapular nerve [115,116]. Passive abduction of the weak shoulder without appropriate external rotation normally provided by the rotator cuff may compress the subdeltoid bursa or tendon of the supraspinatus muscle or the long head of the biceps brachii, causing tendonitis or bursitis (Figure 21.32) [107]. Spasticity has also been implicated as a contributing factor to shoulder pain [107]. Finally, stroke patients may develop reflex sympathetic dystrophy in the affected arm. The reported incidence varies from 15% to 41% [107,108,117]. The onset is often insidious and delayed, with a peak incidence occurring 1 to 3 months after stroke. Symptoms consist of pain on range of motion of the fingers, wrist, and shoulder, and evidence of autonomic dysfunction with temperature change and edema in the hand (Figure 21.33). Although the diagnosis is usually clinical, bone scans are frequently positive. Most cases of reflex sympathetic dystrophy following stroke are mild and self-limited. Treatment consists of physical therapy for passive range of motion and a trial of nonsteroidal anti-inflammatory agents [117]. More refractory cases may respond to a short

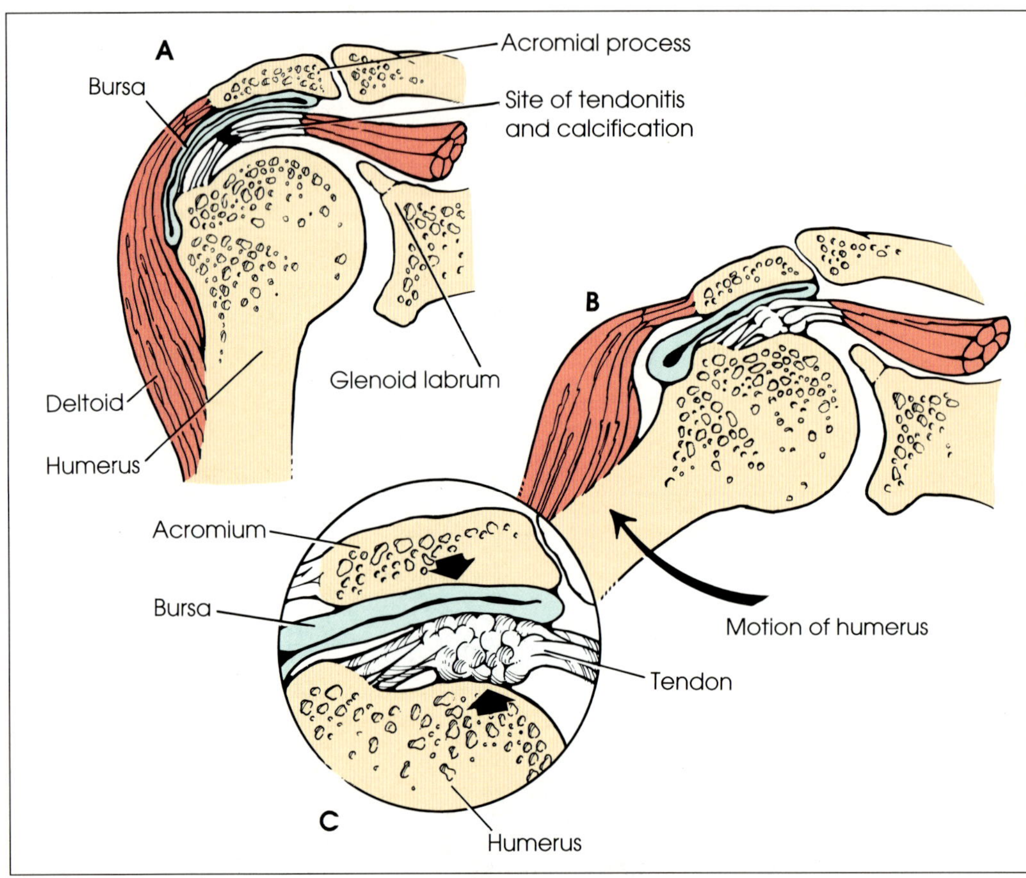

FIGURE 21.32

Impingement of supraspinatus tendon and subdeltoid bursa with adduction of the shoulder. **A**, Shoulder in neutral position. **B**, Shoulder in passive abduction without external rotation. **C**, Impingement of subdeltoid bursa and supraspinatus tendon. (*From* Cailliet [132]; with permission.)

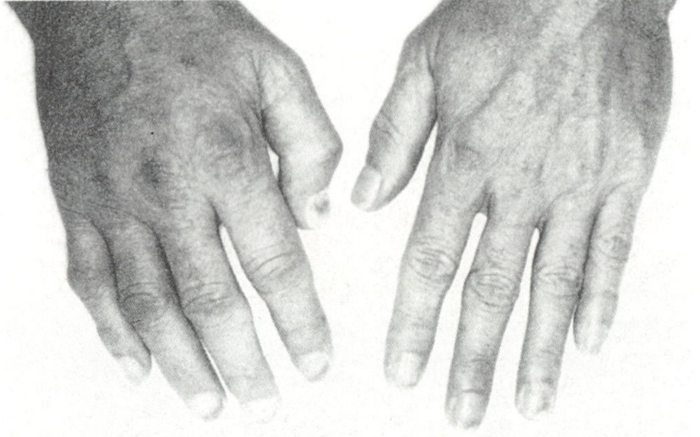

FIGURE 21.33

Example of flushing of the skin over the proximal interphalangeal and metacarpal phalangeal joints of the right hand indicating altered vasomotor control of capillary flow in the plegic right hand. (*From* Chalsen and coworkers [117]; with permission.)

course of oral corticosteroids [117,118], and occasionally superior cervical ganglion blocks are necessary [118].

The multiple possible etiologies of shoulder pain after stroke makes prevention difficult. To prevent unnecessary trauma, the professional staff should be instructed in the proper techniques for range of motion exercises, and should take care to protect the shoulder while turning and transferring the patient. Traction on the shoulder should be avoided. Although the role of subluxation in causing shoulder pain is uncertain, the arm should be supported on a lap tray or arm trough when the patient is sitting (Figure 21.34). When standing or walking for any extended period, the patient should use one of several types of slings (Figure 21.35). If pain develops, an attempt should be made to establish a specific diagnosis and initiate appropriate treatment. Unfortunately, in many individual cases, a definite etiology cannot be determined and treatment consists of continued careful range of motion and symptomatic treatment.

Poststroke Depression

Significant depression following stroke occurs in 25% to 50% of patients [119,120]. Satisfaction with life clearly declines after stroke (Figure 21.36) [72] and depression is a major contributing factor (Figure 21.37) [121]. Although the incidence of depression declines in the first year following stroke [120,122], patients still depressed at 1 year have a high risk for the development of chronic depression [120].

Several studies have indicated an association of poststroke depression with lesions of the left anterior hemisphere [120,122,123], but other investigators have failed to confirm this finding [124,125]. Depression following stroke has been associated with worse functional outcome 2 years after stroke (Figure 21.38) [126]. Fortunately, antidepressant medications are effective in treating poststroke depression [127–129]. Clinical trials have used different drugs, and the relative efficacy of the many medications available to treat poststroke depression is unknown. Therefore, therapeutic choices should be made on the basis of the side-effect profile [119].

CONCLUSIONS

While clinical and research emphasis in stroke has appropriately been directed toward prevention and treatment, the rehabilitation of patients with completed stroke remains an important aspect of total care. Advances in key technical areas, including orthotic design and communication devices, have improved function for some patients. However, clinical rehabilitation for stroke is largely a low-tech, "hands-on" endeavor, largely focused on teaching the patient and family adaptive techniques to compensate for impairment. In the future, emerging knowledge about the neurobiology of recovery is

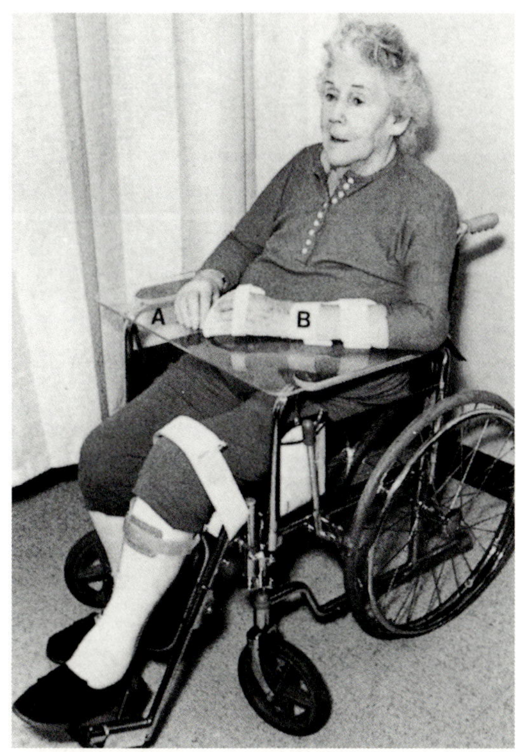

FIGURE 21.34

A, Lap board made of clear plastic to support the hemiplegic shoulder, arm, and hand. **B**, Resting hand splint to prevent progressive finger and wrist flexion deformity. (*From* Reding and McDowell [133]; with permission.)

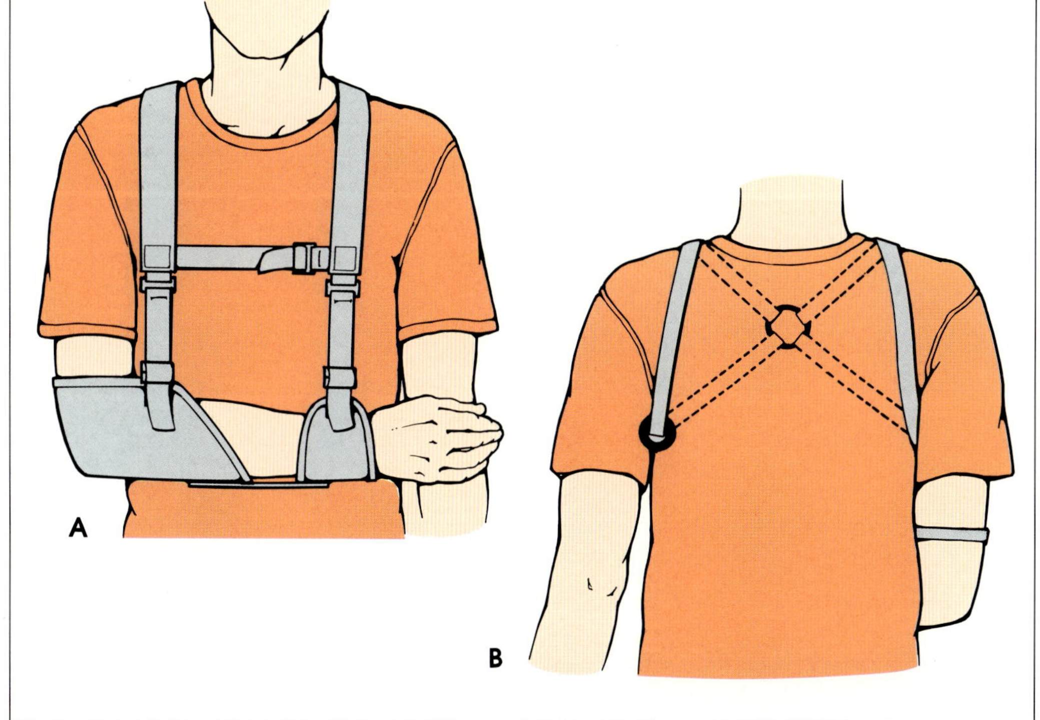

FIGURE 21.35

Slings for support of shoulder in hemiplegia. **A**, Traditional hemisling. **B**, Bobath sling. (*Adapted from* Brooke and coworkers [134]; with permission.)

likely to impact rehabilitation. Sophisticated neuroimaging techniques have resulted in better understanding of task acquisition in normal individuals and the patterns of neural recovery in patients with discrete cerebral injuries. The challenge for rehabilitation is to use this new information to create new treatment paradigms that truly result in improvement beyond natural recovery.

In the meantime, traditional rehabilitation approaches continue to be appropriate. Physicians caring for patients following stroke must also be aware of the special stroke-related problems these patients have and how they affect rehabilitation efforts. A carefully designed rehabilitation program may be the difference between a successful return home and placement in a skilled care facility.

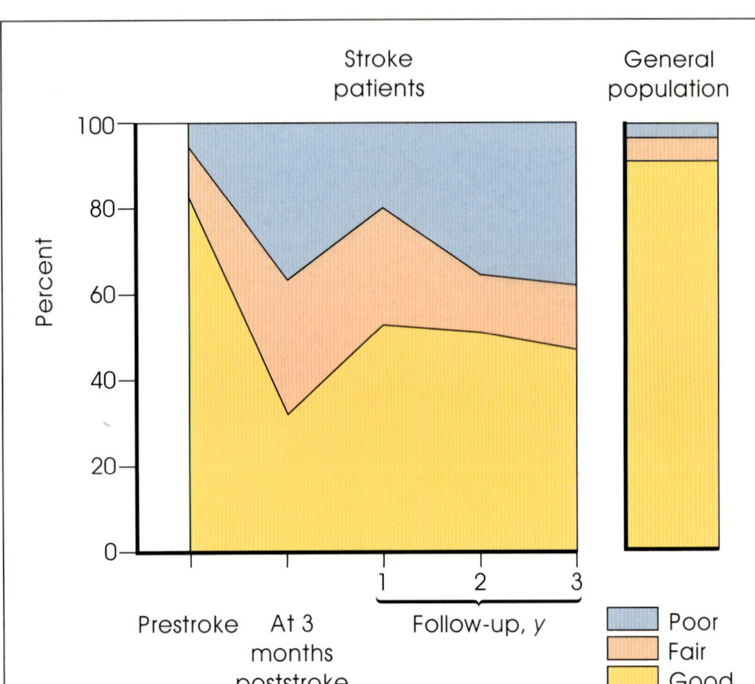

FIGURE 21.36

Global life satisfaction in elderly patients in the general population ($n = 828$) and in long-term survivors after stroke ($n = 50$). (*From* Åström and coworkers [72]; with permission.)

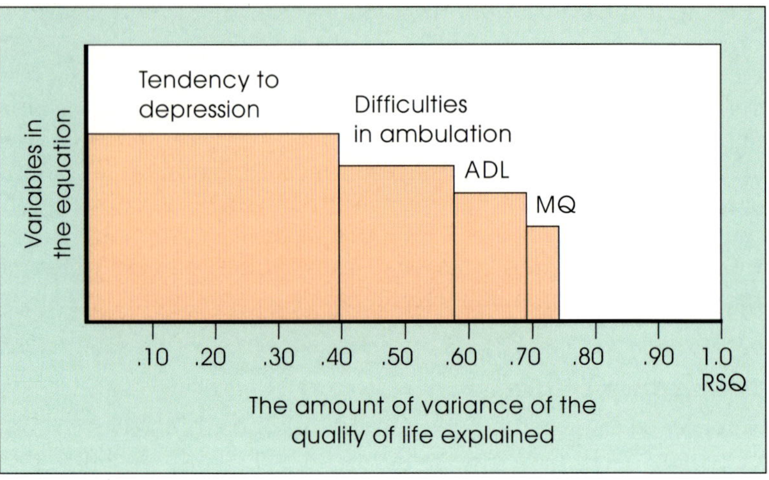

FIGURE 21.37

Variance in quality of life explained (RSQ) by variables in multiple regression equation. The subjective tendency to depression is the most important variable predicting quality of life after stroke, followed by difficulties with ambulation, difficulties with activities of daily living (ADLs), and memory quotient (MQ). (*From* Niemi and coworkers [121]; with permission.)

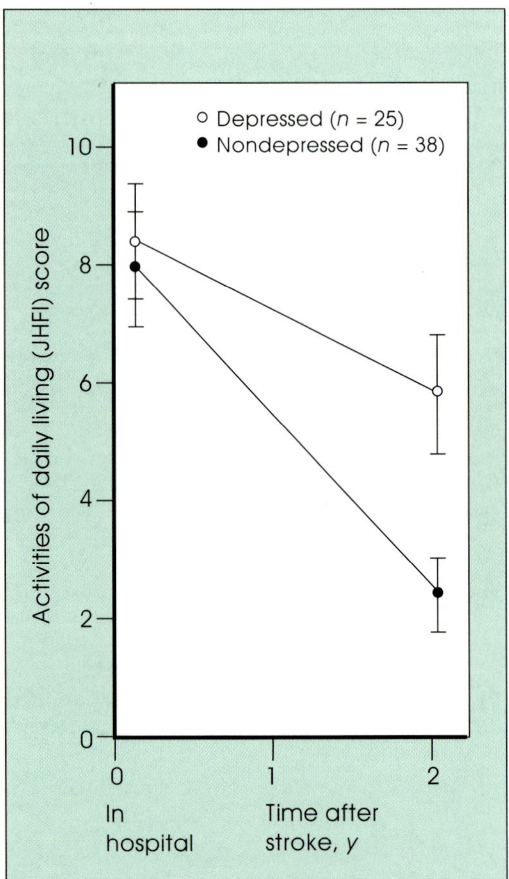

FIGURE 21.38

Depressed patients had greater impairment in activities of daily living (measured as a higher score on the Johns Hopkins Functioning Index [JHFI]) than nondepressed patients, and this persisted at the 2-year follow-up evaluation. (*From* Parikh and coworkers [126]; with permission.)

REFERENCES

1. World Health Organization: *The International Classification of Impairments, Disabilities and Handicaps.* Geneva: World Health Organization; 1980.
2. Asanuma C. Mapping movements within a moving motor map. *Trends Neurosci* 1991, 14:217–218.
3. Pascual-Leone A, Cohen LG, Dang N, *et al.*: Acquisition of fine motor skills in humans is associated with the modulation of cortical motor outputs. *Neurology* 1993, 43(suppl 2):157A.
4. Chollet F, DiPiero V, Wise JS, *et al.*: The functional anatomy of motor recovery after stroke in humans: a study with positron-emission tomography. *Ann Neurol* 1991, 29:63–71.
5. Weiller C, Ramsay SC, Wise RJS: Individual patterns of functional reorganization in the human cerebral cortex after capsular infarction. *Ann Neurol* 1993, 33:181–189.
6. Reding MJ, Potes E: Rehabilitation outcome following initial unilateral hemispheric stroke: life table analysis approach. *Stroke* 1988, 19:1354–1358.
7. Kotila M, Waltimo O, Niemi M, *et al.*: The profile of recovery from stroke and factors influencing outcome. *Stroke* 1984, 15:1039–1044.
8. Lincoln NB, Blackburn M, Ellis S, *et al.*: An investigation of factors affecting progress of patients on a stroke unit. *J Neurol Neurosurg Psych* 1989, 52:493– 496.
9. Garraway WM, Akhtar AJ, Prescott RJ, *et al.*: Management of acute stroke in the elderly: preliminary results of a controlled trial. *BMJ* 1980, 280:1040–1043.
10. Smith DS, Goldenberg E, Ashburn A, *et al.*: Remedial therapy after stroke: a randomized controlled trial. *BMJ* 1981, 282:517–520.
11. Smith ME, Garraway WM, Smith DL, *et al.*: Therapy impact of functional outcome in a controlled trial of stroke rehabilitation. *Arch Phys Med Rehabil* 1982, 63:21–24.
12. Sivenius J, Pyörälä K, Heikonen OP, *et al.*: The significance of rehabilitation of stroke: a controlled trial. *Stroke* 1985, 16:928–931.
13. Indredavik B, Bakke F, Solberg R, *et al.*: Benefit of a stroke unit: a randomized controlled trial. *Stroke* 1991, 22:1026–1031.
14. Johnston MV, Keister M: Early rehabilitation for stroke patients: a new look. *Arch Phys Med Rehabil* 1984, 65:437–441.
15. Novack TA, Satterfield WT, Lyons K, *et al.*: Stroke onset and rehabilitation: time lag as a factor in treatment outcome. *Arch Phys Med Rehabil* 1984, 65:316–319.
16. Ernst E. A review of stroke rehabilitation and physiotherapy. *Stroke* 1990, 21:1081–1085.
17. Wagenaar RC, Meijer OG: Effects of stroke rehabilitation: a critical review of the literature. Part 1. *J Rehabil Sci* 1991, 4:61–73.
18. dePedro-Cuesta J, Widen-Holmqvist L, Bach-y-Rita P: Evaluation of stroke rehabilitation by randomized controlled studies: a review. *Acta Neurol Scand* 1992, 86:433–439.
19. Granger CV, Hamilton BB, Gresham GE: The stroke rehabilitation study: general description. Part 1. *Arch Phys Med Rehabil* 1988, 69:506–509.
20. Granger CV, Dewis LS, Peters NC, *et al.*: Stroke rehabilitation: analysis of repeated Barthel Index measures. *Arch Phys Med Rehabil* 1979, 60:14–17.
21. Good DC: Outcome assessment in chronic neurological disease. In *Handbook of Neurorehabilitation.* Edited by Good DC, Couch JR. New York: Marcel Dekker; 1994:107–128.
22. Fugl-Meyer AR, Jaasko L, Leyman L, *et al.*: The post-stroke hemiplegic patient: a method for evaluation of physical performance. *Scand J Rehabil Med* 1975, 7:13.
23. Bergner M, Bobbitt RA, Carter WB, *et al.*: The sickness impact profile: development and final revision of a health status measure. *Med Care* 1981, 19:787–805.
24. Wade DT, ed.: *Measurement in Neurological Rehabilitation.* Oxford: Oxford University Press; 1992.
25. Lyden PD, Lau GT: A critical appraisal of stroke evaluation and rating scales. *Stroke* 1991, 22:1345–1352.
26. Smith DL, Akhtar AJ, Garraway WM: Motor function after stroke. *Age Ageing* 1985, 14:46–48.
27. Bonita R, Beaglehole R: Recovery of motor function after stroke. *Stroke* 1988, 19:1497–1500.
28. Duncan PW, Goldstein LB, Matchar D, *et al.*: Measurement of motor recovery after stroke. *Stroke* 1992, 23:1084–1089.
29. Andrews K, Brocklehurst JC, Richards B, *et al.*: The rate of recovery from stroke and its measurement. *Int Rehabil Med* 1981, 3:155–161.
30. Kelly-Hayes M, Wolf PA, Kase CS. Time course of functional recovery after stroke: the Framingham study. *J Neurol Rehabil* 1989, 3:65–70.
31. Gresham GE, Phillips TF, Wolf PA, *et al.*: Epidemiologic profile of long-term stroke disability: the Framingham study. *Arch Phys Med Rehabil* 1979, 60:487–491.
32. Price SJ, Reding MJ: Physical therapy philosophies and strategies. In *Handbook of Neurorehabilitation.* Edited by Good DC, Couch JR. New York: Marcel Dekker; 1994:181–196.
33. Knott M, Voss DE: *Proprioceptive Neuromuscular Facilitation: Patterns and Techniques.* New York: Harper & Row; 1956.
34. Bobath B: *Adult Hemiplegia: Evaluation and Treatment.* London: William Heinemann Medical Books; 1970.
35. Brunnstrom S: *Movement Therapy in Hemiplegia: A Neurophysiological Approach.* Philadelphia: Harper & Row; 1970.
36. Carr JH, Shepherd RB: *A Motor Relearning Programme for Stroke.* London: William Heinemann Medical Books; 1982.
37. Taub E, Miller NE, Novack TA, *et al.*: Technique to improve chronic motor deficit after stroke. *Arch Phys Med Rehabil* 1993, 74:347–354.
38. Good DC: Treatment strategies for enhancing motor recovery in stroke rehabilitation. *J Neurol Rehabil,* 1994, 8:177–186.
39. Laven L: Adaptive equipment. In *Handbook of Neurorehabilitation.* Edited by Good DC, Couch JR. New York: Marcel Dekker; 1994:317–341.
40. Good DC, Supan TJ: Basic principles of orthotics in neurologic disorders. In *Orthotics in Neurologic Rehabilitation.* Edited by Aisen ML. New York: Demos; 1992:1–23.
41. Skilbeck CV, Wade DT, Langton Hewer R, *et al.*: Recovery after stroke. *J Neurol Neurosurg Psych* 1983, 46:5–8.
42. Young RR: Treatment of spastic paresis. *N Engl J Med* 1989, 320:1553–1555.
43. Rossi PW: Treatment of spasticity. In *Handbook of Neurorehabilitation.* Edited by Good DC, Couch JR. New York: Marcel Dekker; 1994:197–218.
44. Katz RT: Management of spastic hypertonia after stroke. *J Neurol Rehabil* 1991, 5:S5–S12.
45. Jankovic J, Brin MF: Therapeutic uses of botulinum toxin. *N Engl J Med* 1991, 324:1186–1194.
46. Lazar RB, Rubin SM: Speech therapy and communicative disorders in neurological rehabilitation. In *Handbook of Neurorehabilitation.* Edited by Good DC, Couch JR. New York: Marcel Dekker; 1994:219–241.
47. Kertesz A: What do we learn from recovery from aphasia? *Adv Neurol* 1988, 47:277–292.
48. Albert ML, Helm-Estabrooks N: Diagnosis and treatment of aphasia. Part 2. *JAMA* 1988, 259:1205–1210.
49. Benson DF: Aphasia rehabilitation. *Arch Neurol* 1979, 36:187–189.
50. Wertz RT, Weiss DG, Aten JL, *et al*: Comparison of clinic, home and deferred language treatment for aphasia. *Arch Neurol* 1986, 43:653–658.
51. Hartman J, Landau WM: Comparison of formal language therapy with supportive counseling for aphasia due to acute vascular accident. *Arch Neurol* 1987, 44:646–649.

52. Basso A, Capitani E, Vignolo LA: Influence of rehabilitation on language skills in aphasic patients. *Arch Neurol* 1979, 36:190–196.
53. Lincoln NB, Mulley GP, Jones AC, *et al.*: Effectiveness of speech therapy for aphasic stroke patients. *Lancet* 1984, 1:1197–1200.
54. Yorkston KM, Buekelman DR, Bell KR, eds.: *Clinical Management of Dysarthric Speakers.* Boston: College Hill Press; 1988.
55. Mustonen T, Locke P, Reichle J, *et al.*: An overview of augmentative and alternative communication systems. In *Implementing Augmentative and Alternative Communication.* Edited by Reichle J, York J, Sigafoos J. Baltimore: Paul H. Brooks; 1991:1–37.
56. Tatemichi T, Foulkes M, Mohr J, *et al.*: Dementia in stroke survivors in the stroke data bank cohort. *Stroke* 1990, 21:858–866.
57. Kase C, Wolf P, Kelly-Hayes M, *et al.*: Intellectual decline following stroke. *Neurology* 1987, 37(suppl 1):119.
58. Sohlberg MM, Mateer CA, eds: *Introduction to Cognitive Rehabilitation: Theory and Practice.* New York: Guilford Press; 1989.
59. Richardson JTE: Imagery mnemonics and memory remediation. *Neurology* 1992,42:283–286.
60. Raskin SA, Mateer CA: Rehabilitation of cognitive impairments. In *Handbook of Neurorehabilitation.* Edited by Good DC, Couch JR. New York: Marcel Dekker; 1994:243–259.
61. Chen Sea M-J, Henderson A, Cermak SA: Patterns of visual spatial inattention and their functional significance in stroke patients. *Arch Phys Med Rehabil* 1993, 74:355–360.
62. Denes G, Semenza C, Stoppa E, *et al.*: Unilateral spatial neglect and recovery from hemiplegia: a follow-up study. *Brain* 1982, 105:543–552.
63. Alexander D: Depression and cognition as factors in recovery. In *Handbook of Neurorehabilitation.* Edited by Good DC, Couch JR. New York: Marcel Dekker; 1994:129–152.
64. Carter L, Howard B, O'Neil W: Effectiveness of cognitive skill remediation in acute stroke patients. *Am J Occup Ther* 1983, 37:320–326.
65. Gordon W, Hibbard M, Egelko S, *et al*: Perceptual remediation in patients with right-brain damage: a comprehensive program. *Arch Phys Med Rehabil* 1985, 66:353–359.
66. Söderback I, Bengtsson I, Ginsburg E, *et al.*: Video feedback in occupational therapy: its effect in patients with neglect syndrome. *Arch Phys Med Rehabil* 1992, 73:1140–1146.
67. Robertson IH, Gray JM, Pentland B, *et al.*: Microcomputer-based rehabilitation for unilateral left visual neglect: a randomized controlled trial. *Arch Phys Med Rehabil* 1990, 71:663–668.
68. Rossi PW, Kheyfets S, Reding MJ: Fresnel prisms improve visual perception in stroke patients with homonymous hemianopia or unilateral visual neglect. *Neurology* 1990, 40:1597–1599.
69. Butter CM, Kirsch N: Combined and separate effects of eye patching and visual stimulation on unilateral neglect following stroke. *Arch Phys Med Rehabil* 1992, 73:1133– 1139.
70. Fleet WS, Valenstein E, Watson RT, *et al.*: Dopamine agonist therapy for neglect in humans. *Neurology* 1987, 37:1765–1770.
71. Hier D, Mondlock J, Caplan L: Recovery of behavioral abnormalities after right hemisphere stroke. *Neurology* 1983, 33:345–350.
72. Åström M, Asplund K, Åström T: Psychosocial function and life satisfaction after stroke. *Stroke* 1992, 23:527–531.
73. Dobkin BH: Neuromedical complications in stroke patients transferred for rehabilitation before and after diagnostic related groups. *J Neurol Rehabil* 1987, 1:3–7.
74. Couch JR: Medical complications in the rehabilitation patient. In *Handbook of Neurorehabilitation.* Edited by Good DC, Couch JR. New York: Marcel Dekker; 1994:443–458.
75. Rokey R, Rolak LA, Harati Y, *et al.*: Coronary artery disease in patients with cerebrovascular disease: a prospective study. *Ann Neurol* 1984, 16:50–53.
76. Toole JF, Yuson CP, Janeway R, *et al.*: Transient ischemic attacks: a prospective study of 225 patients. *Neurology* 1978, 28:746–753.
77. Sioson ER: Deep vein thrombosis in stroke patients: an overview. *J Stroke Cerebrovasc Dis* 1992, 2:74–79.
78. Chaudhuri GX, Costa JL: Clinical findings associated with pulmonary embolism in a rehabilitation setting. *Arch Phys Med Rehabil* 1991, 72:671–673.
79. Oczkowski WJ, Ginsberg JS, Shin A, *et al.*: Venous thromboembolism in patients undergoing rehabilitation for stroke. *Arch Phys Med Rehabil* 1992, 73:712–716.
80. Alexander GG, Turpie MD, Gent M, *et al.*: A low-molecular-weight heparinoid compared with unfractionated heparin in the prevention of deep vein thrombosis in patients with acute ischemic stroke. *Ann Intern Med* 1992, 117:353–357.
81. Sioson E, Alexander JT, Mentari A, *et al.*: Effect of elastic compression stockings on venous hemodynamics in hemiplegic patients. *J Stroke Cerebrovasc Dis* 1992, 2:196–201.
82. Goldhaber SZ, Morpurgo M: Diagnosis, treatment and prevention of pulmonary embolism: report of the WHO/International Society and Federation of Cardiology Task Force. *JAMA* 1992, 268:1727–1733.
83. McCarthy ST, Turner JJ, Robertson D, *et al.*: Low dose heparin as a prophylaxis against deep-vein thrombosis after acute stroke. *Lancet* 1977, 2:800–801.
84. McCarthy ST, Turner J: Low-dose subcutaneous heparin in the prevention of deep vein thrombosis and pulmonary emboli following acute stroke. *Age Ageing* 1986, 15:84–88.
85. Gelmers HJ: Effects of low-dose subcutaneous heparin on the occurrence of deep vein thrombosis in patients with ischemic stroke. *Acta Neurol Scand* 1980, 61:313–318.
86. Sandset PM, Dahl T, Stiris M, *et al.*: A double-blind and randomized placebo-controlled trial of low-molecular-weight heparin once daily to prevent deep vein thrombosis in acute ischemic stroke. *Sem Thromb Hemost* 1990, 16(suppl):25–33.
87. Axelsson K, Asplund K, Norberg A, *et al.*: Nutritional status in patients with acute stroke. *Acta Med Scand* 1988, 224:217–224.
88. Baren DH: The natural history and functional consequences of dysphagia after hemispheric stroke. *J Neurol Neurosurg Psych* 1989, 52:236–241.
89. Splaingard ML, Hutchins B, Sutton LD, *et al.*: Aspiration in rehabilitation patients: videofluoroscopy vs. bedside clinical assessment. *Arch Phys Med Rehabil* 1988, 69:637–640.
90. DePippo KL, Holas MA, Reding MJ: Validation of the 3-oz water swallow test for aspiration following stroke. *Arch Neurol* 1992, 49:1259–1291.
91. Horner J, Massey EW, Riski JE, *et al.*: Aspiration following stroke: clinical correlates and outcome. *Neurology* 1988, 38:1359–1362.
92. Walker HE, Robins M, Weinfeld FD: Clinical findings. In *The National Survey of Stroke.* Edited by Weinfeld FD. *Stroke* 1981, 6:12(suppl 1):I13–I37.
93. Bounds JV, Wiebers DO, Whisnant JP, *et al.*: Mechanisms and timing of deaths from cerebral infarction. *Stroke* 1981, 12:474–477.
94. Shanahan TK, Logemann JA, Rademaker AW, *et al.*: Chin-down posture effect on aspiration in dysphagic patients. *Arch Phys Med Rehabil* 1993, 74:736–739.
95. Logemann JA, Kahrilas PJ: Relearning to swallow after stroke-application of maneuvers and indirect biofeedback: a case study. *Neurology* 1990, 40:1136–1138.
96. Palmer JB, DuChane AS: Rehabilitation of dysphagia due to cerebrovascular disease. *Phys Med Rehabil Clin North Am* 1991, 2:529–546.
97. Reding MJ, Winter SW, Hochrein SA, *et al.*: Urinary incontinence after unilateral hemispheric stroke: a neurologic-epidemiologic perspective. *J Neurol Rehabil* 1987, 1:25–30.
98. Borrie MJ, Campbell AJ, Caradoc-Davies TH, *et al.*: Urinary incontinence after stroke: a prospective study. *Age Aging* 1986, 15:177–181.
99. Brocklehurst JC, Andrews K, Richards B, *et al.*: Incidence and correlates of incontinence in stroke patients. *J Am Geriatr Soc* 1985, 33:540–542.
100. Gelber DA, Good DC, Laven LJ, *et al.*: Causes of urinary incontinence after acute hemispheric stroke. *Stroke* 1993, 24:378–382.

101. Granger CV, Hamilton BB, Gresham GE, *et al.*: The stroke rehabilitation outcome study, Part 2: relative merits of the total Barthel Index score and a four-item subscore in predicting patient outcomes. *Arch Phys Med Rehabil* 1989, 70:100–103.

102. Barer DH: Continence after stroke: useful predictor or goal of therapy? *Age Aging* 1989, 18:183–191.

103. Khan Z, Starer P, Yang WC, *et al.*: Analysis of voiding disorders in patients with cerebrovascular accidents. *Urology* 1990, 35:265–270.

104. Garrett VE, Scott JA, Costich J, *et al.*: Bladder emptying assessment in stroke patients. *Arch Phys Med Rehabil* 1989, 70:41–43.

105. Gelber DA, Jozefczyk PB, Good DC, *et al.*: Urinary retention following stroke. *J Neurol Rehabil* 1994, 8:69–74.

106. Schmahmann JD, Leifer D: Parietal pseudothalamic pain syndrome. *Arch Neurol* 1992, 49:1032–1037.

107. van Ouwenaller C, Laplace C, Chantraine A: Painful shoulder in hemiplegia. *Arch Phys Med Rehabil* 1986, 67:23– 26.

108. Griffin J, Reddin G: Shoulder pain in patients with hemiplegia: a literature review. *Phys Ther* 1981, 61:1041–1045.

109. deCourval LP, Barsauskas A, Berenbaum B, *et al.*: Painful shoulder in the hemiplegic and unilateral neglect. *Arch Phys Med Rehabil* 1990, 71:673–676.

110. Joynt RL: The source of shoulder pain in hemiplegia. *Arch Phys Med Rehabil* 1992, 73:409–413.

111. Kumar R, Metter EJ, Mehta AJ: Shoulder pain in hemiplegia: the role of exercise. *Am J Phys Med Rehabil* 1990, 69:205–208.

112. Najenson T, Yacubovich E, Pikielni SS: Rotator cuff injury in shoulder joints of hemiplegic patients. *Scand J Rehabil Med* 1971, 3:131–137.

113. Nepomuceno CS, Miller JM, III: Shoulder arthrography in hemiplegic patients. *Arch Phys Med Rehabil* 1974, 55:49–51.

114. Hakuno A, Sashika H, Ohkawa T, Itoh R: Arthrographic findings in hemiplegic shoulders. *Arch Phys Med Rehabil* 1984, 65:706–711.

115. Chino N: Electrophysiological investigation on shoulder subluxation in hemiplegics. *Scand J Rehabil Med* 1981, 13:17–21.

116. Kaplan PE, Merideth J, Taft G, *et al.*: Stroke and brachial plexus injury: a difficult problem. *Arch Phys Med Rehabil* 1977, 58:415–418.

117. Chalsen GG, Fitzpatrick KA, Navia RA, *et al.*: Prevalence of the shoulder-hand pain syndrome in an inpatient stroke rehabilitation population: a quantitative, cross-sectional study. *J Neurol Rehabil* 1987, 1:137–141.

118. Schwartzman RJ, McLellan TL: Reflex sympathetic dystrophy: a review. *Arch Neurol* 1987, 44:555–561.

119. Alexander D: Depression and cognition as factors in recovery. In *Handbook of Neurorehabilitation.* Edited by Good DC, Couch JR. New York: Marcel Dekker; 1994:129–152.

120. Aström M, Adolfsson R, Asplund K: Major depression in stroke patients: a 3-year longitudinal study. *Stroke* 1993, 24:976–982.

121. Niemi M, Laaksonen MA, Kotila M, *et al.*: Quality of life 4 years after stroke. *Stroke* 1988, 19:1101–1107.

122. Robinson RG, Price TR: Post-stroke depressive disorders: a follow-up study of 103 patients. *Stroke* 1982, 13:635–640.

123. Starkstein SE, Robinson RG, Price TR: Comparison of cortical and subcortical lesions in the production of post-stroke mood disorders. *Brain* 1987, 110:1045–1059.

124. Sinyor D, Amato P, Kalonpek DG, *et al.*: Post-stroke depression: relationships to functional impairment, coping strategies, and rehabilitation outcome. *Stroke* 1986, 17:1102–1107.

125. House A, Dennis M, Warlow C, *et al.*: Mood disorders after stroke and their relation to lesion location. *Brain* 1990, 113:1113–1129.

126. Parikh RM, Robinson RG, Lipsey JR, *et al.*: The impact of post-stroke depression on recovery in activities of daily living over a two-year follow-up. *Arch Neurol* 1990, 47:785–789.

127. Finklestein SP, Weintraub RJ, Karmonz N, *et al.*: Antidepressant drug treatment for post-stroke depression: retrospective study. *Arch Phys Med Rehabil* 1987, 68:772– 776.

128. Robinson RG, Lipsey JR, Price TR: Diagnosis and clinical management of post-stroke depression. *Psychosomatics* 1985, 26:769–778.

129. Reding MJ, Orto LA, Winter SW, *et al.*: Antidepressant therapy after stroke: a double-blind trial. *Arch Neurol* 1986, 43:763–765.

130. Goodglass H, Kaplan E, eds.: *Boston Diagnostic Aphasia Examination Booklet.* Malvern, PA: Lea & Febiger; 1983:6.

131. Lal S: Physiatric complications in stroke syndromes. In *Stroke Rehabilitation.* Edited by Kaplan PE, Cerullo LJ. Boston: Butterworths; 1986:159–181.

132. Cailliet R: Regional pain problems. In *Medical Rehabilitation.* Edited by Basmajian JV, Kirby RL. Baltimore: Williams & Wilkins; 1984:220–229.

133. Reding MJ, McDowell F: Stroke rehabilitation. *Neurol Clin* 1987, 5:601–630.

134. Brooke MM, de Lateur BJ, Diana-Rigby PT: Shoulder subluxation in hemiplegia: effects of three different supports. *Arch Phys Med Rehabil* 1991, 72:582–586.

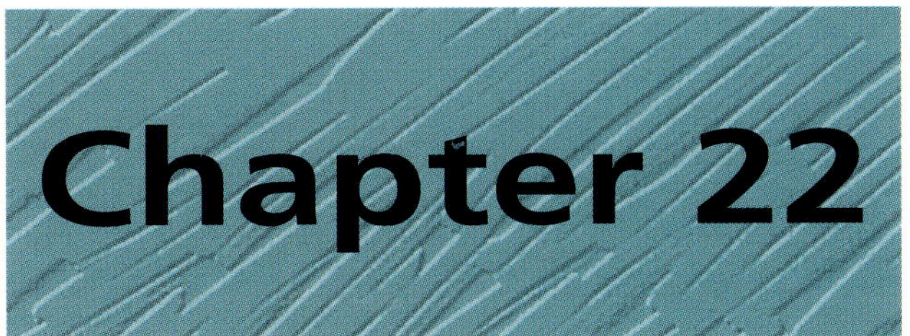

Natural History of Recovery and Influence of Comorbid Conditions on Stroke Outcome

ELLIOT J. ROTH

Stroke often results in some degree of residual disability, but patients usually experience improvements in their ability to perform daily functional skills [1–4]. Several factors determine the extent to which clinically relevant recovery of function will occur [5–9], some of which are listed in Table 22.1. The influence of two of these outcome determinants will be reviewed in this chapter. These are natural spontaneous neurologic recovery and medical comorbidities.

NATURAL SPONTANEOUS NEUROLOGIC RECOVERY AFTER STROKE

There is an important distinction between two different but related types of improvement that are seen after stroke [10]. The first type of recovery reflects a reduction in the degree of neurologic impairment, which may result from spontaneous natural neurologic recovery, the effects of treatments that limit the extent of the stroke, or other interventions that enhance neurologic functioning. This form of clinical improvement is manifested clinically as enhancements in strength, motor control, language ability, or other primary neurologic functions [11].

The other type of recovery experienced by stroke patients is the improved ability to perform daily functions in their environment [1–4], within the limitations of the level and type of physical impairments present. An individual with physical, cognitive, or behavioral deficits resulting from a stroke may regain the capacity to feed, dress, ambulate, control elimination, and carry out other activities of daily living, even with some degree of residual physical impairment. The ability to perform these functional tasks can occur with adaptation and training, either with or without neurologic recovery.

In general, the degree of recovery that occurs in patients with stroke-related functional deficits has been found to be different and greater than that which might be expected by a reduction in neural impairment alone [12–21]. However, the two types of improvements are related in subtle and complex ways [10]. The use of alternative compensatory functional strategies plays a major role in the performance of functional tasks when neurologic improvement is minimal or absent. The present discussion addresses recovery only of neurologic impairments, and not of functional abilities.

Reliable estimates of the extent to which recovery of function occurs are difficult to obtain, but comparisons of the relative frequencies of neurologic deficit between the acute and chronic poststroke stages of recovery provide some limited information on this subject. These comparisons generally show reductions in the frequencies of deficits over time by about one third to one half [11,22,23]. One study documented that the prevalence of hemiparesis declined from 73% to 37%, aphasia from 36% to 20%, dysarthria from 48% to 16%, dysphagia from 13% to 4%, and incontinence from 29% to 9% during the first poststroke year. The time course of recovery is variable. While most improvements in physical functioning occur within the first 3 to 6 months, later recovery is also commonly seen [13,24–27].

Table 22.1. Stroke outcome determinant factors

Factors
Nature, distribution, and severity of physical impairments
Pattern and extent of spontaneous neurologic recovery
Preexisting and acquired comorbid neuromedical conditions
Motivation and determination
Adaptability and coping ability
Family and social supports
Cognition, language, and communication ability
Training and adaptation/rehabilitation
Effects of other treatment interventions

Table 22.2. Components of synergy patterns

Upper extremity flexion synergy	Lower extremity flexion synergy
Scapular retraction	Pelvic protraction
Scalpular elevation	Pelvic depression
Shoulder external rotation	Hip flexion*
Shoulder abduction	Hip abduction
Forearm pronation	Hip external rotation
Elbow flexion*	Knee flexion
Wrist flexion	Ankle dorsiflexion
Finger flexion	Foot inversion
	Toe dorsiflexion
	Great toe extension
Upper extremity extension synergy	**Lower extremity extension synergy**
Scapular protraction	Pelvic retraction
Scalpular depression	Pelvic elevation
Shoulder internal rotation*	Hip extension
Shoulder adduction*	Hip adduction
Forearm pronation	Hip internal rotation
Elbow extension	Knee extension*
Wrist extension	Ankle plantarflexion
Finger extension	Foot inversion
	Toe plantarflexion
	Great toe extension

*Predominant movement in each pattern.

Recovery of Motor Function

For many patients, the pattern of natural spontaneous recovery of motor function follows a relatively predictable sequence of stereotyped events. In the typical patient with a cerebral infarction in the middle cerebral artery distribution, lower extremity function recovers earliest and most completely, followed by upper extremity and hand function. Tone usually returns before voluntary movement, proximal control before distal, and mass movement patterns (or synergy patterns [Table 22.2, Figure 22.1]) before specific isolated coordinated volitional motor functions [28,29]. Synergy patterns are the gross flexion or extension movement combinations of an activated extremity. These patterns are stereotypic, nonselective, and relatively inflexible.

The relative uniformity of these recovery stages was documented systematically by Twitchell [30] in 1951, who observed and recorded the evaluation of motor control in 121 hemiplegic subjects. While there are many exceptions to the sequence that Twitchell outlined, extensive clinical experience and repeated investigations have confirmed that this pattern of motor recovery is a commonly observed phenomenon. Most of the exceptions occur in patients who sustain strokes of a type other than the common middle cerebral artery distribution cerebral infarction. The documentation of these steps in the poststroke motor control evolution process ultimately was formalized in 1970 into stages of motor recovery by Brunnstrom [28,29], who also defined certain specific criteria for classification of patients with particular presentations into specific categories based on stage of recovery (Table 22.3).

Overall prognosis for return of voluntary motor control is variable, but generally is favorable for some degree of improvement in motor function [31–41]. Using the Brunnstrom staging measurement technique, one study [32] reported that lower extremity motor control improved by one stage in 39% of subjects and by two or more stages in 12%, while upper motor extremity control improved by one stage in 24% and by two stages in 8%.

This sequence of recovery may stop at any stage. Ultimately, some hemiparetic patients regain full or nearly complete use of all muscles in an isolated coordinated fashion, independent of synergy patterns. For other patients, the process of recovery is incomplete, and leads to only partial voluntary use of the extremity. Still others make no recovery at all. Bard and Hirschberg [41] found that 40% of all hemiplegic stroke patients regained full upper extremity function, 40% regained partial function, and the remaining 20% had no return of voluntary upper extremity motor control.

Another investigation [31] reported that moderate or severe motor weakness of the arm was present in about two thirds of patients initially and in about one fourth at 3-month follow-up. While it often is tempting to attempt to specify a definitive prognosis in a stroke patient who presents with a particular level of motor function, these expectations for recovery are frequently rendered inaccurate and inadequate by the multiple disparate variables that ultimately determine outcome.

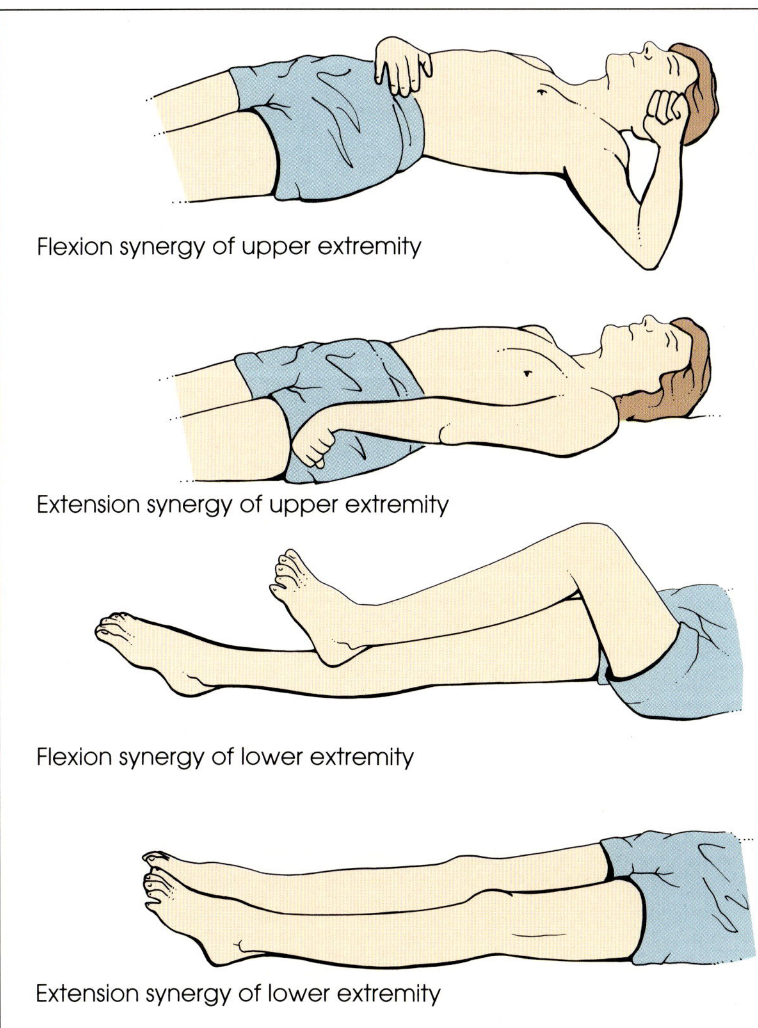

FIGURE 22.1

Limb synergy patterns. Synergy patterns are the mass flexion or extension movement combinations of the activated arm or leg.

Recovery of Language Function

Aphasia is present in about one fourth of patients during the acute phase, and in about one fifth or less of those during the later stages after stroke [42]. The evolution of language function

Table 22.3. Brunnstrom stages of motor recovery

Stage 1
Flaccidity
Phasic stretch reflexes are absent
No volitional or reflex-induced active movement
Stage 2
Spasticity, resistance to passive movement, especially in dominant synergy muscle groups
Appearance of basic limb synergies and associated reactions
Movement patterns stimulated reflexively
Minimal voluntary movement
Stage 3
Spasticity increases to marked degree
Semivoluntary
Volitionally initiates movement of involved limbs, but resulting in basic limb synergies, and not full range
Usually flexion synergy dominates the arm and extension synergy dominates the leg
Stage 4
Spasticity reduced
Synergy patterns still predominant
Some complex movement patterns deviating from synergy, combining antagonistic synergies, when prime movers are synergy components
Stage 5
Spasticity declines more, but still seen with rapid movements and at extremes of range
More difficult movement patterns from synergy, even if movement involves weaker synergy components
Voluntary isolated environmentally specific movements predominate
Stage 6
Spasticity disappearing
Coordination improves to near normal
Individual joint movements possible
Still have abnormal movement patterns with faulty timing during rapid or complex actions
Stage 7
Restoration of normal variety of rapid, complex movement strength patterns with normal timing, coordination, strength, and endurance

after stroke is more difficult to study than changes in motor control, and consequently reports of prognosis in aphasia are more variable. Recovery from aphasia generally occurs at a slower rate, and continues for a longer time course than does motor recovery [26]. While most recovery occurs in the first 3 to 6 months [42–44], at least one group has observed that global aphasic patients show the greatest improvement during the latter half of the first year after stroke [26,44,45].

The amount and pattern of recovery are usually related to initial severity of aphasia and the specific aphasia type [46,47] (Table 22.4). One study of 177 aphasics by Brust and coworkers [47] indicated that nonfluent aphasics generally do not have as favorable a prognosis as fluent aphasics, although it is important to recognize that both groups can and do improve. Comprehension usually returns earlier and to a greater extent than does expression ability [48]. Other factors that have been asserted to influence recovery after aphasia are listed in Table 22.5 [46,47,49–52].

Recovery of Perceptual and Cognitive Functions

Patients with visuospatial perceptual deficits and those with neuropsychologic abnormalities can recover some or all of their cognitive functions. Most of the improvement in perceptual functioning occurs in the first 3 to 6 months after stroke [53–59], but some recovery occurs later. Hier and coworkers [59] observed that recovery of perceptual deficits such as unilateral spatial neglect, denial of illness, loss of facial recognition, and motor impersistence could be seen up to 1 year after stroke, but that most of the improvements occurred within the first 20 weeks. Likewise, a considerable proportion of stroke patients recover from ideomotor apraxia [60]. Statistically significant improvements in memory and other cognitive functioning have been recorded at 3 and 6 months after stroke [61–63].

Factors related to recovery of perceptual disturbances and ideomotor apraxia are listed in Table 22.6 [49,54,55,57,59,60,64]. Interestingly, unilateral spatial neglect [57,59] and degree of memory function loss [63] have been found to be related to the

Table 22.4. Typical evolution of specific aphasia syndromes

Initial presentation	Typical outcomes	Usual overall prognosis
Global	Global Broca's	Fair-Poor
Broca's	Anomic	Good-Fair-Poor
Wernicke's	Wernicke's Conduction Anomic Recovery	Good-Fair-Poor
Conduction	Anomic	Good-Fair
Transcortical	Anomic	Good-Fair
Anomic	Anomic Recovery	Good-Fair

Table 22.5. Factors that may affect language recovery

Age	Lesion location
Gender	Stroke type
Handedness	Presence of hemiplegia
Intelligence level	Presence of other physical deficits
Education	Time from onset
Occupation	Aphasia type
Personality	Specific function studied
General health	Initial language performance
Family and environment	Treatment effects
Lesion size	

Table 22.6. Prognostic factors for recovery of perceptual deficits and ideomotor apraxia

Perceptual deficits	Ideomotor apraxia
Factors related to good recovery:	Factors related to good recovery:
Hemorrhagic stroke	Neuropsychologic test performance
Small size	Factors unrelated to recovery:
Sparing of right frontal and parietal lobes	Age
Factors unrelated to recovery:	Sex
Sex	Education
Age (except unilateral, spatial, neglect, and prosopagnosia)	Initial severity
	Lesion size
	Presence and type of aphasia

level of functional independence in performance of activities of daily living, but not with degree of motor weakness from stroke or its recovery.

Mechanisms of Recovery of Neurologic Function

A number of mechanisms have been proposed to explain the clinically observed phenomenon of spontaneous recovery of neurologic function [65–75]. Some of these mechanisms are listed in Table 22.7, and schematic representations of two of the most important ones, collateral sprouting and unmasking of previously latent pathways, are shown in Figure 22.2. The relative amount that each of these mechanisms contributes to overall outcome is difficult to specify, but it is likely that a combination of factors are operating to produce clinically observed natural neurologic recovery. These mechanisms generally can be divided into two broad categories: 1) resolution of local harmful factors, which usually accounts for early spontaneous improvement after stroke (usually considered within the first 3–6 months); and 2) neuroplasticity, which can take place early or late. Brain plasticity refers to the capacity of the nervous system to modify its structural and functional organization. Experimental evidence indicates that plasticity can be altered by several external conditions, including pharmacologic agents, electrical stimulation, and environmental stimulation [76]. The reported structural and functional changes that have been reported to result from experimental and environmental stimulation are listed in Table 22.8.

Table 22.7. Mechanism of neurologic recovery

Resolution of vascular and metabolic factors
Resolution of edema
Resorption of local toxins
Improved local circulation
Recovery of partially damaged ischemic (not infarcted) neurons
Neuroplasticity
Collateral sprouting of new synaptic connections
Unmasking of previously latent functional pathways
Assumption of function by undamaged redundant pathways
Reversibility from diaschisis: (temporary deactivation of intact brain regions remote from but connected to the injured area)
Denervation supersensitivity: (increased sensitivity of denervated target cells to remaining afferent input)
Regenerative proximal sprouting of transected axons

INFLUENCE OF COMORBIDITIES ON RECOVERY AFTER STROKE

Among the many factors that may inhibit poststroke functional recovery, associated medical conditions frequently cause as much disability as, or at times even more disability than, the stroke itself [23]. Medical comorbidities may adversely affect the length [77,78] and quality of survival after stroke for some patients. Numerous reports indicate that coexisting medical conditions contribute to early and late poststroke mortality [77,78]. There also is growing evidence that these medical problems may limit the ability of the patient to participate in a therapeutic exercise program, to care for oneself independently, and to achieve favorable outcomes

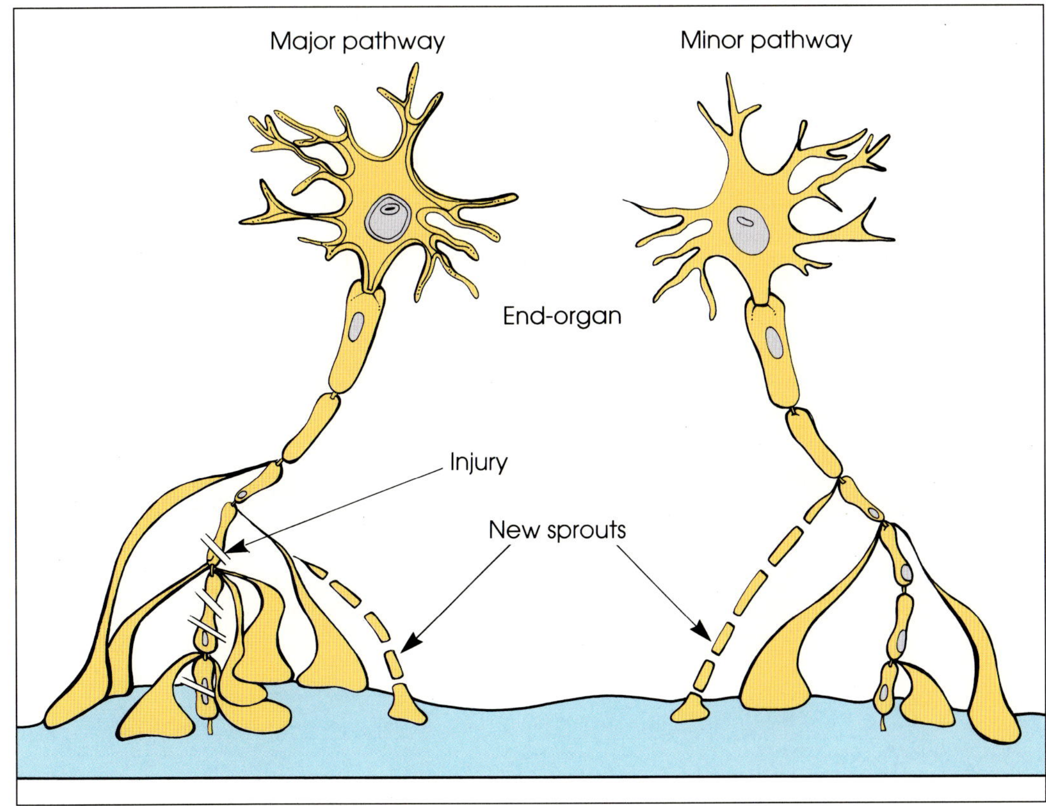

FIGURE 22.2

Mechanisms of brain plasticity. *Collateral sprouting* refers to the development of new connections from remaining nerves to the denervated region. *Unmasking* occurs when anatomically established but previously latent pathways and synapses are called upon to substitute for lost inputs.

after stroke [2,7,23,79–84]. Real and potential implications of medical comorbidities that are relevant during the management of patients during and after the acute and rehabilitation phases of stroke are enumerated in Table 22.9.

Medical problems that may influence the patient's course and outcome can be either chronic medical conditions that predate the stroke (many of which are also risk factors for stroke), secondary complications that follow the stroke, or both. Examples of preexisting medical conditions include hypertension, diabetes, cardiac disease, arthritis, and others. The Framingham Heart Study [23] and other reports [85,86] have documented that many of these diseases are significantly more common among survivors of stroke than among age- and gender-matched control subjects.

Only a few studies have reported the incidence of secondary poststroke medical complications [81,87–95]. These are reviewed in Table 22.10. Examples of complications that present as new problems after stroke include deep venous thrombosis, pneumonia, seizures, pressure sores, shoulder dysfunction, and falls. Other poststroke problems reflect acute manifestations or exacerbations of preexisting chronic disease, such as angina in patients with ischemic heart disease or hyperglycemia in diabetic patients. Still other physiologic functions that require ongoing medical management include hydration, nutrition [96], tolerance to upright posture and to activity [97], and bowel and bladder elimination. Factors that have been found predictive of the occurrence of secondary complications include history of congestive heart failure [81,94], hypoalbuminemia [95], and severity of disability on rehabilitation admission [87].

Several recent reviews, including those by Roth [98], Schmidt and Reding [99], Siegler and Whitney [100], Brott [101], and others have enumerated the common neuromedical comorbidities associated with stroke and reviewed their reported incidence figures, preventive measures, assessment techniques, management strategies, implications for rehabilitation, and effect on outcome. At times, both diagnosis and treatment of ongoing and acute medical problems are difficult during rehabilitation and long-term care. Table 22.11 reviews the factors that interfere with assessment of acute medical illness in stroke patients.

Table 22.8. Structural and functional effects of experimental stimulation on plasticity

Increase in number of dendrites, spine density, spine volume
Alteration in size of synapses
Change in number and distribution of synaptic vesicles
Increase in size and number of synapses
Remodeling of synapses
Potentiation of synaptic transmission
Changes in excitability of terminal dendrites
Increase in receptive fields, enhanced excitability
Alteration in diameter of nerve fibers
Alteration in intracellular and extracellular ions
Sustained increased activity of noradrenergic neurons
Increase in acetylcholine release and concentration
Increase in glia

Deconditioning

The poststroke course may be complicated by physiologic deconditioning, which often accompanies both acute medical illness and the prolonged bed rest that may be enforced immediately after onset of illness. The term *deconditioning* refers to the state of limited endurance that often results from inactivity and illness. Easy fatigueability and orthostatic intolerance are common features of this condition. The state of deconditioning, often unrecognized by clinicians, consists of a number of characteristics that are listed in Table 22.12 [102–104]. Deconditioning can contribute to the problems of fatigue, endurance limitations, lack of motivation and drive, depression, and poor exercise tolerance, all of which may adversely affect the course of recovery and rehabilitation.

Endurance and its limitations are difficult to quantify, rendering inaccurate the measurement of the potential effects that deconditioning exerts on outcome. Nonetheless, clinical experience indicates that many of the medical rehabilitative interventions routinely employed during stroke patient care are directed toward addressing the problem of deconditioning [104].

Heart Disease

Of all of the associated medical conditions that can affect the course and care of the stroke patient, heart disease is the one comorbidity that has been studied most extensively for its impact on outcome [105,106]. Cardiac disease may be a cause, a risk factor, a consequence, or a coincidental condition of stroke [105–107]. Up to three fourths of stroke patients have evidence of some form of heart disease [23,105–114]. The frequencies of specific types of heart diseases are provided in Table 22.13.

Cardiac comorbidity is the second most common cause of death during the first month after stroke [115] and the most common cause of death thereafter [116]. It has been demonstrated that associated heart disease reduces long-term survival following stroke [77,78], but the influence of cardiac disease on morbidity is less clear. Lehmann and coworkers [2], Gresham and coworkers [23], Sheikh and coworkers [80], and Roth and coworkers [81] found that cardiac disease adversely affects func-

Table 22.9. Potential influence of medical comorbidities and complications

Delay initiation of a therapeutic exercise program
Limit participation in therapeutic exercise regimen
Inhibit functional skill performance
Prolong and increase the need for hospitalization
Reduce levels of independence in daily activities
Reduce other functional outcomes
Necessitate additional medical monitoring and management

tional outcome following stroke, but two other groups of investigators [8,92] found no relationship between the presence of heart disease and functional ability. Roth and coworkers [81] reported that coronary artery disease, and especially congestive heart failure (CHF), adversely influence some aspects of mobility functioning in stroke patients. It was also reported that CHF is a predictor of cardiac complications encountered during poststroke rehabilitation [94], as listed in Table 22.14. Effective management of acute exacerbations of heart disease during the poststroke course of care depends on prompt recognition of cardiac symptoms and on appropriate modification of the therapeutic medical or exercise regimen.

Table 22.10. Incidence of medical complications in stroke rehabilitation

Study	Patients, *n*	Incidence of complications, %	Predictors of complications
Alder and coworkers [91]	100	5	—
McClatchie [89]	174	55	—
Dobkin [88]	100	40	Prospective payment system
Roth and coworkers [81]	132	26 (cardiac only)	Coronary heart disease; congestive heart failure
Dromerick and Reding [87]	100	96	Barthel score; length of stay
Aptaker and coworkers [95]	79	53	Hypoalbuminemia
Roth and Green [94]	106	32 (cardiac only)	Congestive heart failure and related factors

Table 22.11. Factors that interfere with diagnosis of acute medical complications in stroke patients

- Inability to exercise
- Endurance limitations
- Sensory changes
- Cognitive deficits
- Communication difficulties

Table 22.12. Effects of physiologic deconditioning

- Loss of postural reflexes
- Orthostatic hypotension
- Increased resting heart rate
- Venous stasis
- Decreased stroke volume
- Decreased blood volume
- Decreased plasma volume
- Decreased extracellular fluid volume
- Decreased maximal oxygen uptake
- Decreased exercise stroke volume
- Increased exercise heart rate
- Reduced cardiac reserve, decreased exercise tolerance
- Deep venous thrombosis and pulmonary embolism
- Decreased pulmonary ventilation
- Lower vital capacity
- Impaired cough mechanism
- Decreased clearance of respiratory tract secretions
- Atelectasis and pnemonia
- Urinary stasis
- Urinary retention
- Urinary incontinence
- Decreased sexual function
- Negative nitrogen and calcium balance
- Urinary stones, infections
- Increased diuresis and natriuresis
- Hypercalciuria
- Slowing of gastrointestinal tract
- Constipation
- Catabolic nutritional state
- Anorexia
- Skin atrophy
- Pressure sores
- Soft tissue contracture
- Muscle weakness
- Muscle atrophy
- Osteoporosis
- Confusion, disorientation
- Psychologic depression
- Decreased sensory functions
- Decreased intellectual functions
- Decreased motor coordination
- Decreased balance

Table 22.13. Types of heart diseases in stroke

Type	Frequency, %	Study
Hypertension	50–84	Wallace and Levy [112]
		Barker and coworkers [113]
Coronary artery disease	32–62	Gresham and coworkers [23]
		Rokey and coworkers [108]
		Hertzer and coworkers [110]
Arrhythmia (atrial fibrillation, ventricular ectopy)	40–70	Myers and coworkers [85]
		Tallman [114]
Congestive heart failure	12–18	Gresham and coworkers [23]
		Roth and coworkers [81]

Table 22.14. Potential poststroke cardiovascular complications

- Angina
- Pulmonary edema
- Hypertension
- Hypotension
- Arrythmia
- Tachycardia
- Bradycardia
- Myocardial infarction
- Silent ischemia
- Sudden death

Deep Venous Thrombosis and Pulmonary Embolism

Estimates for the frequency of deep venous thrombosis (DVT) vary between 22% and 73%, with the most carefully conducted studies suggesting an incidence of 40% to 50% [117–119]. Pulmonary embolism (PE) occurs in about 10% to 15% of stroke patients [117]. While the peak incidence for DVT and PE occurs during the first week after onset [117,120], the risk persists thereafter [117,121].

Because clinical findings of DVT are present in less than one half of patients [117], laboratory evaluation often is needed (Table 22.15). Clinical diagnosis of PE is also unreliable, but the combination of ventilation-perfusion scanning and noninvasive lower extremity venous flow studies usually establishes the diagnosis. When present, treatment of DVT or PE consists of intravenous or subcutaneous high-dose heparin, followed by warfarin for 3 to 6 months [117,122,123].

Deep vein thrombosis prophylaxis is recommended for all patients with stroke who have muscle weakness [117,124]. The various prophylaxis methods of DVT prevention are listed in Table 22.16. The optimal duration of prophylaxis is not known, but increased time since stroke, greater muscle strength, and ambulatory ability generally are associated with reduced DVT risk [117,118,121,125,126].

Pulmonary embolism is the fourth most common cause of death in the first month following stroke [115]. The impact of DVT or PE on measures of functional outcome has not been studied in a systematic way, but it is likely that DVT and its treatment may prolong in-patient hospitalization because of the need for bedrest and relative immobilization.

Pneumonia and Ventilatory Dysfunction

Pneumonia is a major cause of morbidity and mortality [115], occurring in about one third of all patients in the National Survey of Stroke [111]. Table 22.17 lists factors that contribute to the occurrence of pneumonia in stroke patients [127], of which dysphagia with aspiration is thought to be the most important [128–130]. In addition, reduced intercostal muscle activity on the hemiplegic side (recorded on electromyographic testing) [131] results in decreased thoracic movement (as seen on mechanical testing) [132–134]. In turn, these changes cause restrictive ventilatory changes, as detected on pulmonary function testing [135–137] (Table 22.18).

Table 22.15. Assessment of deep venous thrombosis

Clinical features	Differential diagnosis	Laboratory testing
Leg pain (usually in calf and popliteal fossa)	Muscle injury with strain, tear, or hematoma	Impedence plethysmography
Leg swelling	Cellulitis	Doppler ultrasound
Leg erythema	Superficial thrombophlebitis	I-125 fibrinogen scanning
Homan's sign	Ruptured Baker's cyst	Venography
Superficial venous distension	Achilles tendonitis	
Palpable cord	Bursitis	
Fever	Heterotopic ossification	

Table 22.16. Prophylactic measures for deep vein thrombosis and pulmonary embolism in stroke

- Subcutaneous injections of low-dose standard heparin*
- Subcutaneous injections of low-dose low molecular weight heparin*
- Dextran†
- Antiplatelet agents†
- Oral anticoagulants‡
- External pneumatic compression devices‡
- Passive range of motion exercise‡
- Electrical stimulation‡
- Other physical measures‡

*Effective.
†Ineffective.
‡Unknown.

Table 22.17. Factors contributing to pneumonia in stroke patients

- Dysphagia with aspiration
- Cognitive deficits
- Dehydration and malnutrition
- Decreased cough reflex
- Expiratory muscle weakness
- Chest wall muscle spasticity and contracture immobility

Table 22.18. Ventilatory dysfunction in stroke

Decreases in:
- Vital capacity
- Total lung capacity
- Inspiratory capacity
- Expiratory reserve volume

Degree of restrictive ventilatory dysfunction is related to:
- Severity of hemiparesis

Recognition of pneumonia may be difficult, as patients may present with only low-grade fever or minor mental status changes with minimal laboratory findings [138]. Treatment consists of prompt administration of fluids and antibiotics, oxygen, aggressive tracheobronchial hygiene, and rapid remobilization. Whether the occurrence of pneumonia adversely affects overall outcome is difficult to assess. However, it appears that respiratory infections may delay the initiation of, or interfere with participation in, an active therapeutic exercise program, and possibly reduce the level of functional independence that might be achieved during rehabilitation.

Seizures

Seizures occur in less than 10% of all stroke patients [139], but some authors report that the incidence may be greater among patients with certain types of stroke [111], and also greater among those whose stroke involves the cerebral cortex than among those with deeper lesions [139,140]. Factors that increase the risk of seizure in specific stroke types are listed in Table 22.19 [139–146]. Most seizures occur during the first year after stroke. While most poststroke seizures are focal motor, other types are common as well [139]. The 1981 National Survey of Stroke [111] reported that the presence of seizures increases mortality after stroke, but it is not known whether seizure disorder or its treatment are associated with reduced functional outcomes.

Table 22.19. Risk factors for poststroke seizures

In ischemic stroke:
Embolic stroke
Hemorrhagic transformation
Cortical location
In intracerebral hemorrhage:
Early time period after stroke
Lobar location
Structural lesions (*eg*, arteriovenous malformation, aneurysm)
Subarachnoid hemorrhage:
Middle cerebral artery aneurysm
Vasospasm on angiogram
Rebleeding
Infarction on computed tomography scan
Increased cisternal blood on computed tomography scan

Central Poststroke Pain Syndrome

Although it is present in only less than 5% of all stroke patients, central poststroke pain syndrome can be extremely severe and disabling. Formerly known as "Dejerine-Roussy Thalamic Pain Syndrome" because of its past association with thalamic strokes, its nomenclature has been changed recently to reflect the observation that 50% or more of the patients with this condition have strokes in other locations. The clinical presentation is summarized in Table 22.20 [147–152].

Response to treatment is usually either minimal or incomplete [147,148,153,154]. A number of treatment modalities have been attempted, but there is a paucity of randomized controlled clinical trials to test the efficacy of any of these methods. Common interventions used for this syndrome are listed in Table 22.21. The general treatment strategy is step-wise and empiric, starting with methods associated with few side effects and adding or substituting other modalities depending on response. The true adverse impact of this syndrome on functional outcome after stroke has not been studied in a formal way, but is apparently significant for those few individuals who are affected by this condition. The pain can interfere with the sleep-wake cycle, with ability to carry out activities of daily living, and with participation in a therapeutic exercise program. Its management usually requires a long-term effort.

Table 22.20. Common clinical features of central poststroke pain syndrome

Quality of pain	Characteristics of pain	Response to external agents
Severe	Burning	Refractory to most treatment modalities
Persistent	Tingling	Worsened by movement or noxious stimuli
Intractable	Stabbing	Improved by distraction or psychologic preoccupation
Constant	Shooting	
Disabling	"Dysesthetias"	
	"Pins and needles"	
	"Like a knife"	
	Hyperpathia	

Table 22.21. Management of central poststroke pain

Avoid noxious stimuli
Prevent and treat infections
Prevent and treat symptomatic spasticity
Prevent and reduce contracture
Prevent and treat bowel and bladder complications
Prevent pressure sores
Preoccupation therapy
Psychotherapy
Relaxation training
Biofeedback
Mobilization
Passive range of motion exercises
Aerobic exercises
Tricyclic antidepressant medications
Anticonvulsant medications
Transcutaneous electrical nerve stimulation
Neurosurgical procedures

Urinary Dysfunction

Urinary tract dysfunction is experienced by more than one half of patients during the early phase after stroke, with estimates as high as 70% in the first month [155–158]. Control over micturition generally improves, so that one study indicated that urinary incontinence occurred in 51% of stroke patients within the first year, and in 23% after 2 years [157].

Incontinence is more common than retention. The major factors that contribute to both of these problems are listed in Table 22.22 [98,159–161]. The neurogenic bladder that is typically associated with stroke usually is of the spastic disinhibited type, but without urinary retention or detrusor sphincter dyssynergy. This occurs because there is an intact connection with the pontine micturition center, which coordinates detrusor and urinary sphincter function (Figure 22.3) [162]. Exceptions may occur in patients with pontine or medullary strokes.

Urinary tract infection can be a cause or result of both urinary incontinence and retention [98,160,163]. Other potential implications of voiding dysfunction are listed in Table 22.23. Urinary incontinence has been reported in numerous studies to be a predictor of poor functional outcome after stroke [1,6,157,164]. The focus of treatment of incontinence is on providing patients with a planned timed toileting program, and only rarely on the use of medications (Table 22.24) [98,160,164]. Treatment of retention is directed toward insuring bladder emptying [160].

Pressure Sores

The National Survey of Stroke [111] reported a 14.5% incidence of pressure sores, with an even greater incidence in patients who developed coma. Risk factors for pressure sores are reviewed in Table 22.25. Pressure ulcers can be classified according to severity and depth using the Shea Classification (Figure 22.4) [165] or other systems [166]. These sores usually result from prolonged pressure over areas adjacent to bony prominences [167,168], as illustrated in Figure 22.5. Methods of pressure sore prevention, as outlined in guidelines developed by the United States Agency for Health Care Policy and Research, are reviewed in Table 22.26 [169,170]. The full impact of pressure sores on outcome after stroke is not known, but since their treatment often necessitates bedrest and relative immobilization, it is likely that this complication results in increased hospitalization, deconditioning, and additional disability.

Table 22.22. Causes of urinary tract dysfunction in stroke patients

Causes of incontinence
Urinary tract infection
Disinhibited spastic bladder
Mobility limitation
Lack of sensation of bladder fullness
Cognitive dysfunction (*eg*, disorientation, apraxia)
Causes of retention
Diabetic autonomic neuropathy
Other cause of hypotonic bladder (*eg*, lumbar spinal stenosis)
Prostatic enlargement
Other cause of bladder outlet obstruction (*eg*, bladder lithiasis)
Cervical spondylotic myelopathy
Other cause of external sphincter spasticity (*eg*, any spinal cord lesion)
Medications:
Anticholingerics, antihistamines, sympathomimetics
Fecal impaction
Abdominal muscle weakness

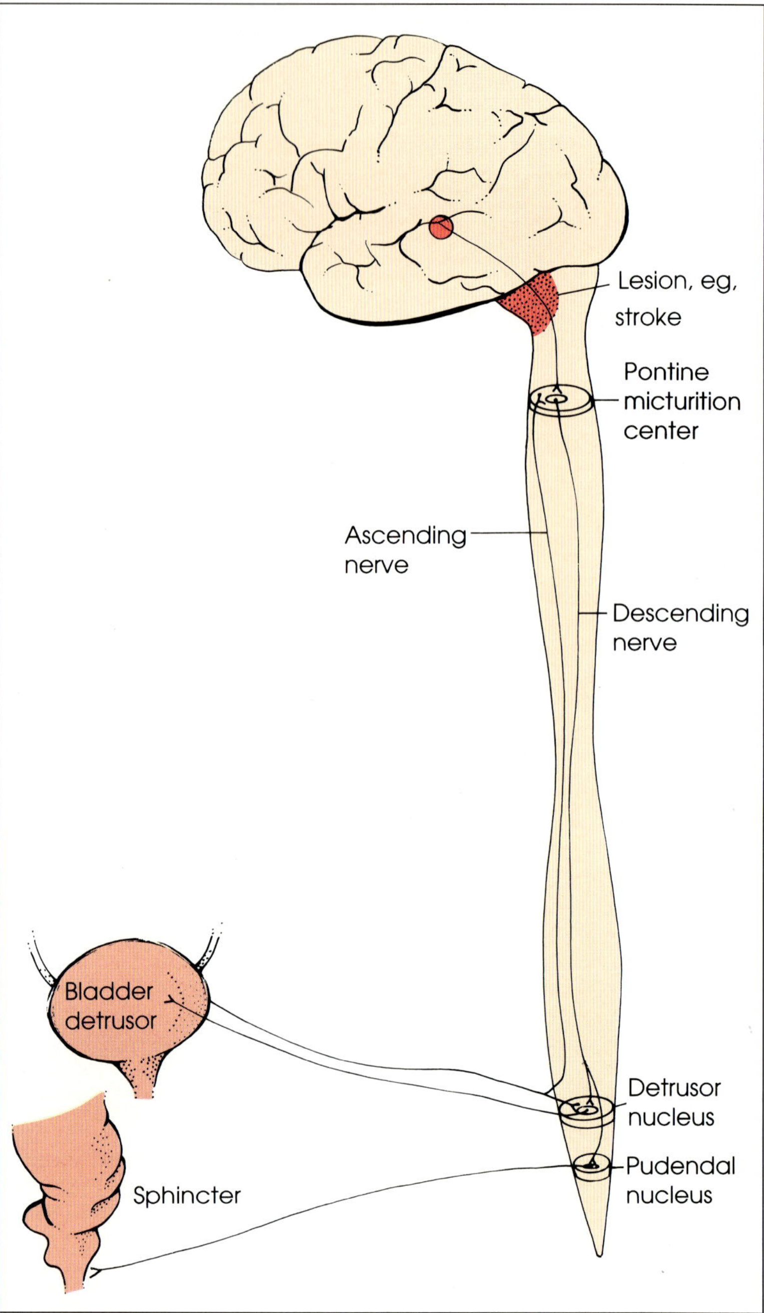

FIGURE 22.3

Central nervous system pathways and centers involved with micturition. Strokes that occur above the pons allow continued connection of the spinal and peripheral micturition mechanism with the pontine micturition center. The coordinating function of the pontine micturition center insures synergistic activity of the detrusor and external sphincter.

Table 22.23. Potential implications of voiding dysfunction
Sepsis
Kidney failure
Local skin breakdown
Falls with injuries en route from bed to toilet
Social embarrassment
Predictor of poorer outcome

Table 22.24. Management of urinary tract dysfunction in stroke patients
Treat infections
Regulate fluid intake
Timed or scheduled toileting program
Medications:
Anticholinergics, antihistamines, sympathomimetics

Table 22.25. Risk factors for pressure sores in stroke patients
Sensory loss
Loss of mobility
Bladder or bowel dysfunction
Cognitive deficits
Tone abnormalities
Nutritional deficiencies

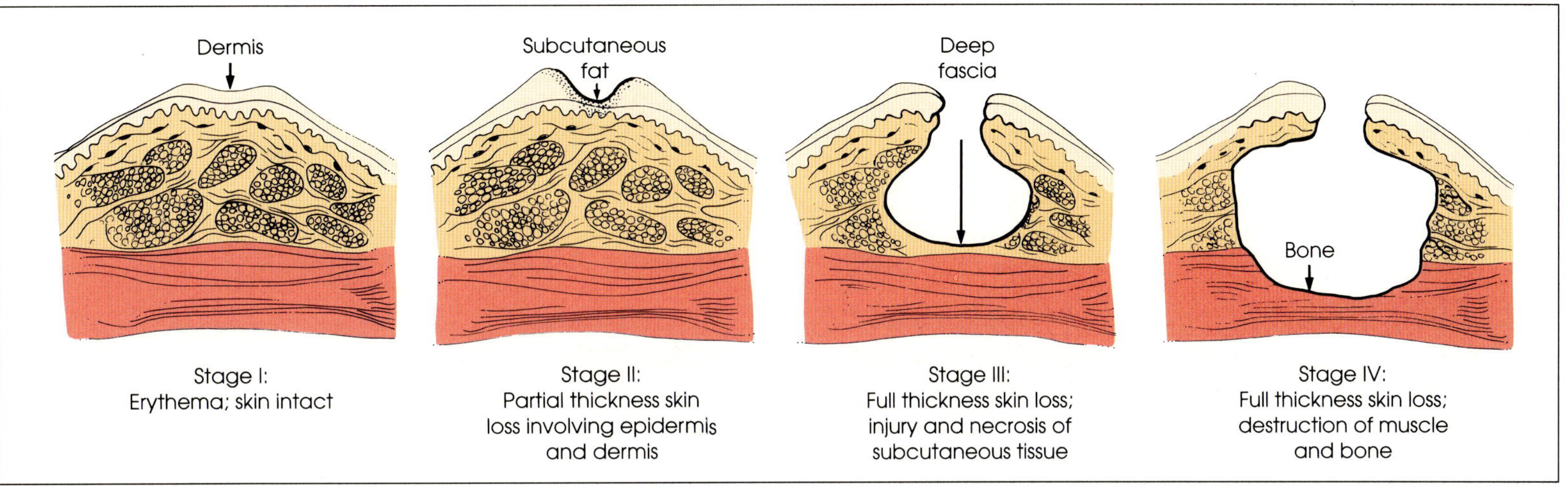

FIGURE 22.4

Pressure sore grading system. Stage I involves epidermis, stage II dermis, stage III subcutaneous tissue, and stage IV muscle and bone.

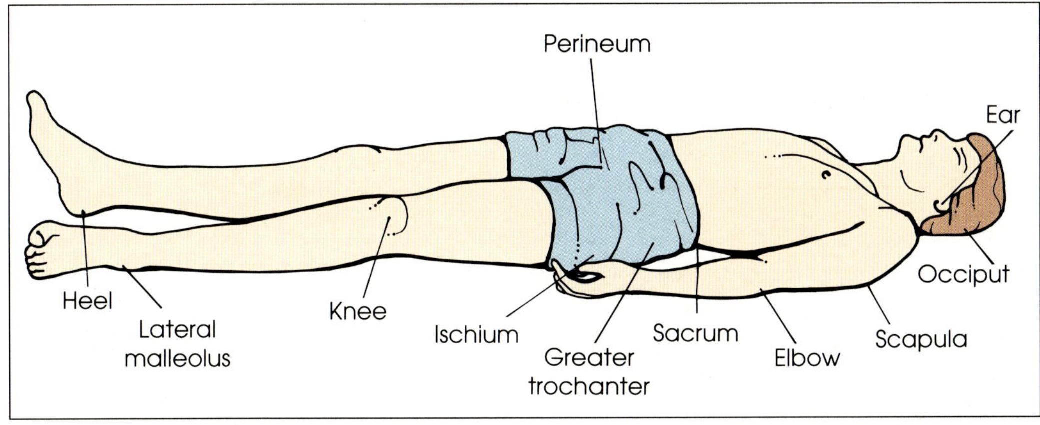

FIGURE 22.5

Common pressure sore locations. Sacral and heel sores are most common in patients who are lying supine; ischial sores are most common in those who are in the sitting position for prolonged durations.

Table 22.26. Pressure sore prevention and management interventions	
Remove source of irritation	Frequent visual skin inspection
Prevent and treat infections	Equipment adjustments
Provide adequate nutrition and hydration	Coordination of sitting schedules
Frequent body position changes	Patient and family education
Pressure-reducing bed and chair surfaces	Local topical wound care
Bladder and bowel management regimens	Surgical skin closure

Other Neuromedical Comorbidities

Many other comorbidities occur commonly, and these have the potential to affect the course and care of the stroke patient. Chronic obstructive pulmonary disease, chronic renal insufficiency, malignant disease, anemia, and other chronic illnesses may adversely affect activity tolerance. Arthritis and other musculoskeletal conditions may reduce ability to perform certain exercises, as might concomitant neurologic illnesses. Because of similarity of pathogenesis, dysvascular amputation is common in stroke patients, and might reduce ability to achieve favorable outcomes.

Among patients with diabetes mellitus, exercise may reduce insulin requirements during rehabilitation. Although hyperglycemia has been shown to adversely affect stroke severity, there is no definitive evidence to date that diabetes affects functional outcome. Similarly, physical activity may reduce the need for antihypertensive agents among patients with high blood pressure, but hypertension has not been shown to affect outcome from rehabilitation.

Among the most common complications of stroke are shoulder dysfunction and falls resulting in injuries. Many excellent reviews and reports are available on these topics [171–187].

PERSPECTIVE

The complex and multifactorial nature of the problems and outcomes after stroke underscores the importance of specialized care of acute and chronic stroke patients by a team of experienced professionals. While the exact role of spontaneous natural recovery of neurologic function in determining overall outcome is difficult to discern, it is likely that reductions in the extent of the stroke-induced impairments account for much but not all of the improvement seen in stroke patients. The influence of associated comorbidities on short-term and long-term outcomes has been studied even less than has natural recovery. To the extent that these problems have been examined, most of the studies demonstrate that some of these preexisting and acquired medical conditions exert some effect on the course and care of the stroke patient. Additional observation and investigation will help to elucidate the ways in which stroke patients are affected by these medical and neurologic factors.

REFERENCES

1. Wade DT, Langton-Hewer R: Functional abilities after stroke: measurement, natural history and prognosis. *J Neurol Neurosurg Psychiatr* 1987, 50:177–182.
2. Lehmann JF, DeLateur BJ, Fowler RS, *et al.*: Stroke rehabilitation: outcome and prediction. *Arch Phys Med Rehabil* 1975, 56:383–389.
3. Granger CV, Hamilton BB, Fiedler RC: Discharge outcome after stroke rehabilitation. *Stroke* 1992, 23:978–982.
4. Heinemann AW, Roth EJ, Cichowski K, Betts HB: Multivariate analysis of improvement and outcome following stroke rehabilitation. *Arch Neurol* 1987, 44:1167–1172.
5. Johnston MV, Kirshblum S, Zorowitz R, Shiflett SC: Prediction of outcomes following rehabilitation of stroke patients. *Neurol Rehabil* 1992, 2:72–97.
6. Jongbloed L: Prediction of function after stroke: a critical review. *Stroke* 1986, 17:765–776.
7. Shah S, Vanclay F, Cooper B: Predicting discharge status at commencement of stroke rehabilitation. *Stroke* 1989, 20:766–769.
8. Anderson TP, Bourestom N, Greenberg FR, *et al.*: Predictive factors in stroke rehabilitation. *Arch Phys Med Rehabil* 1974, 55:545–553.
9. Allen CMC: Predicting the outcome of acute stroke: a prognostic score. *J Neurol Neurosurg Psychiatr* 1984, 47:475–480.
10. Brandstater ME: An overview of stroke rehabilitation. *Stroke* 1990, 21(suppl II):II-40–II-42.
11. Kotila M, Waltimo O, Niemi M-L, *et al.*: The profile of recovery from stroke and factors influencing outcome. *Stroke* 1984, 15:1039–1044.
12. Ferruci L, Bandinelli S, Guralnik JM, *et al.*: Recovery of functional status after stroke: a postrehabilitation follow-up study. *Stroke* 1993, 24:200–205.
13. Andrews K, Brocklehurst JC, Richards B, *et al.*: The rate of recovery from stroke—and its measurement. *Int Rehabil Med* 1981, 3:155–161.
14. Lehmann JF, DeLateur BJ, Fowler RS, *et al.*: Stroke: does rehabilitation affect outcome? *Arch Phys Med Rehabil* 1975, 56:375–382.
15. Smith DS, Goldenberg E, Ashburn A, *et al.*: Remedial therapy after stroke: a randomized controlled trial. *BMJ* 1981, 282:517–520.
16. Indredavik B, Bakke F, Solberg R, *et al.*: Benefit of a stroke unit: a randomized controlled trial. *Stroke* 1991, 22:1026–1031.
17. Edmans JA, Towle D: Comparison of stroke unit and non-stroke unit in patients on independence in ADL. *Br J Occupat Ther* 1990, 53:415–418.
18. Garraway WM, Akhtar AJ, Prescott RJ, Hockey L: Management of acute stroke in the elderly: preliminary results of a controlled trial. *BMJ* 1980, 280:1040–1043.
19. Wood-Dauphinee S, Shapiro S, Bass E, *et al.*: A randomized trial of team care following stroke. *Stroke* 1984, 15:864–872.
20. Kalra L: The influence of stroke unit rehabilitation on functional recovery from stroke. *Stroke* 1994, 25:821–825.
21. Reding MJ, McDowell FH: Focused stroke rehabilitation programs improve outcome. *Arch Neurol* 1989, 46:700–711.
22. Foulkes MA, Wolf PA, Price TR, *et al.*: The Stroke Data Bank: design, methods, and baseline characteristics. *Stroke* 1988, 19:547–554.
23. Gresham GE, Phillips TF, Wolf PA, *et al.*: Epidemiologic profile of long-term disability: the Framingham study. *Arch Phys Med Rehabil* 1979, 60:487–491.
24. Skilbeck CE, Wade DT, Langton-Hewer R, *et al.*: Recovery after stroke. *J Neurol Neurosurg Psychiatr* 1983, 46:5–8.
25. Bjorneby ER, Reinvang IR: Acquiring and maintaining self-care skills after stroke. *Scand J Rehabil Med* 1985, 17:75–80.
26. Sarno MT, Levita E: Some observations on the nature of recovery in global aphasia after stroke. *Brain Lang* 1981, 13:1–12.
27. Fugl-Meyer AR: Assessment of motor function in hemiplegic patients. In *Neurophysiological Aspects of Rehabilitation Medicine.* Edited by Buerger AA, Tobis JS. Springfield, IL: Chas. C. Thomas; 1976, pp. 231–250.
28. Sawner K, LaVigne J, eds.: *Brunnstrom's Movement Therapy in Hemiplegia: A Neurophysiological Approach*. Second Edition. Philadelphia: J. B. Lippincott; 1992.
29. Gowland C, Stratford P, Ward M, *et al.*: Measuring physical impairment and disability with the Chedoke-McMaster Stroke Assessment. *Stroke* 1993, 24:58–63.
30. Twitchell TE: The restoration of motor function following hemiplegia in man. *Brain* 1951, 74:443–480.
31. Parker VM, Wade DT, Langton-Hewer R: Loss of arm function after stroke: measurement, frequency, and recovery. *Int Rehabil Med* 1986, 8:69–73.
32. Gowland C: Recovery of motor function following stroke: profile and predictors. *Physiother Can* 1982, 34:77–84.
33. Wade DT, Langton-Hewer R, Wood VA, *et al.*: The hemiplegic arm after stroke: measurement and recovery. *J Neurol Neurosurg Psychiatr* 1983, 46:521–524.

34. Bonita R, Beaglehole R: Recovery of motor function after stroke. *Stroke* 1988, 19:1497–1500.

35. Warabi T, Inoue K, Noda H, Murakami S: Recovery of voluntary movement in hemiplegic patients: correlation with degenerative shrinkage of the cerebral peduncles in CT images. *Brain* 1990, 113:177–189.

36. Wing AM, Lough S, Turton A, *et al.*: Recovery of elbow function in voluntary positioning of the hand following hemiplegia due to stroke. *J Neurol Neurosurg Psychiatr* 1990, 53:126–134.

37. Bohanon RW, Smith MB: Assessment of strength deficits in eight paretic upper extremity muscle groups of stroke patients with hemiplegia. *Phys Ther* 1987, 67:522–525.

38. Shah S: Reliability of the original Brunnstrom recovery scale following hemiplegia. *Am Occupat Ther J* 1984, 31:144–151.

39. Bohanon RW: Muscle strength changes in hemiparetic stroke patients during inpatient rehabilitation. *J Neurol Rehabil* 1988, 2:163–166.

40. Shah SK, Corones J: Volition following hemiplegia. *Arch Phys Med Rehabil* 1980, 61:523–528.

41. Bard G, Hirschberg GG: Recovery of voluntary motion in upper extremity following hemiplegia. *Arch Phys Med Rehabil* 1965, 46:567–572.

42. Wade DT, Langton-Hewer R, David RM, Enderby PM: Aphasia after stroke: natural history and associated deficits. *J Neurol Neurosurg Psychiatr* 1986, 49:11–16.

43. Kertesz A, McCabe P: Recovery patterns and prognosis in aphasia. *Brain* 1977, 100:1–18.

44. Pickersgill MJ, Lincoln NB: Prognostic indicators and the pattern of recovery in aphasic stroke patients. *J Neurol Neurosurg Psychiatr* 1983, 46:130–139.

45. Sarno MT, Levita E: Recovery in treated aphasia in the first year post-stroke. *Stroke* 1979, 10:662–670.

46. Kertesz A: What do we learn from recovery from aphasia? In *Advances in Neurology, Volume 47: Functional Recovery in Neurological Disease.* Edited by Waxman SG. New York: Raven Press; 1988:277–292.

47. Brust JCM, Shafer SQ, Richter RW, Bruun B: Aphasia in acute stroke. *Stroke* 1976, 7:167–174.

48. Prins RS, Snow CE, Wagenaar E: Recovery from aphasia: spontaneous speech versus language comprehension. *Brain Lang* 1978, 6:192–211.

49. Kertesz A, Lau WK, Polk M: The structural determinants of recovery in Wernicke's aphasia. *Brain Lang* 1993, 44:153–164.

50. Wade DT, Langton-Hewer R, Skilbeck CE, David RM, eds.: *Stroke: A Critical Approach to Diagnosis, Treatment, and Management.* Chicago: Year Book Medical Publishers; 1985.

51. Sarno MT: Recovery and rehabilitation. In *Acquired Aphasia.* Edited by Sarno MT. New York: Academic Press; 1981, pp. 485–529.

52. Nicholas MJ, Helm-Estabrooks N, Ward-Lonergan J, Morgan AR: Evolution of severe aphasia in the first two years post onset. *Arch Phys Med Rehabil* 1993, 74:830–836.

53. Meerwaldt JD: Spatial disorientation in right hemisphere infarction: a study of the speed of recovery. *J Neurol Neurosurg Psychiatr* 1983, 46:426–429.

54. Stone SP, Patel P, Greenwood RJ, Halligan PW: Measuring visual neglect in acute stroke and predicting its recovery: the visual neglect recovery index. *J Neurol Neurosurg Psychiatr* 1992, 55:431–436.

55. Kotila M, Niemi M-L, Laaksonen R: Four-year prognosis of stroke patients with visuospatial inattention. *Scand J Rehabil Med* 1986, 18:177–179.

56. Egelko S, Simon D, Riley E, *et al.*: First year after stroke: tracking cognitive and affective deficits. *Arch Phys Med Rehabil* 1989, 70:297–302.

57. Sunderland A, Langton-Hewer R: The natural history of visual neglect after stroke: indications from two methods of assessment. *Int Rehabil Med* 1987, 9:55–59.

58. Friedman PJ, Leong L: Perceptual impairment after stroke: improvements during the first 3 months. *Disabil and Rehabil* 1992, 14:136–139.

59. Hier DB, Mondlock J, Caplan LR: Recovery of behavioral abnormalities after right hemisphere stroke. *Neurology* 1983, 33:345–350.

60. Basso A, Capitani E, Sala SD, *et al.*: Recovery from ideomotor apraxia: a study on acute stroke patients. *Brain* 1987, 110:747–760.

61. Meier MJ, Ettinger MG, Arthur L: Recovery of neuropsychological functioning after cerebrovascular infarction. In *Neuropsychology and Cognition, Volume II.* Edited by Malatesha RN, Hartlage LC. Boston: Martinus Nuhoff Publishers; 1982:552–563.

62. Vartanian GA: Memory function and recovery after brain lesion. In *Central Nervous System Plasticity and Repair.* Edited by Bignami A. New York: Raven Press; 1985:97–104.

63. Wade DT, Parker V, Langton-Hewer R: Memory disturbance after stroke: frequency and associated losses. *Int Rehabil Med* 1986, 8:60–64.

64. Levine DN, Warach JD, Benowitz L, Calvanio R: Left spatial neglect: effects of lesion size and premorbid brain atrophy on severity and recovery following right cerebral infarction. *Neurology* 1986, 36:362–366.

65. Dombovy ML, Bach-y-Rita P: Clinical observations on recovery from stroke. In *Advances in Neurology, Volume 47: Functional Recovery in Neurological Disease.* Edited by Waxman SG. New York: Raven Press; 1988:265–276.

66. Bach-y-Rita P: Process of recovery from stroke. In *Stroke Rehabilitation.* Edited by Brandstater ME, Basmajian JV. Baltimore: Williams and Wilkins; 1987:80–108.

67. Bach-y-Rita P, Baillet R: Recovery from stroke. In *Motor Deficits Following Stoke.* Edited by Duncan PW, Badke MB. New York: Year Book Medical Publishers; 1987:79–107.

68. Bach-y-Rita P, ed.: *Recovery of Function: Theoretical Considerations for Brain Injury Rehabilitation.* Baltimore: University Park Press; 1980.

69. Kaplan MS: Plasticity after brain lesions: contemporary concepts. *Arch Phys Med Rehabil* 1988, 69:984–991.

70. Wainberg MC: Plasticity of the central nervous system: functional implications for rehabilitation. *Physiother Can* 1988, 40:224–232.

71. Bach-y-Rita P: Brain plasticity as a basis of the development of rehabilitation procedures for hemiplegia. *Scand J Rehabil Med* 1981, 13:73–83.

72. Feeney DM, Baron JC: Diaschisis. *Stroke* 1986, 17:817–830.

73. Marshall JF: Neural plasticity and recovery of function after brain injury. *Int Rev Neurobiol* 1985, 26:201–247.

74. Boyeson MG, Bach-y-Rita P: Determinants of brain plasticity. *J Neurol Rehabil* 1989, 3:35–57.

75. Bach-y-Rita P: Central nervous system lesions: sprouting and unmasking in rehabilitation. *Arch Phys Med Rehabil* 1981, 62:41–47.

76. Illis LS: The effects of repetitive stimulation in recovery from damage to the central nervous system. *Int Rehabil Med* 1982, 4:178–184.

77. Sacco RL, Wolf PA, Kannel WB, McNamara PM: Survival and recurrence following stroke: the Framingham study. *Stroke* 1982, 13:290–295.

78. Solzi P, Ring H, Najenson T, Luz Y: Hemiplegics after a first stroke: late survival and risk factors. *Stroke* 1985, 4:703–709.

79. Dombovy ML, Basford JR, Whisnant JP, Bergstrahl EJ: Disability and use of rehabilitation services following stroke in Rochester, Minnesota, 1975-1979. *Stroke* 1987, 18:830–836.

80. Sheikh K, Brennan PJ, Meade TW, *et al.*: Predictors of mortality and disability in stroke. *J Epidemiol Commun Health* 1983, 37:70–74.

81. Roth EJ, Mueller K, Green D: Stroke rehabilitation outcome: impact of coronary artery disease. *Stroke* 1988, 19:42–47.

82. Topic E, Pavlicek I, Brinar V, Korsick M: Glycosylated haemoglobin in clarification of the origin of hyperglycaemia in acute cerebrovascular accident. *Diabetic Med* 1989, 6:12–15.

83. Gray CS, Taylor R, French JM, *et al.*: The prognostic value of stress hyperglycaemia and previously unrecognized diabetes in acute stroke. *Diabetic Med* 1987, 4:237–240.

84. Woo E, Chan YW, Yu YL, Huang CY: Admission glucose level in relation to mortality and morbidity outcome in 252 stroke patients. *Stroke* 1988, 19:185–191.
85. Myers MG, Norris JW, Hachinski VC, *et al.*: Cardiac sequelae of acute stroke. *Stroke* 1982, 13:838–842.
86. Nishide M, Irino T, Gotoh M, *et al.*: Cardiac abnormalities in ischaemic cerebrovascular disease studied by two-dimensional echocardiography. *Stroke* 1983, 14:541–545.
87. Dromerick A, Reding M: Medical and neurologic complications during inpatient stroke rehabilitation. *Stroke* 1994, 25:358–361.
88. Dobkin BH: Neuromedical complications in stroke patients transferred for rehabilitation before and after diagnostic related groups. *J Neurol Rehabil* 1987, 1:3–7.
89. McClatchie G: Survey of the rehabilitation outcome of strokes. *Med J Aust* 1980, 1:649–651.
90. Feigenson J, Gitlow H, Greenberg S: The disability oriented rehabilitation unit: a major factor influencing stroke outcome. *Stroke* 1979, 10:5–7.
91. Adler M, Hamaty D, Brown CC, Potts H: Medical audit of stroke rehabilitation: a critique of medical care review. *J Chron Dis* 1977, 30:461–471.
92. Feigenson JS, McDowell FH, Meese P, *et al*: Factors influencing outcome and length of stay in a rehabilitation unit: Part 1: analysis of 248 unscreened patients: medical and functional prognostic indicators. *Stroke* 1977, 8:651–656.
93. Feigenson JS, McCarthy M, Greenberg S, Feigenson W: Factors influencing outcome and length of stay in a rehabilitation unit: Part II: comparison of 318 screened and 248 unscreened patients. *Stroke* 1977, 8:657–662.
94. Roth EJ, Green D: Cardiac complications during stroke rehabilitation. *Top Stroke Rehabil* 1994, 2:241–249.
95. Aptaker RL, Roth EJ, Reichardt G, *et al.*: Serum albumin level as a predictor of geriatric stroke rehabilitation outcome. *Arch Phys Med Rehabil* 1994, 75:80–84.
96. Axelsson K, Asplund K, Norberg A, Alafuzoff I: Nutritional status in patients with acute stroke. *Acta Med Scand* 1988, 224:217–224.
97. Asberg KH: Orthostatic tolerance training of stroke patients in general medical wards. *Scand J Rehabil Med* 1989, 21:179–185.
98. Roth EJ: Medical complications encountered in stroke rehabilitation. *Phys Med Rehabil Clin North Am* 1991, 2:563–578.
99. Schmidt J, Reding M: Recognition and management of medical and specific associated neurological complications in stroke rehabilitation. *Top Geriatr Rehabil* 1991, 7:1–14.
100. Siegler EL, Whitney FW: Prevention and other special management issues in the postacute care of the geriatric stroke patient. *Neurol Rehabil* 1993, 3(1):1–11.
101. Brott T: Prevention and management of medical complications of the hospitalized elderly stroke patient. *Clin Geriatr Med* 1991, 7:475–482.
102. Steinberg FU, ed.: *The Immobilized Patient: Functional Pathology and Management.* New York: Plenum Medical Book Co.; 1980.
103. St. Pierre D, Gardiner PF: The effect of immobilization and exercise on muscle function: a review. *Physiother Can* 1987, 39:24–36.
104. Reddy MP: A guide to early mobilization of bedridden elderly. *Geriatrics* 1986, 41:59–70.
105. Roth EJ: Heart disease in patients with stroke: incidence, impact, and implications for rehabilitation. Part I: classification and prevalence. *Arch Phys Med Rehabil* 1993, 74:752–760.
106. Roth EJ: Heart disease in patients with stroke: Part II: impact and implications for rehabilitation. *Arch Phys Med Rehabil* 1994, 75:94–101.
107. Hachinski V, Norris JW, eds.: *The Acute Stroke.* Philadelphia: F. A. Davis; 1985.
108. Rokey R, Rolak LA, Harati Y, *et al.*: Coronary artery disease in patients with cerebrovascular disease: a prospective study. *Ann Neurol* 1984, 16:50–53.
109. DiPasquale G, Andreoli A, Carini G, *et al.*: Noninvasive screening for silent ischemic heart disease. *Acta Med Scand* 1979, 205:425–428.
110. Hertzer NR, Young JR, Beren EG, *et al.*: Coronary angiography in 506 patients with extracranial cerebrovascular disease. *Arch Intern Med* 1985, 145:849–852.
111. Walker AE, Robins M, Weinfeld FD: The National Survey of Stroke: clinical findings. *Stroke* 1981, 12(suppl 1):I-13–I-31.
112. Wallace JD, Levy LL: Blood pressure after stroke. *JAMA* 1981, 246:2177–2180.
113. Barker WH, Feldt KS, Feibel JH: Community surveillance of stroke in persons under 70 years old: contributions of uncontrolled hypertension. *Am J Public Health* 1983, 73:260–265.
114. Tallman WT: Cardiovascular regulation and lesions of the central nervous system. *Ann Neurol* 1985, 18:1–12.
115. Bounds JV, Wiebers DO, Whisnant JP, *et al.*: Mechanisms and timing of deaths from cerebral infarction. *Stroke* 1981, 12:474–477.
116. Matsumoto N, Whisnant JP, Kurland LT, *et al.*: Natural history of stroke in Rochester, Minnesota 1955 through 1969: an extension of a previous study 1945 through 1954. *Stroke* 1973, 4:20–29.
117. Brandstater ME, Roth EJ, Siebens HC: Venous thromboembolism in stroke: literature in review and implications for clinical practice. *Arch Phys Med Rehabil* 1992, 73(suppl):S-379–S-391.
118. Turpie AGG, Hirsh J, Jay RM, *et al.*: Double-blind randomised trial of ORG 10172 low-molecular weight heparinoid in prevention of deep-vein thrombosis in thrombotic stroke. *Lancet* 1987, 1:523–526.
119. McCarthy ST, Turner J: Low-dose subcutaneous heparin in the prevention of deep-vein thrombosis and pulmonary emboli following acute stroke. *Age Ageing* 1986, 15:84–88.
120. Warlow C, Ogston D, Douglas AS: Deep venous thrombosis of the legs after stroke (parts I and II). *BMJ* 1976, 1:1178–1183.
121. Oczkowski WJ, Ginsberg JS, Shin A, Panju A: Venous thromboembolism in patients undergoing rehabilitation for stroke. *Arch Phys Med Rehabil*, 1992.
122. Hirsh J: Heparin. *N Engl J Med* 1991, 324:1568–1574.
123. Hirsh J, Levine M: Therapeutic range for the control of oral anticoagulant therapy. *Arch Neurol* 1986, 43:1162–1164.
124. Office of Medical Applications of Research, NIH: Consensus conference: prevention of venous thrombosis and pulmonary embolism. *JAMA* 1986, 256:744–749.
125. Sioson ER, Crowe WE, Dawson NV: Occult proximal deep vein thrombosis: its prevalence among patients admitted to a rehabilitation hospital. *Arch Phys Med Rehabil* 1988, 69:183–185.
126. Bromfield EB, Reding MJ: Relative risk of deep venous thrombosis or pulmonary embolism post-stroke based on ambulatory status. *J Neurol Rehabil* 1988, 2:51–57.
127. Couser JI: Diagnosis and management of pneumonia and ventilatory disorders in patients with stroke. *Top Stroke Rehabil* 1994, 1(2):106–118.
128. Horner J, Massey EW, Riski JE, *et al.*: Aspiration following stroke: clinical correlates and outcome. *Neurology* 1988, 38:1359–1362.
129. Martin BJW, Corlew MM, Wood H, *et al.*: The association of swallowing dysfunction and aspiration pneumonia. *Dysphagia* 1994, 9:1–6.
130. Schmidt J, Holas M, Halvorson K, Reding M: Videofluoroscopic evidence of aspiration predicts pneumonia and death but not dehydration following stroke. *Dysphagia* 1994, 9:7–11.
131. Przedborski S, Brunko E, Hubert M, *et al.*: The effect of acute hemiplegia on intercostal muscle activity. *Neurology* 1988, 38:1882–1884.
132. Fluck DC: Chest movements in hemiplegia. *Clin Sci* 1966, 31:383–388.
133. Korczyn AD, Herman G, Don R: Diaphragmatic involvement in hemiplegia and hemiparesis. *J Neurol Neurosurg Psychiatr* 1969, 32:588–594.
134. Smith M: The effect of hemiplegia on the diaphragm. *Am Rev Respir Dis* 1964, 89:450–452.
135. Haas A, Rusk HA, Pelosof H, Adam JR: Respiratory function in hemiplegic patients. *Arch Phys Med Rehabil* 1967, 48:174–179.

136. Odia GI: Spirometry in convalescent hemiplegic patients. *Arch Phys Med Rehabil* 1978, 59:319–321.

137. Fugl-Meyer AR, Linderholm H, Wilson AF: Restrictive ventilatory dysfunction in stroke: its relation to locomotor function. *Scand J Rehabil Med* [suppl] 1983, 9:118–124.

138. Scherzer HH, Nurse BA: Pneumonia in the elderly stroke patient. In *Medical Management of the Elderly Stroke Patient: Physical Medicine State of the Art Reviews.* Edited by Erickson RV. Philadelphia: Hanley & Belfus Medical Publishers; 1989, 3:519–536.

139. Wiebe-Velazquez S, Blume WT: Seizures. In *Long-Term Consequences of Stroke. Physical Medicine and Rehabilitation State of the Art Reviews.* Edited by Teasell RW. 1993, Philadelphia: Hanley & Belfus Publishers; 7(1):73–87.

140. Olsen TS, Hogenhaven H, Thage O: Epilepsy after stroke. *Neurology* 1987, 37:1209–1211.

141. Black SE, Norris JW, Hachinski VC: Post-stroke seizures. *Stroke* 1983, 14:134.

142. Cocito L, Favale E, Reni L: Epileptic seizures in cerebral arterial occlusive disease. *Stroke* 1982, 13:189–195.

143. DeRueck J, Krahel N, Sieben G, *et al.*: Epilepsy in patients with cerebral infarcts. *J Neurol* 1980, 224:101–109.

144. Faught E, Peters D, Bartolucci A, *et al.*: Seizures after primary intracerebral hemorrhage. *Neurology* 1989, 39:1089–1093.

145. Lesser RP, Luders H, Dinner DS, Morris HH: Epileptic seizures due to thrombotic and embolic cerebrovascular disease in older patients. *Epilepsia* 1985, 26:622–630.

146. Saver JL: Poststroke seizures. *Top Stroke Rehabil* 1994, 1:109–130.

147. Teasell RW: Pain following stroke. *Crit Rev Phys Med Rehabil* 1992, 3:205–217.

148. Garrison SJ: Post-stroke pain. *Physical Medicine and Rehabilitation State of the Art Reviews* 1991, 5:83–88.

149. Boivie J, Leijon G: Clinical findings in patients with central poststroke pain. In *Pain and Central Nervous System Disease: Central Pain Syndromes.* Edited by Casey KL. New York: Raven Press; 1991:65–75.

150. Leijon G, Boivie J, Johansson I: Central post-stroke pain-neurological symptoms and pain characteristics. *Pain* 1989, 36:13–25.

151. Holmgren H, Leijon G, Boivie J, *et al.*: Central post-stroke pain: somatosensory evoked potentials in relation to location of the lesion and sensory signs. *Pain* 1990, 40:43–52.

152. Boivie J, Leijon G, Johansson I: Central post-stroke pain: a study of mechanisms through analysis of the sensory abnormalities. *Pain* 1989, 36:173–185.

153. Leijon G, Boivie J: Central post-stroke pain: the effect of high and low frequency TENS. *Pain* 1989, 38:187–191.

154. Leijon G, Boivie J: Central post-stroke pain: a controlled trial of amitriptyline and carbamazepine. *Pain* 1989, 36:27–36.

155. Borrie MJ: Urinary incontinence after stroke. In *Long-Term Consequences of Stroke. Physical Medicine and Rehabilitation State of the Art Reviews.* Edited by Teasell RW. 1993, 7(1):101–112.

156. Hoogasian S, Walzak MP, Wurzel R: Urinary incontinence in the stroke patient: etiology and rehabilitation. In *Medical Management of the Elderly Stroke Patient. Physical Medicine and Rehabilitation State of the Art Reviews.* Edited by Erickson RV. Philadelphia: Hanley and Belfus; 1989:581–594.

157. Brocklehurst JC, Andrews K, Richards B, Laycock PJ: Incidence and correlates of incontinence in stroke patients. *J Am Geriatr Soc* 1985, 33:540–542.

158. Reding MJ, Winter SW, Hochrein SA, *et al.*: Urinary incontinence after unilateral hemispheric stroke: a neurologic epidemiologic perspective. *J Neurorehabil* 1987, 1:25–30.

159. Gelber DA, Good DC, Laven LJ, Verhulst SJ: Causes of urinary incontinence after acute hemispheric stroke. *Stroke* 1993, 24:378–382.

160. Sedarat SM, Hecht JS: Urologic problems after stroke (Parts I and II). *Stroke Clin Updates* 1993, 4:17–24.

161. Linsenmeyer TA, Zorowitz RD: Urodynamic findings in patients with urinary incontinence after cerebrovascular accident. *Neurol Rehabil* 1992, 2(2):23–26.

162. Krane RJ, Siroky MB: Classification of neuro-urologic disorders. In *Clinical Neurourology.* Edited by Krane RJ, Siroky MB. *Clinical Neurourology.* Boston: Little Brown; 1979:143–158.

163. Garrett VE, Scott JA, Costich J, *et al.*: Bladder emptying assessment in stroke patients. *Arch Phys Med Rehabil* 1989, 70:41–43.

164. Barer DH: Continence after stroke: useful predictor or goal of therapy? *Age Aging* 1989, 18:183–191.

165. Shea JD: Pressure sores: classification and management. *Clin Orthop Rel Res* 1975, 112:89–100.

166. Yarkony GM, Kirk P, Carlson C, *et al.*: Classification of pressure ulcers. *Arch Dermatol* 1990, 126:1218–1219.

167. Melcher RE, Longe RL, Gelbart AO: Pressure sores in the elderly: a systematic approach to management. *Postgrad Med* 1988, 83:299–308.

168. Reuler J, Cooney T: The pressure sore: pathophysiology and principles of management. *Ann Intern Med* 1981, 94:661–666.

169. Panel for the Prediction and Prevention of Pressure Ulcers in Adults: *Pressure Ulcers in Adults: Prediction and Prevention. Clinical Practice Guideline, Number 3.* AHCPR Publication No. 92-0047. Rockville, MD: Agency for Health Care Policy and Research, Public Health Service, U.S. Department of Health and Human Services; 1992.

170. Perez ED: Pressure ulcers: updated guidelines for treatment and prevention. *Geriatrics* 1993, 48:39–44.

171. Caillet R, ed.: *The Shoulder in Hemiplegia.* Philadelphia: F.A. Davis Co.; 1980.

172. Totta M, Beneck S: Shoulder dysfunction in stroke hemiplegia. *Phys Med Rehabil Clin North Am* 1991, 2(3):627–641.

173. Griffin J, Reddin G: Shoulder pain in persons with hemiplegia: a literature review. *Phys Ther* 1981, 61:1041–1045.

174. Kozin F, *et al.*: The reflex sympathetic dystrophy syndrome. Parts 1,2, and 3. *Am J Med* 1976, 60:321–338; 1981, 70:23–30.

175. Moodie NB, Brisbin J, Morgan AMG: Subluxation of the glenohumeral joint in hemiplegia: evaluation of supportive devices. *Physiother Can* 1986, 38:151–157.

176. Najenson T, Yacubovich E, Pikielini S: Rotator cuff injury in shoulder joints of hemiplegic patients. *Scand J Rehabil Med* 1971, 3:131–137.

177. Smith RG, Cruikshank JG, Dunbar S: Malalignment of the shoulder after stroke. *BMJ* 1982, 284:1224–1226.

178. Teasell RW, Gillen M: Upper extremity disorders and pain following stroke. In *Long-Term Consequence of Stroke. Physical Medicine and Rehabilitation State of the Art Reviews.* Edited by Teasell RW. 1993, 7(1):133–146.

179. Tepperman PS, Greyson ND, Hilbert L, *et al.*: Reflex sympathetic dystrophy in hemiplegia. *Arch Phys Med Rehabil* 1984, 65:442–447.

180. Van Ouenaller C, Laplace PM, Chantraine A: Painful shoulder in hemiplegia. *Arch Phys Med Rehabil* 1986, 67:23–36.

181. Werner RA, Priebe MM, Davidoff GN: Reflex sympathetic dystrophy syndrome associated with hemiplegia. *Neuro Rehabil* 1992, 2(2):16–22.

182. Mion LC, Gregor S, Buettner M, *et al.*: Falls in the rehabilitation setting: incidence and characteristics. *Rehabil Nurs* 1989, 14:17–21.

183. Tinetti ME, Speechley M: Prevention of falls among the elderly. *N Engl J Med* 1989, 320:1055–1059.

184. DeVincenzo DK, Watkins S: Accidental falls in a rehabilitation setting. *Rehabil Nurs* 1987, 12:248–252.

185. Mayo NE, Korner-Bitensky N, Kaizer F: Relationship between response time and falls among stroke patients undergoing physical rehabilitation. *Int J Rehabil* 1990, 13:47–55.

186. Poplingher AR, Pillar T: Hip fracture in stroke patients. Epidemiology and rehabilitation. *Acta Orthop Scand* 1985, 56:226–227.

187. Tinetti ME, Speechley M, Ginter S: Risk factors for falls among elderly persons living in the community. *N Engl J Med* 1988, 319:1701–1707.

Chapter 23

Commonly Prescribed Medications and Novel Pharmacologic Approaches in Stroke Rehabilitation

LARRY B. GOLDSTEIN

A variety of factors may influence functional recovery after stroke. Recent laboratory studies show that the recovery process can be modulated by certain drugs that affect the activities of central neurotransmitters. Although some of these drug effects may be beneficial, others may be detrimental. This chapter reviews the emerging pharmacology of behavioral recovery and presents data from preliminary clinical studies in humans recovering from stroke.

Enhancement of functional recovery is one of the major goals of treatment after the acute phase of stroke (Table 23.1). Working towards this objective is traditionally undertaken by rehabilitative and neurorehabilitative specialists, including physicians, nurses, physical therapists, occupational therapists, psychologists, and speech pathologists. Facilitation of motor recovery is particularly important because motor function is one of the major determinants of independence in activities of daily living [1]. Conventional therapy aimed at decreasing disability after stroke depends on a variety of physical training techniques based on different philosophies. These include those that are designed to either provide optimal compensation for particular impairments, such as the traditional approach, or to specifically improve lost function, such as the neurodevelopmental technique, Brunnstrom approach, or integrated behavioral-physical therapy. Regardless of the treatment methodology, stroke patients appear to benefit at least marginally from rehabilitation with physiotherapy, although definitive evidence is lacking [2]. Recently, advances in the neurosciences indicate that drugs that influence the activity of specific central neurotransmitters can modulate the recovery process. These data not only suggest that pharmacotherapy may enhance recovery of lost function, but that some commonly prescribed medications used to treat coincident medical conditions may be harmful. Thus, the primary physician caring for the acute stroke patient is a critical member of the neurorehabilitative team.

DEFINITIONS OF FUNCTIONAL RECOVERY AFTER STROKE

The functional impact of stroke may be considered at several levels (Table 23.2) [3]. At the level of *impairment*, stroke affects specific physiologic functions. *Disability* is the result of physiologic impairments and is reflected in specific activities. *Handicap* results from impairment or disability and refers to loss of function at a societal level. It is important to recognize that progress at the impairment level may not be mirrored by improvement in a disability or handicap and that diminished disability or handicap may not reflect decreased impairment. For example, limb paresis may subside after stroke, but the patient may still be unable to walk without assistance (disability) or ride a bicycle (handicap). A patient with an upper limb amputation may learn to use the remaining arm to dress (improved disability) or operate a motor vehicle (reduction of handicap). Therefore, in considering functional recovery, the level of function must be understood. Similarly, in laboratory studies, the level of deficit and its measurement are critical. As with humans, laboratory animals may use behavioral substitution to compensate for a specific impairment to perform a particular task (Figure 23.1) [4]. Rather than enhancing this functional compensation, certain drugs may influence the neurophysiologic processes underlying specific behavioral recovery.

Table 23.1. Goals of treatment in stroke

Stroke prevention
  Identification and management of general risk factors
    Hypertension
    Cigarette smoking
    Hyperlipidemia
    Cardiac disease
  Medical management
    Platelet antiaggregants, anticoagulants
  Surgical management
    Endarterectomy (minor hemispheric stroke)
	Prevention of complications
	  Infection
	  Aspiration pneumonia
	  Urinary tract infection
	  Pulmonary embolism
	  Contractures
	Improved functional recovery
	  Physical, occupational, and speech therapy

Table 23.2. Functional impact of stroke

Impairment	Disability	Handicaps
Language	Bathing	Loss of employment
Spatial perception	Physical activity (*eg*, walking, biking)	
Sensation	Dressing	
Strength	Driving	
Coordination	Using telephone	

GENERAL FACTORS INFLUENCING THE RECOVERY PROCESS

Regardless of the initial severity of the deficit, most stroke patients exhibit some degree of specific behavioral recovery (Figure 23.2) [5–7]. However, clinicians recognize that patients with acute brain lesions of similar size, location, and etiology may experience different degrees of recovery. This is true because a variety of factors, in addition to the lesion itself, influence the recovery process. These factors, some of which are amenable to therapeutic intervention, may be either environmental and extrinsic to the individual, or biologic and intrinsic (Figure 23.3). Recognition of these factors provides a framework for the rational consideration of the effects of drugs.

Both laboratory and clinical evidence point to the importance of extrinsic environmental factors in the recovery process (Figure 23.4). For example, with regard to motor deficits, rats reared in enriched environments in which toys, tunnels, and running wheels are provided show less severe deficits after motor cortex lesions than control rats housed in standard laboratory cages [8]. Task-specific postlesion training is also quite effective in enhancing motor recovery [9]. Rats given specific motor training after sensorimotor cortex injury recover motor function more rapidly than rats not given this training. Non–task-specific postle-

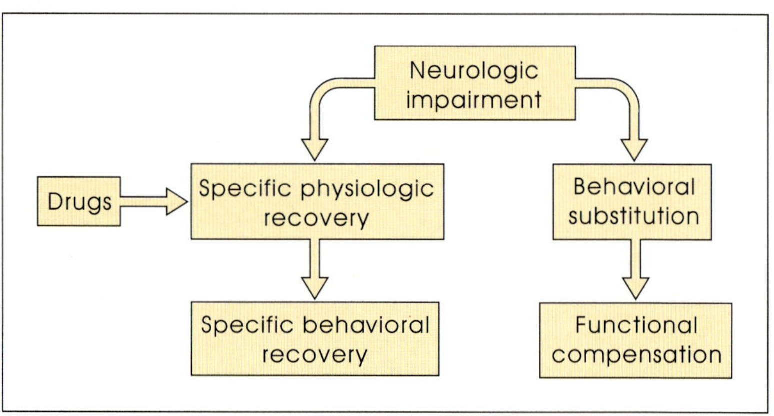

FIGURE 23.1

"Functional" recovery. Behavioral substitution may result in functional compensation without specific physiologic recovery of a specific impairment.

sion environmental enrichment is also effective in improving the motor deficit in these animals, albeit to a somewhat lesser degree than animals given environmental enrichment before the lesion [8]. The interested reader is referred to a recent review of experimental environmental approaches to recovery of function from brain damage [10]. Similarly, in humans, the various physiotherapeutic approaches may be considered types of task-specific or non–task-specific postlesion environmental experience. Nonspecific environmental factors, such as social support mechanisms, can also have a clinically important impact on recovery after stroke [1,11].

General intrinsic or biologic factors clearly affect the capacity of the individual to recover from brain injury (Figure 23.5). These factors may be divided into those that are fixed and those that are potentially amenable to treatment. Fixed factors that may influence recovery include the individual's age [12], sex [13],

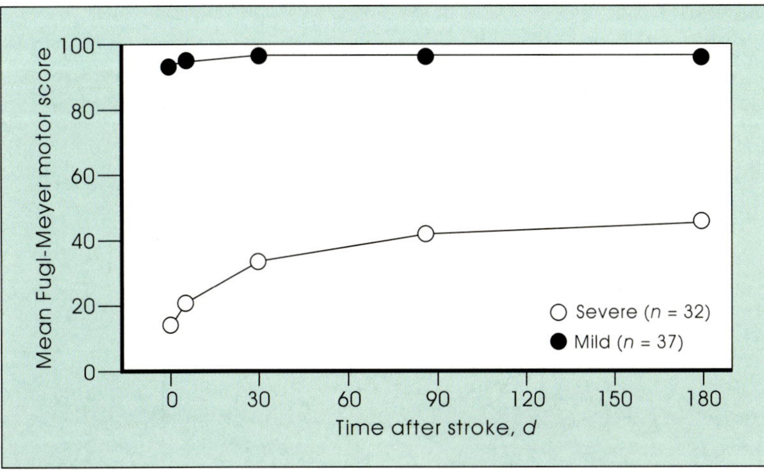

FIGURE 23.2

Recovery of motor function after stroke. In this study, motor recovery in a cohort of patients with carotid-distribution ischemic stroke was measured with the Fugl-Meyer assessment, a reliable and validated measure of motor impairment [130,131]. Recoveries of patients with mild and severe initial motor deficits are shown. Regardless of initial severity, both groups of stroke patients recovered to some degree. The most dramatic recovery occurred over the first 30 days. (*Adapted from* Duncan and coworkers [5]; with permission.)

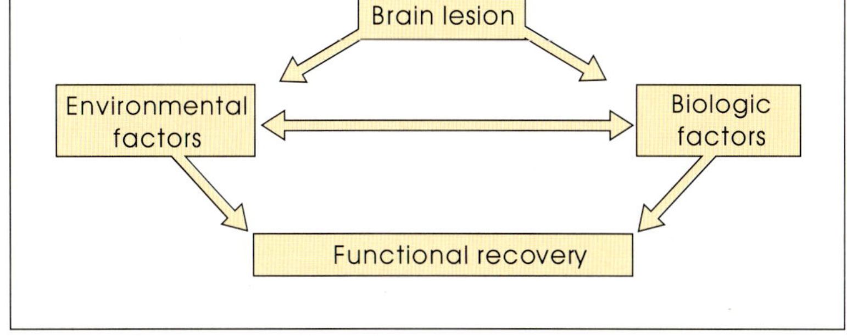

FIGURE 23.3

Factors influencing the stroke recovery process. Both extrinsic environmental factors and intrinsic biologic factors may influence recovery.

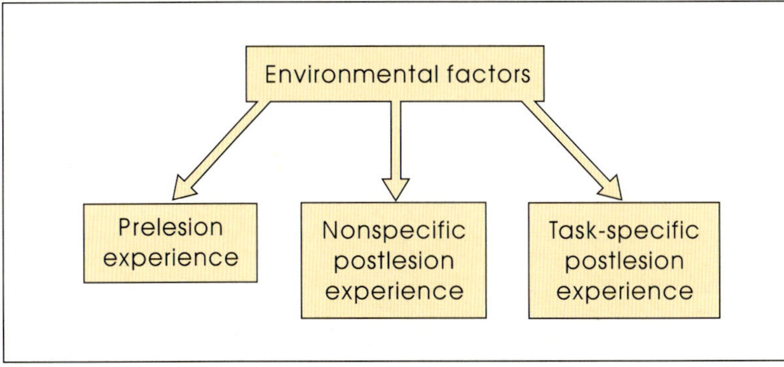

FIGURE 23.4

Stroke experience and recovery. Both prelesion and postlesion environmental factors may influence recovery.

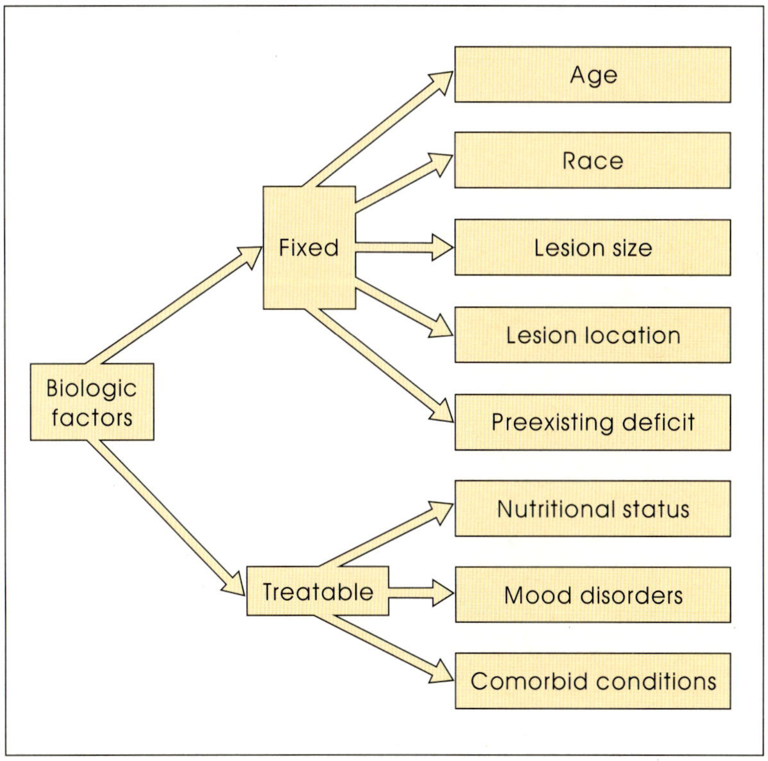

FIGURE 23.5

Biologic factors of stroke and recovery. The final degree of recovery may be influenced by a variety of factors, some of which are fixed and others of which are amenable to treatment.

racial group [14,15], lesion size [16,17], lesion location [17,18], and preexisting neurologic (*eg*, cognitive, motor, perceptual, and so forth) [13] and nonneurologic (*ie*, limb amputation, severe arthritis, refractory congestive heart failure, and so forth) deficits. General factors that are potentially treatable from the standpoint of the recovery period include nutritional status [19], mood disorders [20], and certain comorbid conditions (*ie*, infection, pulmonary or cardiac conditions). Certain drugs that may be used to treat these coincident medical problems may have significant effects on specific behavioral recovery.

THE NEUROBIOLOGY OF RECOVERY

Despite major advances, knowledge of the fundamental neurophysiologic processes underlying specific behavioral recovery remains rudimentary. We have considered these processes in two major groups [21,22] (Figure 23.6). These adaptive responses may occur either rapidly or develop more slowly over time.

The development and resolution of pathologic sequelae of focal brain injury such as cerebral edema [23], local inflammation [24], and diaschisis [25] may be reflected in the functional deficit. The potential effects of certain drugs on diaschisis forms the basis of an attractive hypothesis for considering their effects on recovery after focal cortical injury [26]. Diaschisis entails a "remote functional depression" of brain regions distant from the site of

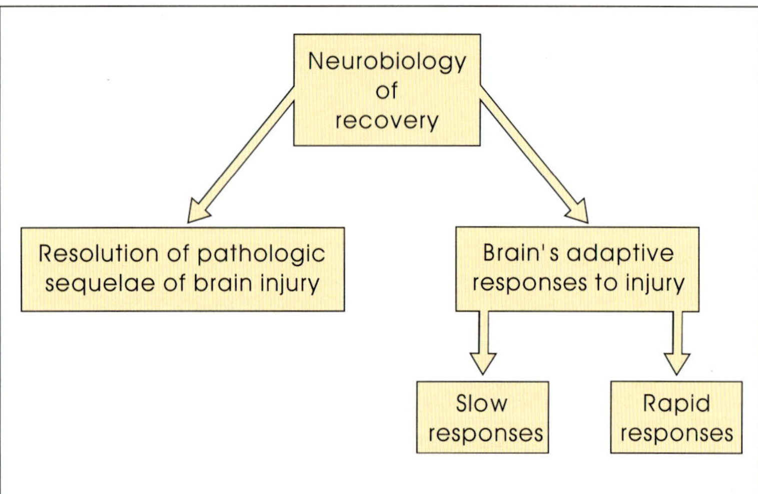

FIGURE 23.6

Neurobiology of stroke recovery. Recovery may occur due to a resolution of the pathologic sequelae of brain injury or to the brain's adaptive responses.

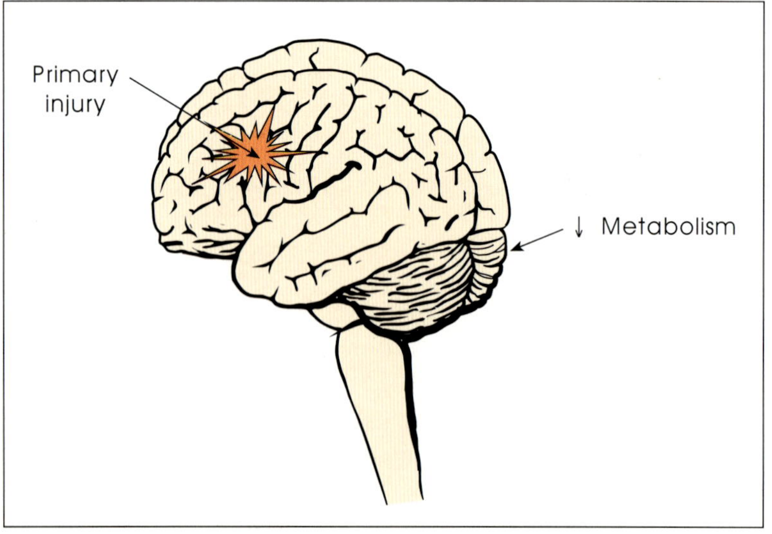

FIGURE 23.7

Diaschisis. A lesion in one area of the nervous system can have remote effects on distant areas of the brain. In this example, crossed cerebellar diaschisis is illustrated.

Table 23.3. Examples of possible rapid adaptive responses

Unmasking
Redundant neural networks might take over functions lost due to brain injury
Long-term potentiation
Putative cellular mechanism of learning and memory

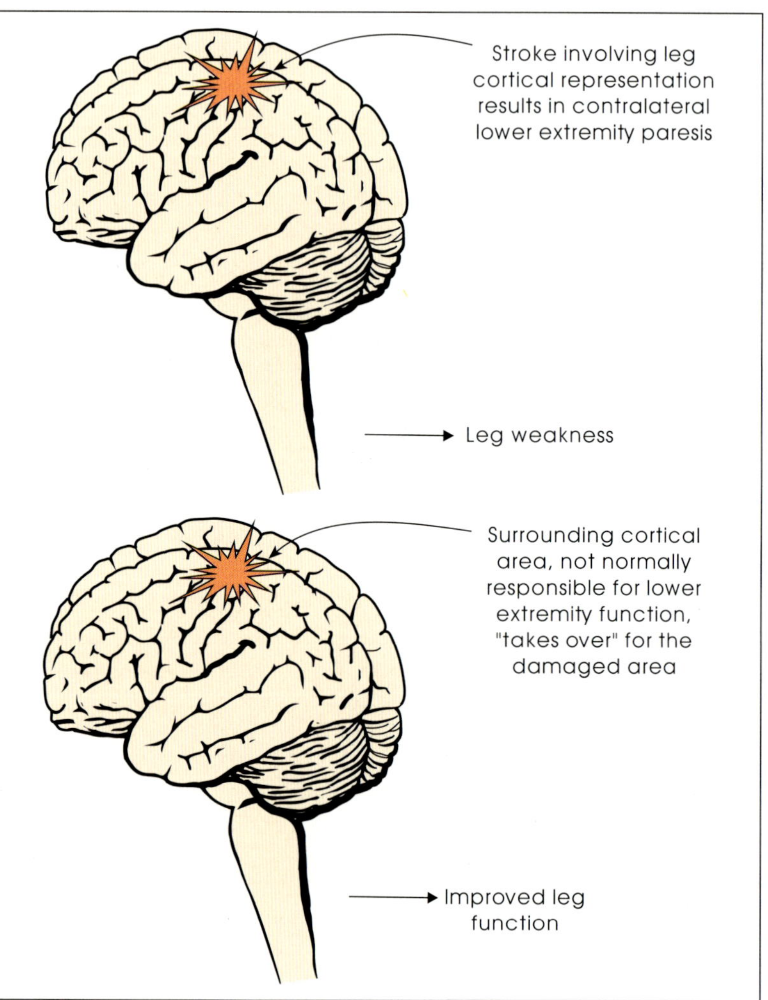

FIGURE 23.8

Theoretical example of "unmasking." The *upper panel* indicates an injury to the area of cerebral cortex involved in the control of motor function in the contralateral lower extremity. *Unmasking* entails the "activation" of redundant neural networks that are not normally responsible for a given function. In the *lower panel*, an area of surrounding undamaged cortex, not normally responsible for the control of lower extremity motor function, takes over for the damaged area of cortex.

primary injury (Figure 23.7). Diaschisis has been demonstrated experimentally in a variety of laboratory animal models [27–29]. In human stroke patients, diaschisis-like changes in metabolism have been demonstrated by positron emission tomography (PET) in the noninjured ipsilateral cerebral hemisphere, the contralateral cerebral hemisphere, and the contralateral cerebellum [30–32]. Crossed cerebellar-cortical diaschisis occurs in patients with unilateral cerebellar infarction [33]. Deep hemispheric strokes can have remote effects on metabolism in both the cerebral cortex and cerebellum [34]. The pathophysiologic mechanism underlying diaschisis is not understood [25,28]. The observed depression of metabolic activity in distant brain regions might be the direct result of regional changes in cerebral blood flow, or decreased regional cerebral blood flow (rCBF) might be secondary to locally depressed cerebral metabolism. Drugs that promote the resolution of diaschisis could facilitate recovery, whereas those that prolong or worsen diaschisis could be detrimental.

From the standpoint of specific behavioral recovery, rapid adaptive responses to brain injury may also be considered as forms of relearning (*ie*, with stroke-associated motor impairment the individual "relearns" how to use the affected limb) (Table 23.3). The physiologic mechanism by which this relearning occurs remains uncertain. For example, Lashley [35] and Luria [36] suggested that redundant neural networks might take over for functions lost due to brain injury. PET studies in human stroke patients show metabolic changes consistent with this phenomenon (also termed *unmasking*) (Figure 23.8) [37]. In uninjured humans, motor movement is associated with increases in rCBF in a circumscribed region in the contralateral primary sensorimotor cortex. However, in patients who have recovered from stroke-associated limb paresis, movement of the previously affected extremity is associated with significant changes in rCBF in widespread areas of the brain, including both the ipsilateral and contralateral sensorimotor cortex and cerebellar hemispheres [38–40].

It is also possible that the normal neuronal processes responsible for learning might underlie the relearning that occurs after brain injury. Long-term potentiation (LTP) is the best understood putative cellular mechanism of learning and memory (Figure

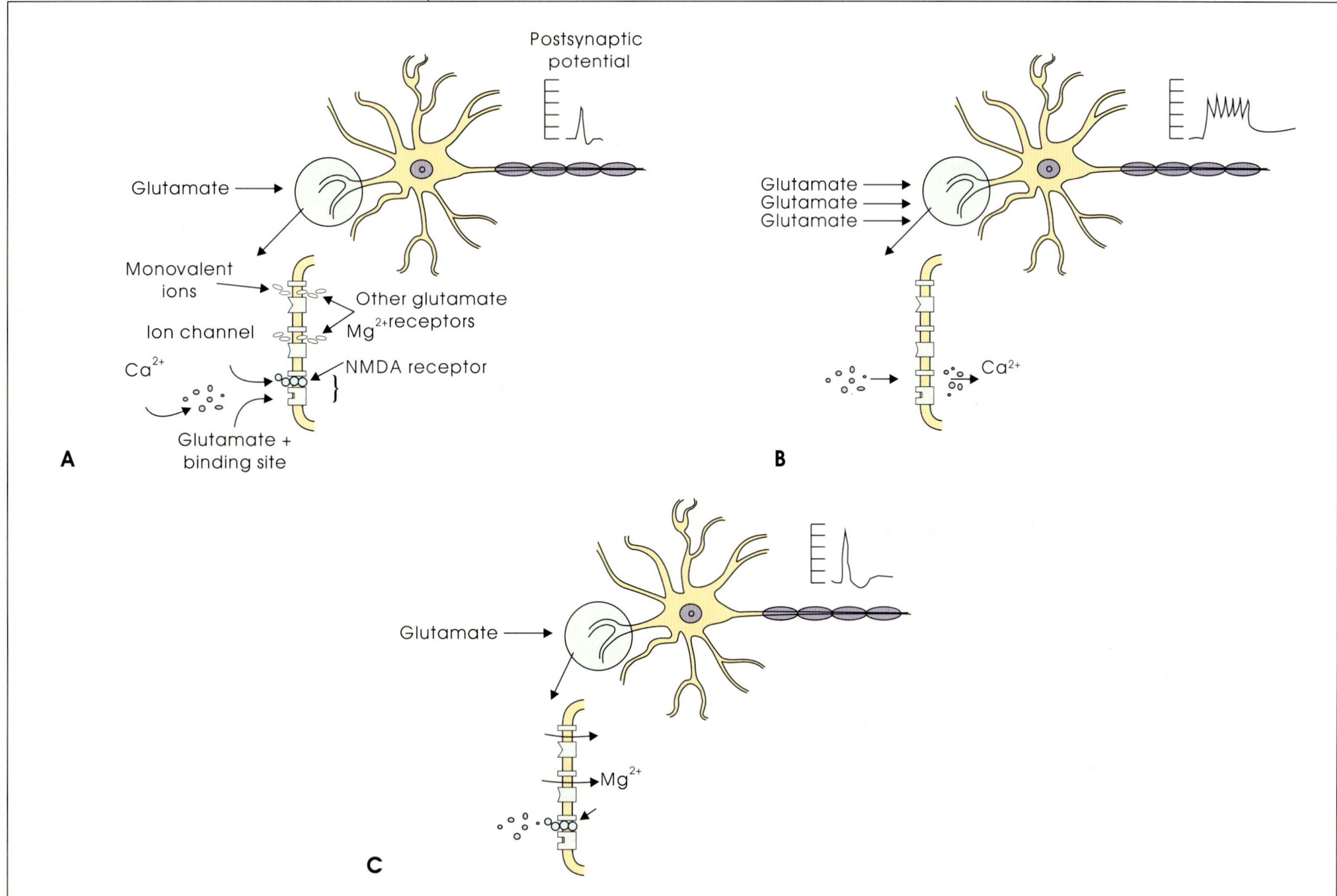

FIGURE 23.9

Long-term potentiation. **A**, Glutamate acts at non–*N*-methyl-D-aspartate (NMDA) receptors to generate an excitatory postsynaptic response. The ion channel of the NMDA subtype of glutamate receptor is blocked by Mg^{2+} ions. **B**, When large amounts of glutamate are released (*ie*, tetany), depolarization reduces the Mg^{2+} block of the NMDA receptor, allowing both monovalent and Ca^{2+} ions to enter the neuron. **C**, Subsequently, Mg^{2+} blocks the NMDA receptor and the excitatory postsynaptic response is again generated by opening ion channels of non-NMDA receptors. The excitatory postsynaptic response is enhanced. (*Adapted from* Collingridge and Bliss [42]; with permission.)

23.9) [41]. LTP entails a change in synaptic efficacy that is assumed to provide the physiologic basis of information storage in the brain [42]. LTP occurs in diverse brain regions, including those not typically associated with memory including hypothalamus [43], visual cortex [44], and motor cortex [45]. Under experimental conditions, the development of LTP is mediated by the *N*-methyl-D-aspartate (NMDA) subtype of glutamate receptor [42]. Tetanic stimulation activates the NMDA receptor, resulting in an opening of its associated ion channel that is normally blocked by Mg^{2+} permitting the entry of Ca^{2+} into the neuron. Subsequent presentation of nontetanic stimulation results in an enhanced postsynaptic potential that persists. NMDA–receptor antagonists block the induction of LTP and disrupt learning and memory [46,47]. Other neurotransmitters, such as catecholamines [48], γ-aminobutyric acid (GABA) [49,50], and acetylcholine [51,52] can modulate the induction of LTP. Drugs that either promote the activation of redundant neural networks or facilitate the induction of LTP could hasten recovery. In contrast, drugs that either inhibit the activation of alternative neural pathways or impair the induction of LTP could interfere with the recovery process.

The slow adaptive responses (Figure 23.6) involve anatomic neuronal rearrangements that occur after many types of brain injury [53–55]. Some of these neuronal reorganizations are potentially beneficial, others are potentially maladaptive [53]. For a drug to enhance behavioral recovery by influencing these types of neuronal alterations, it would have to selectively facilitate favorable rearrangements or retard potentially harmful ones. A variety of specific growth factors that may improve functional recovery after brain injury including nerve growth factor (NGF) and GM_1 gangliosides, are now being studied [56]. Drugs that influence central neurotransmitters may also have neuronotrophic effects [57].

LABORATORY AND CLINICAL DATA ON DRUG EFFECTS ON RECOVERY

The majority of prestroke patients are already receiving medications to treat a variety of coincident medical conditions (Figure 23.10) [58]. In one study, 77% of patients were receiving at least one medication at the time of their stroke (Figure 23.11) [58] and 65% were receiving multiple drugs. By the time of hospital discharge, 95% of patients were receiving medications, and 86% were prescribed multiple drugs. A vast experimental and rudimentary clinical literature about potential drug effects on recovery after stroke is developing. As should be clear from the previous discussion, an awareness of this literature is essential because certain drugs now used to treat concurrent medical conditions may have a detrimental effect on recovery. Table 23.4 and the following sections review the effects of various classes of drugs that influence behavioral recovery after focal brain lesions in laboratory-based studies. Where applicable, preliminary clinical data is presented.

Sympathomimetic and Related Drugs

Amphetamine is one of the most extensively studied drugs that may influence recovery after focal brain injury. Experimental reports of favorable effects of amphetamine administration have been recognized since the 1940s. More recently, Feeney and coworkers [59] found that the administration of a single dose of dextroamphetamine to a rat the day after unilateral injury to its sensorimotor cortex resulted in an enduring enhancement of motor recovery. Other laboratory studies have replicated this effect [60,61]. Postlesion treatment with amphetamine also enhances motor recovery in cats after unilateral or bilateral frontal cortex ablation [62,63]. The beneficial effect of amphetamine is

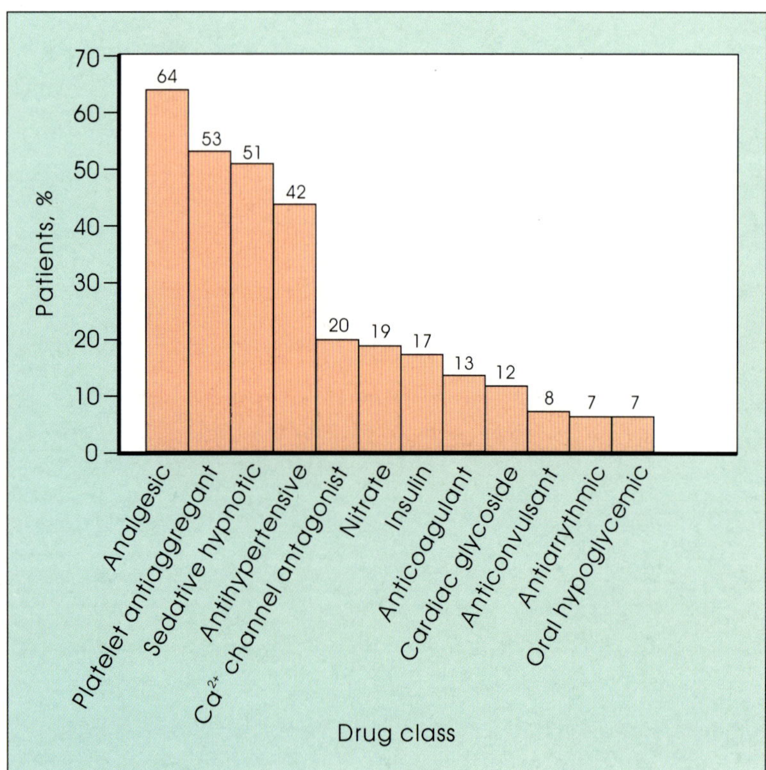

FIGURE 23.10

Classes of drugs prescribed for patients with ischemic stroke. (*From* Goldstein and Davis [58]; with permission.)

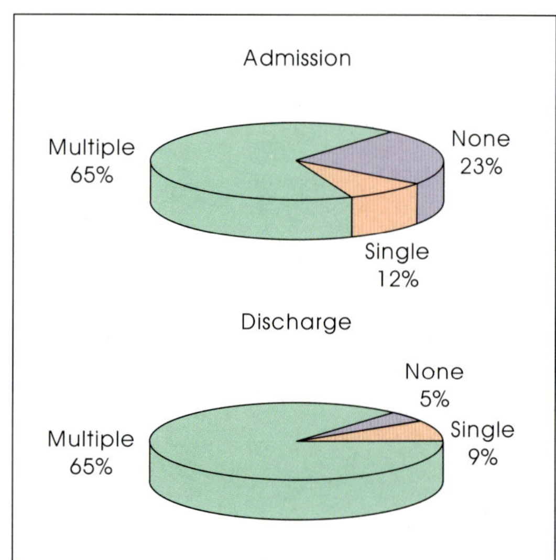

FIGURE 23.11

Frequency of medication use in patients hospitalized with ischemic stroke. Percentages of patients receiving a single drug, multiple drugs, or no drugs at the times of hospital admission and discharge are given. (*From* Goldstein and Davis [58]; with permission.)

also observed in functional deficits that occur following focal lesions involving other areas out of the cortex. For example, an enduring recovery of stereopsis has been demonstrated in cats that had bilateral visual cortex ablations [64,65]. Furthermore, amphetamines facilitate relearning of a visual discrimination task in visually decorticated rats and behavioral recovery after infarction of the barrel cortex in rats [66,67]. However, the animal's behavior after drug administration was critical. For motor recovery, if rats were restrained rather than given motor practice after drug administration, the amphetamine effect was not observed [59]. The recovery of stereoscopic vision in visually decorticated cats also depends on visual experience after drug administration [64,65]. Although the beneficial effect of amphetamine on motor recovery is clearly greater in animals given motor training after drug administration, a smaller independent positive effect of amphetamine may be observed in rats that are not given specific training [9]. Experiments testing the effect of amphetamine on behavioral recovery after more diffuse, nonfocal brain injury have shown conflicting results [68,69].

Although amphetamine is hypothesized to have its beneficial effect on recovery mediated by its action on central noradrenergic neurons, a variety of other mechanisms are possible (Table 23.5). Amphetamine's central actions may be mediated through dopaminergic, serotonergic, or noradrenergic neurons [70]. In addition, systemic administration of amphetamine may increase blood pressure, produce behavioral arousal, and cause hypermotility [71]. Dextroamphetamine induces increases in rCBF and metabolism [72,73]. In addition, amphetamine may cause a disaggregation of brain polysomes, thereby influencing protein synthesis [74]. The importance of concomitant motor training as described above suggests that amphetamine may enhance the relearning process. For example, amphetamine treatment in rats decreases spatial learning deficits caused by bilateral lesions of the neostriatum and improves maze acquisition in rats with unilateral aspiration lesions of the frontal cortex. Also, amphetamine both facilitates the development of LTP in a dose-dependent manner [75] and enhances memory retrieval [76]. Finally, amphetamine may also facilitate unmasking (Figure 23.8). Amphetamine administration results in a widespread increase in glucose metabolism following sensory activation after barrel field infarction in the rat [77], and amphetamine may also act to reverse diaschisis [26].

Table 23.4. Classes of drugs with effects on behavioral recovery

Sympathomimetic and related drugs	Tricyclic antidepressants
Antihypertensives	Benzodiazepines
Major tranquilizers	Anticonvulsants
	Anticholinergics

Table 23.5. Possible mechanisms of action of amphetamine

Increased neurotransmitter actions	Increased relearning
Norepinephrine	Long-term potentiation
Dopamine	Unmasking
Serotonin	Decreased diaschisis
Increased blood pressure	Decreased protein synthesis
Increased cerebral blood flow	

Although the experimental data is quite convincing, only preliminary clinical data concerning the effects of amphetamine on recovery after stroke are known. One study found that the administration of amphetamine, when combined with physical therapy (*eg*, task-specific experience) improved motor function [78]. Because this study involved only a small group of highly selected patients, the results may not be applicable to stroke patients with nonmotor types of deficits. Because only short-term motor recovery was measured, the long-term effectiveness of amphetamine treatment is unknown. A small, double-blind, placebo-controlled study was designed to determine whether treatment with amphetamine would enhance motor recovery in stroke rehabilitation patients [79]. Patients were treated with amphetamine or a placebo daily for 3 weeks, with a final assessment 1 week after discontinuation of the drug. Although the motor performances of amphetamine-treated patients were better than those of the control group, the difference was not statistically significant. However, study patients did not receive physical therapy in conjunction with amphetamine administration. This may have limited the potential benefit of the drug.

Finally, speech pathologists have begun to study the effects of amphetamine on language recovery after stroke [80,81]. In one study, a group of aphasic patients with stroke were given amphetamine just prior to speech therapy for several weeks. Overall, the patients met or exceeded their predicted 6-month language functions by the time of their 3-month evaluations.

The effects of other selected sympathomimetic agents have been studied in the laboratory and are shown in Table 23.6. Phentermine, an amphetamine analogue, accelerates motor recovery in both rats and cats [82]. Similarly, phenylpropanolamine at high doses facilitates recovery in a rat hemiplegia model [83,84]. However, the administration of a single dose of methylphenidate, a piperidine derivative structurally similar to amphetamine, has only a transient beneficial effect on locomotor function after injury to the sensorimotor cortex of rats [85]. The lack of effectiveness of methylphenidate may be due to its short half-life. Repeated dosing of the drug has not been studied, but could be beneficial. Although both yohimbine and idazoxan (centrally acting α_2-adrenergic receptor antagonists) are not classified as sympathomimetics, they increase norepinephrine

Table 23.6. Effects on recovery after focal brain injury of sympathomimetic and related drugs

Drug	Effect
Amphetamine	Beneficial
Phentermine	Beneficial
Phenylpropanolamine	Beneficial
Methylphenidate	None
Yohimbine	Beneficial
Idazoxan	Beneficial

release and enhance motor recovery when given as a single dose after unilateral sensorimotor cortex injury [86–89]. The effects of these other drugs on motor recovery after stroke in humans have not been investigated.

Antihypertensives

Because of abnormal cerebral autoregulation, antihypertensives should always be used cautiously in the setting of acute ischemic stroke [90]. However, hypertension is common in stroke patients, and antihypertensives are among the most frequently prescribed drugs (Figure 23.10). A variety of classes of antihypertensives are in widespread use and their effects on recovery after focal brain injury have been examined experimentally (Table 23.7). As noted above, centrally acting α_2-adrenergic receptor antagonists enhance recovery in the rat hemiplegia model. Therefore, it is not surprising that a centrally acting α_2-adrenergic receptor agonist would be deleterious. Clonidine, when given even as a single dose the day after cortex injury, has a prolonged detrimental effect on motor recovery [91]. When clonidine is given to rats that had recovered motor function, the motor deficit reappears [89,92]. Prazosin [89,93] and phenoxybenzamine [93,94], centrally acting α_1-adrenergic receptor antagonists, are also harmful. However, propranolol, a nonselective β-adrenergic receptor antagonist, has no effect on motor recovery [93]. Both clonidine and prazosin are frequently used to treat stroke patients (Figure 23.12) [58].

The effect of specific antihypertensives on motor recovery after stroke in humans needs to be further clarified. Phenoxybenzamine caused slight transient worsening of the neurologic deficit in several stroke patients, but this might be due to the hypotensive or other hemodynamic effects of the drug [95]. One retrospective study found that both thiazide diuretics and a mixed group of antihypertensives were associated with impaired language recovery in aphasic stroke patients [96]. Interestingly, propranolol, a drug that had no effect on motor recovery in experimental studies, also had no effect on language recovery in these patients. Given the available data, the use of a β-adrenergic receptor antagonist is preferable to either an α_1-adrenergic receptor antagonist or α_2-adrenergic receptor agonist in the treatment of hypertension after stroke.

Major Tranquilizers

Major tranquilizers are occasionally used for agitated stroke patients. In one study, approximately 4% of stroke patients were given a major tranquilizer during the first 2 days of hospitalization [58]. In laboratory studies, the effect of the butyrophenone haloperidol on recovery after focal cortex injury has been extensively investigated. Coadministration of haloperidol blocks amphetamine-promoted motor recovery in rats and haloperidol impairs motor recovery when given alone [59]. When given to rats that had recovered, haloperidol, as well as other butyrophenones (*eg*, fluanisone, droperidol), transiently reinstate the motor deficit (Table 23.8) [97]. Haloperidol administration also blocks amphetamine-facilitated recovery of stereopsis in visually decorticated cats [65,98]. Although haloperidol is a butyrophenone, it has antagonist effects at noradrenergic receptors in addition to its action as a dopamine-receptor antagonist [99]. The available pharmacologic data suggest that the detrimental effect of haloperidol is mediated nonadrenergically rather than through dopaminergic blockade. Intraventricular administration of dopamine does not affect recovery from hemiplegia after sensorimotor cortex injury in rats [100]. If a dopamine-β-hydroxylase inhibitor (blocking the conversion of dopamine to norepinephrine) is given in conjunction with intraventricular dopamine, the weak beneficial effect is blocked [100]. Until the pharmacology of the effects of major tranquilizers is better understood, they should be withheld whenever possible in patients recovering from stroke.

Table 23.7. Effects on recovery after focal brain injury of antihypertensives

Drug	Effect
Clonidine	Detrimental
Prazosin	Detrimental
Phenoxybenzamine	Detrimental
Propranolol	None
Thiazides	Uncertain or detrimental

Table 23.8. Effects on recovery after focal brain injury of major tranquilizers

Drug	Effect
Haloperidol	Detrimental
Fluanisone	Detrimental
Droperidol	Detrimental

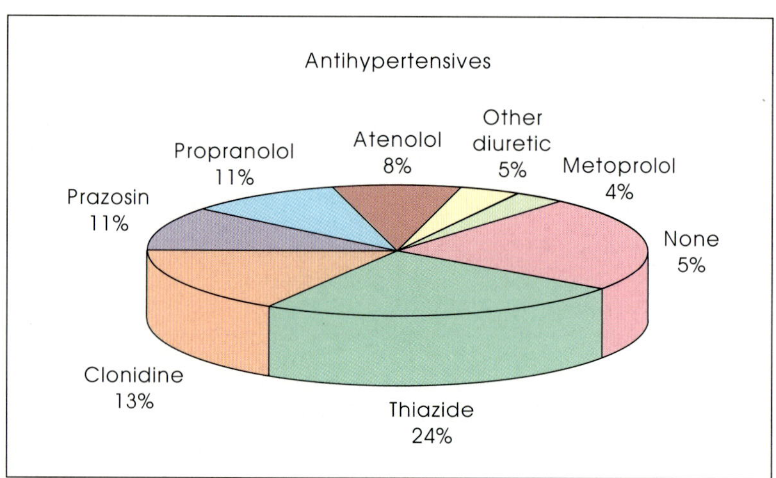

FIGURE 23.12

Antihypertensive drugs. The frequency of use of antihypertensives in patients with acute ischemic stroke. The percentage of patients who were taking each drug at the time of stroke, or were prescribed each drug during the acute hospitalization are shown.

Tricyclic Antidepressants

Clinical depression is associated with impaired recovery after stroke in humans [101]. Tricyclic antidepressants (TCAs) are commonly used to treat mood disorders in stroke patients. Because of their effects on central neurotransmitters, these drugs may have a considerable impact on specific behavioral recovery. The administration of a single dose of trazodone transiently slows motor recovery in rats with sensorimotor cortex injury and reinstates the hemiparesis in recovered animals [102]. In contrast, when rats are given a single dose of desipramine, a facilitation of motor recovery is observed [102].

The precise mechanisms underlying these effects in the hemiplegia model are uncertain. Although desipramine acts by inhibiting the reuptake of norepinephrine, it causes a decrease in the firing of presynaptic noradrenergic neurons through a feedback mechanism [103]. Repeated administration of desipramine actually reduces brain norepinephrine content [104]. Thus, given the hypothesis that enhanced noradrenergic transmission underlies amphetamine's beneficial effect, despite the apparently beneficial effect of desipramine when given as a single dose, repeated administration should probably be avoided. Trazodone, a drug that impairs recovery from hemiplegia in rats, was found to improve outcome when measured with the Barthel Index in depressed stroke patients [20]. However, the Barthel Index provides a measure of disability, not specific motor impairments. Motor function was not specifically measured in the study. Therefore, recommendations concerning the choice of specific TCAs in stroke patients must await further laboratory and clinical evaluation (Table 23.9).

Anxiolytics

The impact of benzodiazepines on recovery after focal injury to the cerebral cortex has been studied extensively. The anxiolytics and sedative-hypnotics are also frequently prescribed for stroke patients (Figure 23.10) [58]. In one study, the number of stroke patients prescribed sedative-hypnotic agents more than doubled over the first 2 days of hospitalization (17% to 44%), including a doubling of the number receiving benzodiazepines (10% to 20%) [58]. Benzodiazepines act as indirect agonists of the inhibitory neurotransmitter GABA. The short-term administration of diazepam permanently impedes recovery from the sensory asymmetry caused by anteromedial neocortex damage in the rat [105,106]. This sensory asymmetry is measured by a task similar to the double simultaneous stimulation used clinically. Rats are trained to remove adhesive pads attached to their forepaws. Rats without a cortex lesion have a 50% chance of removing either the left or right adhesive pad first. After a unilateral lesion to the sensory cortex, rats preferentially remove the ipsilateral pad. The magnitude of the sensory asymmetry can be quantitated by systematically decreasing the size of the ipsilateral pad and increasing the size of the contralateral pad over a series of trials until the ipsilateral bias is removed. The long-term deleterious effect of diazepam is mimicked by short-term infusion of the GABA agonist muscimol into the sensorimotor cortex adjacent to the lesion [107] and is blocked by coadministration of the benzodiazepine antagonist Ro 15-1788 [108]. Ro 15-1788 transiently facilitates recovery [109]. Intracortical infusion of GABA itself increases hemiparesis produced by a small motor cortex lesion in rats [110]. Anxiolytics that do not act through the GABA-benzodiazepine receptor complex may not interfere with recovery [109]. Gepirone is an anxiolytic with no activity at the benzodiazepine receptor site. Chronic administration of this drug does not impair recovery from the sensory asymmetry caused by anteromedial neocortex injury in the rat [109].

The harmful effects of benzodiazepines after anteromedial cortex injury has implications for understanding the processes underlying recovery (Figure 23.6). For example, benzodiazepines impair learning and memory [111] and may suppress the induction of LTP [112,113]. However, unlike motor recovery after sensorimotor cortex injury, the sensory asymmetry after anteromedial cortex damage is not influenced by practice, suggesting a mechanism other than interference with relearning [114]. Chronic administration of diazepam in rats with anteromedial cortex injury led to a significant loss in size of the ipsilateral striatum [115,116]. It has also been hypothesized that benzodiazepines might exert their detrimental effects by prolonging diaschisis and causing metabolically depressed regions to persist [109]. Regardless of the mechanism of action, benzodiazepines should be avoided in patients recovering from stroke as described in Table 23.10.

Anticonvulsants

In addition to their anxiolytic effects, benzodiazepines are also potent anticonvulsants. Anticonvulsants are used frequently in the treatment of poststroke seizure disorders. In one study, 8% of stroke patients received the anticonvulsant phenytoin during the acute phase of hospitalization [58]. The deleterious effect of GABA on motor recovery after motor cortex injury is enhanced by the systemic administration of phenytoin [117], which may act through a GABA-mediated mechanism [118]. Phenobarbital also delays behavioral recovery after injury to the cerebral cortex in laboratory studies [119,120]. In contrast, chronic administration of carbamazepine in anticonvulsant doses did not affect sensory recovery after anteromedial cortex injury [121].

Table 23.9. Effects on recovery after focal brain injury of tricyclic antidepressants

Drug	Effect
Trazodone	Detrimental or beneficial
Desipramine	Uncertain or beneficial

Table 23.10. Effects on recovery after focal brain injury of anxiolytics

Drug	Effect
Diazepam	Detrimental
Gepirone	None

MK-801 is a noncompetitive NMDA-receptor antagonist with anticonvulsant activity that has been under intense study as a neuroprotective agent. The administration of NMDA-receptor antagonists either before or after focal ischemia reduces the volume of cerebral infarction in rats [122], cats [123], and rabbits [124]. However, because NMDA-receptor antagonists disrupt both the induction of LTP [42] and learning and memory [46,47], they may be detrimental if given during the recovery period. MK-801 had no effect on either motor recovery in the rat hemiplegia model [125] or on recovery of limb placing, but it facilitated recovery of the sensory asymmetry caused by anteromedial cortex injury [126]. The drug also had no effect on sensory function but reinstated forelimb-placing deficits in rats that recovered from anteromedial cortex injury [126]. This observation led to the hypothesis that the NMDA receptor is involved in maintenance of motor relearning because recovery of limb placing, unlike sensory asymmetries, is dependent on practice [126]. However, NMDA-receptor antagonists interfere with the acquisition rather than the retention of learned behavior, and MK-801 had no effect on rats that recovered from hemiplegia (a behavior also dependent on practice) [125].

As with other drugs, there is a paucity of data concerning the impact of anticonvulsants on recovery after stroke in humans. As in the animal studies, a randomized clinical study in victims of head trauma showed that phenytoin had a detrimental effect on neurobehavioral recovery [127]. Of the anticonvulsants experimentally tested during the recovery period, carbamazepine was the only drug that was not harmful. Unfortunately, carbamazepine cannot be given intravenously and therefore cannot be used in the emergent treatment of status epilepticus. However, this drug should be considered in nonemergent treatment of seizure disorders in stroke patients (Table 23.11).

Anticholinergics

Russian literature on cholinergic drugs and functional recovery is outdated by current standards [84]. In 1942, Ward and Kennard [128] reported that cholinergic agonists increased the rate of motor recovery in monkeys with motor cortex lesions. The beneficial effects of cholinergic agonists were blocked by administration of phenytoin [120]. More recent data suggest that the anticholinergic drug scopolamine interferes with motor recovery following infarction of the cortex in rats [129]. There is very limited data regarding the effects of cholinergic agents on recovery after stroke in humans.

DETRIMENTAL EFFECTS OF DRUGS ON RECOVERY AFTER STROKE IN HUMANS

Ethical considerations limit the likelihood of a prospective randomized trial to determine whether the hypothesized detrimental drug effects on recovery after stroke actually occur in humans. Retrospective studies must be interpreted cautiously because they may not fully take into account other comorbid conditions that could influence recovery and warrant the use of a specific drug. We performed a retrospective study that tested the hypothesis that drugs that are harmful during recovery in laboratory animals would interfere with motor recovery in human stroke patients [15]. The drugs that were studied included clonidine, prazosin, neuroleptics, benzodiazepines, and phenytoin. The motor recoveries of stroke patients who received one or a combination of these drugs were compared with those of a group of patients who were not given these agents. The two groups of patients were similar with respect to a variety of characteristics, including age, blood pressure, sex, and comorbid conditions. Patients who received one or a combination of the potentially detrimental drugs at the time of stroke or during subsequent hospitalization had significantly slower motor recoveries than patients who did not receive one of these drugs. A multivariate analysis indicated an independent effect of the drugs.

CONCLUSIONS

Certain drugs influence behavioral recovery following focal brain injury in laboratory animals. These drug effects can be either beneficial or harmful to the recovery process. Similar drug effects may occur in humans. When choosing a drug to treat coincident medical problems in stroke patients, this emerging pharmacology should be kept in mind. The use of a β–adrenergic receptor antagonist is preferable to either an α_1–adrenergic receptor antagonist or α_2–adrenergic receptor agonist in the treatment of hypertension after stroke. Thiazide diuretics should be used cautiously. Haloperidol is potentially harmful and should be withheld whenever possible in patients recovering from stroke. Recommendations concerning the choice of specific TCAs in stroke patients must await further laboratory and clinical evaluation. Benzodiazepines should generally be avoided. Among anticonvulsants, carbamazepine was the only drug not found to be harmful. The use of drugs to enhance recovery after stroke may be possible in the future.

Table 23.11. Effects on recovery after focal brain injury of anticonvulsants

Drug	Effect
Phenytoin	Detrimental
Phenobarbital	Detrimental
Carbamazepine	None
MK-801	Uncertain, detrimental, or none

REFERENCES

1. Lincoln NB, Blackburn M, Ellis S, *et al.*: An investigation of factors affecting progress of patients on a stroke unit. *J Neurol Neurosurg Psych* 1989, 52:493–496.
2. Ernst E: A review of stroke rehabilitation and physiotherapy. *Stroke* 1990, 21:1081–1085.
3. Granger CV, Gresham GE: International classification of impairments, disabilities, and handicaps (ICIDH) as a conceptual basis for stroke outcome research. *Stroke* 1990, 21(suppl II):II-66–II-67.
4. Finger S, Stein DG: Behavioral compensation and response and cue theories. In *Brain Damage and Recovery.* New York: Academic Press, Inc.; 1982:303–317.
5. Duncan PW, Goldstein LB, Divine GW, *et al.*: Measurement of motor recovery after stroke: outcome assessment and sample size requirements. *Stroke* 1992, 23:1084–1089.
6. Wade DT, Wood VA, Hewer RL: Recovery after stroke: the first three months. *J Neurol Neurosurg Psych* 1985, 48:7–13.
7. Kinsella G, Ford B: Acute recovery patterns in stroke patients. *Med J Aust* 1980, 2:662–666.
8. Held JM, Gordon J, Gentile AM: Environmental influences on locomotor recovery following cortical lesions in rats. *Behav Neurosci* 1985, 99:678–690.
9. Goldstein LB, Davis JN: Post-lesion practice and amphetamine-facilitated recovery of beam-walking in the rat. *Restorative Neurol Neurosci* 1990, 1:311–314.
10. Will B, Kelche C: Environmental approaches to recovery of function from brain damage: a review of animal studies (1981 to 1991). *Adv Exp Med Biol* 1992, 325:79–103.
11. Glass TA, Matchar DB, Belyea M, *et al.*: Impact of social support on outcomes in first stroke. *Stroke* 1993, 24:64–70.
12. Granger CV, Hamilton BB, Fiedler RC: Discharge outcome after stroke rehabilitation. *Stroke* 1992, 23:978–982.
13. Novack TA, Haban G, Graham K, *et al.*: Prediction of stroke rehabilitation outcome from psychologic screening. *Arch Phys Med Rehabil* 1987, 68:729–734.
14. Horner RD, Matchar DB, Divine GW, *et al.*: Racial variations in ischemic stroke-related physical and functional impairments. *Stroke* 1991, 22:1497–1501.
15. Goldstein LB, Matchar DB, Morgenlander JC, *et al.*: The influence of drugs on the recovery of sensorimotor function after stroke. *J Neuro Rehabil* 1990, 4:137–144.
16. Irle E: Lesion size and recovery of function: some new perspectives. *Brain Res Rev* 1987, 12:307–320.
17. Irle E: An analysis of the correlation of lesion size, localization, and behavioral effects in 283 published studies of cortical and subcortical lesions in old-world monkeys. *Brain Res Rev* 1990, 15:181–213.
18. Lundgren J, Flodstrom K, Sjogren K, *et al.*: Site of brain lesion and functional capacity in recovered hemiplegics. *Scand J Rehabil Med* 1982, 14:141–143.
19. Finger S, Stein DG, eds.: *Brain Damage and Recovery.* New York: Academic Press; 1982.
20. Reding MJ, Orto LA, Winter SW, *et al.*: Antidepressant therapy after stroke: a double-blind trial. *Arch Neurol* 1986, 43:763–765.
21. Goldstein LB: Pharmacologic enhancement of recovery. In *The Handbook of Neurorehabilitation.* Edited by Good DC, Couch JR. New York: Marcel Dekker, Inc.; 1994.
22. Goldstein LB: Basic and clinical studies of pharmacologic effects on recovery from brain injury. *J Neurol Transplant Plast* 1993, 3:175–192.
23. Katzman R, Clasen R, Klatzo I, *et al.*: Report of Joint Committee on Stroke Resources. Part 4: brain edema in stroke. *Stroke* 1977, 8:512–540.
24. Dereski MO, Chopp M, Kight RA, *et al.*: Focal cerebral ischemia in the rat: temporal profile of neutrophil responses. *Neurosci Res Commun* 1992, 11:179–186.
25. Feeney DM, Baron JC: Diaschisis. *Stroke* 1986, 17:817–830.
26. Feeney DM: Pharmacologic modulation of recovery after brain injury: a reconsideration of diaschisis. *J Neurol Rehabil* 1991, 5:113–128.
27. Jaspers RMA, Van Der Sprenkel JWB, Tulleken CAF, *et al.*: Local as well as remote functional and metabolic changes after focal ischemia in cats. *Brain Res Bull* 1990, 24:23–32.
28. Castella Y, Dietrich WD, Watson BD, *et al.*: Acute thrombotic infarction suppresses metabolic activation of ipsilateral somatosensory cortex: evidence for functional diaschisis. *J Cereb Blood Flow Metab* 1989, 9:329–341.
29. Feeney DM, Sutton RL, Boyeson MG, *et al.*: The locus-coeruleus and cerebral metabolism: recovery of function after cortical injury. *Physiol Psych* 1985, 13:197–203.
30. Martin WRW, Raichle ME: Cerebellar blood flow and metabolism in cerebral hemisphere infarction. *Ann Neurol* 1983, 14:168–176.
31. Fiorelli M, Blin J, Bakchine S, *et al.*: PET studies of cortical diaschisis in patients with motor hemineglect. *J Neurol Sci* 1991, 104:135–142.
32. Tanaka M, Kondo S, Hirai S, *et al.*: Crossed cerebellar diaschisis accompanied by hemiataxia: a PET study. *J Neurol Neurosurg Psych* 1992, 55:121–125.
33. Botez MI, Leveille J, Lambert R, *et al.*: Single photon emission computed tomography (SPECT) in cerebellar disease: cerebello-cerebral diaschisis. *Eur Neurol* 1991, 31:405–412.
34. Pappata S, Mazoyer B, Dinh T, *et al.*: Effects of capsular or thalamic stroke on metabolism in the cortex and cerebellum: a positron tomography study. *Stroke* 1990, 21:519–524.
35. Lashley KS, ed.: *Brain Mechanisms and Intelligence.* Chicago: University of Chicago Press; 1929.
36. Luria AR, ed. *Restoration of Function After Brain Injury.* New York: MacMillan; 1963.
37. Wall PD: Mechanisms of plasticity of connection following damage in adult mammalian nervous systems. In *Recovery of Function: Theoretical Considerations for Brain Injury Rehabilitation.* Edited by Bach-y-Rita P. Baltimore: University Park Press; 1978:91–105.
38. Chollet F, DiPiero V, Wise RJS, *et al.*: The functional anatomy of motor recovery after stroke in humans: a study with positron-emission tomography. *Ann Neurol* 1991, 29:63–71.
39. Weiller C, Chollet F, Friston KJ, *et al.*: Functional reorganization of the brain in recovery from striatocapsular infarction in man. *Ann Neurol* 1992, 31:463–472.
40. Weiller C, Ramsay SC, Wise RJS, *et al.*: Individual patterns of functional reorganization in the human cerebral cortex after capsular infarction. *Ann Neurol* 1993, 33:181–189.
41. Bliss TVP, Dolphin AC: What is the mechanism of long-term potentiation in the hippocampus? *Trends Neurol Sci* 1982, 5:289–290.
42. Collingridge GL, Bliss TVP: NMDA receptors: their role in long-term potentiation. *T I N S* 1987, 10:288–293.
43. Corbett D: Long-term potentiation of lateral hypothalamic self-stimulation following parabrachial lesions in the rat. *Brain Res Bull* 1980, 5:637–642.
44. Aroniadou VA, Teyler TJ: The role of NMDA receptors in long-term potentiation (LTP) and depression (LTD) in rat visual cortex. *Brain Res* 1991, 562:136–143.
45. Keller A, Iriki A, Asanuma H: Identification of neurons producing the long-term potentiation in the cat motor cortex: intracellular recordings and labeling. *J Comp Neurol* 1990, 300:47–60.
46. Benvenga MJ, Spaulding TC: Amnesic effect of the novel anticonvulsant MK-801. *Pharmacol Biochem Behav* 1989, 30:205–207.
47. Handelmann GE, Contreras PC, O'Donohue TL: Selective memory impairment by phencyclidine in rats. *Eur J Pharmacol* 1987, 140:69–73.
48. Dahl D, Sarvey JM: Norepinephrine induces pathway-specific long-lasting potentiation and depression in the hippocampal dentate gyrus. *Proc Natl Acad Sci U S A* 1989, 86:4776–4780.

49. Wigstrom H, Gustafsson B: Facilitation of hippocampal long-lasting potentiation by GABA antagonists. *Acta Physiol Scand* 1985, 125:159–172.

50. Olpe HR, Karlsson G: The effects of baclofen and two GABA B-receptor antagonists on long-term potentiation. *Naunyn Schmiedebergs Arch Pharmacol* 1990, 342:194–197.

51. Ito T, Miura Y, Kadokawa T: Effects of physostigmine and scopolamine on long-term potentiation of hippocampal population spikes in rats. *Can J Physiol Pharmacol* 1988, 66:1010–1016.

52. Williams S, Johnston D: Muscarinic depression of long-term potentiation in CA3 hippocampal neurons. *Science* 1988, 242:84–87.

53. Davis JN: Neuronal rearrangements after brain injury: a proposed classification. In *NIH Central Nervous System Trauma Status Report.* Edited by Becker DP, Povlishock JT. Washington, D.C.: National Institutes of Health; 1985:491–501.

54. Cotman CW, Nieto-Sampedro M, Harris EW: Synapse replacement in the nervous system of adult vertebrates. *Physiol Rev* 1981, 61:684–784.

55. Jones TA, Schallert T: Overgrowth and pruning of dendrites in adult rats recovering from neocortical damage. *Brain Res* 1992, 581:156–160.

56. Lipton SA: Growth factors for neuronal survival and process regeneration: implications for the mammalian central nervous system. *Arch Neurol* 1989, 46:1241–1248.

57. Lipton SA, Kater SB: Neurotransmitter regulation of neuronal outgrowth, plasticity and survival. *T I N S* 1989, 12:265–270.

58. Goldstein LB, Davis JN: Physician prescribing patterns after ischemic stroke. *Neurology* 1988, 38:1806–1809.

59. Feeney DM, Gonzalez A, Law WA: Amphetamine haloperidol and experience interact to affect the rate of recovery after motor cortex injury. *Science* 1982, 217:855–857.

60. Goldstein LB: Pharmacology of recovery after stroke. *Stroke* 1990, 21(suppl III):139–142.

61. Dunbar GL, Smith GA, Look SK, *et al.*: d-Amphetamine attenuates learning and motor deficits following cortical injury in rats. *Soc Neurosci Abstr* 1989, 15:132.

62. Hovda DA, Feeney DM: Amphetamine with experience promotes recovery of locomotor function after unilateral frontal cortex injury in the cat. *Brain Res* 1984, 298:358–361.

63. Sutton RL, Hovda DA, Feeney DM: Amphetamine accelerates recovery of locomotor function following bilateral frontal cortex ablation in cats. *Behav Neurosci* 1989, 103:837–841.

64. Feeney DM, Hovda DA: Reinstatement of binocular depth perception by amphetamine and visual experience after visual cortex ablation. *Brain Res* 1985, 342:352–356.

65. Hovda DA, Sutton RL, Feeney DM: Amphetamine-induced recovery of visual cliff performance after bilateral visual cortex ablation in cats: measurements of depth perception thresholds. *Behav Neurosci* 1989, 103:574–584.

66. Braun JJ, Meyer PM, Meyer DR: Sparing of a brightness habit in rats following visual decortication. *J Comp Physiol Psych* 1986, 61:79–82.

67. Hurwitz BE, Dietrich WD, McCabe PM, *et al.*: Amphetamine-accelerated recovery from cortical barrel-field infarction: pharmacological treatment of stroke. In *Cerebrovascular Diseases. The Sixteenth Research (Princeton) Conference.* Edited by Ginsberg MD, Dietrich WD. New York: Raven Press; 1989:309–318.

68. Dunbar GL, Hecht SA, Merbaum SL, *et al.*: Use of gangliosides and amphetamines to promote behavioral recovery following bilateral caudate nucleus lesions. In *Neuroplasticity: A New Therapeutic Tool in the CNS.* Edited by Masland RL, Portera-Sanchez A, Toffano G. Padova: Liviana Press; 1987:117–124.

69. Colbourne F, Corbett D: Effects of d-amphetamine on the recovery of function following cerebral ischemic injury. *Pharmacol Biochem Behav* 1992, 42:705–710.

70. Fuxe K, Ungerstedt U: Histochemical, biochemical, and functional studies on central monamine neurons after acute and chronic amphetamine administration. In *Amphetamines and Related Compounds.* Edited by Costa E, Garattini S. New York: Raven Press; 1970:257–288.

71. Weiner N: Norepinephrine, epinephrine, and the sympathomimetic amines. In *The Pharmacological Basis of Therapeutics.* Edited by Bilman AG, Goodman LS, Rall TW, *et al.* New York: MacMillan Publishing Company, Inc.; 1985.

72. Mathew RJ, Wilson WH: Dextroamphetamine-induced changes in regional cerebral blood flow. *Psychopharmacology* 1985, 87:298–302.

73. McCulloch J, Harper AM: Cerebral circulatory and metabolism changes following amphetamine administration. *Brain Res* 1977, 121:196–199.

74. Moskowitz MA, Weiss BF, Lytle LD, *et al.*: D-amphetamine disaggregates brain polysomes via a dopaminergic mechanism. *Proc Natl Acad Sci U S A* 1975, 72:834–836.

75. Gold PE, Delanoy RL, Merrin J: Modulation of long-term potentiation by peripherally administered amphetamine and epinephrine. *Brain Res* 1984, 305:103–107.

76. Altman HJ, Quartermain D: Facilitation of memory retrieval by centrally administered catecholamine stimulating agents. *Behav Brain Res* 1983, 7:51–63.

77. Dietrich WD, Alonso O, Busto R, *et al.*: Influence of amphetamine treatment on somatosensory function of the normal and infarcted rat brain. *Stroke* 1990, 21(suppl):147–150.

78. Crisostomo EA, Duncan PW, Propst MA, *et al.*: Evidence that amphetamine with physical therapy promotes recovery of motor function in stroke patients. *Ann Neurol* 1988, 23:94–97.

79. Borucki SJ, Langberg J, Reding M: The effect of dextroamphetamine on motor recovery after stroke. *Neurology* 1992, 42(suppl 3):329–330.

80. Homan R, Panksepp J, Mcsweeny J, *et al.*: d-Amphetamine effects on language and motor behaviors in a chronic stroke patient. *Soc Neurosci Abstr* 1990, 16:439.

81. Walker-Batson D, Unwin H, Curtis S, *et al.*: Use of amphetamine in the treatment of aphasia. *Restorative Neurol Neurosci* 1992, 4:47–50.

82. Hovda DA, Bailey B, Montoya S, *et al.*: Phentermine accelerates recovery of function after motor cortex injury in rats and cats. *Fed Am Soc Exp Biol* 1983, 42:1157.

83. Chen MJ, Sutton RL, Feeney DM: Recovery of function after brain injury in rat and cat: beneficial effects of phenylpropanolamine. *Soc Neurosci Abstr* 1986, 12:881.

84. Feeney DM, Sutton RL: Pharmacotherapy for recovery of function after brain injury. *CRC Crit Rev Neurobiol* 1987, 3:135–197.

85. Kline AE, Flores TP, Tso-Olivas DY, *et al.*: Effects of methylphenidate on recovery from ablation-induced hemiplegia. *Soc Neurosci Abstr* 1988, 14:1152.

86. Goldstein LB: Amphetamine facilitated functional recovery after stroke. In *Cerebrovascular Diseases. Sixteenth Research (Princeton) Conference.* Edited by Ginsberg MD, Dietrich WD. New York: Raven Press; 1989:303–308.

87. Goldstein LB, Poe HV, Davis JN: An animal model of recovery of function after stroke: facilitation of recovery by an alpha2-adrenergic receptor antagonist. *Ann Neurol* 1989, 26:157.

88. Weaver MS, Farmer LJ, Feeney DM: Norepinephrine receptor agonists and antagonists influence rate and maintenance of recovery of function after sensorimotor cortex contusion in the rat. *Soc Neurosci Abstr* 1987, 13:477.

89. Sutton RL, Feeney DM: α-Noradrenergic agonists and antagonists affect recovery and maintenance of beam-walking ability after sensorimotor cortex ablation in the rat. *Restorative Neurol Neurosci* 1992, 4:1–11.

90. Powers WJ: Acute hypertension after stroke: the scientific basis for treatment decisions. *Neurology* 1993, 43:461–467.

91. Goldstein LB, Davis JN: Clonidine impairs recovery of beam-walking rats. *Brain Res* 1990, 508:305–309.

92. Stephens J, Goldberg G, Demopoulos JT: Clonidine reinstates deficits following recovery from sensorimotor cortex lesion in rats. *Arch Phys Med Rehabil* 1986, 67:666–667.

93. Feeney DM, Westerberg VS: Norepinephrine and brain damage: alpha noradrenergic pharmacology alters functional recovery after cortical trauma. *Can J Psych* 1990, 44:233–252.

94. Hovda DA, Feeney DM, Salo AA, *et al.*: Phenoxybenzamine but not haloperidol reinstates all motor and sensory deficits in cats fully recovered from sensorimotor cortex ablations. *Soc Neurosci Abstr* 1983, 9:1002.

95. Meyer JS, Miyakawa Y, Welch KMA, *et al.*: Influence of adrenergic receptor blockade on circulatory and metabolic effects of disordered neurotransmitter function in stroke patients. *Stroke* 1976, 7:158–167.

96. Porch BE, Feeney DM: Effects of antihypertensive drugs on recovery from aphasia. *Clin Aphasiology* 1986, 16:309–314.

97. Van Hasselt P: Effect of butyrophenones on motor function in rats after recovery from brain damage. *Neuropharmacology* 1973, 12:245–247.

98. Hovda DA, Feeney DM: Haloperidol blocks amphetamine-induced recovery of binocular depth perception after bilateral visual cortex ablation in the cat. *Proc West Pharmacol Soc* 1985, 28:209–211.

99. Peroutka SJ, U'Pritchard DC, Greenberg DA, *et al.*: Neuropleptic drug interactions with norepinephrine alpha receptor-binding sites in rat brain. *Neuropharmacology* 1977, 16:549–556.

100. Boyeson MG, Feeney DM: Intraventricular norepinephrine facilitates motor recovery following sensorimotor cortex injury. *Pharmacol Biochem Behav* 1990, 35:497–501.

101. Morris PLP, Raphael B, Robinson RG: Clinical depression is associated with impaired recovery from stroke. *Med J Aust* 1992, 157:239–242.

102. Boyeson MG, Harmon RL: Effects of trazodone and desipramine on motor recovery in brain-injured rats. *Am J Phys Med Rehabil* 1993, 72:286–293.

103. Svensson TH, Usdin T: Feedback inhibition of brain noradrenaline neurons by tricyclic antidepressants: alpha-receptor mediation. *Science* 1978, 202:1089–1091.

104. Roffler-Tarlov S, Schildkraut JJ, Draskoczy PR: Effects of acute and chronic administration of desmetylimipramine on the content of norepinephrine and other monamines in the rat brain. *Biochem Pharmacol* 1973, 22:2923–2926.

105. Schallert T, Hernandez TD, Barth TM: Recovery of function after brain damage: severe and chronic disruption of diazepam. *Brain Res* 1986, 379:104–111.

106. Hernandez TD, Kiefel J, Barth TM, *et al.*: Disruption and facilitation of recovery of behavioral function: implication of the γ aminobutyric acid/benzodiazepine receptor complex. In *Cerebrovascular Diseases. The Sixteenth Research (Princeton) Conference.* Edited by Ginsberg MD, Dietrich WD. New York: Raven Press; 1989:327–334.

107. Hernandez TD, Schallert T: Long-term impairment of behavioral recovery from cortical damage can be produced by short-term GABA-agonist infusion into adjacent cortex. *Restorative Neurol Neurosci* 1990, 1:323–330.

108. Hernandez TD, Jones GH, Schallert T: Coadministration of Ro 15-1788 prevents diazepam-induced retardation of recovery of function. *Brain Res* 1989, 487:89–95.

109. Schallert T, Jones TA, Weaver MS, *et al.*: Pharmacologic and anatomic considerations in recovery of function. *Phys Med Rehabil* 1992, 6:375–393.

110. Brailowsky S, Knight RT, Blood K: Gamma-aminobutyric acid-induced potentiation of cortical hemiplegia. *Brain Res* 1986, 362:322–330.

111. Lister R: The amnesic action of benzodiazepines in man. *Neurosci Biobehav Rev* 1985, 9:87–93.

112. Riches IP, Brown MW: The effect of lorazepam upon hippocampal long-term potentiation. *Neurosci Lett* 1986, S42–S50.

113. Satoh M, Ishihara K, Iwama T, *et al.*: Aniracetam augments, and midazolam inhibits, the long-term potentiation in guinea pig hippocampal slices. *Neurosci Lett* 1986, 68:216–220.

114. Schallert T, Whishaw IQ: Bilateral cutaneous stimulation of the somatosensory system in hemidecorticate rats. *Behav Neurosci* 1984, 98:518–540.

115. Schallert T, Jones TA, Lindner MD: Multilevel transneuronal degeneration after brain damage: behavioral events and effects of GABAergic drugs. *Stroke* 1990, 21(suppl):143–157.

116. Jones TA, Schallert T: Subcortical deterioration after cortical damage: effects of diazepam and relation to recovery of function. *Behav Brain Res* 1992, 51:1–13.

117. Brailowsky S, Knight RT, Efron R: Phenytoin increases the severity of cortical hemiplegia in rats. *Brain Res* 1986, 376:71–77.

118. Chweh AY, Swinyard EA, Wolf HH: Involvement of a GABAergic mechanism in the pharmacologic action of phenytoin. *Pharmacol Biochem Behav* 1986, 24:1301–1304.

119. Hernandez TD, Russell LC: Phenobarbital delays recovery from cortex damage. *Soc Neurosci Abstr* 1992, 18:870.

120. Watson CW, Kennard MA: The effect of anticonvulsant drugs on recovery of function following cerebral cortical lesions. *J Neurophysiol* 1945, 8:221–231.

121. Fulton RL, Schallert T: Effects of carbamazepine on recovery after cortical damage. *Soc Neurosci Abstr* 1989, 15:782.

122. Park CK, Nehls DG, Graham DI, *et al.*: The glutamate antagonist MK-801 reduces focal ischemic brain damage in the rat. *Ann Neurol* 1988, 24:543–551.

123. Ozyurt E, Graham DI, Woodruff GN, *et al.*: Protective effect of the glutamate antagonist, MK-801 in focal cerebral ischemia in the cat. *J Cereb Blood Flow Metab* 1988, 8:138–143.

124. Steinberg GK, Saleh J, Kunis D, *et al.*: Protective effect of *N*-methyl-D-aspartate antagonists after focal cerebral ischemia in rabbits. *Stroke* 1989, 20:1247–1252.

125. Goldstein LB, Coviello A: Postlesion administration of the NMDA receptor antagonist MK-801 does not impair motor recovery after unilateral sensorimotor cortex injury in the rat. *Brain Res* 1992, 580:129–136.

126. Barth TM, Grant ML, Schallert T: Effects of MK-801 on recovery from sensorimotor cortex lesions. *Stroke* 1990, 21(suppl):153–157.

127. Dikmen SS, Temkin NR, Miller B, *et al.*: Neurobehavioral effects of phenytoin prophylaxis of posttraumatic seizures. *JAMA* 1991, 265:1271–1277.

128. Ward AA, Jr, Kennard MA: Effect of cholinergic drugs on recovery of function following lesions of the central nervous system in monkeys. *Yale J Biol & Med* 1942, 15:189–228.

129. De Ryck M, Duytschaever H, Janssen PAJ: Ionic channels, cholinergic mechanisms, and recovery of sensorimotor function after neocortical infarcts in rats. *Stroke* 1990, 21(suppl):158–163.

130. Duncan PW, Propst MA, Nelson SG: Reliability of the Fugl-Meyer assessment of sensorimotor recovery following cerebrovascular accident. *J Am Phys Ther Assn* 1983, 63:1606–1610.

131. Fugl-Meyer AR, Jaasko L, Leyman I, *et al.*: The poststroke hemiplegic patient: I: a method for evaluation of physical performance. *Scand J Rehab Med* 1975, 7:13–31.

Index

Page numbers followed by f and t indicate figures and tables, respectively.

A

B

C

D

E

F

G

H

I

K

L

M

N

O

P

Q

R

S

T

U

V

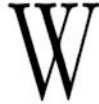

X

Y